Unintended Thought

Unintended Thought

Edited by

James S. Uleman
John A. Bargh

THE GUILFORD PRESS
New York London

© 1989 The Guilford Press
A Division of Guilford Publications, Inc.
72 Spring Street, New York, NY 10012

Printed in the United States of America

Last digit is print number: 9 8 7 6 5 4 3 2 1

Library of Congress Cataloging-in-Publication Data

Unintended thought / edited by James S. Uleman and John A. Bargh.
    p.   cm.
  Includes bibliographies and index.
  ISBN 0-89862-379-0
  1. Thought and thinking. 2. Will. I. Uleman, James S.
II. Bargh, John A.
BF441.U54 1989
153.4′2—dc20   89-7582
                                         CIP

Contributors

JOHN A. BARGH, Ph.D., Department of Psychology, New York University, New York, New York

SHELLY CHAIKEN, Ph.D., Department of Psychology, New York University, New York, New York

GREGORY ANDRADE DIAMOND, M.A., Department of Psychology, University of Michigan, Ann Arbor, Michigan

ALICE H. EAGLY, Ph.D., Department of Psychological Sciences, Purdue University, West Lafayette, Indiana

SUSAN T. FISKE, Ph.D., Department of Psychology, University of Massachusetts at Amherst, Amherst, Massachusetts

DANIEL T. GILBERT, Ph.D., Department of Psychology, University of Texas at Austin, Austin, Texas

E. TORY HIGGINS, Ph.D., Department of Psychology, Columbia University, New York, New York

ALICE M. ISEN, Ph.D., Department of Psychology, Cornell University, Ithaca, New York

GORDON D. LOGAN, Ph.D., Department of Psychology, University of Illinois, Champaign, Illinois

AKIVA LIBERMAN, M.A., Department of Psychology, New York University, New York, New York

LEONARD L. MARTIN, Ph.D., Department of Psychology and Institute for Behavioral Research, University of Georgia, Athens, Georgia

MARLENE M. MORETTI, Ph.D., Department of Psychology, University of Waterloo, Waterloo, Ontario, Canada

LEONARD S. NEWMAN, M.A., Department of Psychology, New York University, New York, New York

JAMES W. PENNEBAKER, Ph.D., Department of Psychology, Southern Methodist University, Dallas, Texas

MICHAEL I. POSNER, Ph.D., Department of Psychology, University of Oregon, Eugene, Oregon

MARY K. ROTHBART, Ph.D., Department of Psychology, University of Oregon, Eugene, Oregon

DAVID J. SCHNEIDER, Ph.D., Department of Psychology, Rice University, Houston, Texas

BRIAN F. SHAW, Ph.D., Departments of Psychiatry and Behavioural Science, University of Toronto, and Department of Psychology, Toronto General Hospital, Toronto, Ontario, Canada

ROXANE COHEN SILVER, Ph.D., Department of Psychology, University of Waterloo, Waterloo, Ontario, Canada

ROSEMARY TAIT, M.A., Department of Psychology, University of Waterloo, Waterloo, Ontario, Canada

ABRAHAM TESSER, Ph.D., Department of Psychology and Institute for Behavioral Research, University of Georgia, Athens, Georgia

JAMES S. ULEMAN, Ph.D., Department of Psychology, New York University, New York, New York

DANIEL M. WEGNER, Ph.D., Department of Psychology, Trinity University, San Antonio, Texas

Contents

Introduction

JOHN A. BARGH
JAMES S. ULEMAN
New York University

To what extent are our conscious intentions and strategies in control of the way information is processed in our minds? This seems to be a question of importance to us both as psychologists and as human beings.

—Posner and Snyder (1975, p. 55)

How two social–personality psychologists came to edit a volume on the unintentionality of thought does perhaps merit a bit of explanation. It seems safe to say that the notion of thought being outside of one's ability to control it is usually identified with the study of abnormal rather than normal psychological functioning. Obsessional, delusional, schizoid, and other maladaptive modes of thought that produce emotional suffering and an inability to function in society typically are considered to be unintended. For many years, it was assumed that when unintended thought processes and contents did occur, they were the markers of abnormal functioning; but in the normal and far more common case, an individual was in control of his or her perceptual interpretations, judgments, and behavior.

Up to the mid-1970s or so, information processing approaches to the study of learning and memory, and the cognitive psychology that emerged from them, did essentially assume that a person had a rational, logical, and intentional control over the flow of thought and decisional output (see review by Lachman, Lachman, & Butterfield, 1979). Social psychology, which had been cognitive in its orientation for far longer (see Zajonc, 1980), also implicitly or explicitly assumed that the mediating cognitive processing was conscious and intentional in nature (Bargh, 1984). But by the time Posner and Snyder posed their question in the opening of their 1975 Loyola Symposium chapter, these assumptions were under attack. Cognitive models were being developed in which the information processing involved in reading or in answering questions about category membership were seen as largely uncontrolled, automatic "spreading activation" phenomena (e.g., Anderson & Bower, 1973; Collins & Quillian, 1969; La-Berge & Samuels, 1974). The assumption of rationality in decision making was coming under attack as well from demonstrations of illogical or at least nonoptimal use of available information (Chapman & Chapman, 1967; Langer & Abelson, 1972; Nisbett & Borgida, 1975; Tversky & Kahneman, 1974). Given this ferment at the time, what was it about Posner and Snyder's chapter that made it so influential, such a turning point in the study of intentionality in cognitive processing?

For one thing, the assumption of control was still alive and well in the research that appeared to challenge it. Models of semantic memory that posited a mechanistic spreading activation process assumed that such processing was instigated by an intention to search memory or to answer the experimentally given question (e.g., Is a penguin a bird?). The uncontrolled activation of a word's meaning was considered a consequence of the larger intentional act of reading. And the demonstrations of irrational decision making were taken as evidence of short-cut, heuristic decision *strategies*. None of these areas of research ever explicitly challenged the assumption of intentional control over the way information is processed in one's mind. It was Posner and Snyder's explicit recognition that the existing evidence implied that intentional control may not always exist, and that the degree to which one could control one's own thoughts and decisions was an *empirical* question, that opened the gates for research on the role of intention. By framing it up front as an empirical question, and not as an assumption a model could make or could not make, the longstanding implicit assumption of intentionality was transformed into an explicit empirical question. More than this, Posner and Snyder specifically discussed the importance of studying the role of intentionality in the domains of emotional experience and impression formation, and in the areas of perception and memory retrieval processes more generally.

As most social psychological models implicitly assumed the role of deliberate, calculated, conscious, and intentional thought, the degree to which such thought did occur in naturalistic social settings became of critical importance. In a chapter perhaps as influential as Posner and Snyder's, and maybe more so within social psychology, Langer (1978) emphatically rejected the assumption of deliberative, conscious thought as typically underlying social behavior, and provided several demonstrations from her work on social scripts (e.g., Langer & Abelson, 1972). Our own research programs have followed in this tradition by addressing the extent to which impressions of others are formed and dispositional attributions are made without the person's intention that such processing occurs.

From our own interest in these issues of automaticity, control, awareness, and intention, we noticed how these issues kept coming up, implicitly as well as explicitly, with increasing frequency during this decade in the cognitive, social–personality, clinical, and health psychology literatures. We were also struck by how little one area of this research seemed aware of research going on in the other domains. Consequently, we set out to organize a symposium at a national psychology conference to bring everyone together as a first step in opening lines of communication between people interested in the same set of fundamental issues, albeit applied to different substantive concerns. We were pleasantly surprised by the enthusiastic reaction the idea received, and the timeliness of the project became obvious to us through nearly everyone's interest and eagerness to participate. It was also clear that a single, brief symposium could hardly contain the number of centrally relevant researchers who expressed a desire to participate.

To give credit where credit is due, when he heard of our dilemma, Tory Higgins helpfully suggested that we forget the symposium and instead edit a book on the topic. Our embarrassment of riches for the symposium turned into as stellar a lineup of chapter contributors as one could wish. Still, we hasten to add that there are many potential contributors doing interesting and innovative research related to the themes of the book, in addition to the present set of contributors. Only our concern with keeping the cost of the volume reasonable prevented us from asking another dozen or so to contribute. Although we are in fact quite proud of the breadth of perspectives and issues covered by the chapters in this book, we must also emphasize that the present coverage by no means represents a complete and exhaustive treatment of unintentional thought, its causes, and its consequences. There is much relevant and provocative work being done in the areas of metacognition, industrial–organizational psychology, and psycholinguistics, as well as in philosophical inquiries into the nature of free will. It is one of our hopes for this book that it might open the door to further volumes integrating these additional perspectives on the vagaries and varieties of unintended thought.

As this was the first time either of us had edited a volume, perhaps we did not deserve the lack of complications and headaches that are supposed to be part and parcel of the editor's lot. But the cause of our good fortune was not so much beginner's luck as the enthusiasm of our contributors and their promptness (some more than others) in getting their chapters to us. Equally important, our publisher, Seymour Weingarten, has been supportive of this project from the outset and exceptionally helpful and patient with us novices throughout the entire process.

MAJOR THEMES

The importance of investigating the question of whether influences on thought and behavior are unintended, and its centrality to so many issues in all areas of psychology, is illustrated by the diversity of backgrounds of the contributors and the specific issues they address. We can identify several themes running through the various chapters. One is a concern with ecological validity, with the extent to which previous research findings in the areas of impression formation, causal attribution, stereotyping, and persuasion, in which subjects typically had a restricted set of information and ample time to consider it and the goal or *instructions* to use it in a certain way—generalize to more natural settings in which (1) people may not have that goal or purpose, (2) may not have the motivation to engage in the necessary effortful thought, or (3) have many other things to attend to. Other chapters on ruminations and the self-control of thought, and clinical interventions to *regain* lost control, are equally concerned with naturally occurring problematic cognitive processes that are unintended and at least not fully controlled.

A second theme is the growth of sophistication in terminology, reflecting the complexity of the basic issue of whether one can and does control one's own thought. Although the title of the book focuses on the issue of intentionality, the concerns of the chapters encompass a wide spectrum of facets to the question of intentionality and degrees of control. What constitutes an act of control—namely, the ability to stop an ongoing process at will—is directly addressed by Logan (Chapter 2) and by Wegner and Schneider (Chapter 9). The difference between an *unintended* influence over judgment and an *uncontrollable* influence is the primary focus of the Fiske (Chapter 8) and the Uleman (Chapter 14) contributions: Both point out that the unintended influences that a person becomes aware of may be controllable, but only if the effort is made to do so. From this it is clear that whether one is *aware* of the operation of an interpretational bias (such as in stereotyping and prejudice: Fiske, Chapter 8) or goal-directed ruminations (as in an unresolved personal dilemma: Martin & Tesser, Chapter 10; Pennebaker, Chapter 11) is critical for whether there is even the possibility of controlling that process (see Bargh, Chapter 1; Moretti & Shaw, Chapter 13; Higgins, Chapter 3; and Isen & Diamond, Chapter 4). Finally, as unintended perceptual influences and streams of conscious thoughts occur easily, without much if any mental effort, they constitute a rather *efficient* mode of thought. Gilbert (Chapter 6) concentrates on the greater efficiency by which people make dispositional rather than situational attributions and the implications that this has for social situations in which attention may likely be spread thin. In those cases the more efficient forms of social perception that are not knocked out by concurrent attentional demands will have primary influence over the course of subsequent attributional and evaluative judgments.

Yet a third theme pervading this volume has to do with whether self-control over the various forms of unintended thought is even possible, and if it is possible, what determines when a person will *exert* that control? There appears to be a healthy debate on the possibility of control over the relatively automatic output of perceptual, interpretational mechanisms (see Fiske, Chapter 8; Gilbert, Chapter 6; Bargh, Chapter 1; Isen & Diamond, Chapter 4; Newman & Uleman, Chapter 5; Posner & Rothbart, Chapter 15; and Moretti & Shaw, Chapter 13). However, even if such control is in fact possible, there is still a question as to whether such control will be exercised, and the determinants of when it will be. This is a much less researched topic than the first, and both Fiske (Chapter 8) and Chaiken, Liberman, and Eagly (Chapter 7) provide valuable insights on which situational factors are critical in motivating a person to exert the necessary effort for more deliberate processing.

There appears to be more of a consensus among researchers that unbidden conscious thoughts are quite difficult to control, even *with* the intention and desire to stop them (see Wegner & Schneider, Chapter 9; Tait & Silver, Chapter 12; Martin & Tesser, Chapter 10; and Pennebaker, Chapter 11), as anyone who has a jingle from a commercial persistently running through their head can testify. These contributors, along with Moretti and Shaw (Chapter 13), provide valuable ideas about how best to go about reestablishing control over those unintended thoughts. However, there does seem to be some disagreement, at least on the surface, about whether it is preferable from a therapeutic standpoint to attempt to suppress such thoughts in the first place. Wegner and Schneider (Chapter 9) are quite lucid as to the potential dangers of attempts at thought suppression—that those attempts might well backfire and exacerbate the problem—and Pennebaker discusses the stress involved in constant inhibition of unwanted memories and the potential benefits of finally talking about the precipitating traumatic event. Of course, the matter is not so simple as whether ruminations are "good" or "bad," but these basic differences in how the contributors approach the topic do underscore the potential downside of exerting control over the natural course of one's stream of thought.

CHAPTER SUMMARIES

These summaries are designed to give you a quick idea of each chapter's viewpoint and the major topics covered. They are by no means exhaustive, but merely present our slightly idiosyncratic view of highlights. Photocopying these summaries is no substitute for buying the book, to say nothing of actually reading it.

Part I (Chapters 1 to 4) deals with basic processes and issues central to understanding what unintended thought may be, how it may operate, and how it may interact with other important aspects of mental life such as the self concept and affect.

Bargh (Chapter 1) takes up the concept of automatic social perception and cognition—that is, mental processes that are unintended, involuntary, effortless, autonomous, and nonconscious. He presents a strong argument that while purely automatic processes do exist, classifying processes in this all-or-none fashion omits many of the most important cases, and hinders recognition of some of the most interesting questions. In place of the simple automatic/not-automatic dichotomy, he offers "a taxonomy of automaticities" based on their necessary preconditions, and demonstrates this taxonomy's utility in classifying an impressive array of phenomena. "Preconscious automaticity" has the fewest preconditions, though it has some. "Postconscious automaticity" additionallly requires awareness of the initiating stimulus. And "goal-dependent automatic processes" (both unintended and intended) have more preconditions, and are shown not to be oxymorons but essential categories for understanding the influence of automatic processes in daily life. Bargh then discusses how these processes seem to affect consciousness, focusing on salience effects, the nature of phenomenal experience and consciousness, and how much control we ultimately have over our own thoughts and actions. As the lead chapter in this collection, I (J.U.) think that it provides an excellent overview and introduction to the central issues and phenomena.

Logan (Chapter 2) challenges one of the characteristics usually attributed to automatic processes—their autonomy or uncontrollability. He begins his persuasive case that automatic processes are controllable by reviewing research on intentions' influence in the Stroop task, priming, and reflexes. Then, noting that the ability to stop a process is a sine qua non of control, he reviews evidence from his "stop signal" paradigm that a simple arithmetic calculation is easier to stop in midcourse than a rhyming or category judgment, even though all of these are automatic in some respects. A brief review of obsessive thought and everyday slips and errors further supports his conclusion that automatic activities are not beyond control, except in pathological hyperactivity and obsessive disorders. Finally, he outlines his provocative "instance theory" of automaticity as memory processes, and shows how it naturally implies five kinds of control over automatic processes or their consequences.

Higgins (Chapter 3) presents his most extensive theoretical integration to date of theory and research on automatic concept activation and accessibility, and also describes how concept activation can be an unconscious source of emotional distress and suffering. He first reviews research on variation in the accessibility of knowledge, whether declarative, episodic, or procedural. This leads to presentation and further development of the synapse model of knowledge accessibility and activation; a discussion of some of the implications of knowledge applicability, and of multiple sources of knowledge activation; and the suggestion of a possible basis for hallucinations. He then reviews the latest evidence on whether self-knowledge forms an interconnected cognitive structure and concludes that although it does not, there are subsystems of self-knowledge that do, organized around mismatches with self-standards. These subsystems are described by his self-concept discrepancy theory and, being subject to automatic activation, constitute vulnerability factors for suffering. Finally he describes an impressive series of research findings demonstrating that "it is this unconscious activation of *psychologically significant patterns* that is a major source of subjectivity and suffering."

Isen and Diamond's chapter (Chapter 4) on affect and automaticity focuses on two affective phenomena in which research has implicated automatic processes: valence and feeling states. They begin with an extended review of some of automaticity's most relevant features including parallel processing, the capture of attention, effects of intentions and goals on automatic processes, extraction of meaning (in dichotic listening, the Stroop effect, and semantic priming), the difficulty of assessing awareness, and problems posed by multiple criteria for automaticity. Their review of available studies on automatic valence activation ends with a conclusion that they "fall short of establishing unambiguously that affect is activated or perceived automatically." Research on feeling states—including affect as a retrieval cue, affect's influences on encoding, state-dependent learning, and asymmetries between positive and negative affect—suggests to them that automatic processing is more the exception than the rule. They explore the utility of viewing relations between automaticity and affect in terms of overlearning, and outline a challenging research agenda that follows from this. The importance of chunking, hierarchical organization, and cognitive load is described, and is developed for positive affect and cognitive organization. They close with an invitation to view affect not as something apart from cognition, but "as a factor that is similar in fundamental ways to other factors that influence thought and behavior."

Part II of the book brings together four chapters on unintended thought about particular content that is common in social life: thought about people's traits, thought about persuasive messages, and stereotyped thinking about others.

Newman and Uleman (Chapter 5) focus on thought about others' traits. They begin with evidence that people sometimes spontaneously infer other's traits from their behavior without intending to, or even being aware that they have done so. This raises three general questions. First, what kinds of inference processes generate traits, particularly spontaneously? They suggest that although attribution theorists have traditionally treated traits as causes, trait inferences need not result from causal thinking, and both traits and causes may be embedded in the implicit knowledge structures we routinely activate to understand events. Second, what do traits describe, and what kinds of traits are most likely to be inferred spontaneously? They consider traits as causes, traits as dispositions that only become apparent under particular conditions, and traits as summary behavioral frequencies; and review empirical evidence on when people use traits to refer to behavioral stability, predictability, and causality. They suggest that for laypeople, traits usually refer to dispositions, and present evidence that more "confirmable" traits are inferred spontaneously. Third, what consequences might spontaneous trait inferences have? They make a case for their role in self-perception, including the perseverance of misperceptions; self-fulfilling prophecies in social interaction; stereotype confirmation and persistence; and vividness effects. Finally, they discuss developmental and cross-cultural limits on the ubiquity of spontaneous trait inferences.

Gilbert (Chapter 6) examines intentional inferences about another's traits (and attitudes and moods) and finds that they occur in two stages: a relatively automatic "characterization" stage in which the person and focal behavior are similarly described, and a more deliberate "correction" stage in which the characterization may be modified in light of situational constraints on the person. He then describes an ingenious series of experiments that supports this formulation. The "Sexual Fantasies" experiment showed that a demanding concurrent task prevents subjects from correcting their initial impressions of another's anxiousness; the "Preoccupied Listener" experiment showed the same effect of "cognitive busyness" on attitude ratings. In "Don't Look Now," subjects rated another's mood, and failed to correct initial characterizations because they were too busy *not* doing something. The "Mr. Smile and Mr. Sneer" experiment replicated this effect with a demanding concurrent task we have all performed: ingratiating the other person. The "Hungry Chameleon" and "Silly Faces" experiments suggested that nonverbal information may be processed more efficiently than verbal information. Gilbert concludes with an attempt to answer the musical question. "How is the inferential system designed to employ conscious attention and why is it designed this way?" In addition to being one of the wittiest chapters in the book, this chapter draws on the ideas of a thinker who has been dead longer than anyone else cited.

Chaiken, Liberman, and Eagly (Chapter 7) present the latest and most fully developed version of the heuristic–systematic model (HSM) of how people assess the validity of persuasive messages. "Systematic" processing is the more methodical, effort- and data-intensive, explicit mode; "heuristic" processing depends more on implicit rules and schemata, and requires less effort and cognitive capacity. Heuristic cues include message length ("length implies strength") and source likability. The model describes what determines how extensively each mode is used, including heuristics' cognitive availability, accessibility, and reliability; available capacity; the sufficiency principle; beliefs about one's own systematic processing ability; and personal relevance. Other topics include the interactional and additive effects of concurrent use of these two processing modes, and sources of biased processing. The authors expand the model from its initial accuracy motivation context to include effects of other motives: the defense of current beliefs, and impression management. Finally, they suggest ways in which the HSM is applicable to other judgment and decision-making tasks, including impression formation and social prediction. Altogether, this chapter presents an extremely rich synthesis of established findings from the persuasion literature, the latest theorizing on underlying cognitive and motivational processes, and bold hypotheses to guide future research on both attitudinal and nonattitudinal social judgment.

Fiske (Chapter 8) analyzes the meaning of the book's central concept—intent—in the context of stereotyping and discrimination. "That stereotyping is unintentional and perhaps inevitable is a mistaken assumption, at worst, and an inadequately examined one, at best." She reviews classical (James; Freud; Tolman; Lewin; and Miller, Galanter, and Pribram) as well as contemporary psychological theorists; evidence on lay usage of intent; and legal conceptions of intent. This last is particularly relevant to stereotyping because unintended discrimination is usually not illegal. This analysis leads to identifying the central defining feature of intent—having cognitively available options—and two other features important in attributing intent: making the hard or difficult choice, and motivated attention. In addition, she discusses the relationship of intention to the automatic/controlled processing dichotomy, the ideas of conscious and unconscious intent, and how intent distinguishes between conservative and liberal readings of the law on discrimination. Her conclusion that "people can help it when they stereotype and prejudge" is disarmingly simple in light of the sophisticated scholarship that supports it.

Part III of the book consists of five chapters in which regaining control of unintended thought, both normal and pathological, is the central issue. In contrast to earlier chapters, these discuss more long-term, "real world" phenomena that are distinguished by their phenomenology. These chapters are particularly relevant to depression, to psychological and physiological stress responses to traumatic life events, and even to obsessional and anxiety disorders.

Wegner and Schneider (Chapter 9) focus on the suppression of thoughts about particular things (e.g., white bears). How can people keep things out of mind while keeping in mind what to keep out of mind? Although this question seems to tie concepts of will and consciousness into a Gordian knot (or, using their phrase, a "phantom of the ganglia"), they cut through it by simply asking subjects to avoid particular thoughts and report when they occur nonetheless. So unlike Logan (Chapter 2), they track control over minutes, rather than milliseconds, rely largely on self-report, and look at inhibiting conscious content rather than halting process. After reviewing some of Freud's and their own ideas on why and how people suppress, they distinguish between two methods: unfocused and focused self-distraction. Unfocused self-distraction is more common, and their research suggests that it is one basis for a reliable "rebound effect." After subjects suppress for 5 minutes and are then free to think about anything, they think more about the suppressed content than subjects who have never suppressed. Focused self-distraction, as well as changing the physical environment after suppression, reduces rebound. They discuss the processes that may underlie these effects, and tentatively suggest some "home remedies and nostrums." Finally, they summarize some fascinating preliminary evidence on differences between depressed and nondepressed college students' suppression strategies for emotional content.

Martin and Tesser (Chapter 10) advance a set of ideas on the nature of ruminations, which they characterize as (1) occurring over days or years rather than merely minutes, (2) usually counterproductive, and (3) involving both automatic and controlled processes. What starts them? What stops them? And what determines their content? Their ideas are organized in terms of three assumptions, supported by a wealth of classical (e.g., Zeigarnik) and contemporary research. First, "people's thoughts and actions are directed by goals." Second, "goals are structured hierarchically," and there are known determinants of which hierarchy levels one is aware of at any time. And third, there is "a relatively specific sequence of behaviors following frustration of an important goal," consisting of repetition, problem solving, end-state thinking, negotiation, channelization, and learned helplessness. They discuss the challenging problems of conceptualizing control that result from their view that conscious behavior is directed by unconscious goals, and that "rumination will continue until the individual correctly identifies (either deliberately or fortuitously) the goal that has been frustrated." Finally, they discuss a variety of methods for doing empirical research on ruminations, and present promising preliminary results from their laboratory employing recognition reaction times.

Pennebaker (Chapter 11) also employs the idea of levels of thought, in terms not of goal hierarchies but of breadth of content. Low (vs. high) "level of thought" (LoT) involves narrowed perspective, lack of self-reflection and self-consciousness, and impoverished affect. Pennebaker's research shows that major uncontrollable stressors (e.g., traumatic life events) lower LoT. He describes how to measure LoT from stream of consciousness transcripts, and discusses relationships between LoT and Vallacher and Wegner's action identification, Langer's mindlessness, cognitive complexity, and the repressive coping style. But his major focus is on the remarkable effects of chronic and changing LoT on physiological and cognitive functioning. Chronically low LoT may increase hemispheric lateralization in the brain's processing of verbal and emotional information. His own research shows interactions between people's chronic LoT, current LoT, and skin conductance. And it shows long-term effects of manipulating LoT on immune system functioning (T-lymphocyte activity), frequency of minor illnesses, blood pressure, and heart rate. He suggests that low LoT is associated with less complex social judgments, and notes similarities between low LoT and the clinical disorder of alexithymia. Finally, while chronically high LoT is also associated with health problems, these do not seem to be as severe as those associated with chronic low LoT.

Tait and Silver (Chapter 12), like Martin and Tesser (Chapter 10), are concerned with involuntary, intrusive ruminations. However, they focus not on frustrated and often unconscious goals, but on the attempt to give meaning to past traumatic life events. Past research shows that the frequency of such ruminations correlates with reported levels of stress and negative affect, and that they occur in Posttraumatic Stress Disorder. The authors describe results of their extensive interview study, among senior citizens, of ruminations about "the worst thing that ever happened" to them. These included the loss of family members and the onset of health problems, and occurred an average of 23 years earlier. Although ruminations' frequency, intensity, and intrusiveness correlated with current life dissatisfaction and self-assessed lack of recovery, these features of ruminations were unrelated to when the trauma occurred (2 to 50 years earlier). The same was true for ruminations about the event's continuing negative implications for their lives, the event's meaninglessness, and the need to discuss it. Understanding these findings entails a theoretical analysis of obstacles to giving personal meaning to traumatic life events, and integrating them into a coherent assumptive world view. Tait and Silver are insightful and compassionate in discussing the importance of relations between the nature of the events and the belief systems that must accommodate them, as well as characteristics of the social milieu, including divergent effects of others' empathetic distress and empathetic concern. Finally, they note the irony that time alone does *not* heal psychological wounds, but the common belief that it does may actually keep them from healing.

Moretti and Shaw (Chapter 13) focus on the intrusive, self-disparaging, self-reproachful, and apparently automatic thoughts that characterize clinical depression. They begin by noting that automatic cognition can be quite functional, and that dysfunctional automatisms are more likely to develop when people are not aware of their dysfunctions or their consequences; when they are embedded in complex processes, making it harder to isolate the source of dysfunction; when affective arousal is high and cognitive resources are limited; and when dysfunctional constructs are highly accessible. These conditions appear to obtain in depression. They critically review current theories of depression, including Beck's, and then experimental research on the role of dysfunctional automatic processing in depression. The latter includes Moretti's own research on depressed and nondepressed subjects' response latencies for self- and other-referent judgments, as well as work by Bargh, Higgins, and Wegner. Their lucid review highlights questions for future research, and generally supports their thesis that "self-referent information processing in depression is automatic and dysfunctional." Finally they discuss clinical interventions in light of this evidence, noting that psychodynamic approaches do not consider negative self-referential thoughts per se to be an appropriate treatment focus, and that behavior therapy's "thought-stopping" technique does not have reliably enduring effects. Thus they concentrate on convincingly enumerating the probable reasons for cognitive therapy's demonstrated effectiveness with depression, and the likely role of stable individual differences in vulnerability to depression.

The last section of the book (Part IV) is devoted to perspectives on the preceding chapters. It does not provide the kind of authoritative integration that reviewers, readers, and even contributors often crave. That, as always, is left to the future "as an exercise for the interested student." But its two chapters do champion broader integrations, across the other chapters' remarkable range of phenomena (which span ten orders of magnitude in duration alone), and across subdiscipline boundaries. And they offer some suggestions and illustrations of how these integrations might look.

Uleman's chapter (Chapter 14) and whimsical diagram distinguish among five kinds of cognitive processes, in terms of extent of personal control. Automatic processes (including Bargh's preconscious and postconscious varieties) are uncontrolled (autonomous) after they are triggered, though the triggering stimuli and subsequent processing may be controlled. Spontaneous processes produce unintended and usually nonconscious results, but they seem to require other intentional processing goals (Bargh's unintended goal-dependent automaticity). Intentional processes are under the control of conscious goals, which involve conscious choices among optional routes to envisioned end states. Ruminative processes fall between spontaneous and intentional processes because they are neither nonconscious byproducts of intended processing nor consciously goal directed. Finally, responsible processes are those governed by others' goals as well as strictly personal goals. These rough categories emerge from reviewing the meanings of "automatic" and "control," and the range of phenomena to which personal control seems relevant. The categories' utility is illustrated in a review of some of the cognitive processes known to occur when comprehending text.

Posner and Rothbart (Chapter 15) discuss the book's major topics from the unique but happily congenial perspective of neuropsychology. They note that the extremely complex cognitive processing found in split brain and amnesic patients, without benefit of consciousness, is consistent with many chapters' claims of complex nonconscious processing. They discuss several of the chapters' proffered alternatives to a dichotomous conception of automaticity, calling the purely automatic process "a convenient fiction" and joining in suggesting ways that automatic processes are controlled. They enumerate the functions of attention, and focus on attention as the psychological control system. Recent data on cerebral blood flow, during dual task versions of repetition and semantic priming, point to the exciting discovery of two anatomically distinct but functiallly integrated attentional control centers. Disorders of the anterior center, which seems to be involved in controlling semantic memory and language, may underlie schizophrenics' illusion that their thoughts are controlled by external agents. The authors present a view of affect as not "just another node within a cognitive network, but as a system with its own separate neural basis and rules of operation," and describe some of the difficulties with giving either the cognitive or affective system priority. Finally, they illustrate the benefits of studying the development of central control systems, at both neural and cognitive levels, with research on developing control of eye movements, of temperament, and of visually guided reaching and grasping.

ACKNOWLEDGMENTS

We've already noted our gratitude to the contributors and the publisher for their splendid contributions to this project. In addition (and just a bit redundantly), we must thank our generous and supportive colleagues in the Social–Personality Program at New York University. They have all worked at creating a collegial atmosphere that could not be better. Finally, the preparation of this book was facilitated by NIMH grant BSR-1-R01-MH43959 to Uleman and NIMH grant BSR-1-R01-MH43265 to Bargh.

REFERENCES

Anderson, J. R., & Bower, G. H. (1973). *Human associative memory.* Washington, DC: Winston and Sons.

Bargh, J. A. (1984). Automatic and conscious processing of social information. In R. S. Wyer, Jr. & T. K. Srull (Eds.), *Handbook of social cognition* (Vol. 3, pp. 1–43). Hillsdale, NJ: Erlbaum.

Chapman, L. J., & Chapman, J. P. (1957). Genesis of popular but erroneous diagnostic observations. *Journal of Abnormal Psychology, 72,* 193–204.

Collins, A. M., & Quillian, M. R. (1969). Retrieval time from semantic memory. *Journal of Verbal Learning and Verbal Behavior, 8,* 240–247.

LaBerge, D., & Samuels, S. J. (1974). Toward a theory of automatic information processing in reading. *Cognitive Psychology, 6,* 293–323.

Lachman, R., Lachman, J. L., & Butterfield, W. C. (1979). *Cognitive psychology and information processing: An introduction.* Hillsdale, NJ: Erlbaum.

Langer, E. J. (1978). Rethinking the role of thought in social interaction. In J.H. Harvey, W. J. Ickes, & R. F. Kidd (Eds.), *New directions in attribution research* (Vol. 2). Hillsdale, N.J: Erlbaum.

Langer, E. J., & Abelson, R. P. (1972). The semantics of asking a favor: How to succeed in getting help without really dying. *Journal of Personality and Social Psychology, 24,* 26–32.

Nisbett, R. E., & Borgida, E. (1975). Attribution and the psychology of prediction. *Journal of Personality and Social Psychology, 32,* 932–943.

Posner, M. I., & Snyder, C. R. R. (1975). Attention and cognitive control. In R. L. Solso (Ed.), *Information processing and cognition: The Loyola symposium.* Hillsdale, NJ: Erlbaum.

Tversky, A., & Kahneman, D. (1974). Judgment under uncertainty: Heuristics and biases. *Science, 185,* 1124–1131.

Zajonc, R. B. (1980). Cognition and social cognition: A historical perspective. In L. Festinger (Ed.), *Retrospections on social psychology.* New York: Oxford.

PART I

BASIC PROCESSES

1

Conditional Automaticity: Varieties of Automatic Influence in Social Perception and Cognition

JOHN A. BARGH
New York University

Although the notion of automatic cognitive processing has a tradition as old as the field of psychology itself (see review by James, 1890; also Bargh, 1984; Gilbert, Chapter 6, this volume), the widespread application of the concept to social perception, judgment, and behavior is a relatively recent occurrence. Its renaissance can be traced to the introduction of a theoretical distinction between "automatic" and "conscious" or "controlled" processes in the mid-1970s—a distinction that since has become increasingly important for an ever-wider range of social phenomena.

An automatic thought process was initially defined as one that is capable of occurring without the need for any intention that it occur, without any awareness of the initiation or operation of the process, and without drawing upon general processing resources or interfering with other concurrent thought processes (LaBerge & Samuels, 1974; Posner & Snyder, 1975; Shiffrin & Schneider, 1977). In other words, an automatic process was defined as satisfying the criteria of being *unintentional, involuntary, effortless* (i.e., not consumptive of limited processing capacity), *autonomous*, and occurring *outside of awareness*. Currently, the consensus definition of automaticity remains that it possess all of these features (see reviews by Johnson & Hasher, 1987; Kahneman & Treisman, 1984; Logan & Cowan, 1984; Zbrodoff & Logan, 1986); this unitary nature is what distinguishes the concept of automaticity from each of its defining qualities (see also Fiske, Chapter 8, this volume).

Conscious or controlled processes, on the other hand, were defined as those that are under the flexible, intentional control of the individual, that he or she is consciously aware of, and that are effortful and constrained by the amount of attentional resources available at the moment (see also Atkinson & Shiffrin, 1968; Logan, 1980; Neely, 1977; Shallice, 1972). Any single cognitive process, then, was thought to be either controlled or automatic (although most processing *tasks* are sufficiently complex to involve a combination of automatic and controlled components; e.g., Shiffrin & Schneider, 1977), according to this dual-mode model of cognition.

AUTOMATICITY AND ITS DISCONTENTS

It is a central aim of this chapter to persuade the reader that the assumption that a given cognitive process is either automatic or controlled by these definitional criteria is incorrect. What is more, my thesis is that this assumption is misleading, resulting in faulty conclusions regarding the nature of social-cognitive processing. Let us start with the assumption that a cognitive process is either automatic or controlled, according to the definitional criteria of the two types. It logically follows that if a process fails to meet one or more of the criteria for one type, then it must be, by default, an instance of the other form of processing. For example, if a process is found to occur effortlessly, or outside of awareness, then it may be concluded that the process is automatic because, by definition, it is *not* a controlled process. On the assumption that the automatic and controlled processing modes are mutually exclusive and exhaustive, if a process does not meet all of the criteria for an automatic process, then it must be of the controlled variety. Ascribing the quality of automaticity or control to a process by default in this manner is therefore a direct consequence of assuming that the automatic–controlled dichotomy exhausts the universe of cognitive processes.

What Does It Mean for a Social-Cognitive Process to Be "Automatic"?

Because, by definition, a controlled process is not unintentional, or effortless, or autonomous, or involuntary, or occurring outside of conscious awareness, this "automaticity by default" has meant in practice that a social-cognitive process has been considered to be automatic if it possesses *any* of these qualities. Thus, automaticity has been invoked to explain the following processing effects:

1. Effects of which a person is *unaware* (in making attributions—Taylor & Fiske, 1978; during impression formation—Higgins & King, 1981; that result in emotional experience—Strauman & Higgins, 1987).

2. Effects that are relatively *effortless,* such that they will operate even when attentional resources are scarce (e.g., Bargh & Thein, 1985; Bargh & Tota, 1988; Gilbert, Pelham, & Krull, 1988).
3. Effects that are *unintentional* and occur even in the absence of explicit intentions and goals (e.g., Winter & Uleman, 1984).
4. Effects that are *autonomous,* in that they will run by themselves to completion, without the need of conscious attentional monitoring (e.g., Smith, Branscombe, & Bormann, 1988; Smith & Lerner, 1986).
5. Effects that are *involuntary* or uncontrollable even when one is aware of them (e.g., Bargh & Pratto, 1986; Higgins, Chapter 3, this volume; Wegner & Schneider, Chapter 9, this volume).

It is clear from these examples that the concept of automaticity has become important in understanding a wide variety of social-perceptual and social-judgmental phenomena. It is also apparent that several of the component criteria of automaticity have been investigated in their own right because of their relevance for these research domains. But as the present review of the social research into automatic phenomena indicates, most of these findings meet only one or two of the defining criteria of automaticity, and not the others.

A few examples may illustrate the point to be developed more completely later. Several studies of automaticity in impression formation (e.g., Bargh & Thein, 1985; Gilbert & Krull, 1988) and social judgment (e.g., Smith & Lerner, 1986) have shown subjects to be able to engage in task-relevant forms of processing very efficiently, even when attentional resources are scarce. Because these routinized modes of thought are relatively independent of the availability of conscious attention, they are automatic in the "efficient" or "effortless" sense. But in these studies, subjects were given explicit instructions by the experimenter to form an impression or make the judgment. Thus, it could not be said that the subjects performed these cognitive operations unintentionally or involuntarily, or that they were not aware of doing so or could not stop themselves.

By the same token, many processing effects that have been shown to be unintentional depend on conscious and attentional processing of some form for their occurrence. Examples of these unintended outcomes of intended and aware thought are the activation of accessible attitudes upon perception of the attitude object (Fazio, Sanbonmatsu, Powell, & Kardes, 1986), trait categorizations of behavioral information (Uleman, 1987; Winter & Uleman, 1984), and most category-priming demonstrations (e.g., Higgins & King, 1981; Wyer & Srull, 1986).

Intention, Awareness, Efficiency, and Control as Separate Issues

These examples, and the other research to be reviewed herein, illustrate that there is a problem both with the unitary definition of automaticity and with the assumption that automatic and controlled processes, as consensually defined, exhaust all possibilities. These difficulties with the concept of automaticity are not unique to social-cognitive research by any means, having been noted and debated for several years within cognitive psychology. Whereas in social cognition the research emphasis in this decade has been on documenting the automatic (albeit single-criterion—unintended or efficient) aspects of perceptual and judgmental processes previously assumed to be conscious and deliberate, in cognitive psychology just the reverse has been true. Processes previously believed to be prototypic examples of automaticity—for instance, the activation of a word's meaning during reading; effects of semantic priming and spreading activation; the Stroop color–word interference effect; and well-practiced visual target detection—have all been shown to require some attentional resources (and thus not to be completely effortless), and not to occur if the subject has certain processing goals (e.g., Dark, Johnston, Myles-Worsley, & Farah, 1985; Hoffman & MacMillan, 1985; Kahneman & Henik, 1981; Ogden, Martin, & Paap, 1980). In addition, as Logan and Cowan (1984) have pointed out, most processes that are popularly considered to be automatic, such as typing, reading, driving, and walking, are actually highly controlled, in that they are intentional and stoppable. Furthermore, one is usually aware of such routinized action sequences while they are occurring, although one does not need to pay active attention to them because of their autonomous nature (Norman & Shallice, 1986). It sometimes happens that people are aware of performing complex actions, even though they did not intend them, as in the "action slips" documented by Norman (1981).

Thus, attention, awareness, intention, and control do not necessarily occur together in an all-or-none fashion. They are to some extent independent qualities that may appear in various combinations. As there is ample evidence that automatic processing is not unitary, such that all of its component properties do not co-occur, so also are there no compelling theoretical reasons to believe in its unitary nature (Zbrodoff & Logan, 1986). On these grounds, Zbrodoff and Logan (1986) concluded that it would be more profitable to investigate the individual properties separately.

It is clear that continuing to treat intentionality, awareness, efficiency, and control as a composite, all-or-none package may well confuse rather than clarify these component issues, which are of great importance in their own right to the study of social perception, judgment, and behavior. Take, for example, the conclusion that stereotyping is "automatic" because one finds that it is an efficient and easily activated process. As Fiske (Chapter 8, this volume) argues, consumers of such research in the legal arena may quite logically take this conclusion to mean that there is evidence that stereotyping is uncontrollable as well, and there would be important and far-reaching consequences for findings of responsibility in discrimination cases. More than that, studies that have found stereotype activation to be efficient have at the same time found the use of such stereotypes in making judgments about others to be controllable, given values or motivation not to do so (Devine, 1987).

Another example is the proposal that dispositional attributions are made "automatically" because they are made more easily and efficiently than situational ones (e.g., Gilbert, Chapter 6, this volume; Smith & Miller, 1983; Winter, Uleman, & Cunniff, 1985); this conclusion has been interpreted to mean that such judgments often are made unintentionally and involuntarily (e.g., Hastie & Park, 1986; Trope, 1986). Whether attributions are made with little or no conscious consideration, or only through a deliberate weighing of evidence following certain rules, has been an issue of great theoretical importance within attribution theory and research for many years (e.g., Hansen, 1980; Jones, 1979; Kruglanski, 1980; Langer, 1978; Winter & Uleman, 1984).

All Automatic Processing Is Conditional

If one examines the uses of the label "automatic" within social psychology, one finds that some of the processes are intended, whereas others require recent conscious and intentional processing of related informational input, or attentional resources. Still others are not intended, but do depend on goal-driven processing of a certain kind. As discussed in this chapter, the obtained automatic effects fall into certain regular classes: those that occur prior to conscious awareness ("preconscious" automaticity); those that require some form of conscious processing but that produce an unintended outcome ("postconscious" automaticity); and those that require a specific type of intentional, goal-directed processing ("goal-dependent" automaticity). Subtypes within each of these major classes can also be delineated, based on variations in their necessary instigating conditions. These types of processes clearly vary as to the conditions needed to produce the effect in question: whether subject's awareness of certain stimuli is a requirement, whether focal–spatial attention is necessary, and whether a certain goal or intention must be operative.

All automaticity is conditional; it is dependent on the occurrence of some specific set of circumstances. A cognitive process is automatic *given* certain enabling circumstances, whether it be merely the presence of the triggering proximal stimulus, or that plus a specific goal-directed state of mind and sufficient attentional resources. The various phenomena labeled as "automatic" within social psychology vary greatly in the number and quality of the conditions explicitly required for them to occur. Moreover, there are many such "automatic" effects that may have implicit or "hidden" preconditions, due to the specifics of the experimental procedures. Numerous studies administer mood or attitude or personality inventories just prior to experimental tests of the "automaticity" of the subject's cognitive processing in the domain of the questionnaire. Given what is known about the residual effects of recent conscious thought (see below; also Higgins & Bargh, 1987; Wyer & Srull, 1986), one cannot tell from such experimental designs whether the obtained effect would occur *without* the extensive prior thought (see Bargh, 1984; Bargh & Tota, 1988). Another difficulty in interpretation results from the specific instructions given the subjects. If one instructs them to form an impression of a target person, for example, and then finds that they do so even when operating under severe attentional shortage (Bargh & Thein, 1985; Gilbert et al., 1988), one cannot conclude that such impression formation, however efficient and effortless, would have occurred in the absence of the explicit goal. If subjects have the task of differentiating between various stimuli, and then learn to do so (e.g., Lewicki, 1986b), their pattern identification abilities have not yet been shown to be independent of the intention and goal of learning the patterns.

When such implicit assumptions are put to the test, they are often found to be invalid. For example, impressions are not always formed in the absence of an impression formation goal (see Bargh & Thein, 1985, p. 1143; Sherman, Zehner, Johnson, & Hirt, 1983; Wyer & Gordon, 1982; Wyer & Srull, 1986), and implicit pattern learning does not occur unless one attends to the task and attempts to learn the target pattern (Nissen & Bullemer, 1987).

Johnson and Hasher (1987) concluded from their review of automaticity research that one must be very careful to specify all of the necessary conditions for producing a given effect (instructions, attention availability, direction of focal–spatial attention, etc.), because "theoretical ideas based on incomplete task analyses are likely to be wrong" (p. 655). If such task analyses are important to a complete understanding of the operation of the relatively simple cognitive tasks reviewed by Johnson and Hasher (e.g., lexical decision, word pronunciation), then they are even more critical for phenomena of interest in social perception and cognition.

The Ecology of Automaticity

Deconstructing the concept of automaticity into its component features also facilitates an assessment of the ecological validity of the phenomenon in question by focusing attention on the extent to which the phenomenon possesses each of the separate qualities, instead of just one or two. Among the issues that this would help to address are the following:

1. If the effect requires an explicit intention or goal on the part of the subject, how likely is the person to have such a goal outside the laboratory? Are there individual differences in motivation, values, or interests, for example, that would make it more or less likely for a person to have this goal or intention in the first place, and if so, to have it to a greater or lesser degree? And does the effect depend on not only the specific intention, but one of a certain minimal strength? Are there situational factors that are likely to produce such intentions?

2. If the effect requires the availability of attentional capacity, then will such capacity be available in natural settings? For example, findings in the area of person memory (Srull, 1981, Experiment 4), causal attribution (see Gilbert et al., 1988), impression formation (Bargh & Thein, 1985; Strack, Erber, & Wicklund, 1982), and stereotyping (Pratto & Bargh, 1988) are different under a shortage of attentional resources than with ample attention available, and such minimal attention allocation may be the norm outside the laboratory.

3. Is the effect controllable, or will it occur even when the person does not intend it and is trying to stop it (see Tait & Silver, Chapter 12, this volume; Wegner & Schneider, Chapter 9, this volume)? If a person is not aware of the effect, will making the person aware allow him or her to control it (see Moretti & Shaw, Chapter 13, this volume)?

Clearly, the fewer the conditions that have to be in place to produce an effect, and the more likely those conditions are to occur in the social environment, the more general and constant the effect will be. Cognitive processes that require only registration of the triggering proximal stimulus pattern, and that will occur even if the person is trying to prevent them, will be the most generally influential in ongoing and subsequent judgment and behavior. These have been referred to by Fodor (1983) as "input processes"; they are unavoidable and uncontrollable (e.g., basic sensory encoding). For example, try as one might, it is not possible to see the oranges in a bowl as actually being purple, or the sky at noon as a vivid red. On the other hand, processes that require intention and attentional resources in addition to the triggering stimulus pattern are less general, because attention may not be available and other intentions might be in place when the proximal stimulus event occurs. The prediction and understanding of any given phenomenon will be greatly enhanced by the discovery of those component processes that automatically occur given the least provocation.

In summary, the concept of automaticity continues to be important to understanding social perception, judgment, and interaction, but it has assumed a variety of meanings that correspond to its separate defining qualities. If one is not aware of a process, or does not need to consciously monitor its operation, or does not intend it, the process often is considered to be automatic in nature, despite the fact that it is manifestly controlled and conscious in all other respects. This problem can be traced to the underlying assumptions that the defining features of automaticity will necessarily co-occur, and that the automatic–controlled dichotomy comprises the entire set of cognitive processes. However, it is becoming ever more obvious that these assumptions are inherently invalid.

As noted elsewhere in this volume as well (e.g., see the chapters by Fiske, Gilbert, Logan, and Uleman), the multiple meanings of the concept of "automaticity" that are currently in use have resulted in some confusion as to what one means by the term. Because social-psychological research is not really concerned with the question of whether automatic processing exists in its purest form, but rather with the individual component issues of intentionality, awareness, autonomy, and efficiency, the field would be better served if research explored these separate issues in their own right. Namely, does a process require attention? Does it require one's intention that it occur? Does it occur involuntarily? Does it depend on recent preactivating or priming experience? In other words, theory should conceptualize the judgment or behavior process of interest as automatic *given* certain necessary conditions, and research should focus on establishing those minimal conditions needed to produce the effect.

VARIETIES OF AUTOMATICITY

The several demonstrations of automatic processing of social stimuli have varied widely as to their necessary conditions. Some require conscious awareness and attentional processing; some need preactivation alone without necessarily any awareness of the preactivating event; some are dependent on specific processing goals; and some require the intention that the

TABLE 1.1.   Necessary Conditions for Each of the Several Varieties of Automatic Processing

	Precondition				
Variety of automaticity	Awareness of instigating stimulus	Specific processing goal in place	Intention that effect occur	Allocation of focal attention to process	Conscious guidance to completion
Preconscious					
Construct activation	No	No	No	No	No
Evaluation and affect	No	No	No	No	No
Postconscious					
Reverberatory	Yes	No	No	No	No
Residual	Yes	No	No	No	No
Goal-dependent					
Unintended					
Side effect	Yes	Yes	No	Yes	No
Context-dependent	Yes	Yes	No	No	No
Intended					
Autonomous procedures	Yes	Yes	Yes	No	No
Incubation	Yes	Yes	Yes	No	No

effect itself occur. Technically speaking, all of these effects are quasi-automatic, but each of them nonetheless captures some essence of what it means to be automatic. A review of these findings follows, organized in terms of necessary conditions and ordered from the fewest to the greatest number of them. Table 1.1 contains a summary of the prerequisites for each of the varieties of automaticity delineated in this section.

Preconscious Automaticity

Preconscious processes require only the triggering proximal stimulus event, and occur prior to or in the absence of any conscious awareness of that event. In these forms of environmental analysis reside the interpretative analyses that produce the "givens" of consciousness and the starting point of controlled processing. Preconscious processes operate uncontrollably, autonomously, involuntarily, and nearly effortlessly. Fodor (1983) has likened preconscious input analyses to reflexes, as "they are automatically triggered by the stimuli they apply to" (p. 55).

To be precise, inside the precondition of the presence of the relevant proximal stimulus event is the additional one that the environmental event to be preconsciously analyzed be detected by the sensory apparatus. This requires, at least in the case of vision, the allocation of spatial attention to the relevant part of the environmental field (Kahneman & Treisman, 1984). In other words, a modicum of attention allocation may be necessary for registration of the proximal stimuli, even though the analysis of the stimulus takes place prior to conscious awareness (see Kahneman & Treisman, 1984, and Norman & Shallice, 1986, for more on the distinction between attention and awareness). Because many such preawareness and involuntary processes have been shown to require some minimal amount of attentional processing (Dark et al., 1985; Kahneman & Treisman, 1984), the term "preconscious" is preferred here to the term "preattentive" (e.g., Neisser, 1967), and the strong claim of completely effortless preconscious processing is not made here (see Kahneman & Treisman, 1984).

The importance of the preconscious variety of automaticity is twofold. First of all, the validity of the interpretations and evaluations that are made prior to awareness and that constitute one's subjective experience are then trusted as accurate and valid, precisely because the person is not aware of any inferential activity (Johnson & Raye, 1981; Jones & Nisbett, 1971). Thus, these interpretations are not questioned, but are seen as undoubtedly valid sources of information, and are as a result a prime source of judgments and decisions (Andersen, 1984; Andersen & Ross, 1984; Bargh, 1988; Jacoby & Kelley, 1987; Jones & Nisbett, 1971). Second, there is an increasingly influential model of consciousness (to be discussed presently), to the effect that consciousness is a *construction* of the world that integrates all current sources of activated memory locations, both those preconsciously and those intentionally activated. Thus, preconscious analyses also may play an indirect role in memory and judgmental processes, even when the output or products of such analyses are not expressed in phenomenal awareness, through their influence on the outcome of the judgment or interpretation that is made consciously.

Chronically Accessible Social Constructs

Two major forms of chronic preconscious interpretative influences have been studied in social cognition: social construct activation and evaluation extraction. Through frequent and consistent activation by the environment, social constructs representing types of behavior (e.g., honesty, selfishness, aggressiveness) become capable of being activated by the relevant proximal stimulus information itself, without the need for conscious intention or goals or attention, or any awareness that the information has been thus categorized (Bargh, 1984; Higgins & King, 1981). As a consequence, chronically accessible constructs are more likely to become activated by relevant information than are constructs that require intentional, goal-directed processing to be used. Considerable individual differences emerge in the content of the chronically accessible constructs one possesses (Higgins, King, & Mavin, 1982); these are presumably due to differences in idiosyncratic life experiences (i.e., long-term social environment).

The interpretative influence of chronically accessible constructs was demonstrated in one study (Bargh, Bond, Lombardi, & Tota, 1986). We found that subjects with a chronically accessible construct for kind or shy behavior were more likely to interpret ambiguously kind or shy target behaviors in terms of that trait than were other subjects, in the absence of any priming or preactivation of these constructs, and in an experimental session held 2 months after the assessment of chronicity was made.

The implication that chronically accessible constructs should exert a preconscious influence on the selection of social information, so that chronic construct-relevant information would be more likely to influence conscious judgments, has found empirical support as well. Higgins et al. (1982) found that subjects were more likely to later remember those behaviors of a target person that corresponded to the subjects' chronically accessible constructs than those that did not. Using the Stroop color–word technique to test the involuntary and uncontrollable aspects of preconscious construct activation (see Logan, 1980; Kahneman & Treisman, 1984), we (Bargh & Pratto, 1986) found that subjects required more time to name the color of trait adjectives that corresponded to their chronically accessible constructs than those that corresponded to their inaccessible constructs. As the word meanings were irrelevant to the color-naming task, it was in the subjects' interest to ignore them, yet the chronically accessible material proved more of an involuntary distraction. And information relevant to subjects' self-concept also caused greater distraction from the conscious and intentional task (i.e., shadowing a list of words in the dichotic listening task), even when subjects were unaware of the presence of that information (Bargh, 1982). As self-relevant information is among the most frequently experienced, it is likely that individuals possess chronically accessible constructs for such domains of social information (Bargh, 1984; Higgins et al., 1982). Fitting the defining criteria of a preconscious process, therefore, the activation of such constructs by relevant environmental events is involuntary, is uncontrollable, and occurs prior to and even in the absence of conscious awareness of the activating information.

Preconscious social information processes are also important for their efficiency, such that in the common environmental situation of attentional or informational overload, these preconscious processes will still furnish their output to conscious judgment processes. Social interactions are rich in information content as well as in such attention-demanding tasks as self-presentation, impression management, action planning, and action execution, not to mention the more routine operation of comprehending the environment and reacting to it. Consequently, preconsciously supplied data will tend to have a proportionately greater impact on judgments and behavioral decisions under these overload conditions, as many of the conscious and attention-demanding information-gathering procedures will not be possible (see Bargh & Thein, 1985; Gilbert, Chapter 6, this volume).

We (Bargh & Thein, 1985) simulated such a situation by presenting information about a target person very quickly to some subjects, so that they had just enough time to read the information; the remaining subjects had control over how long they could examine each of the target's ascribed behaviors. The target was described either as behaving mainly honestly (12 honest and 6 dishonest behaviors) or mainly dishonestly (12 dishonest and 6 honest behaviors). Within each of these conditions, some subjects had a chronically accessible construct relevant to the target behaviors ("chronics"), and the other subjects did not ("nonchronics"). Subjects were instructed to form an impression of the target, and all subjects (chronics and nonchronics alike) in the self-paced condition did so easily, on line, at the time they read through and considered the target's behavior, and these impressions were in accord with the proportion of honest to dishonest behaviors the subjects had been shown. In the overload condition, however, only subjects with a chronically accessible construct for honesty were able to form an impression of the target person on line; the patterns of their free-recall and impression results were, in fact, not distinguishable from subjects in the self-paced (nonoverload) condition. Overloaded subjects without this efficient construct showed no evidence of being able to form an on-line impression of the target person, and were the only group who later had to rely on their memory for the behaviors to compute their impression ratings (see also Hastie & Park, 1986).

Several writers have argued that group stereotypes may be easily activated by the presence of identifying features, such as skin color or gender characteristics (e.g., Brewer, 1988; Deaux & Lewis, 1984; Rothbart, 1981).

These structures would thus constitute a preconscious influence on the interpretation of target behaviors and on decisions about the targets (see Bodenhausen & Wyer, 1985). Several studies have documented the unintentional aspects of stereotype activation (e.g., McArthur & Friedman, 1980; Mills & Tyrrell, 1983), and others have shown the efficient and relatively effortless nature of stereotype operation (Devine, 1987; Pratto & Bargh, 1988).

Evaluation and Affect

The second major form of preconscious meaning extraction that has been investigated is affect or evaluation (see Bargh, 1988; Spielman, Pratto, & Bargh, 1988, for reviews). Johnson (1983), Gordon and Holyoak (1983), Jacob and Kelley (1987), and Mandler and Nakamura (1987) have discussed how liking for a person or other environmental object or event may be due to the buildup of a sensory representation of the physical features of the stimulus that is not available to conscious introspection. Theoretically, the greater ease or fluency with which the sensory representation enables the stimulus to be perceived results in a positively valenced feeling of familiarity that is misattributed by the subject to qualities of the stimulus itself (Zajonc, 1968, 1980; but see Mandler, Nakamura, & Van Zandt, 1987). Thus, the mere exposure effect of frequency of experience on liking may be produced entirely preconsciously (Kunst-Wilson & Zajonc, 1980; Seamon, Brody, & Kauff, 1983; Wilson, 1979). The importance of such automatic and preconsciously extracted affect has been demonstrated for concurrent and subsequent consciously made social judgments and behavioral decisions. Bornstein, Leone, and Galley (1987) subliminally presented a photograph of a confederate repeatedly to subjects in a first task, and then the subjects interacted with him and another confederate in a subsequent group decision-making task. During the group discussion, subjects expressed agreement with the confederate whose photograph they had been exposed to reliably more often than they did with the other confederate, apparently because they had greater liking for the target confederate due to their prior subliminal processing of his facial features.

Postconscious Automaticity

Another variety of automaticity is that which depends on recent conscious experience and attentional processing of some type for its occurrence. This postconscious influence on processing can be defined as the nonconscious consequences of conscious thought. The conscious experience may be intentional, or it may be unintentional—what is important is that the material be in awareness. Much of the contents of awareness are driven by the environment, and one does not intend or control the flood of these perceptual experiences, yet they should still result in postconscious effects.

Postconscious influences take two forms. One is a "spreading" or *re-verberatory* influence, as in the effect of a recent positive or negative experience on the accessibility of similarly valenced material in memory (e.g., Clark & Isen, 1982; Isen, 1984). This increased accessibility results in influences on judgment, phenomenal experience (e.g., mood), and behavior that the person does not intend and of which he or she is not aware.[1] The second form of postconsciousness is a *residual* influence of material recently in awareness, as in priming effects in which the activation resulting from processing information in one context persists long enough to affect subsequent interpretation in an unrelated context (see Bargh, 1984; Higgins, Chapter 3, this volume; Wyer & Srull, 1986, for reviews). The difference between reverberatory and residual postconscious influences lies in whether spreading activation to related memory locations is involved, or whether the effect is produced by the same construct originally activated during conscious thought.

Reverberatory Effects

Postconscious influences on judgments and decisions may occur when a recent positive or negative experience carries over to influence consciously made decisions in unrelated domains and to spread throughout memory to activate similarly valenced material. Postman and Brown (1952), for example, showed that activating the concept "good" lowered subjects' recognition threshold for words related to success, and activating the concept "bad" made subjects more sensitive to failure-related words. People who have recently thought about a positive event believe that they are less likely to contract fatal diseases or have other unpleasant events in their future, whereas people who have just thought about a negative event believe that these events are more likely to happen to them (Johnson & Tversky, 1983). Forgas and Moylan (1987) found that individuals interviewed outside a theater after seeing a film made more positive or negative judgments across a variety of domains (e.g., politics, expectations for the future, quality of life), in line with the emotional tone of the film (i.e., happy vs. aggressive or sad). And Isen, Shalker, Clark, and Karp (1978) found that experimentally manipulated positive experiences resulted in subjects' being more able to recall positive events from their past. Clark and Isen (1982) concluded from their review of this area of research that "there are automatic processes initiated by feeling-state including events," and that "this increased accessibility of material related to a person's current affective state may then affect his or her impression of the world and behavior" (p. 87).

Another manifestation of postconscious affect is the automatic activation of a consciously made and stored evaluation associated with a specific mental representation, as an immediate consequence of conscious attention to the relevant object or event in the environment. Fazio et al. (1986) have argued that social stimuli for which one has a strong attitude (with strength defined in terms of speed of evaluation) automatically activate that evaluation upon the mere perception of the object, person, or event in the environment. Fazio et al. (1986) demonstrated the automatic evaluation effect by employing the names of subjects' strong-attitude objects as primes in an evaluative decision task. Subjects were instructed to attend to each prime in order to be able to repeat it out loud at the end of the trial.[2] When presented immediately before adjectives of the same valence, the names of these strong-attitude objects facilitated the task of evaluating the adjectives, compared to a baseline prime condition; when the object names were presented before oppositely valenced adjectives, decision times were slowed. Such priming influences did not accrue for weak-attitude objects (i.e., objects to which subjects were slow to respond). Apparently, conscious attention to a strong-attitude object name automatically activated the evaluation associated with it, so that subjects were faster to make that evaluative response for the target adjective and slower to make the opposite evaluative response (presumably due to the need to inhibit the primed evaluation from becoming the [incorrect] response; see Logan, 1980; Neely, 1977).

There was some indication in the Fazio et al. (1986) study that the automatic evaluation effect might not be restricted to just the most strongly held attitudes. In their Experiment 3, the evaluative priming effect was obtained even for attitude objects that were relatively weak (i.e., slowly evaluated). In a recent series of experiments, we (Bargh, Chaiken, Pratto, & Govender, 1988) found that at least 70% of the attitude objects in the Fazio et al. (1986) study showed the automatic evaluation effect, with the size of the effect nearly identical throughout the range of attitude response speeds. The only attitude objects that did *not* show the effects were the very weakest, and even these were found to show the effect under certain experimental conditions. Thus, the automatic and preconscious activation of evaluations may be a very general and pervasive phenomenon.

An intriguing aspect of these findings is that activation was found to spread from one activated representation to others of similar valence. Thus, even though Johnson and Tversky (1983) varied the degree of similarity between the event that subjects were asked to think about in order to induce the desired affective state, and the event of which they judged the likelihood, the degree of similarity did not affect the results. For example, subjects were more likely than a control group to believe they would get cancer, whether they had just read about someone who had cancer or someone who died in a fire. Moreover, the preconscious evaluative priming effects obtained in the Fazio et al. (1986) and Bargh, Chaiken, et al. (1988) studies, as well as by Greenwald, Liu, and Klinger (1986), occurred for *randomly* paired attitude objects and adjectives of the same valence, such that no other features besides valence were shared. On the basis of these findings, in which evaluative similarity was the only linking feature between prime and target concepts, it seems that there may exist separate positive and negative affective networks that are independent from other semantic and lexical networks (see Bargh, 1988; Clark & Isen, 1982).

Postconscious effects due to mood-congruent spreading activation often involve declarative knowledge as well as episodic memories; temporary construct accessibility may be increased either by recent activation by construct-relevant features or by activation spreading to that construct from other representations to which it is linked by evaluative valence (see Bargh, 1988). For example, subjects are most likely to incidentally recall those self-relevant trait adjectives that are congruent in valence with their experimentally induced mood state (Brown & Taylor, 1986). And not only can mood states influence construct accessibilities, but the reverse is true as well: Strauman and Higgins (1987) showed that presenting a subject with trait adjectives in a sentence completion task that were related to that subject's specific emotional vulnerabilities (e.g., agitation, depression) automatically activated those emotions on line, as indicated by physiological reactions.

Residual Effects ("Priming")

The best-known example of residual postconscious influences is the demonstration of temporary category accessibility effects. In these experiments, a social construct such as *hostile* or *independent* is activated by relevant information in one context, and the subject is then shown to be more likely to use that construct to interpret the behavior of a target person in an apparently unrelated second task (see Higgins, Chapter 3, this volume; see also reviews by Higgins & Bargh, 1987; Wyer & Srull, 1986). The activation of the construct in the "priming" task is typically nonsocial in nature, such as having subjects use construct-related words in a sentence construction task (e.g., Srull & Wyer, 1979), or presenting the priming stimuli as "memory words" to hold in mind while performing another task (Higgins, Rholes, & Jones, 1977).

Recent category-relevant conscious experience thus increases the accessibility (and likelihood of use) of that category in subsequent processing for some time thereafter, after the relevant input is no longer in conscious awareness (see Higgins, Bargh, & Lombardi, 1985; Lombardi, Higgins, & Bargh, 1987). The primed constructs, while active, exert a contextually preconscious influence on the selection and interpretation of relevant proximal stimuli.

Residual postconscious or priming effects have been obtained for more abstract memory representations as well. The self-concept may be primable; Fenigstein and Levine (1984), for example, found that subjects who were instructed to use the pronouns "I" and "me" in a preliminary task subsequently made more self-attributions in an ostensibly unrelated task than did subjects who had earlier used third-person pronouns (see also Higgins, Bond, Klein, & Strauman, 1986, Study 2; Pyszczynski & Greenberg, 1987; Rhodewalt & Agustsdottir, 1986). And Chaiken (1987) and her colleagues have shown in a series of studies that simple decision rules for use in processing persuasive messages may be primable by recent experience. Subjects were exposed to a "rule of thumb" (e.g., "More is better," "Experts can be trusted") as the theme of a message in a first experiment. In an ostensibly unrelated second experiment that followed immediately, subjects were presented with a persuasive message, and those who had been primed with a decision rule were more likely to use it to evaluate the validity of the message than were nonprimed subjects. It should be noted that what was postconsciously automatic in these studies was not the processing of the persuasive message per se, which was clearly intentional, but the adoption of a particular heuristic strategy (as opposed to a more controlled and systematic mode) with which to evaluate the message (Sherman, 1987, pp. 80–81).

Postconscious Sources of Preconscious Influence

The preconscious automatic influences discussed earlier are structural interpretative biases that operate on the relevant informational input even when in a dormant (i.e., not recently active) state. What might be termed "contextual preconscious" influences result from the priming or preactivation of social constructs or knowledge structures, so that the temporarily active structures simulate the chronically active, preconscious processes in their effects on selection and interpretation of environmental information. The only difference between chronic and contextual preconscious automaticity in terms of their necessary preconditions is therefore that the latter and not the former requires an activating stimulus event prior to the automatic influence on subsequent interpretation of informational input. To the extent that such priming or preactivation requires the intervention of conscious processing and attention, the consequence influence on processing is properly considered as postconscious in nature.

Postconscious states thus can result in preconscious influences on subsequent processing. The similarity of chronic and contextual preconscious influences is shown by the fact that they independently produce the same effects on the interpretation of ambiguously relevant social events. The Bargh et al. (1986) experiment was designed to assess how chronic and contextual sources of preconscious construct accessibility influences interacted. Thus, half of the chronic and half of the nonchronic subjects were also primed outside of their awareness with trait-relevant adjectives; the remaining subjects were not primed. Both the chronic and the temporary accessibility (priming) factors demonstrated reliable main effects on the impression ratings of the target person: The chronics considered the person to be more kind (shy) than did the nonchronics, even in the no-priming condition, and subjects who were subliminally primed thought the target to be more kind (shy) than nonprimed subjects, even within the nonchronic group. Thus, for a given construct, chronic and contextual sources of preconscious influence appear to combine additively, and both sources have the same quality of influence over interpretation of construct-relevant information (see also Bargh, Lombardi, & Higgins, 1988).[3] In addition, contextual salience effects occur when the person or event is inconsistent either with the postconscious effects of the current situation (e.g., Taylor & Fiske, 1978) or with the preconscious effects of normative long-term knowledge (e.g., McArthur, 1981). And activation appears to spread among evaluatively similar memory representations, whether the initial activation is preconscious (e.g., Greenwald et al., 1986) or conscious (e.g., Isen et al., 1978). For the duration of their residual or reverberatory activation, postconscious processes may simulate preconscious effects on subjective experience and conscious judgments (see review by Higgins & Bargh, 1987).

Despite these functional similarities, the distinction between preconscious and postconscious processing is an important one. The two forms of automaticity differ in a fundamental way—the necessity of conscious awareness of the activating event—and this difference has important implications for their relative powers to influence subsequent judgment and behavior. As argued elsewhere in this chapter, the importance of preconscious automaticity lies in the fact that one implicitly trusts in the veracity of the interpretation made, because one is not aware of any processing effort being applied. In the case of postconscious effects, however, conscious awareness of and attention to the stimulus event are necessary, so that one is much more likely to be aware of the *possible* influence of that event on concurrent inferences and judgments (e.g., Jacoby & Kelley, 1987; Johnson, 1983). There is thus a greater probability in the postconscious case that when later considering their opinions or feelings about the person or event they have encountered, people will realize that the consciously noted occurrence might have an influence over their judgment. Moreover, it has been found that the residual postconscious effects of priming social constructs on subsequent judgments are dramatically different when the activating information still resides in consciousness at the time the judgment is made, compared to when the material is no longer in consciousness (Lombardi et al., 1987). As the likelihood of the activating event's remaining in conscious awareness at the time of its influence over judgment or behavior is necessarily greater for automatic effects that require conscious awareness of the event than for those that do not, the quality of the automatic influence as well as one's ability to control for it may depend on whether the effect is preconscious or postconscious.

Goal-Dependent Automaticity

A third major variety of automaticity in social psychology is that which is goal-dependent, because not only does it require conscious processing in order to occur, it depends on the person's having a particular processing goal. There are two important forms of such goal-dependent automaticity, differing as to whether the *outcome* of the processing is intended or not. One form is goal-directed processing that produces concomitant effects that are not intended by the person. One example of such unintended goal-dependent automaticity is the encoding of target behaviors in terms of personality trait constructs by subjects who are instructed merely to memorize the sentences containing the behaviors (Winter & Uleman, 1984; Winter et al., 1985).

Intended goal-dependent automaticity, on the other hand, occurs autonomously and outside of awareness, and its output is what was intended by the current processing goal. Well-practiced procedures that one intentionally employs in social judgment (Smith & Lerner, 1986) or pattern discrimination (Lewicki, 1986b), or as part of a complex skilled action (Norman & Shallice, 1986), qualify as this type of automaticity.

Unintended Goal-Dependent Automaticity

Unintended goal-dependent automatic effects have as a necessary precondition the instantiation of specific processing contexts, but they are unintended consequences of those intentional thought processes. There are two major varieties: (1) the storage in memory of abstract encodings as unintended "side effects" of another, intended process; and (2) the unintended activation and subsequent influence of social constructs and construct systems as a consequence of the current processing context.

Perhaps the best-known form of side-effect encodings when social information is being processed is the encoding of behaviors in terms of personality trait concepts. Several studies have shown that exposure to behaviors in a task in which trait inferences are not necessary or relevant (e.g., constructing grammatical sentences from a randomly ordered word string) activates the abstract trait concept to which the behavior is relevant, which then is more likely to be used to encode subsequent ambiguously relevant information (e.g., Bargh, Lombardi, & Higgins, 1988; Higgins et al., 1985; Srull & Wyer, 1979). Winter and Uleman (1984; Winter et al., 1985) showed that subjects trying to memorize sentences that contained trait-relevant behaviors encoded that trait concept as part of the episodic memorial representation of the sentence, as demonstrated by the effectiveness of adjectives related to the trait concept as retrieval cues for the sentence (see Uleman, 1987).

A study by Moskowitz and Uleman (1987) showed that the trait-encoding effect depended on the subjects' particular processing goal. Subjects had to at least intend to comprehend the meaning of the sentence; if they focused on the physical (i.e., the typeface) or the phonemic aspects of the sentence, the effect did not occur. (This finding is similar to that in the area of semantic priming, in which activation does not spread between related concepts if subjects are instructed to search for a particular letter in the priming word; e.g., Henik, Friedrich, & Kellogg, 1983; Hoffman & MacMillan, 1985.) Moreover, an impression formation goal resulted in the strongest effect (see also Bassili & Smith, 1986).

It may be, however, that such encodings are the default state, and occur *unless* a relatively unusual, overriding processing goal is in place. That is, these encodings may not depend on a specific goal state as much as they may be interfered with by a special type of processing. This distinction is important for ecological considerations, as in natural settings these special processing goals may rarely if ever occur. What the findings of Winter, Uleman, and their colleagues imply, therefore, is that an automatic and unintended way in which people understand and encode social behavioral information is in terms of personality trait dimensions, even when they are processing behaviors for purposes unrelated to their social aspects. A precondition for this effect is that one must be intending to understand the *meaning* of the behavioral information for such spontaneous encodings to occur; yet it may be that this comprehension goal is nearly always in place (see Srull & Wyer, 1986). The importance of the processing-context-dependent automaticity of trait encodings from behavioral input is that it is probably a major contributor to the tendency of people to make dispositional trait attributions from behavioral evidence, especially when their ability or inclination to consciously undertake an attributional analysis is precluded in some way (see Gilbert, Chapter 6, this volume; Trope, 1986).

Another form of side-effect encoding is the phenomenon known as "implicit learning" (e.g., Gordon & Holyoak, 1983; Reber, 1967). One is capable of picking up patterns in incoming information that one is attending to, even when one is not trying to learn that pattern. Gordon and Holyoak (1983, Experiment 1), for example, found that subjects trying to memorize letter strings nonetheless learned repeated pattern sequences, as shown by subjects' performance in classifying subsequently presented novel strings as being similar or dissimilar to the earlier set of strings. In a second experiment, the investigators found that subjects' liking judgments of test stimuli they had not seen before were a function of the stimuli's similarity to previously shown patterns that subjects were instructed only to "look at."

Does implicit learning such as this occur for social stimuli? Recently, Lewicki (1986a) has argued that the detection of covariation between personality traits and physical features (such as hair length and voice pitch) is "nonconscious." The pairing of these traits and features in the first part of the experiments was shown to influence the subsequent evaluation of novel target persons, with subjects evidencing no awareness of the relation between the traits and features in the earlier part of the study, nor of the influence of the features on their later judgments. That subjects were not able to report on the sensory features guiding their response in these ex-

periments is consistent with considerable recent research on the dissociation of sensory storage from conscious access to it (see reviews by Graf &
Mandler, 1984; Jacoby & Kelley, 1987; Johnson, 1983; Johnson & Hasher,
1987).

It is important to note, however, that in all of Lewicki's demonstrations of covariation detection using social stimuli (Lewicki, 1982, 1985,
1986a, 1986b), subjects were instructed to form an impression of the target person to whom they were paying conscious attention, and were also
informed that the study was an examination of their personality assessment abilities. As Nissen and Bullemer (1987) have shown, such implicit
pattern learning does *not* occur unless one attends to the task and attempts
to learn the target pattern. Nissen and Bullemer concluded that their findings "emphasize the importance of distinguishing between attending to the
task itself and being aware of information carried by the task. Subjects
could learn the sequence without being aware of it, but not without attending to the task itself" (1987, p. 29). Thus, the influence of the feature–
trait exposure on the subsequent evaluation of novel target persons in the
Lewicki experiments may have depended on the explicit impression formation instructions and the framing of the experiment in terms of "personality assessment." Yet the outcome of the processing—the encoding of
feature–trait relations and their later influence—was not intended by subjects, and so these effects satisfy the criteria for side-effect automaticity.

Recently, some assumed processing effects of the side-effect, unintended variety of encoding have been found not to occur. Smith and Kihlstrom (1987) found that a subject's "implicit personality theory" of how
traits covary did not affect the organization of personality-relevant material about a target person encoded into memory (see also Lewicki, 1986a,
p. 111). Moreover, the evidence frequently cited to support the assumption
that social perceivers routinely go beyond the information given and encode schema-consistent information that was not actually present has been
found lacking, and the assumption of internally generated intrusions at
encoding has been found to be unsubstantiated (Higgins & Bargh, 1987;
see also Johnson & Raye, 1981). Another widely held assumption has been
that during reading, material is automatically associated if it shares a common overarching theme. Seifert, McKoon, Abelson, and Ratcliff (1986)
showed that different stories that shared a common underlying theme were
not associated together in terms of the common theme in subjects' memory
for the information, unless subjects had the goal of detecting the abstract
similarity. Seifert et al. (1986) concluded that such thematic connections
are not made automatically in reading narrative material, but are strategy-
dependent. These studies highlight the importance of testing the conditions
under which effects assumed to be automatic do and do not occur.

The second type of unintended goal-dependent automatic processing,
context-dependent automaticity, is the unintended activation of memory
locations by the intended instantiation of a specific processing goal, so that

the constructs or schemata activated exert an influence on on-line interpretation or judgmental processes. According to Fiske and Pavelchak's (1986) model of category-based affect, impressions and evaluations of other people may be unintentionally influenced by the evaluation stored within social categories, given the intentional act of comprehending an event or person. Subsequent evaluation of and behavior toward that person or event may then proceed in line with the context-driven evaluation, even when there is other information present that might lead to a different conclusion.

Just as an evaluation may be unintentionally and automatically activated, given that the category it is associated with has been activated as part of an intentional process, so too can social constructs become active unintentionally, given the goal of self-referential thought. The unintended consequences of such activation are shown most clearly in depression, in which a negative self-concept is automatically activated in self-judgment (Bargh & Tota, 1988), leading to unwanted feelings of worthlessness, despair, and dejection (Beck, 1967; Beck, Rush, Shaw, & Emery, 1979; Moretti & Shaw, Chapter 13, this volume). We (Bargh & Tota, 1988) had depressed and nondepressed subjects judge themselves and the average other person on each of a series of depressed-content and nondepressed-content adjectives. While making these judgments, half of the subjects also tried to keep sets of six digits in mind, severely limiting the amount of attention they had for the judgment task. As subjects were instructed to make their judgments as quickly as they could, the extent to which the judgment was facilitated by an automatic, non-attention-consuming activation of the relevant construct would be indicated by a smaller increase in judgment latencies by the load manipulation. It was found that depressives thought much more efficiently in terms of negative, depression-related constructs when judging themselves, but in terms of positive constructs when judging the average other person. Nondepressives made both self- and other-judgments more efficiently in terms of positive constructs.

The automatic activation of negative constructs for depressives therefore depended on the judgment context. Given self-referential thought, negative constructs were triggered; given thought about the features of other people, positive constructs were activated. The set of constructs that became active relatively automatically for the depressed subjects was different, depending on the current processing goal. But depressives are not aware of and do not intend such fluency in negative self-judgment (e.g., Beck, 1967; Ingram & Kendall, 1987), and so the negative content constitutes an unintentional consequence of an intentional thought process.

Another example of context-dependent automaticity is the "action slip," an unintended action that results from not paying sufficient attention to the completion of an intended action (Norman, 1981). This unintended consequence of intentional behavior occurs during a routinized, well-learned behavior (e.g., driving, walking) that, once the initial behavioral goal is set in motion, operates with little or no attentional involvement. Sometimes the less frequent behavioral variations on such routine themes default into the routine actions themselves, because the needed attentional control and direction are not asserted. William James's (1890) example of the man who goes upstairs to dress for dinner and winds up in bed after undressing illustrates this point.

Intended Goal-Dependent Automaticity

According to the most recent edition of Webster's *New International Dictionary*, the central meaning of the term "automatic" is "involuntary" or "unintentional." Thus it is somewhat paradoxical to refer to an "intentional" form of automaticity—one for which both the instigation and the outcome of the process are desired and controlled. However, the notion of a form of automaticity that requires an intentional instigation follows logically from the present thesis of conditional automaticities. Such processes are autonomous, not needing to be controlled once started, and "autonomy" perhaps may be what most people (other than Webster) mean when they use the term "automatic" (Zbrodoff & Logan, 1986). (Note that all of the varieties of automaticity outlined in Table 1.1 are autonomous, as none of them require conscious guidance to run to completion.) Well-learned situational scripts (Abelson, 1980; Langer, 1978) and routinized complex action sequences (Norman & Shallice, 1986), such as those involved in driving or athletic skills, are perhaps the best-known examples of these autonomous processes. The automatized memory structures guide attention, make behavioral decisions, and direct action within the situation with a minimum of attentional control necessary (Langer & Abelson, 1972; Langer, Blank, & Chanowitz, 1978).

Because these processes are directed toward a current conscious goal, they are flexible in their application. The same general restaurant script, for example, can be applied at most restaurants within a given culture (Schank & Abelson, 1977), and the "subroutine" knowledge structures involved in the complex skill of driving can be invoked to achieve whatever is the desired destination (Norman & Shallice, 1986; see also Vallacher & Wegner, 1987). The relative autonomy of these processes is determined by how well the environmental features match the input sought by the autonomous structures. More attentional control and conscious decision making are needed when the situation has novel characteristics, such as finding one's way while driving through a new city, or encountering an unusual occurrence in a familiar setting (e.g., when the waiters in a restaurant surround your table and sing "Happy Birthday").

The fact that such processes immediately demand and attract conscious attention at these nonroutine junctures indicates how closely controlled they are, despite their otherwise autonomous nature (Logan & Cowan, 1984). Scripts and action sequences have as components conscious decision steps when the given situation typically calls for attentional processing, such as checking the rear-view mirror and deciding whether it is safe to switch lanes, or making one's selection from the menu (Abelson, 1980; Norman & Shallice, 1986).

These processes are more properly termed "semiautomatic" than "automatic," because of their intentional and controlled nature, and because they continually require reinitiation by an intentional process to continue. Logan and Cowan (1984) noted that such autonomous phases of otherwise intended and controlled processes, once started, will run to completion no matter what. An act of control is needed to initiate the next autonomous phase, however, and an act of control may stop the process after such a phase has been completed. For semiautomatic processes, the duration of such autonomous processing phases has been found to be quite short (about half a second or less) across a variety of mental and motor tasks—even for complex processing sequences that are routinized and well practiced (Logan & Cowan, 1984). Examples of such processes are the finger, hand, and arm movements involved in typing, which only occur given the intentional goal to type, but which do not need conscious attention and control for the skilled typist. Other examples are the foot and leg movements that occur when one is driving and a stop sign suddenly appears around a corner in the road—the act of hitting the brake occurs reflexively and without conscious deliberation. However, the same stop sign when one is walking up to the intersection, and the goal of driving a car is thus not currently in place, does not result in the reflexive leg and foot movements. Thus, what is needed for this type of goal-dependent automaticity is the relevant goal's being currently active, plus the presence of the triggering proximal stimulus (see Norman & Shallice, 1986).

In addition to the performance of skilled behaviors (Abelson, 1980; Norman & Shallice, 1986; Vallacher & Wegner, 1987) and nonsocial mental operations (Logan & Cowall, 1984; Zbrodoff & Logan, 1986), there are two other types of intentional goal-directed automaticity. One consists of procedural knowledge structures that have become autonomous with practice or frequent application (e.g., Anderson, 1983; Smith, 1984). The second type, "incubational automaticity," is goal-directed thought that continues after one's conscious attention has moved on to other concerns, typically when the goal was not satisfied during the material's residence in consciousness.

Smith and his colleagues (Smith, 1984; Smith et al., 1988; Smith & Lerner, 1986) have studied the development of autonomous procedures that perform social inferences from relevant sets of behavioral data. Given the intention to do so, such procedures take a relevant input and perform a transformation or apply an inferential decision rule to it. Smith and Lerner (1986) showed that components of social judgments decreased in their attentional demands to an asymptotic level after only a small amount of practice. The generality of these efficient classificatory procedures to other content domains was evidenced by the lesser amount of practice a person skilled in making one type of inference (e.g., a waitress stereotype) needed to transfer that skill to a different content area (e.g., a librarian stereo-type), compared to control subjects with no practice in making the judgment.

In incubational processing, goal-directed processes that have not achieved their goal of a problem solution nonetheless continue to operate subconsciously, after the conscious mind has moved on to other matters. This second variety of intentional goal-dependent automaticity is thus less closely controlled by the individual than is procedural automaticity, but it nonetheless satisfies the definitional criteria, as it is unintentional and autonomous once initiated. A well-known example of this situation is the "tip-of-the-tongue" phenomenon (Brown & McNeill, 1966): One is trying to remember something, definitely feels as though one knows it and is very close to remembering it, but cannot. Later, when one is thinking about something else entirely, the answer pops into consciousness (e.g., Norman & Bobrow, 1976; Yaniv & Meyer, 1987). Apparently, the search for the answer goes on in these cases autonomously without conscious awareness or control, to achieve the desired goal after all. Ghiselin (1952) has assembled examples of such nonconscious problem solving and creativity in the writings of scientists, poets, and artists. The common theme suggested by these excerpts is that such nonconscious solutions appeared only after a great deal of conscious thought and effort had gone into the attempts.

Apparently, then, processing goals that have been frequently activated over a substantial period of time can become themselves capable of operating outside of awareness. This is not surprising, considering the evidence of the subconscious operation of complex subgoals in skilled action, given the initiating intention (Norman & Shallice, 1986); in the process of developing the complex skill, the component skill originally required considerable attentional monitoring and control (see Newell & Rosenbloom, 1981). But the implications of chronically activated goal structures (Srull & Wyer, 1986) that can operate autonomously are considerable. It is possible that chronic motivations may manifest themselves in a totally automatic way, beginning with preconscious activation by triggering situational features of the overarching goal structure (see Bargh, in press; Srull & Wyer, 1986). (Note that this is very different from the Freudian notion of "unconscious" goals and motivations, in which the person is never aware of having such goals in the first place.)

This tendency for goals to continue operating after the individual has made a deliberate choice to move on to other things may result in abnormal thought patterns under certain circumstances. Several chapters in this volume (those by Moretti & Shaw, Tait & Silver, and Wegner & Schneider) are concerned with uncontrollable ruminations or obsessive thinking about negative and traumatic events. Martin and Tesser (Chapter 10, this volume) argue that this intrusive and uncontrollable conscious thinking may in fact be attributable, at least in part, to the operation of unsatisfied goals of long-standing importance to the person. Tait and Silver (Chapter

12, this volume) also contend that these unwanted ruminations may be due to the attempt to find some explanation or resolution of the traumatic event.

To summarize, the varieties of automatic processing documented by recent social-cognitive research fall into distinct groupings as a function of their necessary conditions. The three major types—preconscious, postconscious, and goal-dependent—can be distinguished by whether or not the automatic process requires recent conscious processing of the relevant stimulus, and whether a certain processing goal must be in place. Postconscious automaticity, which requires conscious awareness of the relevant stimulus event, can be further analyzed into residual effects of the specific construct activated by conscious processing, and reverberatory effects, in which the effect is attributable to spreading activation from that construct to others associated with it. The effects produced by goal-dependent automatic processing may be either unintended or intended. An unintended representation of the stimulus information may be encoded into memory as a side effect of an intended processing of the information, or knowledge structures may become activated without the person's awareness or intent due to the current conscious processing context. Finally, efficient processing procedures may operate autonomously, given one's intent to obtain their output; sometimes this output is not available immediately, but must first "incubate" for some time subconsciously.

Figure 1.1 is presented as a guide to this classification scheme. With fond memories of summer camp field guides to the identification of birds and trees, I have organized Figure 1.1 as a series of yes–no questions based on distinguishing features. These questions progressively narrow down the alternatives until only one remains.

In developing the present taxonomy of automaticities, I have found it necessary to discuss each type of process separately and in isolation from the others. Yet automatic processes, of whatever variety, do not occur in a vacuum, but in parallel or in combination with other ongoing automatic and controlled cognitive work (Logan, 1980; Posner, 1978; Shiffrin & Schneider, 1977). In present terms, this interaction is most apparent with goal-dependent automaticities, as the occurrence of the automatic effect requires specific forms of controlled processing. Postconscious effects as well are a function of the current or recent contents of conscious awareness. Thus, conscious awareness and goals in part determine the nature and course of automatic processing.

But, as alluded to already in this chapter, the reverse is true as well: There is an interface between preconscious/postconscious processing and consciousness, such that the latter is very much a function of the former. In the next section, I focus on the ways in which conscious experience and judgments are influenced by preconscious and postconscious processing, and the extent of this influence.

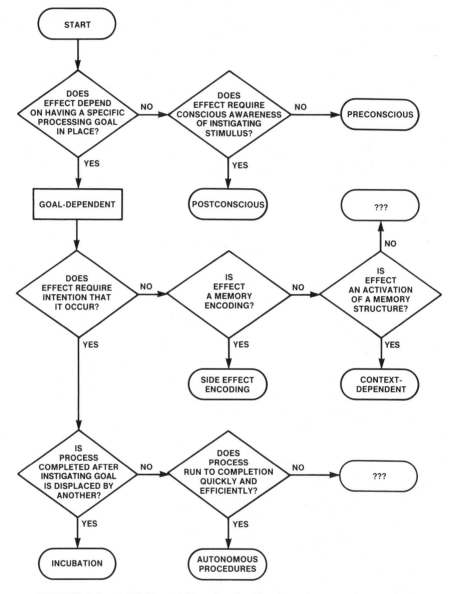

FIGURE 1.1. A "field guide" to the classification of automatic processes.

HOW PRECONSCIOUS AND POSTCONSCIOUS PROCESSING SHAPE CONSCIOUSNESS

Conscious experience is shaped by preconscious and postconscious influences in three ways: through an influence on the direction and allocation of conscious attention to environmental events; through a direct impact on

phenomenal experience via interpretative and evaluative processing of input; and through an indirect effect on consciously made decisions and judgments by preconsciously and postconsciously activated memory locations that do not themselves attain conscious awareness.

Attentional Salience Effects

Preconscious Determinants

The focus of conscious attention is to an extent under the direction of the preconscious analysis mechanism. Friedman (1979), for example, found the duration of first fixations of the eyes to elements in common scenes to be much longer for those aspects that are not usually features of such scenes (e.g., a hippopotamus in a farm pond); the mental "frame" for each scene was activated preconsciously, so that the very first time the incongruent input fell upon the retina, it required greater processing effort to be comprehended. (The importance of the measurement of *first* eye fixations is that the greater attention allocation was immediate, and was not a function of a conscious, attentional process that would have taken longer to note the inconsistencies; see Neely, 1977.) The greater attention allocated to social events that are unexpected or unusual, given long-term knowledge such as social norms (Fiske, 1980) and the typical physical features of people (McArthur, 1981), is well established, as are the judgmental consequences of the differential attention allocation (see Fiske & Taylor, 1984; Higgins & Bargh, 1987, for reviews).

A more direct preconscious influence on attention consists of automatic attention responses (Shiffrin & Schneider, 1977), in which conscious attention is automatically drawn to stimuli upon the detection of the relevant stimulus. There is very little research on such a phenomenon with regard to social stimuli, despite the fact that the original demonstration of the effect used the subject's name as the attention-grabbing stimulus (Moray, 1959). Recently, however, Hansen and Hansen (1988) showed that subjects with the task of picking out the emotionally discrepant face from an array of faces were able to detect angry faces in happy "crowds" very efficiently, such that angry faces appeared to "pop out" of the arrays. In showing that subjects' speed in detecting angry faces in happy crowds was relatively independent of the size of the crowds, Hansen and Hansen (1988) provided strong evidence of an automatic attention response to the angry face, as the time needed for a controlled, sequential search of the arrays would be necessarily increased by the number of faces to be searched (Shiffrin & Schneider, 1977).

It should be noted that in the Hansen and Hansen (1988) study, as in the Shiffrin and Schneider (1977) experiments, subjects were given the goal of detecting a target from an array. In studies in which subjects were not trying to attend consciously to targets assumed to be automatically processed, but instead to ignore them, we (Bargh, 1982; Bargh & Pratto, 1986)

showed that such stimuli (adjectives relevant to the self-concept and to chronically accessible constructs, respectively) attracted processing resources automatically; however, in both studies subjects were able to inhibit this activation from affecting their actual task responses (although the necessity of inhibition did result in slower response times). Clearly, then, if automatic attention responses to social stimuli exist, they are at least partially controllable with an intention to exert such control. Thus, whether conscious, focal attention is automatically drawn to specifiable classes of social stimuli in the absence of an explicit intention to attend to them—or, in the stronger case, despite attempts to ignore them—must remain an open question at present.

Postconscious Determinants

Salience effects in which certain environmental features or events unintentionally and autonomously attract conscious attention are also attributable to residual postconscious processing. Aspects of the current situation activate their corresponding memory representations, with this activation persisting as a background state of perceptual readiness against which the foreground of focal attentional processing takes place. Greater attention is then automatically allocated to people or events that are inconsistent with the representations activated postconsciously in this manner, such as the one male in an otherwise all-female group, or the few aggressive behaviors in a set of passive acts (Bargh & Thein, 1985; Hastie & Kumar, 1979; Higgins & King, 1981, Study 5; Taylor, Crocker, Fiske, Sprinzen, & Winkler, 1979; Taylor & Fiske, 1978). Whereas the natural direction of attention in this way is unintended and autonomous, requiring no top-down deliberative control, it is not uncontrollable, as it can be overriden by intentional concentration of attention. Of course, such concentration is more or less difficult, depending on the strength of the automatic attention response (James, 1890; Shiffrin & Schneider, 1977). As is discussed in the section to follow, preconscious and postconscious sources of activation together constitute an activated, working memory model of the environment as it usually is and recently has been.

The Social Reality Monitor

The working model of the current environment that is set up by the "social reality monitor"[4] of preconscious and postconscious processes appears to be tuned to both the long-term and the short-term expected features of that environment, in that the corresponding mental representations of those features are more accessible and easily triggered in comprehending subsequent input. We (Bargh, Lombardi, & Higgins, 1988) pitted a chronically accessible construct against a competing temporarily accessible construct to examine which would capture an event relevant to both. It was found

that the postconscious, temporarily accessible construct more often captured the ambiguous behavior after a short delay (15 seconds) between the priming and the labeling tasks, whereas the preconscious, chronically accessible construct emerged as the majority choice after a longer postpriming delay (2 minutes). Apparently, a recently primed construct is more accessible than a chronic, unprimed one for a brief time, after which the longer-term accessibility influence reasserts itself.

A similar pattern occurs for competing sources of postconscious priming influences: the more frequently a construct has been recently activated, the longer the duration of its influence (see also Bargh & Pietromonaco, 1982; Srull & Wyer, 1979), but the more recently activated construct is more accessible and likely to be used than the frequently activated one for a short time after it has been primed (Higgins et al., 1985; Lombardi et al., 1987). Moreover, the social reality monitor is flexible and not rigidly locked into a certain exclusive set of preconscious interpretative biases, because one is more likely to interpret an event in line with what has just happened instead of one's relevant chronic construct if the two suggest conflicting meanings (Bargh, Lombardi, & Higgins, 1988). Thus, the preconscious filter of social experience is automatically tuned to interpret events on the basis of the probabilities of those events, given past and recent experience.

It may be that the operation of the social reality monitor to process efficiently those aspects of the environment that are consistent with the current working model has the natural consequence of causing conscious attention to be drawn to those features of the environment that are inconsistent with that model, the constructs associated with which would not be as accessible (see Hastie, 1981; Logan, 1980), and perhaps even inhibited (see Shallice, 1972). Those aspects of the environment that are consistent with the working model (see Yates, 1985) do not require as many attentional resources to activate their already activated representations, but to the extent that an environmental event does not match this model, it requires a greater amount of attentional processing to activate its corresponding memory location (Logan, 1980). What should receive the greatest amount of attention allocation in this automatic fashion are those events that contradict an aspect of the chronically or contextually activated model. These events not only require enough attention to activate their own representation; they also require the additional amount of processing effort needed to inhibit the competing representation, as only one of the two can capture the input (see Bruner, 1957; Logan, 1980; Shallice, 1972).

Phenomenal Experience

Subjective experience is shaped by the hidden operation of input analyses of which a person is not aware. The interpretation of a behavior in line with a chronically accessible or primed social construct is seen by the subject to be due to a property of the behavior; there is no awareness of the interpretative work done by the capturing construct (e.g., Bargh, 1984; Higgins & Bargh, 1987; Higgins & King, 1981). The effect of previous exposure to a stimulus is to make that stimulus easier to perceive in the future; however, a person often misattributes this feeling of perceptual fluency to qualities of the stimulus rather than to the previous experience (Jacoby & Kelley, 1987; Johnson, 1983; Mandler et al., 1987). From their review of these and similar findings, Jacoby and Kelley (1987) concluded that "people do not develop a general ability to distinguish between what is given in a stimulus and what is an interpretation" (p. 332). And earlier, from a quite different vantage point, Jones and Nisbett (1971) argued that the different attributional tendencies of actors and observers are "amplified by bias from . . . the tendency to regard one's reactions to entities as based on accurate perceptions of them. Rather than humbly regarding our impressions of the world as interpretations of it, we see them as understandings or correct apprehensions of it" (p. 86).

Perhaps the most important consequence of preconscious input to conscious processes, therefore, is the confidence one has in the validity and accuracy of such input, given the effortless way it comes to our attention (Bargh, 1988). Such "social-perceptual fluency" is often misunderstood as being due to the clarity or obviousness of the data; the unquestioning way in which we accept preconscious interpretations, beyond the fact that we are not aware of them, may go a long way toward explaining the resistance to change of our preconceptions and stereotypes, and the strength of our convictions about people.

The history of social psychology is replete with demonstrations of people's lack of awareness or knowledge of the true influences on their judgment or behavior. Cognitive dissonance experiments relied on the fact that subjects would not be aware of the power of the social influence exerted by the experimenter or other features of the task environment, and so would have the "illusion" that they had free choice in how they behaved (e.g., Festinger & Carlsmith, 1959; Wicklund & Brehm, 1976). Exactly this notion of a lack of introspective access was embraced by self-perception theorists (e.g., Bem, 1972) as an alternative explanation for the same phenomena. In bystander intervention studies, subjects are not aware of and dismiss the possibility that the number of other people present influenced their own decision to help or not (Latane & Darley, 1970). Attributional research has uncovered a myriad of misattributional tendencies—for example, that people can easily mistake the source of their emotional arousal (e.g., Schachter & Singer, 1962; Zillman & Bryant, 1974). Furthermore, Nisbett and his colleagues (e.g., Nisbett & Bellows, 1977; Nisbett & Wilson, 1977) have demonstrated how people might not have access to the real influence on their judgments of both social and nonsocial stimuli. And Lewicki (1982, 1985, 1986a) has provided similar evidence that people can be influenced in their social judgments without their knowledge by recently encountered covariations between personality traits and physical features of target persons. Thus, there is a tradition of social-psychological research documenting the myriad of hidden influences on phenomenal experience and judgments based on it.

The Constructive Nature of Consciousness

One is consciously aware of only a subset of all of the memory representations currently activated by perceptual and cognitive activity (Bowers, 1985; Johnston & Dark, 1986; Mandler & Nakamura, 1987; Posner, 1978; Posner & Snyder, 1975). This dissociation between activation and one's awareness of that activation has been demonstrated in a wide variety of contexts, in addition to the studies of subliminal mere exposure already described. Recent exposures to words may influence perceptual thresholds and identification ability for them, independently of recognition memory (Jacoby & Dallas, 1981; Tulving, Schacter, & Stark, 1982). Several studies have found subjects to be able to discriminate stimuli of which they are not aware on the basis of lexical and semantic characteristics of the words (Balota, 1983; Cheesman & Merikle, 1986; Fowler, Wolford, Slade, & Tassinary, 1981; Marcel, 1983; Posner, 1978). Such preconscious semantic activation seems to be general across subjects, as the average person fluent in his or her native language has sufficiently frequent and consistent experience in mapping a given word to its meaning(s) for such automatic encoding pathways to develop (see Posner, 1978; Shiffrin & Dumais, 1981). Experiments in our laboratory have shown that such general preconscious effects also hold for categories of social behavior with which people have had considerable experience (Bargh et al., 1986; Bargh & Pietromonaco, 1982). We (Bargh & Pietromonaco, 1982) presented synonyms of the concept "hostile" to subjects in such a way that they were not aware of the presentation. The greater the frequency of such presentation, the more hostile were subjects' subsequent impressions of a target person who performed ambiguously hostile behaviors. We (Bargh et al., 1986) replicated this finding for the trait concepts of *kindness* and *shyness,* and Erdley and D'Agostino (1988) replicated it for *honesty* and *meanness.* Apparently, the presentation of trait-relevant words outside of awareness activates the trait construct, making it more accessible and likely to be used subsequently to interpret the ambiguous behaviors.

Finally, the "feeling-of-knowing" phenomenon documented by several recent studies (Blake, 1973; Glucksberg & McCloskey, 1981; Metcalfe, 1986; Nelson, Gerler, & Narens, 1984; Schacter, 1983; Yaniv & Meyer, 1987) refers to subjects' ability to predict accurately their subsequent ability to recognize material they cannot currently recall. Metcalfe (1986), for example, found that subjects' feeling-of-knowing ratings for trivia questions they could not answer predicted their later correct recognition of those answers. Thus, something about the degree of activation of the relevant memory location gave people the "feeling"of knowing in the absence of actual awareness of the answer, documenting the potential independence of activation from awareness.

In addition to the automatic interpretations experienced by the perceiver as stimulus properties (i.e., not as inferences), preconscious sources of activation that do not attain conscious awareness and postconscious sources that have receded from consciousness influence judgments and decisions as well. Recently, there have been a growing number of theoretical and empirical arguments in support of the constructive nature of consciousness (Fodor, 1983; Mandler & Nakamura, 1987; Marcel, 1983; Trope, 1986; Yates, 1985). Consciousness is considered to be an integration of all sources of activation relevant to current goals and purposes. People may be aware of some information, such as the products of intentional retrieval of reasoning processes; however, other sources may be nonconscious, and their influence on judgment may thus be hidden from the individual. Lewicki (1986a, Experiment 7.8), for example, has demonstrated a postconscious effect of a recent negative experience with an experimenter, resulting in avoidance behavior in an ostensibly unrelated experiment toward another experimenter having similar physical features. Niedenthal and Cantor (1986) showed that the favorability of subjects' impressions of target persons is influenced by the dilation of the targets' pupils, with subjects apparently unaware of this influence on their judgments.

The "Eternal Vigilance" of Preconscious Input Analysis

The importance of preconscious automatic input processes for consciousness is also increased by the fact that such input will always be present to influence conscious decisions, whereas input that relies on intentional and attention-demanding processes will not. Fodor (1983) postulated that mandatory input processes transform the proximal stimuli and furnish the results to central (i.e., controlled or conscious) processes, which are optional and which operate on any and all available activated memory locations that might be relevant to their goals. Trope's (1986) model of dispositional attribution similarly posits an automatic (preconscious) *identification* process, which transforms the relevant informational input into attribution-relevant features (e.g., situational influences, behavioral features), with these features serving as the input for optional and intentional inferential processes. Controlled processes, on the other hand, only occur if they are intended, and if there are sufficient attentional resources at the time to sustain them (Bargh & Thein, 1985). If the intention or motivation is not present, or if there are insufficient attentional resources because of time constraints or the focusing of attention elsewhere, then conscious reasoning and information-gathering processes will not have an influence on the judgment or decision, which will consequently be based only on the automatic input.

Thus, without sufficient motivation to engage in the effortful evaluation of a persuasive message, only the efficient and relatively effortless relevant information concerning superficial aspects of the message source, such as his or her attractiveness or expertise, will be present as input into the attitude judgment (e.g., Chaiken, 1980, 1987; Chaiken, Liberman, & Eagly, Chapter 7, this volume). Langer et al. (1978) showed that the amount of attention paid to a routine request was minimal when the personal cost of compliance was low, resulting in a decision to comply that did not take into account the nonroutine features of the request. However, when the personal cost was greater, the consequent additional conscious and effortful processing of the request resulted in detection of those unusual features and a lower compliance rate (see also Kitayama & Burnstein, 1988). When one is making attributional judgments about a person's actions and attention is loaded or scarce, preventing the effortful and intentional computation of the possible role of situational influences, the only information available is that of the actor performing a trait-like behavior, and so a dispositional attribution is made solely on the basis of this information (Gilbert et al., 1988; see also Trope, 1986). And when one is trying to form an impression of another person, attentional scarcity restricts the information available for the judgment to only those aspects of the person that can be extracted preconsciously—that is, those that are salient and automatically draw attention (Higgins & Bargh, 1987; Taylor et al., 1979), or that correspond to one's chronically accessible constructs (Bargh & Thein, 1985). Strack et al. (1982) found that judgments of a salient target's influence in a social situation were a function of prior beliefs about the target's general ability to influence others, but only when those judgments were made under time pressure, thus restricting the ability to perform a controlled search of memory for relevant evidence. When subjects had sufficient time to make the judgment, the effects of salience and prior knowledge dissipated.

As Rothbart (1981, p. 178) noted, it is often the case that we must make "snap" decisions under certainty because of an immediate need to act. Once made, these decisions and judgments are used as the basis for further decisions and judgments (e.g., Carlston, 1980; Hastie & Park, 1986) as well as the actions necessary to implement those decisions (Beckmann & Gollwitzer, 1987). Therefore, it is essential for models of social judgment, memory, and behavior to include an account of the preconscious mechanisms that transform sensory data into the stuff that conscious experience and judgments are made of.

The Limits of Preconscious Processing

What are the limits to preconscious processing's influence over the course of social cognition? Given the necessity of conscious involvement and attention for material other than sensory features (Johnson, 1983) to be stored permanently in memory (Bargh, 1984; Carlson & Dulany, 1985; Fisk & Schneider, 1984; see review by Johnson & Hasher, 1987), preconscious processes themselves are unlikely to result in the production of judgments or attributions and their storage in memory. Still, it has been argued that dispositional attributions are made automatically from behavioral input alone (see Gilbert, Chapter 6, this volume; Smith & Miller, 1983; Winter & Uleman, 1984; Winter et al., 1985). There is no convincing evidence as yet that attributions are made without conscious and intentional intervention, however; the evidence often cited for this effect is problematic because subjects did not actually make attributional judgments (see Higgins & Bargh, 1987; Uleman, 1987), or the effect required an intentional goal on the part of subjects.

Moreover, if attributions or impressions are made given only the relevant behavioral data, then they should be made at the time a person encounters such behaviors—that is, on line, at the time of information acquisition, whether or not the person has the intention of making any judgments. It has been shown that when a judgment is made (intentionally) on line, at the time of information acquisition, subsequent relevant judgments are based on that original judgment instead of being recomputed from the information accessible in memory on which the initial judgment was based (see Bargh & Thein, 1985; Carlston, 1980; Hastie & Park, 1986; Lingle & Ostrom, 1979). This holds true even when the original information is re-presented to the subject prior to the second judgment (Schul & Burnstein, 1985). Yet there are many documented circumstances when such initial judgments during information acquisition are *not* made, forcing subjects to rely on whatever information about the event is accessible in memory by that time (Bargh & Thein, 1985; Hastie & Park, 1986; Wyer & Srull, 1986). In addition, the failure to make on-line judgments, and subjects' consequent later dependence on memory for the behaviors, occur even when subjects are instructed to form impressions and are presented with very diagnostic behavioral information, but do not have sufficient attentional resources to compute an impression (Bargh & Thein, 1985). On-line judgments also are not always formed when subjects have sufficient attention but are instructed to memorize the information (i.e., not instructed to form an impression; Sherman et al., 1983; Wyer & Gordon, 1982). In short, if social judgments and attributions were made automatically and on line upon the mere presence of the relevant proximal stimuli, such judgments would not need to be based on subsequent memory for the original information.

Still, all of the studies that found that no on-line judgments were made under conditions of a lack of intention or attention presented the stimulus information to subjects in a verbal form, and it may be that in naturalistic social-interactive settings, judgments are indeed made automatically. Gilbert and Krull (1988), for example, found that subjects watching a target person on videotape formed more accurate impressions of the target when they were prevented from paying much attention to what the target was saying. As the authors concluded, it may be that dispositions are more easily inferred from nonverbal than from verbal behavior (but see Krauss, Apple, Morency, Wenzel, & Winton, 1981). Thus, a definitive conclusion as to whether impressions and dispositional attributions are formed and stored entirely preconsciously must await studies of the necessity of intention and attention that employ nonverbal as well as verbal stimulus materials.

As for whether social behavior could be under preconscious control (e.g., Langer, 1978), the evidence is fairly consistent that overt actions are under conscious control (Abelson, 1980; Logan & Cowan, 1984; Norman & Shallice, 1986; Vallacher & Wegner, 1987).[5] However, the behavioral decision itself may be based only on automatically supplied sources of information. In the theories of action control recently proposed by Vallacher and Wegner (1987) and Norman and Shallice (1986), skilled and highly practiced actions are capable of being performed autonomously and without the need for conscious monitoring, but even these (as well as all others) must be initially set in motion by an overarching intention (see "Goal-Dependent Automaticity" section).

In summary, there is frequently a confusion between the preconsciously or automatically supplied input that may influence a consciously made judgment, and this judgment itself, as if it did not need the intention or goal to occur. Preconscious processing categorizes, evaluates, and imputes the meaning of social input, and this input is available for conscious and controlled judgment and behavioral decisions; however, those judgments and decisions are not mandatory and uncontrollable, given the proximal stimulus event alone. Similarly, the uncontrollable and mandatory nature of preconscious analyses should not be mistaken for the impossibility of counteracting or adjusting their influence on judgment and behavior when one is aware of them, if that is what one wishes to do. When one knows that input processes are misleading and leading one astray, as in perceptual illusions, one does not *have* to make judgments or act as though what is apparent is real. One can grit one's teeth and drive through what one's senses insist is a lake ahead on the desert highway. Or one can prevent one's stereotypically generated preconceptions of a person from affecting one's judgments, *if* one wishes to (Devine, 1987; see also Fiske, Chapter 8, this volume) *and* if one has the attentional capacity and time to monitor the judgment process (Bargh & Thein, 1985; Pratto & Bargh, 1988). In other words, although the operation and output of preconscious processes are uncontrollable, this does not mean that the use of the output in consciously made judgments is mandatory (see Bargh, 1988; Jacoby & Kelley, 1987).

CONCLUSIONS: THE POWER BEHIND THE THRONE
OF JUDGMENT

The phenomena discussed in this chapter vary greatly in the conditions needed to produce them. Some require intention or goals; some require conscious attention or awareness; some are controllable and some are not. What all seem to have in common is that they are autonomous, not requiring conscious control (at least to some extent) once they are initiated. But the fact that many of the phenomena do require an act of control to begin, and that some even require periodic monitoring and control to be completed, suggests that the automatic–controlled processing dichotomy, especially as applied in social psychology, is misleading. On the basis of the widely held assumption that this dichotomy is composed of mutually exclusive and exhaustive types of information processing, a process that is found not to meet one or more of the criteria for one form of processing can be properly concluded to possess all of the defining qualities of the opposite form. The review of research in this chapter shows very clearly that this assumption is incorrect. Intention, awareness, attention, and control do not covary in many social-perceptual and social-cognitive phenomena, but are distinct qualities that may or may not be necessary to produce a given effect.

Whether an effect occurs unintentionally, or in the absence of awareness, or efficiently without needing many attentional resources, or autonomously once set into motion is a question of fundamental importance, especially to the ecological validity of laboratory and experimental phenomena. If an effect only occurs when the subject is instructed to think in a certain way, then whether or not he or she ever or usually has the intention to think that way outside of the laboratory should be a question of primary importance. The methodological corollary is not to assume that a processing effect would occur without the types of conditions needed to produce it in the laboratory, but to assess the extent to which those conditions of intention, attention availability, or priming, for example, are necessary to produce the effect. The fewer the preconditions, the more general, pervasive, and important the influence of the process in question.

The classification of extant research into the categories of preconscious, postconscious, and goal-dependent processing in this chapter should not be taken as the definitive word on the phenomena discussed. Further research could well determine that effects that seem today to require specific goals or instructions, for example, may only require awareness of the triggering stimuli (i.e., to be postconscious); effects that appear to require recent conscious experience may not require awareness, but preactivation alone (i.e., to be contextually preconscious). Of course, such research may instead demonstrate that effects previously believed to occur automatically, given only the triggering relevant environment event (i.e., to be preconscious), actually require a specific processing goal. This was the case with Uleman's (1987) reinterpretation of the Winter and Uleman (1984) findings, given the result of the Moskowitz and Uleman (1987) study, in which the possible influence of processing goals was tested.

Preconscious processes (and, to a somewhat lesser extent, the postconscious effects that simulate them) are important both because of the automatic selective and interpretive work they perform, and also because of the unhesitating way in which people tend to use preconsciously supplied information about the environment in constructing subjective experience and in computing judgments and decisions. The interaction of preconsciousness and consciousness can be conceptualized as "automatic input for controlled output" (Bargh, 1988), with the implication that to the extent that other information is not being supplied concurrently by intentional information-gathering processes, judgments and decisions will be largely determined by the preconscious input (Bargh & Pratto, 1986; Chaiken, 1987; Chaiken et al., Chapter 7, this volume; Gilbert, Chapter 6, this volume). Goal-dependent effects that generate unintended encodings and inferences as a side effect of an intended process are yet another important source of hidden influence.

Is this to say that one is usually not in control of one's own judgments and behavior? If by "control" over responses is meant the *ability* to override preconsciously suggested choices, then the answer is that one *can* exert such control in most cases (see Fiske, Chapter 8, this volume; Logan & Cowan, 1984). The occurrence of preconscious influences on interpretation of input and generation of evaluations is probably not controllable in the immediate, on-line sense (but is perhaps alterable through extensive and controlled rechanneling of unwanted interpretative biases, as through cognitive therapy; see Beck et al., 1979; Moretti & Shaw, Chapter 13, this volume). However, one can reduce or perhaps eliminate such preconscious influences on judgments by an intentional search for and examination of relevant evidence. Such effortful processes require the availability of sufficient attentional capacity (Bargh & Thein, 1985; Gilbert, Chapter 6, this volume) and the motivation to exert the needed effort, such as when one's own outcomes depend on the person one is evaluating (Erber & Fiske, 1984), or when an issue has important personal consequences (e.g., Chaiken, 1980; Chaiken et al., Chapter 7, this volume; Petty & Cacioppo, 1981). And even highly routinized and habitual behavior is controllable in this sense of intentionally stopping or changing it (Logan & Cowan, 1984; Norman & Shallice, 1986).

But if by "control" is meant the actual *exercise* of that ability, then the question remains open. The assertion of control over preconscious, postconscious, and context-dependent automatic influences—the three types discussed in this chapter that produce unintended outcomes—can only occur if one is aware of those influences. My own hunch is that control over automatic processes is not usually exercised, not so much because of a lack of motivation as because people tend not to accept the idea that there are many ways in which awareness, judgment, and behavior may be influenced without one's knowledge. As long as most people believe that they are aware of all such influences, that subjective awareness is an objective reflection of reality, and that their introspective ability is fully capable of sorting out the true causes of one's emotions and evaluations, then they will not take care to counteract the hidden preconscious biases and other unintended influences upon thought and behavior that are discussed in this chapter. Furthermore, the constructive nature of consciousness will result in the use of whatever sources of activation information are available and relevant at that moment, whether or not the person is aware of those sources of information.

Finally, there is the bedrock trust that people place in the validity of their subjective experience, and especially those forms of information that are the "givens" of conscious awareness (i.e., for which people do not feel that much active inferential work was needed or done). The confidence that people have in the accuracy and validity of input selection and analyses can therefore cause the pieces of evidence furnished by preconscious interpretations to awareness to be weighted more heavily than other sources of data in conscious judgmental and decision-making processes, even when a person is motivated to be deliberate and "objective" in making judgments and decisions.

For all of these reasons, it would appear that only the illusion of full control is possible, as the actual formation of a judgment or decision is intended and controllable, although the inputs and influences largely may not be. A fitting metaphor for the influence of automatic input on judgment, decisions, and behavior is that of the ambitious royal advisor upon whom a relatively weak king relies heavily for wisdom and guidance. The actual power of decision always rests with the king, who by no means has to follow the proferred advice; yet the counselor who "has the king's ear" wields the real power over decisions and the policy of the kingdom. Preconscious, postconscious, and context-dependent automatic influences have this behind-the-scenes power over judgments and action, to the extent that the conscious and intentional processes that actually make those decisions trust the automatically supplied information and do not seek to supplement it with advice from other quarters.

ACKNOWLEDGMENTS

Preparation of this chapter was supported in part by National Science Foundation Grant No. BNS-8404181 and National Institute of Mental Health Grant No. MH-43265. The extensive and insightful comments of Susan Andersen, Shelly Chaiken, Susan Fiske, Dan Gilbert, Doug Hazlewood, Tory Higgins, Len Newman, Jamie Pennebaker, Felicia Pratto, Eliot Smith, Yaacov Trope, Dan Wegner, Joanne Wood, and Jim Uleman on a previous draft are greatly appreciated. I am also indebted to the participants in my seminar on Automaticity and Social Cognition for many thought-provoking discussions of these issues.

NOTES

1. When discussing the mediating role of awareness, it is important to be explicit as to what the awareness is *of* (Bargh, 1984; Uleman, 1987). Postconscious effects require awareness of the stimulus events, not awareness of the subsequent influence of the activation resulting from them.

2. It may be that the amount of attentional effort required to hold the prime word in working memory in order to be able to repeat it after the evaluation of the adjective is a necessary precondition of the automatic evaluation effect (see Bargh, Chaiken, et al., 1988). If so, the effect would not be classifiable as a reverberatory, spreading-activation effect needing merely conscious awareness of the relevant stimulus event. It would more accurately be considered as "context-dependent"— that is, as unintended but conditional on the goal of memorizing the prime (see "Unintended Goal-Dependent Automaticity" section).

3. The duration of the priming effect, on the other hand, does appear to be a function of the extent of processing of the prime (see Bargh & Pratto, 1986, p. 301).

4. This phrase is derived from the work of Johnson and Raye (1981), whose research on "reality monitoring" concerned how one knows the difference between memories driven by sensory experience and those generated by imagination and other internal sources of thought.

5. The validity of this assertion, of course, depends on at what level one defines "behavior." It appears that behavior in the form of facial expressions and visceral reactions to affectively laden stimuli may not be as controllable, for example (Winton, Putnam, & Krauss, 1984). But it seems reasonable in light of present evidence to state that verbal behavior and bodily motion, and even facial expression to a considerable extent—in short, the components of social-interactive behavior—are never under the direct control of the environment (see also Bargh, 1984).

REFERENCES

Abelson, R. P. (1980). Psychological status of the script concept. *American Psychologist, 36*, 715–729.

Andersen, S. M. (1984). Self-knowledge and social inference: II. The diagnosticity of cognitive/affective and behavioral data. *Journal of Personality and Social Psychology, 46*, 294–307.

Andersen, S. M., & Ross, L. (1984). Self-knowledge and social inference: I. The impact of cognitive/affective and behavioral data. *Journal of Personality and Social Psychology, 46*, 280–293.

Anderson, J. R. (1983). *The architecture of cognition.* Cambridge, MA: Harvard University Press.

Atkinson, R. C., & Shiffrin, R. M. (1968). Human memory: A proposed system and its control processes. In K. W. Spence & J. T. Spence (Eds.), *Advances in the psychology of learning and motivation research and theory* (Vol. 2). New York: Academic Press.

Balota, D. A. (1983). Automatic semantic activation and episodic memory encoding. *Journal of Verbal Learning and Verbal Behavior, 22,* 88–104.

Bargh, J. A. (1982). Attention and automaticity in the processing of self-relevant information. *Journal of Personality and Social Psychology, 43,* 425–436.

Bargh, J. A. (1984). Automatic and cognitive processing of social information. In R. S. Wyer, Jr., & T. K. Srull (Eds.), *Handbook of social cognition* (Vol. 3, pp. 1–43). Hillsdale, NJ: Erlbaum.

Bargh, J. A. (1988). Automatic information processing: Implications for communication and affect. In L. Donohew, H. E. Sypher, & E. T. Higgins (Eds.), *Communication, social cognition, and affect* (pp. 9–37). Hillsdale, NJ: Erlbaum.

Bargh, J. A. (in press). Preconscious activation of goal-structures as a cognitive basis of chronic motivational states. In E. T. Higgins & R. M. Sorrentino (Eds.), *Handbook of motivation and cognition* (Vol. 2). New York: Guilford Press.

Bargh, J. A., Bond, R. N., Lombardi, W. J., & Tota, M. E. (1986). The additive nature of chronic and temporary sources of construct accessibility. *Journal of Personality and Social Psychology, 50,* 869–878.

Bargh, J. A., Chaiken, S., Pratto, F., & Govender, R. (1988). *The automatic activation of attitudes revisited.* Unpublished manuscript, New York University.

Bargh, J. A., Lombardi, W. J., & Higgins, E. T. (1988). Automaticity of chronically accessible constructs in Person × Situation effects on person perception: It's just a matter of time. *Journal of Personality and Social Psychology, 55,* 599–605.

Bargh, J. A., & Pietromonaco, P. (1982). Automatic information processing and social perception: The influence of trait information presented outside of conscious awareness on impression formation. *Journal of Personality and Social Psychology, 43,* 437–449.

Bargh, J. A., & Pratto, F. (1986). Individual construct accessibility and perceptual selection. *Journal of Experimental Social Psychology, 22,* 293–311.

Bargh, J. A., & Thein, R. D. (1985). Individual construct accessibility, person memory, and the recall–judgment link: The case of information overload. *Journal of Personality and Social Psychology, 49,* 1129–1146.

Bargh, J. A., & Tota, M. E. (1988). Context-dependent automatic processing in depression: Accessibility of negative constructs with regard to self but not others. *Journal of Personality and Social Psychology, 54,* 925–939.

Bassili, J. N., & Smith, M. C. (1986). On the spontaneity of trait attribution: Converging evidence for the role of cognitive strategy. *Journal of Personality and Social Psychology, 50,* 239–245.

Beck, A. T. (1967). *Depression: Clinical, experimental and theoretical aspects.* New York: Harper & Row.

Beck, A. T., Rush, A. J., Shaw, B. F., & Emery, G. (1979). *Cognitive therapy of depression.* New York: Guilford Press.

Beckmann, J., & Gollwitzer, P. M. (1987). Deliberative versus implemental states of mind: The issue of impartiality in predecisional and postdecisional information processing. *Social Cognition, 5,* 259–279.

Bem, D. J. (1972). Self-perception theory. In L. Berkowitz (Ed.), *Advances in experimental social psychology* (Vol. 6, pp. 1–62). New York: Academic Press.

Blake, M. (1973). Prediction of recognition when recall fails: Exploring the feeling-of-knowing phenomenon. *Journal of Verbal Learning and Verbal Behavior, 12,* 311–319.

Bodenhausen, G. V., & Wyer, R. S., Jr. (1985). Effects of stereotypes on decision making and information-processing strategies. *Journal of Personality and Social Psychology, 48,* 267–282.

Bornstein, R. F., Leone, D. R., & Galley, D. J. (1987). The generalization of subliminal mere exposure effects: Influence of stimuli perceived without awareness on social behavior. *Journal of Personality and Social Psychology, 53,* 1070–1079.

Bowers, K. S. (1985). On being unconsciously influenced and informed. In K. S. Bowers & D. Meichenbaum (Eds.), *The unconscious reconsidered.* New York: Wiley.

Brewer, M. B. (1988). A dual process model of impression formation. In T. K. Srull & R. S. Wyer, Jr. (Eds.), *Advances in social cognition* (Vol. 1, pp. 1–36). Hillsdale, NJ: Erlbaum.

Brown, J. D., & Taylor, S. E. (1986). Affect and the processing of personal information: Evidence for mood-activated self-schemata. *Journal of Experimental Social Psychology, 22,* 436–452.

Brown, R., & McNeill, D. (1966). The "tip of the tongue" phenomenon. *Journal of Verbal Learning and Verbal Behavior, 5,* 325–337.

Bruner, J. S. (1957). On perceptual readiness. *Psychological Review, 64,* 123–152.

Carlson, R. A., & Dulany, D. E. (1985). Conscious attention and abstraction in concept learning. *Journal of Experimental Psychology: Learning, Memory, and Cognition, 11,* 45–58.

Carlston, D. E. (1980). The recall and use of traits and events in social inference processes. *Journal of Experimental Social Psychology, 16,* 303–329.

Chaiken, S. (1980). Heuristic versus systematic information processing and the use of source versus message cues in persuasion. *Journal of Personality and Social Psychology, 39,* 752–766.

Chaiken, S. (1987). The heuristic model of persuasion. In M. P. Zanna, J. M. Olson, & C. P. Herman (Eds.), *Social influence: The Ontario Symposium* (Vol. 5, pp. 33–39). Hillsdale, NJ: Erlbaum.

Cheesman, J., & Merikle, P. M. (1986). Distinguishing conscious from unconscious perceptual processes. *Canadian Journal of Psychology, 40,* 343–367.

Clark, M. S., & Isen, A. M. (1982). Toward understanding the relationship between feeling states and social behavior. In A. H. Hastorf & A. M. Isen (Eds.), *Cognitive social psychology* (pp. 73–108). New York: Elsevier.

Dark, V. J., Johnston, W. A., Myles-Worsley, M., & Farah, M. J. (1985). Levels of selection and capacity limits. *Journal of Experimental Psychology: General, 114,* 472–497.

Deaux, K., & Lewis, L. L. (1984). Structure of gender stereotypes: Interrelationships among components and gender label. *Journal of Personality and Social Psychology, 46,* 991–1004.

Devine, P. G. (1987). *Stereotypes and prejudice: Their automatic and controlled components.* Unpublished manuscript, University of Wisconsin.

Erber, R., & Fiske, S. T. (1984). Outcome dependency and attention to inconsistent information. *Journal of Personality and Social Psychology, 47,* 709–726.

Erdley, C. A., & D'Agostino, P. R. (1988). Cognitive and affective components of automatic priming effects. *Journal of Personality and Social Psychology, 54,* 741–747.

Fazio, R. H., Sanbonmatsu, D. M., Powell, M. C., & Kardes, F. R. (1986). On the automatic activation of attitudes. *Journal of Personality and Social Psychology, 50,* 229–238.

Fenigstein, A., & Levine, M. P. (1984). Self-attention, concept activation, and the causal self. *Journal of Experimental Social Psychology, 20,* 231–245.

Festinger, L., & Carlsmith, J. M. (1959). Cognitive consequences of forced compliance. *Journal of Abnormal and Social Psychology, 58,* 203–210.

Fisk, A. D., & Schneider, W. (1984). Memory as a function of attention, level of processing, and automatization. *Journal of Experimental Psychology: Learning, Memory, and Cognition, 10,* 181–197.

Fiske, S. T. (1980). Attention and weight in person perception: The impact of negative and extreme behavior. *Journal of Personality and Social Psychology, 38,* 889–906.

Fiske, S. T., & Pavelchak, M. (1986). Category-based versus piecemeal-based affective responses: Developments in schema-triggered affect. In R. M. Sorrentino & E. T. Higgins (Eds.), *Handbook of motivation and cognition* (pp. 167–203). New York: Guilford.

Fiske, S. T., & Taylor, S. E. (1984). *Social cognition.* Reading, MA: Addison-Wesley.

Fodor, J. A. (1983). *The modularity of mind.* Cambridge, MA: MIT Press.

Forgas, J. P., & Moylan, S. (1987). After the movies: Transient mood and social judgments. *Personality and Social Psychology Bulletin, 13,* 467–477.

Fowler, C. A., Wolford, G., Slade, R., & Tassinary, L. (1981). Lexical access with and without awareness. *Journal of Experimental Psychology: General, 110,* 341–362.

Friedman, A. (1979). Framing pictures: The role of knowledge in automatized encoding and memory for gist. *Journal of Experimental Psychology: General, 108,* 316–355.

Ghiselin, B. (Ed.). (1952). *The creative process.* New York: New American Library.

Gilbert, D. T., & Krull, D. S. (1988). Seeing less and knowing more: The benefits of perceptual ignorance. *Journal of Personality and Social Psychology, 54,* 193–202.

Gilbert, D. T., Pelham, B. W., & Krull, D. S. (1988). On cognitive busyness: When person perceivers meet persons perceived. *Journal of Personality and Social Psychology, 54,* 733–740.

Glucksberg, S., & McCloskey, M. (1981). Decisions about ignorance: Knowing that you don't know. *Journal of Experimental Psychology: Human Learning and Memory, 7,* 311–325.

Gordon, P. C., & Holyoak, K. J. (1983). Implicit learning and generalization of the "mere exposure" effect. *Journal of Personality and Social Psychology, 45,* 492–500.

Graf, P., & Mandler, G. (1984). Activation makes words more accessible, but not necessarily more retrievable. *Journal of Verbal Learning and Verbal Behavior*, 23, 553–568.

Greenwald, A. G., Liu, T. J., & Klinger, M. (1986). *Unconscious processing of word meaning*. Unpublished manuscript, Ohio State University.

Hansen, C. H., & Hansen, R. D. (1988). Finding the face in the crowd: An anger superiority effect. *Journal of Personality and Social Psychology*, 54, 917–924.

Hansen, R. D. (1980). Commonsense attribution. *Journal of Personality and Social Psychology*, 39, 996–1009.

Hastie, R. (1981). Schematic principles in human memory. In E. T. Higgins, C. P. Herman, & M. P. Zanna (Eds.), *Social cognition: The Ontario Symposium* (Vol. 1, pp. 39–88). Hillsdale, NJ: Erlbaum.

Hastie, R., & Kumar, P. (1979). Person memory: Personality traits as organizing principles in memory for behaviors. *Journal of Personality and Social Psychology*, 37, 25–38.

Hastie, R., & Park, B. (1986). The relationship between memory and judgment depends on whether the judgment task is memory-based or on-line. *Psychological Review*, 93, 258–268.

Henik, A., Friedrich, F. J., & Kellogg, W. A. (1983). The dependence of semantic relatedness effects upon prime processing. *Memory & Cognition*, 11, 366–373.

Higgins, E. T., & Bargh, J. A. (1987). Social perception and social cognition. *Annual Review of Psychology*, 38, 369–425.

Higgins, E. T., Bargh, J. A., & Lombardi, W. (1985). The nature of priming effects on categorization. *Journal of Experimental Psychology: Learning, Memory, and Cognition*, 11, 59–69.

Higgins, E. T., Bond, R. N., Klein, R., & Strauman, T. (1986). Self-discrepancies and emotional vulnerability: How magnitude, accessibility, and type of discrepancy influence affect. *Journal of Personality and Social Psychology*, 51, 5–15.

Higgins, E. T., & King, G. (1981). Accessibility of social constructs: Information-processing consequences of individual and contextual variability. In N. Cantor & J. F. Kihlstrom (Eds.), *Personality, cognition, and social interaction* (pp. 69–122). Hillsdale, NJ: Erlbaum.

Higgins, E. T., King, G. A., & Mavin, G. H. (1982). Individual construct accessibility and subjective impressions and recall. *Journal of Personality and Social Psychology*, 43, 35–47.

Higgins, E. T., Rholes, W. S., & Jones, C. R. (1977). Category accessibility and impression formation. *Journal of Experimental Social Psychology*, 13, 141–154.

Hoffman, J. E., & MacMillan, F. W. (1985). Is semantic priming automatic? In M. I. Posner & O. S. M. Marin (Eds.), *Attention and performance XI* (pp. 585–599). Hillsdale, NJ: Erlbaum.

Ingram, R. E., & Kendall, P. C. (1987). The cognitive side of anxiety. *Cognitive Therapy and Research*, 11, 523–536.

Isen, A. M. (1984). Toward understanding the role of affect in cognition. In R. S. Wyer, Jr., & T. K. Srull (Eds.), *Handbook of social cognition* (Vol. 3, pp. 179–236). Hillsdale, NJ: Erlbaum.

Isen, A. M., Shalker, T. L., Clark, M., & Karp, L. (1978). Affect, accessibility of material in memory, and behavior: A cognitive loop? *Journal of Personality and Social Psychology, 36,* 1–12.

Jacoby, L. L., & Dallas, M. (1981). On the relationship between autobiographical memory and perceptual learning. *Journal of Experimental Psychology: General, 110,* 306–340.

Jacoby, L. L., & Kelley, C. M. (1987). Unconscious influences of memory for a prior event. *Personality and Social Psychology Bulletin, 13,* 314–336.

James, W. (1890). *The principles of psychology* (2 vols.). New York: Holt.

Johnson, E. J., & Tversky, A. (1983). Affect, generalization, and the perception of risk. *Journal of Personality and Social Psychology, 45,* 20–31.

Johnson, M. K. (1983). A multiple-entry, modular memory system. In G. H. Bower (Ed.), *The psychology of learning and motivation* (Vol. 16, pp. 81–123). New York: Academic Press.

Johnson, M. K., & Hasher, L. (1987). Human learning and memory. *Annual Review of Psychology, 38,* 631–668.

Johnson, M. K., & Raye, C. L. (1981). Reality monitoring. *Psychological Review, 88,* 67–85.

Johnston, W. A., & Dark, V. J. (1986). Selective attention. *Annual Review of Psychology, 37,* 43–75.

Jones, E. E. (1979). The rocky road from acts to dispositions. *American Psychologist, 34,* 107–117.

Jones, E. E., & Nisbett, R. E. (1971). The actor and the observer: Divergent perceptions of the causes of behavior. In E. E. Jones, D. Kanouse, H. H. Kelley, R. E. Nisbett, S. Valins, & B. Weiner (Eds.), *Attribution: Perceiving the causes of behavior* (pp. 79–94). Morristown, NJ: General Learning Press.

Kahneman, D., & Henik, A. (1981). Perceptual organization and attention. In M. Kubovy & J. R. Pomerantz (Eds.), *Perceptual organization.* Hillsdale, NJ: Erlbaum.

Kahneman, D., & Treisman, A. (1984). Changing views of attention and automaticity. In R. Parasuraman & D. R. Davies (Eds.), *Varieties of attention* (pp. 29–61). New York: Academic Press.

Kitayama, S., & Burnstein, E. (1988). Automaticity in conversations: A reexamination of the mindlessness hypothesis. *Journal of Personality and Social Psychology, 54,* 219–224.

Krauss, R. M., Apple, W., Morency, N., Wenzel, C., & Winton, W. (1981). Verbal, vocal, and visible factors in judgments of another's affect. *Journal of Personality and Social Psychology, 40,* 312–320.

Kruglanski, A. W. (1980). Lay epistemologic process and contents: Another look at attribution theory. *Psychological Review, 87,* 70–87.

Kunst-Wilson, W. R., & Zajonc, R. B. (1980). Affective discrimination of stimuli that cannot be recognized. *Science, 207,* 557–558.

LaBerge, D., & Samuels, S. J. (1974). Toward a theory of automatic information processing in reading. *Cognitive Psychology, 6,* 293–323.

Langer, E. J. (1978). Rethinking the role of thought in social interaction. In J. H. Harvey, W. J. Ickes, & R. F. Kidd (Eds.), *New directions in attribution research* (Vol. 2, pp. 36–58). Hillsdale, NJ: Erlbaum.

Langer, E. J., & Abelson, R. P. (1972). The semantics of asking a favor: How to succeed in getting help without really dying. *Journal of Personality and Social Psychology, 24,* 26–32.

Langer, E. J., Blank, A., & Chanowitz, B. (1978). The mindlessness of ostensibly thoughtful action: The role of "placebic" information in interpersonal interaction. *Journal of Personality and Social Psychology, 36,* 635–642.

Latane, B., & Darley, J. M. (1970). *The unresponsive bystander: Why doesn't he help?* New York: Appleton-Century-Crofts.

Lewicki, P. (1982). Trait relationships: The nonconscious generalization of social experience. *Personality and Social Psychology Bulletin, 8,* 439–445.

Lewicki, P. (1985). Nonconscious biasing effects of single instances on subsequent judgments. *Journal of Personality and Social Psychology, 48,* 563–574.

Lewicki, P. (1986a). *Nonconscious social information processing.* New York: Academic Press.

Lewicki, P. (1986b). Processing information about covariations that cannot be articulated. *Journal of Experimental Psychology: Learning, Memory, and Cognition, 12,* 135–146.

Lingle, J. H., & Ostrom, T. M. (1979). Retrieval selectivity in memory-based impression judgments. *Journal of Personality and Social Psychology, 37,* 180–194.

Logan, G. D. (1980). Attention and automaticity in Stroop and priming tasks: Theory and data. *Cognitive Psychology, 12,* 523–553.

Logan, G. D., & Cowan, W. B. (1984). On the ability to inhibit thought and action: A theory of an act of control. *Psychological Review, 91,* 295–327.

Lombardi, W. J., Higgins, E. T., & Bargh, J. A. (1987). The role of consciousness in priming effects on categorization: Assimilation versus contrast as a function of awareness of the priming event. *Personality and Social Psychology Bulletin, 13,* 411–429.

Mandler, G., & Nakamura, Y. (1987). Aspects of consciousness. *Personality and Social Psychology Bulletin, 13,* 299–313.

Mandler, G., Nakamura, Y., & Van Zandt, B. J. S. (1987). Nonspecific effects of exposure to stimuli that cannot be recognized. *Journal of Experimental Psychology: Learning, Memory, and Cognition, 13,* 646–648.

Marcel, A. J. (1983). Conscious and unconscious perception: Experiments on visual masking and word recognition. *Cognitive Psychology, 15,* 197–237.

McArthur, L. Z. (1981). What grabs you? The role of attention in impression formation and causal attribution. In E. T. Higgins, C. P. Herman, & M. P. Zanna (Eds.), *Social cognition: The Ontario Symposium* (Vol. 1, pp. 201–246). Hillsdale, NJ: Erlbaum.

McArthur, L. Z., & Friedman, S. (1980). Illusory correlation in impression formation: Variations in the shared distinctiveness effect as a function of the distinctive person's age, race, and sex. *Journal of Personality and Social Psychology, 39,* 615–624.

Metcalfe, J. (1986). Feeling of knowing in memory and problem-solving. *Journal of Experimental Psychology: Learning, Memory, and Cognition, 12,* 288–294.

Mills, C. J., & Tyrrell, D. J. (1983). Sex-stereotypic encoding and release from proactive interference. *Journal of Personality and Social Psychology, 45,* 772–781.

Moray, N. (1959). Attention in dichotic listening: Affective cues and the influence of instructions. *Quarterly Journal of Experimental Psychology, 11,* 56–60.

Moskowitz, G. B., & Uleman, J. S. (1987, August). *The facilitation and inhibition of spontaneous trait inferences.* Paper presented at the 95th Annual Convention of the American Psychological Association, New York City.

Neely, J. H. (1977). Semantic priming and retrieval from lexical memory: Roles of inhibitionless spreading activation and limited-capacity attention. *Journal of Experimental Psychology: General, 106,* 226–254.

Neisser, U. (1967). *Cognitive psychology.* New York: Appleton-Century-Crofts.

Nelson, T. O., Gerler, D., & Narens, L. (1984). Accuracy of feeling-of-knowing judgments for predicting perceptual identification and relearning. *Journal of Experimental Psychology: General, 113,* 282–300.

Newell, A., & Rosenbloom, P. S. (1981). Mechanisms of skill acquisition and the law of practice. In J. R. Anderson (Ed.), *Cognitive skills and their acquisition* (pp. 1–55). Hillsdale, NJ: Erlbaum.

Niedenthal, P. M., & Cantor, N. (1986). Affective responses as guides to category-based inferences. *Motivation and Emotion, 10,* 217–232.

Nisbett, R. E., & Bellows, N. (1977). Verbal reports about causal influences on social judgments: Private access versus public theories. *Journal of Personality and Social Psychology, 35,* 613–624.

Nisbett, R. E., & Wilson, T. D. (1977). Telling more than we can know: Verbal reports on mental processes. *Psychological Review, 84,* 231–259.

Nissen, M. J., & Bullemer, P. (1987). Attentional requirements of learning: Evidence from performance measures. *Cognitive Psychology, 19,* 1–32.

Norman, D. A. (1981). Categorization of action slips. *Psychological Review, 88,* 1–15.

Norman, D. A., & Bobrow, D. G. (1976). On the role of active memory processes in perception and cognition. In C. N. Cofer (Ed.), *The structure of human memory* (pp. 114–132). San Francisco: W. H. Freeman.

Norman, D. A., & Shallice, T. (1986). Attention to action: Willed and automatic control of behavior. In R. J. Davidson, G. E. Schwartz, & D. Shapiro (Eds.), *Consciousness and self-regulation: Advances in research and theory* (Vol. 4, pp. 1–18). New York: Plenum.

Ogden, W. C., Martin, D. W., & Paap, K. R. (1980). Processing demands of encoding: What does secondary task performance reflect? *Journal of Experimental Psychology: Human Perception and Performance, 6,* 355–367.

Petty, R. E., & Cacioppo, J. T. (1981). *Attitudes and persuasion: Classic and contemporary approaches.* Dubuque, IA: William C. Brown.

Posner, M. I. (1978). *Chronometric explorations of mind.* Hillsdale, NJ: Erlbaum.

Posner, M. I., & Snyder, C. R. R. (1975). Attention and cognitive control. In R. L. Solso (Ed.), *Information processing and cognition: The Loyola Symposium* (pp. 55–85). Hillsdale, NJ: Erlbaum.

Postman, L., & Brown, D. R. (1952). Perceptual consequences of success and failure. *Journal of Abnormal and Social Psychology, 47,* 213–221.

Pratto, F., & Bargh, J. A. (1988). *Sex stereotyping under information overload: Two paths for going beyond the information given.* Unpublished manuscript, New York University.

Pyszczynski, T., & Greenberg, J. (1987). Self-regulatory perseveration and the depressive self-focusing style: A self-awareness theory of reactive depression. *Psychological Bulletin, 102,* 122–138.

Reber, A. S. (1967). Implicit learning of artificial grammars. *Journal of Verbal Learning and Verbal Behavior, 5,* 855–863.

Rhodewalt, F., & Agustsdottir, S. (1986). Effects of self-presentation on the phenomenal self. *Journal of Personality and Social Psychology, 50,* 47–55.

Rothbart, M. (1981). Memory processes and social beliefs. In D. L. Hamilton (Ed.), *Cognitive processes in stereotyping and intergroup behavior* (pp. 145–181). Hillsdale, NJ: Erlbaum.

Schachter, S., & Singer, J. L. (1962). Cognitive, social, and physiological determinants of emotional state. *Psychological Review, 69,* 379–399.

Schacter, D. (1983). Feeling-of-knowing in episodic memory. *Journal of Experimental Psychology: Learning, Memory, and Cognition, 9,* 39–54.

Schank, R. C., & Abelson, R. P. (1977). *Scripts, plans, goals, and understanding.* Hillsdale, NJ: Erlbaum.

Schul, Y., & Burnstein, E. (1985). The informational basis of social judgments: Using past impression rather than the trait description in forming a new impression. *Journal of Experimental Social Psychology, 21,* 421–439.

Seamon, J. G., Brody, N., & Kauff, D. M. (1983). Affective discrimination of stimuli that are not recognized: Effects of shadowing, masking, and cerebral laterality. *Journal of Experimental Psychology: Learning, Memory, and Cognition, 9,* 544–555.

Seifert, C. M., McKoon, G., Abelson, R. P., & Ratcliff, R. (1986). Memory connections between thematically similar episodes. *Journal of Experimental Psychology: Learning, Memory, and Cognition, 12,* 220–231.

Shallice, T. (1972). Dual functions of consciousness. *Psychological Review, 79,* 383–393.

Sherman, S. J. (1987). Cognitive processes in the formation, change, and expression of attitudes. In M. P. Zanna, J. M. Olson, & C. P. Herman (Eds.), *Social influence: The Ontario Symposium* (Vol. 5, pp. 75–106). Hillsdale, NJ: Erlbaum.

Sherman, S. J., Zehner, K. S., Johnson, J., & Hirt, E. R. (1983). Social explanation: The role of timing, set, and recall on subjective likelihood estimates. *Journal of Personality and Social Psychology, 44,* 1127–1143.

Shiffrin, R. M., & Dumais, S. T. (1981). The development of automatism. In J. R. Anderson (Ed.), *Cognitive skills and their acquisition* (pp. 111–140). Hillsdale, NJ: Erlbaum.

Shiffrin, R. M., & Schneider, W. (1977). Controlled and automatic human information processing: II. Perceptual learning, automatic attending, and a general theory. *Psychological Review, 84,* 127–190.

Smith, E. R. (1984). Model of social inference processes. *Psychological Review, 91,* 392–413.

Smith, E. R., Branscombe, N. R., & Bormann, C. (1988). Generality of the effects of practice on social judgment tasks. *Journal of Personality and Social Psychology, 54,* 385–395.

Smith, E. R., & Lerner, M. (1986). Development of automatism of social judgments. *Journal of Personality and Social Psychology, 50,* 246–259.

Smith, E. R., & Miller, F. D. (1983). Mediation among attributional inferences and comprehension processes: Initial findings and a general method. *Journal of Personality and Social Psychology, 44,* 492–505.

Smith, S. S., & Kihlstrom, J. F. (1987). When is a schema not a schema? The "Big Five" traits as cognitive structures. *Social Cognition, 5,* 26–57.

Spielman, L. A., Pratto, F., & Bargh, J. A. (1988). Automatic affect: Are one's moods, attitudes, evaluations, and emotions out of control? *American Behavioral Scientist, 31,* 296–311.

Srull, T. K. (1981). Person memory: Some tests of associative storage and retrieval models. *Journal of Experimental Psychology: Human Learning and Memory, 7,* 440–463.

Srull, T. K., & Wyer, R. S., Jr. (1979). The role of category accessibility in the interpretation of information about persons: Some determinants and implications. *Journal of Personality and Social Psychology, 37,* 1660–1672.

Srull, T. K., & Wyer, R. S., Jr. (1986). The role of chronic and temporary goals in social information processing. In R. M. Sorrentino & E. T. Higgins (Eds.), *Handbook of motivation and cognition: Foundations of social behavior* (pp. 503–549). New York: Guilford Press.

Strack, F., Erber, R., & Wicklund, R. A. (1982). Effects of salience and time pressure on ratings of social causality. *Journal of Experimental Social Psychology, 18,* 581–594.

Strauman, T. J., & Higgins, E. T. (1987). Automatic activation of self-discrepancies and emotional syndromes: When cognitive structures influence affect. *Journal of Personality and Social Psychology, 53,* 1004–1014.

Taylor, S. E., Crocker, J., Fiske, S. T., Sprinzen, M., & Winkler, J. D. (1979). The generalizability of salience effects. *Journal of Personality and Social Psychology, 37,* 357–368.

Taylor, S. E., & Fiske, S. T. (1978). Salience, attention, and attribution: Top of the head phenomena. In L. Berkowitz (Ed.), *Advances in experimental social psychology* (Vol. 11, pp. 249–288). New York: Academic Press.

Trope, Y. (1986). Identification and inferential processes in dispositional attribution. *Psychological Review, 93,* 239–257.

Tulving, E., Schacter, D. L., & Stark, H. A. (1982). Priming effects in word-fragment completion are independent of recognition memory. *Journal of Experimental Psychology: Learning, Memory, and Cognition, 8,* 336–342.

Uleman, J. S. (1987). Consciousness and control: The case of spontaneous trait inferences. *Personality and Social Psychology Bulletin, 13,* 337–354.

Vallacher, R. R., & Wegner, D. M. (1987). What do people think they're doing? Action identification and human behavior. *Psychological Review, 94,* 3–15.

Wicklund, R. A., & Brehm, J. W. (1976). *Perspectives on cognitive dissonance.* Hillsdale, NJ: Erlbaum.

Wilson, W. R. (1979). Feeling more than we can know: Exposure effects without learning. *Journal of Personality and Social Psychology, 37,* 811–821.

Winter, L., & Uleman, J. S. (1984). When are social judgments made? Evidence for the spontaneousness of trait inferences. *Journal of Personality and Social Psychology, 47,* 237–252.

Winter, L., Uleman, J. S., & Cunniff, C. (1985). How automatic are social judgments? *Journal of Personality and Social Psychology, 49,* 904–917.

Winton, W. M., Putnam, L. E., & Krauss, R. M. (1984). Facial and autonomic manifestations of the dimensional structure of emotion. *Journal of Experimental Social Psychology, 20,* 195–216.

Wyer, R. S., Jr., & Gordon, S. E. (1982). The recall of information about persons and groups. *Journal of Experimental Psychology, 18,* 128–164.

Wyer, R. S., Jr., & Srull, T. K. (1986). Human cognition in its social context. *Psychological Review, 93,* 322–359.

Yaniv, I., & Meyer, D. E. (1987). Activation and metacognition of inaccessible stored information: Potential bases for incubation effects in problem solving. *Journal of Experimental Psychology: Learning, Memory, and Cognition, 13,* 187–205.

Yates, J. (1985). The content of awareness is a model of the world. *Psychological Review, 92,* 249–284.

Zajonc, R. B. (1968). Attitudinal effects of mere exposure. *Journal of Personality and Social Psychology Monograph Supplement, 9,* 1–27.

Zajonc, R. B. (1980). Feeling and thinking: Preferences need no inferences. *American Psychologist, 35,* 151–175.

Zbrodoff, N. J., & Logan, G. D. (1986). On the autonomy of mental processes: A case study of arithmetic. *Journal of Experimental Psychology: General, 115,* 118–130.

Zillman, D., & Bryant, J. (1974). Effect of residual excitation on the emotional response to provocation and delayed aggressive behavior. *Journal of Personality and Social Psychology, 30,* 782–791.

2

Automaticity and Cognitive Control

GORDON D. LOGAN
University of Illinois

Much of everyday cognition depends on automatic processing. Attention and motivation may determine who or what is focal in the stream of consciousness, but automatic processing provides the background. Routine events are interpreted automatically, plausible inferences are generated automatically, and even current judgments and attributions are influenced by automatic processing. The information provided by such processing seems to come unbidden; we need only to look at a familiar scene to recognize it and know what to do in it. Moreover, the information sometimes comes unwanted, as when we are plagued by unpleasant memories or, even worse, obsessed by disturbing thoughts. These intuitions raise important questions about the control of automatic processes.

Research on automaticity is as old as experimental psychology (see Bryan & Harter, 1897; James, 1890), but it has flourished in the last decade (for reviews, see Bargh, Chapter 1, this volume; Kahneman & Treisman, 1984; Logan, 1985b; Schneider, Dumais, & Shiffrin, 1984). Much of the research is driven by the phenomenology of automatic processing: One makes a claim about automatic processing, supports it with compelling examples from phenomenology, and performs experiments to confirm the claim in behavioral terms. This approach has provided important data and theoretical insights that have a certain face validity, but it can lead to conflicting conclusions and provides no way to resolve them. The relation between automaticity and control is an important example.

The phenomenological experience that automatic processes come unbidden and unwanted suggests that automatic processes are hard to control. This suggestion is corroborated by Stroop and priming experiments, in which subjects attend to one stimulus or one aspect of it and ignore other stimuli or aspects (e.g., Neely, 1977; Stroop, 1935). Subjects seem unable to ignore familiar stimuli, especially those that are processed automatically. Consequently, many researchers conclude that automatic processes are hard to control. The ubiquity of this conclusion is evident in the contrast, drawn by many researchers, between automatic and controlled processing (e.g., Posner & Snyder, 1975a; Shiffrin & Schneider, 1977). By their definition, automatic processing cannot be controlled.

The conclusion that automatic processing is hard to control conflicts with other aspects of its phenomenology. Automatic processing is reliable and useful. We depend on it in much of our daily lives. The information that becomes available automatically is often just what we need to do the task at hand, as if automatic processes anticipate what will need attention (see, e.g., Reason & Myceilska, 1982). These aspects of the phenomenology of automaticity suggest that automatic processes may be closely controlled.

This suggestion is corroborated in studies of skill acquisition, where the evidence indicates that control and automaticity both increase with skill. On the one hand, skilled practitioners are faster than novices and respond more effectively to perturbations in the input (e.g., Salthouse, 1986), which suggests better control. On the other hand, skilled practitioners are better at time sharing than novices, suffering less interference from concurrent tasks (e.g., Hirst, Spelke, Reeves, Caharack, & Neisser, 1980; Logan, 1979), which suggests greater automaticity. Many researchers argue that automatic processing provides an important basis for skilled behavior (e.g., LaBerge & Samuels, 1974; Logan, 1985b; Schneider, 1985), and skilled behavior is closely controlled. Thus, automatic processes may not be so hard to control; perhaps they are easy to control.

The way out of an impasse like this is not to argue whose phenomenology is better or whose experiments are more appropriate. Phenomenology is hard to debate, because it amounts to denying the validity of what others say about their experience (which can lead to blows), and the appropriateness of the experiments hinges on the phenomenology. A more fruitful approach is to present a theory that explains automaticity and control in terms of underlying processes. Such a theory could resolve the empirical differences and explain the different phenomenologies.

The purpose of this chapter is to review the evidence on automaticity and control and to fit a recent theory of automaticity (Logan, 1988) to the evidence. First, the chapter looks at Stroop and priming tasks, which have been the focus of theoretical debate about automaticity and control, and then at other tasks and other measures of control. Finally, the new theory of automaticity is summarized, and means by which it allows automatic processes to be controlled are described.

CONTROL OF THOUGHT AND ACTION

Many factors, some theoretical and some empirical, contribute to the widespread belief that automatic processes are hard to control. On the theoretical side, the most prominent theories in the 1970s defined automaticity in terms of control: Processes that could not be controlled were automatic; processes that could be controlled were "controlled," "strategic," or "attentional" (see Hasher & Zacks, 1979; LaBerge & Samuels, 1974; Logan, 1978, 1980; Posner & Snyder, 1975a; Schneider & Shiffrin, 1977; Shiffrin & Schneider, 1977). The theories were typically articulated in terms of activation of memory structures: Automatic processing was "spreading activation." Long-term memory nodes were activated by stimulus presentation alone, and activation propagated through the network of associations connected to the initial node. Controlled or strategic processing was a function of attention, and nodes could be activated by attending to them. Control was exerted by attending selectively (activating relevant nodes without activating irrelevant nodes) and by attending to nodes in sequence. Activation from automatic processing was often viewed as noise with respect to controlled processing, perturbing the intended pattern of activation. This trend in theorizing continues today (e.g., Hunt & Lansman, 1986; Schneider, 1985). Few theorists even consider the possibility that automatic and nonautomatic processes can both be controlled (but see Logan, 1985b, 1988; Neumann, 1984).

The theories of the 1970s led to several hypotheses about control of automatic processing: Automatic processing is driven by stimulus presentation alone; automatic processing is independent of attention; automatic processing is independent of intention.[1] A number of experiments addressed these hypotheses, the earlier ones suggesting that they might be true and the later ones raising serious doubts. These experiments are reviewed in the remainder of this section.

Stroop Experiments

Much of the evidence on automaticity and control comes from Stroop experiments, in which subjects report one dimension of a multidimensional stimulus while ignoring others. The main finding is that the other dimensions are hard to ignore. If they convey a meaning that is different from the meaning of the attended dimension, performance suffers; reaction time and error rate increase (for a review, see Logan, 1980). This intrusion of irrelevant information occurs despite subjects' best intentions to ignore it.

Many people interpret the Stroop effect as indicating that the unattended dimension is processed as fully as possible, in much the same manner as it would be processed if it were attended. But this may be overinterpreting the data. Certainly, the Stroop effect would occur if all subjects processed the unattended dimension completely on all trials, but it could also occur (in averaged data) if some subjects processed the unattended dimension to some extent on some trials. Simply finding a Stroop effect does not indicate which of these possibilities underlie it (Kahneman & Treisman, 1984); converging experiments are required to discriminate between them (Zbrodoff & Logan, 1986). The distinction is important: Automatic responses that were the same whether or not the dimension that gave rise to them was attended would be much more difficult to control than automatic responses that were relatively feeble and unreliable without attention to support them.

Experiments have shown that intention can modulate Stroop effects: Subjects are sensitive to the probability that attended and unattended dimensions are compatible, showing stronger facilitation when compatible stimuli are more likely and diminished interference when conflicting stimuli are more likely (Greenwald & Rosenberg, 1978; Logan, Zbrodoff, & Williamson, 1984). The Stroop effect can actually be reversed by this manipulation, producing faster responses to conflicting stimuli than to compatible ones (Logan, 1980; Logan & Zbrodoff, 1979; Zbrodoff & Logan, 1986).

Theoretical analyses suggest that probability manipulations modulate but do not eliminate Stroop effects. Jane Zbrodoff and I (Logan & Zbrodoff, 1979; see also Logan, 1980) modeled these effects in terms of a decision process that weighed information from different sources. Automatic processes received weights that were small in magnitude and were constant across experimental conditions, whereas attentional processes received weights that were large in magnitude and varied across experimental conditions according to the probability of compatible stimuli. The intentional effects (modeled by the attentional weights) did not eliminate automatic effects; rather, they outweighed them in the decision process. Nevertheless, these results suggest that the automatic processes tapped in Stroop experiments are not totally beyond control. At least, they can be modulated by intention.

The automatic processes tapped by Stroop experiments are not independent of attention. In most Stroop experiments, the interfering stimulus is at the spatial focus of attention—it is an irrelevant dimension of an attended object. Experiments that vary the spatial separation between relevant and irrelevant dimensions (e.g., by having subjects name a color bar and presenting a conflicting word some distance from it) show a weaker Stroop effect as spatial separation increases (e.g., Dyer & Severance, 1973; Goolkasian, 1981). Kahneman and Henik (1981) provided a more dramatic demonstration, presenting subjects with two words, one black and one colored, and requiring them to name the color of the colored word. If the colored word named a conflicting color, the usual Stroop effect was observed. But if the colored word was neutral and the black (ignored) word named a conflicting color, there was virtually no Stroop effect. The irrelevant-color word produced Stroop interference only when it was attended. Francolini and Egeth (1980) reported similar results in a version of the Stroop task in which subjects had to count the number of red characters in arrays of red and black characters. On some trials, the red characters were numbers, so subjects had to count five 3's or two 4's. This produced a sizable Stroop effect. However, when the black characters were numbers and the red ones were letters, there was no Stroop effect. The irrelevant numbers produced a Stroop effect only when they were red and subjects focused spatial attention on them. These results provide strong evidence that Stroop effects cannot be independent of attention.

Priming Experiments

Much of the evidence on the control of automatic processes comes from priming experiments. Priming experiments are closely related to Stroop experiments, in that an irrelevant stimulus affects responses to a relevant stimulus; however, in priming experiments, the irrelevant stimulus is usually separate from the relevant one, preceding it in time (for a further discussion of parallels between them, see Logan, 1980). When the irrelevant or priming stimulus is related in meaning to the relevant or target stimulus, performance is facilitated; reaction time and error rate decrease. When prime and target are unrelated in meaning, interference is often observed; reaction time and error rate increase, relative to a neutral control condition. The choice of a neutral control is currently controversial, so facilitation and interference are hard to assess separately (see Jonides & Mack, 1984), but the difference between related and unrelated primes is robust and remains untouched by the controversy.

In priming studies, the controllability of automatic processes is inferred from the effects of the delay between the prime and the target. Priming occurs at delays so short (less than 250 milliseconds) that attention is unlikely to have had time to take effect (Neely, 1977; Posner & Snyder, 1975b; Ratcliff & McKoon, 1981). Moreover, the pattern of priming at these short delays is different from the pattern at longer delays: Often, short delays produce facilitation but no interference, whereas longer delays produce both facilitation and interference (Neely, 1977; Posner & Snyder, 1975b). The interference is interpreted as a concomitant of attention: The unrelated prime directs attention away from the relevant nodes in memory, and time must be taken to reorient attention appropriately. The early facilitation is interpreted as an automatic effect, due to "pathway activation"; that is, the prime activates some of the pathway that the target follows in its journey through the information-processing system (Posner & Snyder, 1975a, 1975b).

The effects of delay and the patterns of facilitation and interference that go with them suggest that automatic processing is beyond control in the sense that it occurs too quickly for attention to affect it. This does not mean that attention *cannot* control automatic processing; it means that sometimes attention may not be fast enough to exert control. Thus, priming effects should be interpreted as indicating a (temporal) limit on the ability to control automatic processes, rather than an inability to control them.[2]

It is commonly believed that priming is an obligatory consequence of stimulus presentation: The prime activates its node or its pathway in memory, regardless of the direction of attention. However, recent evidence suggests that subjects must attend to the prime in a way that makes it relevant to the task requirements in order for priming to occur. Smith (1979; also see Smith, Theodor, & Franklin, 1983) had subjects perform a lexical decision on the prime or search through the prime for a letter before the target stimulus was presented, and found priming only in the first case. Apparently, the prime must be treated as a word to produce a priming effect. Treating the prime as a string of letters apparently prevents it from accessing the lexicon or semantic memory or whatever produces the priming effects. Henik, Friedrich, and Kellogg (1983) found similar results with the Stroop task. These results provide strong evidence that Stroop and priming effects are not driven by mere stimulus presentation. They are not beyond strategic control.

Like the Stroop task, priming tasks are also influenced by cue validity. The higher the probability that the prime is related to the target, the stronger the priming effect; facilitation from related primes and interference from unrelated primes both increase with cue validity (den Heyer, Briand, & Dannenbring, 1983; Posner & Snyder, 1975b; Tweedy, Lapinski, & Schvaneveldt, 1977). As in the Stroop task, these effects could be modeled by a decision process that weighed information from different sources: The weight alotted to the prime could increase strategically as cue validity increased (Logan, 1980). But that model does not explain nonword facilitation, which occurs in these experiments. As cue validity increases, nonwords are rejected more rapidly after word primes than after neutral primes. Neely (1977; Neely & Keefe in press), has explained the cue validity effect and nonword facilitation in terms of a postlexical checking strategy, whereby subjects decide whether or not the target is a word by checking to see whether the prime and the target are related in meaning. If they are, then the target is likely to be a word; if they are not, it is likely to be a nonword. The utility of this strategy increases with cue validity: The higher the cue validity, the lower the probability that targets *un*related to the prime are words, and the higher the probability that they are nonwords. Thus, subjects should be able to respond faster to nonwords as cue validity increases, as is observed in the nonword facilitation effect.

Neely's idea is a special case of a general priming mechanism proposed by Ratcliff and McKoon (1988), in which subjects use the relation between the prime and the target to drive the decision process. Ratcliff and McKoon are concerned with priming in episodic memory tasks as well as lexical decision, and with priming in complex propositional structures as well as simple associations. Their approach uses Gillund and Shiffrin's (1984) "Search of Associative Memory" (SAM) model of memory to retrieve relations between primes and targets, which drive Ratcliff's (1978) random-walk decision process. The details are not important for the present purposes. Rather, it is the general idea that priming is strategic that is important. It suggests that little in priming tasks may be beyond the subject's control.

Stroop and Priming Tasks: Conclusions

Stroop and priming tasks have been the major focus of theoretical controversies over the control of automatic processes. Some data suggest that the automatic processes underlying Stroop and priming effects may be beyond control, but the bulk of the evidence reviewed here suggests that they are closely controlled. The same conclusion—that automatic processes are closely controlled—can be reached, sometimes more clearly, by looking at other tasks and paradigms. That is the purpose of the remainder of this section.

Reflex Modification

The hypothesis that automatic processes are independent of attention is seriously challenged by experiments on the modification of reflexes. In many ways, reflexes are the paradigm case of automaticity; they are triggered by the presence of the eliciting stimulus and require no cognitive involvement or intention to be carried out (Anthony, 1985). Automatic processes are viewed as learned cognitive reflexes, acquired cognitive activity driven by stimulus presentation. So evidence that reflexes can be affected by attention would seriously challenge the idea that automatic processes are independent of attention.

Studies of the blink reflex suggest that reflexes can be modified by attention (for a review, see Anthony, 1985). The blink reflex is part of the startle response elicited by sudden, intense stimulus: The mouth opens; head and shoulders lean forward; knees, elbows, and fingers contract; and the eyes close briefly. The blink reflex is the most reliable of these components, resisting habituation and occurring in babies, children, and adults— even in brain-dead individuals, who by all accounts have no cognitive activity. Yet the blink reflex can be modified by attention. Anthony and Graham (1985) showed that it was stronger when subjects attended to the modality of the eliciting stimulus. Subjects who looked at pictures blinked more intensely to a bright light than to a loud sound, whereas subjects listening to music did the opposite. Other studies, reviewed by Anthony (1985), showed attenuation of the blink reflex if attention was directed to a modality different from that of the eliciting stimulus.

These data challenge the idea that automatic processes are independent of attention. If innate reflexes such as the blink reflex can be modified by attention, then surely learned reflexes (automatic processes) cannot be independent of attention. Automatic processing does not seem so impervious to cognitive control.

The Stop-Signal Paradigm: Stopping Responses

The ability to inhibit thought and action is an important aspect of cognitive control. Sometimes we make errors and must inhibit the erroneous response; at other times, the environment changes unexpectedly and we must inhibit our old thoughts and actions to clear the way for new ones; at still other times, our goals change and we must inhibit courses of thought and action that are no longer relevant to our current goals. Inhibition may be viewed as an act of control that is triggered by events such as errors or changes in goals. It can be studied by presenting an explicit signal to change one's goals and observing the subsequent response. This is the method employed in the "stop-signal" paradigm: Subjects are engaged in a primary task and, on occasion, are presented with a stimulus (a stop signal) that instructs them to inhibit the current response (for a review, see Logan & Cowan, 1984). The idea is that the primary task sets up certain goals for the subject to attain—for example, to decide which of two letters was presented or whether a given word is the name of a mammal. Certain processes are engaged in the service of these goals when a relevant stimulus appears; the stop-signal paradigm allows us to determine whether those processes are controlled. The stop signal indicates that the goals are no longer relevant. Controlled processes, acting in service of the goals, should stop when the goals change; uncontrolled or uncontrollable processes should run on to completion despite the change in goals.

The most straightforward application of the stop-signal paradigm is in studies of the ability to inhibit overt actions. The experimenter presents a stop signal and simply observes whether the overt response occurs. The main dependent variable is the probability of inhibiting the response, or, equivalently, the probability of making the response when given a stop signal. The most important independent variable is the delay between the onset of the primary-task stimulus and the onset of the stop signal: If the stop signal is presented early enough (e.g., well before the primary-task stimulus), subjects will always inhibit their responses; if the stop signal is presented late enough (e.g., after the primary-task response), subjects will always respond. For delays in between these extremes, the probability of responding increases monotonically with delay. This monotonic increase is the "inhibition function," which can be analyzed to reveal the properties of the underlying processes (Logan & Cowan, 1984; Osman, Kornblum, & Meyer, 1986).

William Cowan and I (Logan & Cowan, 1984) have developed a formal "horse race" model of the stopping task, in which primary-task processes race against stop-signal inhibitory processes, that accounts for many aspects of the data. For the purpose of this chapter, the main point of the model is that it allows us to determine how effectively a process can be controlled (i.e., inhibited). It allows us to interpret certain differences in the probability of inhibition as differences in controllability, and it allows us to estimate the latency of the act of control (i.e., the response to the stop signal) in different contexts.

The ability to inhibit has been studied in a wide variety of contexts, from relatively novel reaction time tasks to relatively automatic tasks such as moving one's eyes, speaking, and typing. In general, the effects of context have been minimal. Differences in subjects, tasks, experimental conditions, and strategies have little direct effect on the ability to inhibit (for a review, see Logan & Cowan, 1984). Even highly skilled activities such as speaking and typing can be stopped within 200–300 milliseconds of the occurrence of the stop signal. The most remarkable difference we have found so far is that between hyperactive children and normal children. Hyperactive children are impulsive, and so should have a hard time inhibiting responses. In the stop-signal paradigm, they inhibit less effectively than normal children and other psychiatric controls, who do not differ markedly from adults (Schachar & Logan, 1989). Interestingly, their ability to inhibit improves with the administration of Ritalin, a stimulant drug that improves the behavioral symptoms of hyperactivity (Tannock, Schachar, Carr, Chajczyk, & Logan, in press).

The main point to be taken from these studies is that overt actions, even highly skilled, automatic actions, are closely controlled.

The Stop-Signal Paradigm: Stopping Thought

The stop-signal paradigm can be adapted to study the control of thought, but the chain of inference is more complex. Cognitive psychologists typically study thought by making some response contingent on thought and observing the accuracy and latency of that response. But if the subject inhibits the response, there is no accuracy or latency measure to interpret, and thus no index of thought. The fate of the underlying thought must be inferred from other measures. Aftereffects of thought, such as memory or repetition effects, can provide a useful index. Thoughts usually leave a trace in memory, and it is reasonable to assume that complete thoughts leave more complete (and hence more accessible) traces than incomplete, interrupted thoughts. Thus, one can have the subject inhibit an overt response to a stimulus and can then ask the subject to recall or recognize the stimulus; the subject's memory performance can then be examined to determine whether the underlying thought runs on to completion or is inhibited along with the overt response. Memory should be good if the thoughts run on to completion and poor if they are inhibited. "Good" and "poor" are defined relative to control conditions in which no stop signals are presented and accuracy and latency measures suggest that subjects complete the underlying thoughts. (For a fuller description of this logic, see Logan, 1983, 1985a.)

Only a few studies have investigated the control of thought in this manner, and they have produced mixed results. Thoughts underlying category and rhyme judgments (e.g., is a PROFESSOR a PROFESSION? does SLEIGH rhyme with PLAY?) run on to completion, but thoughts underlying simple arithmetic are inhibited with the overt action. Category and rhyme judgments were investigated with recognition (Logan, 1983) and repetition priming[3] (Logan, 1985a) as measures of memory. Both measures showed no difference between words whose responses were inhibited and words whose responses were executed on the first presentation, suggesting that the underlying thoughts ran on to completion when the overt responses were inhibited. Subsequent experiments required subjects to switch to a new task when the stop signal occurred, to take attention away from the category or rhyme judgment at the time the response was inhibited. This had little effect on the underlying thoughts; memory was about the same whether or not the overt response was inhibited, suggesting that the underlying thoughts ran on to completion. The only way to inhibit the underlying thought was to terminate the display of the word when the stop signal sounded and replace it with another stimulus. Then memory was worse with a stop signal than without one, as if the underlying thoughts stopped when the overt action was inhibited. Altogether, these experiments suggest that the thoughts underlying category and rhyme judgments are beyond control, in that (1) they cannot be inhibited and (2) they are driven by stimulus presentation, like reflexes.

The experiments on arithmetic produced different results. Jane Zbrodoff and I (Zbrodoff & Logan, 1986) had subjects add single-digit numbers or verify equations involving sums of single digits. Stop signals occurred on 40 percent of the trials. In both tasks, memory for the arithmetic problems was worse when the overt response was inhibited than when it was not. In other experiments, we showed that the arithmetic problems were processed automatically to some extent: We found a Stroop-like effect when subjects had to verify problems such as $3 \times 4 = 7$ and $3 + 4 = 12$, which would be true under a different arithmetic operation. However, the automaticity did not imply a lack of control; subjects could inhibit the underlying thoughts if they wanted to.

Why arithmetic should be different from category and rhyme judgments is not clear. Several hypotheses come to mind. It may be an artifact of some difference in experimental procedure (the tasks should be compared in the same experiment). It may be that arithmetic is less automatic than category and rhyme judgments. The cognitive abilities underlying linguistic tasks may be practiced more than those underlying arithmetic. It may be that arithmetic tasks are so automatic that they leave little impact on memory. It may be that arithmetic tasks are less interesting, and hence easier to abandon.

More research will be necessary to converge on an answer. Nevertheless, it is possible to reach some tentative conclusions, if the difference is not artifactual. The category and rhyme results rule out the hypothesis that all automatic processes are closely controlled; the arithmetic results rule out the hypothesis that all automatic processes are beyond control. Some are and some are not.

The evidence of close control over some automatic thoughts is interesting, because the simple processes underlying them should require little control, and failures of control should have little consequence in most cases. We are more responsible for our actions than our thoughts. We can think about jumping off a tall building with impunity, but if we actually jump, we pay with our lives. Control over action should be even more stringent than control over thought. Finding stringent control over some thoughts suggests that action should be very stringently controlled (as it apparently is).

Thought Suppression

Obsessive episodes provide striking examples of thoughts beyond control. An eliciting stimulus, either internal or external, triggers the episode, producing disturbing thoughts that cannot be suppressed. The episode takes about 30 seconds to develop and last for 30 minutes or more, during which the sufferer can think of little else (for a review, see Rachman, 1978). But obsessive episodes are pathological, reflecting dysfunction in some underlying control system. Normally, thoughts are better controlled. We usually can turn our minds away from unpleasant thoughts, often with little effort. Recent experiments by Wegner, Schneider, Carter, and White (1987) suggest that thinking of something else is often sufficient (also see Wegner & Schneider, Chapter 9, this volume).

In Wegner et al.'s experiments, subjects were instructed not to think specific thoughts—namely, not to think about white bears. Subjects apparently succeeded in doing so, reporting fewer white-bear thoughts than control subjects during the period in which they were to be suppressed. Evidence that subjects suppressed white-bear thoughts by thinking of something else came from a "rebound" effect in a subsequent "expression" period: When allowed to express white-bear thoughts, subjects who had previously suppressed them reported more than control subjects who had not suppressed them. According to Wegner et al., the rebound effect occurred because suppression subjects inadvertently associated features of the experimental context with white bears: They would think of white bears and, in attempting to suppress the thought, deliberately think of something that was not a white bear. Consequently, whatever they focused on was categorized as "not-white-bear." The experimental context provided many readily available not-white-bear objects. Later, when tested in expression conditions in the same experimental context, the same readily available objects would evoke white-bear thoughts as subjects retrieved the not-white-bear association.

These experiments suggest that normally thoughts are closely controlled and that a common mechanism of control is deliberately thinking of something else. They corroborate the stop-signal experiments on stopping thoughts, in showing that thoughts can be suppressed by changing the eliciting conditions. However, one could argue that the white-bear thoughts subjects tried to suppress were not automatic, and that truly automatic thoughts would be harder to suppress. Moreover, obsessive thoughts may be hard to suppress because they have become automatic. More research is required before definitive conclusions can be reached.

Slips and Errors

Laypeople are familiar with the idea of running on "automatic pilot"—doing one thing while thinking of another. We may rehearse a lecture while driving to work, plan dessert while making the entrée, or dream of fame and fortune while grading papers. The things we do on automatic pilot are usually very familiar and well practiced—paradigm cases of automatic processing. But, unlike most automatic processing seen in the laboratory, they are usually quite complex (think of the steps involved in making chili or the complex contingencies involved in driving along a familiar route). Moreover, things done on automatic pilot are closely controlled; the intended result is achieved with amazing reliability.

We learn from our mistakes; much of what is known about behavior on automatic pilot was learned from analyses of errors and slips (see Norman, 1981; Reason, 1979, 1984). People put cat food in the teapot, search diligently for the glasses they are wearing, and put their pants on backwards. Reason and Myceilska (1982) collected a corpus of errors like these in a diary study—subjects kept records of their slips and errors, noting the context and the time of occurrence—and analyzed them in several ways. Several findings were noteworthy. First, errors tended to occur in automatic activities. They occurred most often in very familiar activities in very familiar circumstances, especially when a person was distracted. Often, the erroneous activities had been completed successfully in the recent past, and subjects rated them as very automatic. Interestingly, errors were not especially likely to occur when subjects were upset, worried, or tired, or when subjects were rushed or bothered by environmental stressors (heat, cold, noise, etc.).

Second, the errors tended to be very coherent and systematic. A large proportion of them (.88) could be classified into one of four categories: "repetitions," in which some intended action was repeated unnecessarily (e.g., using two spoons of sugar instead of one); "wrong objects," in which the intended action was performed on an unintended object (e.g., eating the cat's food instead of one's cereal); "intrusions," in which other actions appropriate to the object were performed (e.g., putting away the milk when intending to pour it on the cereal); and "omissions," in which intended actions were left out of the sequence (e.g., showering without washing one's hair). Each of these categories reflects fairly sophisticated behavior, done properly under close control, but with something wrong or something missing. None of them reflects random, haphazard, or uncontrolled behavior.

Third, the errors tended to be relatively rare. On the average, subjects reported just under one error each day. This number may not be exactly correct, because diary studies are prone to a number of biases (Reason & Myceilska, 1982); however, even if it is within an order of magnitude of the true value, it indicates that automatic processes are very reliable. There are roughly 1,000 seconds in a waking day, and automatic activities typically take a second or less (Logan, 1988), so there are about 1,000 opportunities per day for automatic activity. Even if we exploit only one-third of them, the error rate would be 1/300, based on Reason and Myceilska's data. That is a very low error rate compared to what is usually observed in the psychological laboratory. Apparently, behavior on automatic pilot is very reliable.

To summarize, studies of everyday errors and slips suggest that automatic processing is very closely controlled. Most often, behavior on automatic pilot is coherent, planful, and accurate. When it goes awry, it remains coherent and planful, though the plans and coherence were not what was intended.

Conclusion: Automatic Processing Is Not Beyond Control

The studies reviewed in this section suggest that automatic processing is not beyond control. Stroop and priming experiments, which provide most of the evidence for uncontrollable automatic processing, show that automatic processing is strongly influenced by intention and attention. Studies of reflex modification suggest that even obligatory reflexes can be modified by attention; the acquired reflexes that underlie automatic processing should be even more modifiable. Studies that require subjects to take control of thought and action, inhibiting it or changing its course, suggest that automatic processing is easy to control. Highly skilled actions can be interrupted easily. Most thoughts can be stopped by changing the eliciting conditions—by thinking of something else. The exceptions to these findings are pathological cases (hyperactive children and obsessives). The norm is close control. Studies of everyday errors suggest that these conclusions generalize to very complex activities—habitual behaviors that take several minutes to complete.

The conclusion that automatic processing can be controlled does not deny the existence of automaticity or challenge other properties associated with it. Automatic processing is often facilitative, providing a path of least resistance, well worn by habit, for us to follow. The path may be difficult to resist, and it may still influence us if we resist it, but we can resist it at will and minimize its influence. The question is, how do we do it? The answer requires specifying in some detail how automatic processing works. That is the purpose of the next section.

Some readers may feel that an attack on one of the properties of automaticity must challenge the concept itself. Showing that automatic processing is controlled just as nonautomatic processing is controlled removes an essential difference. If all of the properties are challenged and all of the differences removed, what will remain of the concept of automaticity? These concerns are valid if one defines automaticity by listing essential or characteristic properties, which is a common practice in the literature (see, e.g., Hasher & Zacks, 1979; Logan, 1980; Posner & Snyder, 1975a; Schneider et al., 1984). But they are not a problem if one defines automaticity in terms of the processes that underlie it, and not by listing its properties. The theory described in the next section describes automaticity in terms of underlying memory processes.

AN INSTANCE THEORY OF AUTOMATICITY

The issue of control must be addressed in the context of a theory of automaticity. Instead of reviewing existing theories or patching up theories of the 1970s, this section presents a new theory that takes a fundamentally different perspective on automaticity and derives the relation between control and automaticity from it. The theory, described more fully elsewhere (Logan, 1988), differs from common approaches in that it makes no assumptions about capacity limitations or resources in explaining automaticity. In essence, the theory assumes that automaticity is a memory phenomenon, governed by the theoretical and empirical principles that govern memory, and that automatic processing is processing based on single-step, direct-access retrieval from memory.

The theory makes three main assumptions. First, it assumes that encoding into memory is an obligatory consequence of attention; whatever is attended is encoded. It may not be encoded well enough to be retrieved later—that depends on prevailing conditions—but it will be encoded nevertheless. Second, the theory assumes that retrieval from memory is an obligatory consequence of attention; whatever is related to the current focus of attention is retrieved. Retrieval may not always be successful, but the process occurs nevertheless. And third, the theory assumes that each object of attention is stored in a separate memory representation; the theory assumes "instance" or "exemplar" representation rather than strength. These assumptions are sufficient to account for the acquisition of automaticity and for many of the qualitative properties that distinguish automatic from nonautomatic processing (see Logan, 1988).

Acquisition of Automaticity

The assumptions of obligatory encoding, obligatory retrieval, and instance representation, coupled with an assumption about retrieval, account for the acquisition of automaticity. In general terms, the theory assumes that automatization involves a strategic shift from reliance on an initial algorithm that is sufficient to perform the task to reliance on memory for past solutions. Such a shift is apparent in children's acquisition of skill at simple addition: They begin with a counting algorithm (increment a counter once for each unit of each addend), but soon retrieve from memory the sum of any pair of digits (Ashcraft, 1982; Siegler, 1987). It is also apparent in a person's acquisition of knowledge of a new city: The person begins by consulting maps, street signs, and friendly strangers, but soon remembers without such aids how to get to the intended destination. In both cases, a person acquires a domain-specific data base that provides the appropriate information without much computation (i.e., by direct-access memory retrieval).

The theory assumes that the data base is built up by encoding each encounter with a stimulus separately. Later, when the stimulus is encountered again, each of the stored representations is (potentially) retrieved independently. In that sense, it is an instance or exemplar theory, like those advanced by Landauer (1975), Hintzman (1976, 1988), and Jacoby and Brooks (1984) to account for memory phenomena; by Brooks (1978), Medin and Schaffer (1978), and Hintzman (1986) to account for categorization and category learning; and by Kahneman and Miller (1986) to account for judgments of normality. All of these theories assume that separate representations are accumulated and retrieved. The instance theory of automaticity focuses on different implications of the accumulation and retrieval.

The theory assumes that memory retrieval takes time, and that each trace has its own retrieval time distribution. When a stimulus appears, each related trace is retrieved. The person can respond as soon as one trace is retrieved, so the separate retrieval processes race against each other, with the winner determining the response. Assuming that each retrieval time distribution has the same form and the same parameters, this amounts to selecting the minimum of n samples for the same distribution, where n is the number of related traces in memory. The minimum of n samples from the same distribution decreases as a power function of n (Logan, 1988), which is important because power functions describe the speed-up in processing that accompanies automatization (Newell & Rosenbloom, 1981). Thus, the theory accounts for the major result in the acquisition of automaticity. The theory also predicts a power function reduction in the standard deviation of reaction times that is constrained to have the same exponent as the power function for the means, which is observed in real data (Logan, 1988). This is a novel prediction not made by other theories of automatization. It predicts a constraint between two properties of automaticity—speed and consistency—that were hitherto unrelated.

Properties of Automaticity

The theory accounts for qualitative differences between automatic and nonautomatic processes by assuming that memory retrieval has different properties from those of the algorithm that governs initial performance. This explains why automatic processing is relatively fast, effortless, obligatory, and so forth. Memory retrieval is fast, effortless, and obligatory; algorithms are not (see Logan, 1988).

On the surface, the approach is similar to conventional approaches to the properties of automaticity, but there are deep underlying differences. Conventionally, theorists construct lists of pairs of opposing properties (e.g., effortful vs. effortless, slow vs. fast, serial vs. parallel) and attribute one member of each pair to automatic processes and the other to nonautomatic processes (e.g., Hasher & Zacks, 1979; Logan, 1978; Posner & Snyder, 1975a; Schneider et al., 1984). There is an implicit assumption that the process stays the same as automaticity develops; only its properties change. The question of automatization, then, is this: How can a process change its properties? There is also an implicit assumption that the properties co-occur—in other words, that all automatic processes possess all of the requisite properties, and no nonautomatic processes possess any of them. This approach cannot handle the many in-between cases in the literature, in which some processes have some automatic and some nonautomatic properties (for reviews, see Bargh, Chapter 1, this volume; Kahneman & Treisman, 1984; Logan, 1985b).

In contrast with conventional approaches, the instance theory is explicit about the properties of automatic processing but not about the properties of nonautomatic processing. This reflects a more fundamental difference: The theory assumes that automatization reflects a change from one kind of process to another, not a change in the properties of a single process. It assumes that all automatic processing is done by the same underlying process—namely, single-step, direct-access memory retrieval. All automatic processing has the properties of memory retrieval. Those properties are reasonably well defined, since memory retrieval is fairly well understood theoretically and empirically. But the properties of nonautomatic processing are not well defined. The class of algorithms that may be replaced by memory retrieval is probably infinite, and it is unreasonable to expect any single property or any set of properties to be common to all of members of the class. Some may be slow, some fast; some may be effortful, others effortless. The diversity of processes makes it unlikely that any single property will have any diagnostic value. The properties of algorithms may often be different from the properties of memory retrieval (hence the observed differences in the literature), but they are not *necessarily* different, as they are in the conventional view.

Control of Automatic Processing

In the instance theory, automatic processing depends on an obligatory retrieval process: Attention to an object causes whatever was associated with it to be retrieved from memory.[4] Automatic processing can be controlled to the extent that this retrieval process can be controlled. Five ways to control it are available, according to the theory.

The first two exploit the idea that memory retrieval does not control the response system directly. Responding on the basis of what was retrieved is a strategic, voluntary act. Thus, automatic responses can be controlled by (1) choosing not to respond on the basis of memory retrieval, basing responses on some algorithmic computation instead (adults can still add by counting on their fingers); or (2) relying on memory retrieval, but editing or inhibiting undesirable responses before they are executed. In the first case, memory retrieval may provide potential responses, but they will have little impact on performance. Possibly, if they are incompatible with the computed response, they may perturb overt behavior, slowing the response a little, but the algorithm will still dominate. Behavior will be closely controlled because it is predominantly algorithmic.

In the second case, performance may be largely automatic, based on memory retrieval most of the time, but it will be closely controlled. The retrieval process provides potential responses, which the person edits, executing responses that are appropriate to current goals and inhibiting ones that are not. An inhibited response may be replaced by another one retrieved from memory or one computed algorithmically. The person's goals act as a filter, selecting the responses to be executed, and this selection is a form of control. Selection and hence control can be quite stringent, even if all of the responses are generated automatically.

The first two means of control address whether the retrieval process will be used instrumentally. The last three control what the process retrieves. The retrieval process is driven by retrieval cues: When a cue is given as input, the retrieval process produces whatever was associated with that cue as output (e.g., Gillund & Shiffrin, 1984). Cuing has very specific effects. Information associated with one cue cannot be accessed with a different cue (cf. Tulving & Thompson, 1973). This specificity of cuing is what the instance theory exploits to control the retrieval process.

In the instance theory, the retrieval process is obligatory, running all the time, so it cannot be turned off. What it retrieves is controlled by manipulating retrieval cues. The retrieval cues can be manipulated in three major ways: (3) by changing the current state, (4) by changing the focus of attention, and (5) by changing goals.

The current state is a major retrieval cue, so changing state can have profound effects on what is retrieved. Locomotion, performing actions on the world, "mental travel" through a problem space, drugs, and illness all change the current state. Many of the ways to change state are voluntary, so state changes provide a ready means of control over automatic processing.

The focus of attention provides another major retrieval cue, bringing to mind knowledge about the object of attention. The focus of attention can be changed easily and relatively quickly, changing retrieval cues even if the environmental input stays the same. The focus of attention may be biased by vivid or sudden stimuli, but it is usually under voluntary control. Consequently, it provides a means of control over automatic processing.

Goals and intentions provide a third major retrieval cue, working together with the current environment and the focus of attention to determine what is retrieved. Changing goals changes the significance of aspects of the environment and causes information relevant to the newly significant aspects to be retrieved. This information may feed back into the system, motivating a change in the focus of attention, which will further change the retrieval cues. Changing goals—even *having* goals—is the essence of volition, so deliberate changes in goals provide another ready means of control over automatic processing.

With five ways to control retrieval, it seems unlikely that automatic processing is ever beyond control. It may not take much to keep it in control, particularly if the task is well practiced and the environment is familiar, but it is controlled even if the task of controlling it is easy.

These means of control need not be unique to the instance theory. Any theory that has obligatory retrieval as the main mechanism of automaticity can control automatic processing in these ways. The instance theory differs from the others primarily in its assumptions about instance representation, and those assumptions are not particularly important for the means of control described here. The main point is that theories must be explicit about the nature of the process that underlies automaticity. When the process is described explicitly, ways in which it can and cannot be controlled are often easy to see.

SUMMARY AND CONCLUSIONS

Phenomenology suggests conflicting intuitions about the control of automatic processing. Automatic reactions come to us whether or not we want them, so they seem beyond control. But often they tell us exactly what to do, so we rely on them, thinking they are well controlled. The dominant theories in the field have endorsed the former intuition, asserting that automatic processing is beyond control. For many, the idea that automatic processing is beyond control is a defining characteristic of automaticity. However, the experimental literature is more consistent with the latter intuition. Automatic reactions can be modulated by attention and intention; they can be inhibited and suppressed; and they can be coherent and planful. The instance theory of automaticity, and other theories that assume obligatory memory retrieval as the process underlying automaticity, provide mechanisms to achieve these kinds of control.

ACKNOWLEDGMENT

This research was supported by Grant No. BNS 87-10436 from the National Science Foundation.

NOTES

1. Bargh (Chapter 1, this volume) distinguishes the three types of automaticity, based on their ability to meet these criteria. "Preconscious" automatic processing is driven by stimulus presentation alone, independent of attention and intention. "Postconscious" automatic processing is not driven by stimulus presentation, but occurs as an inevitable consequence of having been conscious of something (i.e., it is dependent on attention, but not intention). And "goal-dependent" automatic processing is not driven by the presentation or conscious registration of the stimulus; it occurs as an inevitable consequence of having a particular goal in mind (i.e., it is dependent on intention and attention).

2. Automaticity is often discussed in studies of "subliminal priming," in which the priming stimulus is followed by a mask that puts it under the threshold for conscious awareness (e.g., Carr, McCauley, Sperber, & Parmalee, 1982; Marcel, 1983; but see Hollender, 1986). Those studies focus on the relation between awareness and automaticity and have little to say directly about control and automaticity. Subliminal priming effects may be beyond the subject's control, but for reasons peculiar to subliminal primes: "You can't hit what you can't see" (see Bargh, Chapter 1, this volume). Control strategies that involve deliberate responses to the prime (e.g., Logan, 1980) could not be used with subliminal primes (e.g., Cheesman & Merikle, 1985). Thus, subliminal effects might not be representative of supraliminal automaticity.

3. "Repetition priming" refers to a reduction in reaction time to the second presentation of an item. It is interpreted as a measure of *implicit* memory, whereas recognition is a measure of *explicit* memory (for a review, see Schacter, 1987).

4. The model does not require that absolutely everything that was ever associated with the object of attention be retrieved. It is sufficient that some proportion of

the associations be retrieved and that the proportion remain relatively constant as the amount to be retrieved varies (Logan, 1988).

REFERENCES

Anthony, B. J. (1985). In the blink of an eye: Implication of reflex modification for information processing. In P. K. Ackles, J. R. Jennings, & M. G. H. Coles (Eds.) *Advances in psychophysiology* (Vol. 1, pp. 167–218). Greenwich, CT: JAI Press.

Anthony, B. J., & Graham, F. K. (1985). Blink reflex modification by selective attention: Evidence for the modulation of "automatic" processing. *Biological Psychology, 20,* 43–59.

Ashcraft, M. H. (1982). The development of mental arithmetic: A chronometric approach. *Developmental Review, 2,* 213–236.

Brooks, L. R. (1978). Non-analytic concept formation and memory for instances. In E. Rosch & B. B. Lloyd (Eds.), *Cognition and categorization* (pp. 169–211). Hillsdale, NJ: Erlbaum.

Bryan, W. L., & Harter, N. (1897). Studies in the physiology and psychology of telegraphic language. *Psychological Review, 4,* 27–53.

Carr, T. H., McCauley, C., Sperber, R. D., & Parmalee, C. M. (1982). Words, pictures, and priming: On semantic activation, conscious identification, and the automaticity of information processing. *Journal of Experimental Psychology: Human Perception and Performance, 8,* 757–777.

Cheesman, J., & Merikle, P. M. (1985). Word recognition and consciousness. In D. Besner, T. Waller, & G. MacKinnon (Eds.), *Reading research: Advances in theory and practice.* Academic Press.

den Heyer, K., Briand, K., & Dannenbring, G. L. (1983). Strategic factors in a lexical decision task: Evidence for automatic and attention driven processes. *Memory and Cognition, 11,* 374–381.

Dyer, F. N., & Severance, L. J. (1973). Stroop interference with successive presentations of separate incongruent words and colors. *Journal of Experimental Psychology, 98,* 438–439.

Francolini, C. M., & Egeth, H. (1980). On the nonautomaticity of "automatic" activation: Evidence of selective seeing. *Perception and Psychophysics, 27,* 331–342.

Gillund, G., & Shiffrin, R. M. (1984). A retrieval model for both recognition and recall. *Psychological Review, 91,* 1–67.

Goolkasian, P. (1981). Retinal location and its effect on the processing of target and distractor information. *Journal of Experimental Psychology: Human Perception and Performance, 7,* 1247–1257.

Greenwald, A. G., & Rosenberg, K. E. (1978). Sequential effects of distracting stimuli in a selective attention reaction time task. In J. Requin (Ed.), *Attention and performance VII* (pp. 487–504). Hillsdale, NJ: Erlbaum.

Hasher, L., & Zacks, R. T. (1979). Automatic and effortful processes in memory. *Journal of Experimental Psychology: General, 108,* 356–388.

Henik, A., Friedrich, F. J., & Kellogg, W. A. (1983). The dependence of semantic relatedness effects on prime processing. *Memory and Cognition, 11,* 366–373.

Hintzman, D. L. (1976). Repetition and memory. In G. H. Bower (Ed.), *The psychology of learning and motivation* (pp. 47–91). New York: Academic Press.

Hintzman, D. L. (1986). "Schema abstraction" in a multiple-trace model. *Psychological Review, 93,* 411–428.

Hintzman, D. L. (1988). Judgments of frequency and recognition memory in a multiple-trace memory model. *Psychological Review, 95,* 528–551.

Hirst, W., Spelke, E. S., Reaves, C. C., Caharack, G., & Neisser, U. (1980). Dividing attention without alternation or automaticity. *Journal of Experimental Psychology: General, 109,* 98–117.

Hollender, D. (1986). Semantic activation without conscious identification in dichotic listening, parafoveal vision, and visual masking: A survey and appraisal. *Behavioral and Brain Sciences, 9,* 1–66.

Hunt, E., & Lansman, M. (1986). Unified model of attention and problem solving. *Psychological Review, 93,* 446–461.

Jacoby, L. L., & Brooks, L. R. (1984). Nonanalytic cognition: Memory, perception, and concept learning. In G. H. Bower (Ed.), *The psychology of learning and motivation* (pp. 1–47). New York: Academic Press.

James, W. (1890). *The principles of psychology* (2 vols.) New York: Holt.

Jonides, J., & Mack, R. (1984). The cost and benefit of cost and benefit. *Psychological Bulletin, 96,* 29–44.

Kahneman, D., & Henik, A. (1981). Perceptual organization and attention. In M. Kubovy & J. Pomerantz (Eds.) *Perceptual organization.* Hillsdale, NJ: Erlbaum.

Kahneman, D., & Miller, D. T. (1986). Norm theory: Comparing reality to its alternatives. *Psychological Review, 93,* 136–153.

Kahneman, D., & Treisman, A. M. (1984). Changing views of attention and automaticity. In R. Parasuraman & R. Davies (Eds.), *Varieties of attention* (pp. 29–61). New York: Academic Press.

LaBerge, D., & Samuels, S. J. (1974). Toward a theory of automatic information processing in reading. *Cognitive Psychology, 6,* 293–323.

Landauer, T. K. (1975). Memory without organization: Properties of a model with random storage and undirected retrieval. *Cognitive Psychology, 7,* 495–531.

Logan, G. D. (1978). Attention in character classification: Evidence for the automaticity of component stages. *Journal of Experimental Psychology: General, 107,* 32–63.

Logan, G. D. (1979). On the use of a concurrent memory load to measure attention and automaticity. *Journal of Experimental Psychology: Human Perception and Performance, 5,* 189–207.

Logan, G. D. (1980). Attention and automaticity in Stroop and priming tasks: Theory and data. *Cognitive Psychology, 12,* 523–553.

Logan, G. D. (1983). On the ability to inhibit simple thoughts and actions: I. Stop-signal studies of decision and memory. *Journal of Experimental Psychology: Learning, Memory, and Cognition, 9,* 585–606.

Logan, G. D. (1985a). On the ability to inhibit simple thoughts and actions: II. Stop-signal studies of repetition priming. *Journal of Experimental Psychology: Learning, Memory, and Cognition, 11,* 675–691.

Logan, G. D. (1985b). Skill and automaticity: Relations, implications and future directions. *Canadian Journal of Psychology, 39,* 367–386.

Logan, G. D. (1988). Toward an instance theory of automatization. *Psychological Review, 95,* 492–527.

Logan, G. D., & Cowan, W.B. (1984). On the ability to inhibit thought and action: A theory of an act of control. *Psychological Review, 91*, 295–327.

Logan, G. D., & Zbrodoff, N. J. (1979). When it helps to be misled: Facilitative effects of increasing the frequency of conflicting stimuli in a Stroop-like task. *Memory and Cognition, 7*, 166–174.

Logan, G. D., Zbrodoff, N. J., & Williamson, J. (1984). Strategies in the color–word Stroop task. *Bulletin of the Psychonomic Society, 22*, 135–138.

Marcel, A. T. (1983). Conscious and unconscious perception: An approach to the relations between phenomenal experience and perceptual processes. *Cognitive Psychology, 15*, 238–300.

Medin, D. L., & Schaffer, M. M. (1978). Context theory of classification learning. *Psychological Review, 85*, 207–238.

Neely, J. H. (1977). Semantic priming and retrieval from lexical memory: Roles of inhibitionless spreading activation and limited-capacity attention. *Journal of Experimental Psychology: General, 106*, 226–254.

Neely, J. H., & Keefe, D. E. (in press). Semantic context effects on visual word processing: A hybrid prospective/retrospective processing theory. In G. H. Bower (Ed.), *The psychology of learning and motivation: Advances in research and theory* (Vol. 23). New York: Academic Press.

Naumann, O. (1984). Automatic processing: A review of recent findings and a plea for an old theory. In W. Prinz & A. F. Sanders (Eds.), *Cognition and motor processes* (pp. 255–293). Berlin: Springer-Verlag.

Newell, A., & Rosenbloom, P. S. (1981). Mechanisms of skill in acquisition and the law of practice. In J. R. Anderson (Ed.), *Cognitive skills and their acquisition* (pp. 1–55). Hillsdale, NJ: Erlbaum.

Norman, D. A. (1981). Categorization of action slips. *Psychological Review, 88*, 1–15.

Osman, A., Kornblum, S., & Meyer, D. E. (1986). The point of no return in choice reaction time: Controlled and ballistic stages of response preparation. *Journal of Experimental Psychology: Human Perception and Performance, 12*, 243–258.

Posner, M. I., & Snyder, C. R. R. (1975a). Attention and cognitive control. In R. L. Solso (Ed.), *Information processing and cognition: The Loyola Symposium* (pp. 55–85). Hillsdale, NJ: Erlbaum..

Posner, M. I., & Snyder, C. R. R. (1975b). Facilitation and inhibition in the processing of signals. In P. M. A. Rabbitt & S. Pornic (Eds.), *Attention and performance V*. New York: Academic Press.

Rachman, S. J. (1978). An anatomy of obsessions. *Behavioral Analysis and Modification, 2*, 253–278.

Ratcliff, R. (1978). A theory of memory retrieval. *Psychological Review, 85*, 59–108.

Ratcliff, R., & McKoon, G. (1981). Automatic and strategic components of priming in recognition. *Journal of Verbal Learning and Verbal Behavior, 20*, 204–215.

Ratcliff, R., & McKoon, G. (1988). A retrieval theory of priming in memory. *Psychological Review, 95*, 385–408.

Reason, J. T. (1979). Actions not as planned: The price of automatization. In G. Underwood & S. Stevens (Eds.), *Aspects of consciousness* (Vol. 1). London: Academic Press.

Reason, J. T. (1984). Lapses of attention in everyday life. In R. Parasuraman & R.

Davies (Eds.), *Varieties of attention* (pp. 515–549). New York: Academic Press.

Reason, J. T., & Myceilska, K. (1982). *Absent minded: The psychology of mental lapses and everyday errors*. Englewood Cliffs, NJ: Prentice-Hall.

Salthouse, T. A. (1986). Perceptual, cognitive, and motoric aspects of transcription of typing. *Psychological Bulletin, 99*, 303–319.

Schachar, R. J., & Logan, G. D. (1989). *Impulsivity and inhibitory control in normal development and childhood psychopathology*. Manuscript submitted for publication.

Schacter, D. L. (1987). Implicit memory: History and current status. *Journal of Experimental Psychology: Learning, Memory, and Cognition, 13*, 501–522.

Schneider, W. (1985). Toward a model of attention and the development of automatic processing. In M. I. Posner & O. S. Marin (Eds.), *Attention and performance XI* (pp. 475–492). Hillsdale, NJ: Erlbaum.

Schneider, W., Dumais, S. T., & Shiffrin, R. M. (1984). Automatic and control processing and attention. In R. Parasuraman & R. Davies (Eds.), *Varieties of attention* (pp. 1–27). New York: Academic Press.

Schneider, W., & Shiffrin, R. M. (1977). Controlled and automatic human information processing: I. Detection, search and attention. *Psychological Review, 84*, 1–66.

Shiffrin, R. M., & Schneider, W. (1977). Controlled and automatic human information processing: II. Perceptual learning, automatic attending, and a general theory. *Psychological Review, 84*, 127–190.

Siegler, R. S. (1987). The perils of averaging data over strategies: An example from children's addition. *Journal of Experimental Psychology: General, 116*, 250–264.

Smith, M. C. (1979). Contextual facilitation in a letter search task depends on how the prime is processed. *Journal of Experimental Psychology: Human Perception and Performance, 5*, 239–251.

Smith, M. C., Theodor, L., & Franklin, P. E. (1983). The relationship between contextual facilitation and depth of processing. *Journal of Experimental Psychology: Learning, Memory and Cognition, 9*, 697–712.

Stroop, J. R. (1935). Studies of interference in serial verbal reactions. *Journal of Experimental Psychology: 18*, 643–662.

Tannock, R., Schachar, R. J., Carr, R. P., Chajczyk, D., & Logan, G. D. (in press). Effects of methylphenidate on inhibitory control in hyperactive children. *Journal of Abnormal Child Psychology*.

Tulving, E., & Thompson, D. M. (1973). Encoding specificity and retrieval processes in episodic memory. *Psychological Review, 80*, 352–373.

Tweedy, J. R., Lapinski, R. H., & Schvaneveldt, R. W. (1977). Semantic-context effects on word recognition: Influence of varying proportion of items presented in an appropriate context. *Memory and Cognition, 5*, 84–89.

Wegner, D. M., Schneider, D. J., Carter, S., & White, T. (1987). Paradoxical effects of thought suppression. *Journal of Personality and Social Psychology, 53*, 1–9.

Zbrodoff, N. J., & Logan, G. D. (1986). On the autonomy of mental processes: A case study of arithmetic. *Journal of Experimental Psychology: General, 115*, 118–130.

3

Knowledge Accessibility and Activation: Subjectivity and Suffering from Unconscious Sources

E. TORY HIGGINS
Columbia University

For over a century now, the "unconscious" has been portrayed as a dominant, if shadowy, figure in theories of people's suffering and subjective responses to the social world. The proposed role of the unconscious in such theories has varied widely. Perhaps the most commanding, or at least best-known, roles created for the unconscious were those developed by Freud (e.g., 1920/1952), who suggested that mechanisms to prevent threatening impulses from escaping the unconscious underlie suffering, and by Jung (e.g., 1952/1956), who suggested that the "collective unconscious" has causal priority as the critical mental system. More recently, the role of the unconscious has been recast from the star of the drama to a supporting role—no longer the source of the problem but a reinforcer of it, not the focus of therapy but a hurdle along the way. For example, in various forms of cognitive–behavioral therapy, where unconscious beliefs are elicited in order to transform them (e.g., Beck, Rush, Shaw, & Emery, 1979; Ellis, 1973), the central problem is understood to be the nature of the beliefs themselves (e.g., irrational beliefs or dysfunctional attitudes) rather than the fact that they are unconscious.

In one respect, however, both psychodynamic and cognitive–behavioral perspectives agree: The unconscious can be a problem when it is associated with a loss of voluntary control. A concept that captures both the out-of-awareness and out-of-control features of the purported role of the unconscious is "automaticity" (see Bargh, 1984; Posner, 1978; Shiffrin & Schneider, 1977). But automatic thoughts or habitual patterns of thinking are neither necessarily problematic nor necessarily unrealistic (see Higgins & Bargh, 1987). It is not only "dysfunctional attitudes" or "irrational beliefs" that can reside in the unconscious or can function automatically. Positive attitudes and beliefs can do so as well.

Perhaps, as suggested by the cognitive–behavioral perspective, the basic problem is with the negative beliefs themselves rather than with their unconsciousness or automaticity per se. From this perspective, automaticity contributes to vulnerability when it increases the pervasiveness of specific negative beliefs or reduces the likelihood of critically assessing them. On the other hand, the contributory role of automaticity to vulnerability may be greater than this. The purpose of the present chapter is to consider a model of knowledge activation in which automaticity is once again a distinct character in the drama.

The chapter begins with a general discussion of how knowledge accessibility and activation produce *subjective* experiences of social stimuli in the sense of being involuntary, phenomenal, personal, and even illusory. This model is then applied to the issue of how self-beliefs are activated and the role of structural interconnectedness in this activation. Different types of problematic self-belief structures are identified and evidence is presented of their relation to distinct emotional/motivational vulnerabilities. Studies are then described that have directly tested the role of automatic processes in producing suffering.

KNOWLEDGE ACCESSIBILITY AND ACTIVATION

To begin at a beginning, Wertheimer (1923) first described a set of variables, including past experiences and expectations, that influence the grouping of perceptual stimuli. Wertheimer's work with the "phi" phenomenon, in which subjects reported that they saw a light "moving across" an unlighted space when a light was switched off at point A and a light was switched on at a separate point B, demonstrated that people impose some interpretation on external stimuli. Past experience or expectations apparently "fill in" information missing in the external stimuli.

In order to deal with "expectancies" and other significant internal events in psychological functioning, Hebb (1949) proposed the concepts of "cell assembly" and "phase sequence." Hebb suggested that the internal representations of stimuli could be conceptualized as massive interconnections of neural networks. In this conceptualization, an expectancy would involve a set of stimuli that initiate the running off of an established cell assembly. Because of such expectancies, people see things that are not there.

Influenced by various theorists, such as Bartlett, Freud, McDougall,

Murray, Thomas, and Whorf, the "New Look" in perception that emerged in the 1940s proposed that needs, values, and attitudes, as well as expectancies, determine perception and result in people's "going beyond the information given" (Bruner, 1957a). In a study by Proshansky and Murphy (1942), for example, subjects were found to accentuate certain aspects of what they perceived and to reject other aspects as a function of whether these aspects were presented in conjunction with a reward (receiving money) or a punishment (losing money), respectively. In another study, Postman and Brown (1952) found that subjects who had been told that they had "succeeded" (surpassed their level of aspiration) in certain tasks were relatively quicker to perceive words related to success, such as "excellent," "succeed," "perfection," and "winner," than those told they had "failed" (fallen short of their level of aspiration). The latter subjects were found to be quicker than the former to perceive words related to failure, such as "unable," "failure," "defeat," and "obstacle."

Multiple Sources of Accessibility[1]

The general role of expectancies and motivational states on perception was formulated by Bruner (1957b), in his paper "On Perceptual Readiness," in terms of a novel notion—the notion of category "accessibility." For Bruner, "accessibility" denotes the ease or speed with which a given stimulus input is coded in terms of a given category under varying conditions. The two proposed general sets of conditions thought to determine accessibility are expectancies (i.e., subjective probability estimates of the likelihood of a given event) and motivational states (i.e., certain kinds of search sets induced by needs, task goals, etc.). In this model, Bruner postulated that expectancies and motivational states momentarily increase the accessibility of stored categories, and that the greater the momentary accessibility of a stored category, the more likely it is that a stimulus input will be perceived or interpreted in terms of that category rather than a competing alternative category.

A significant implication of the notion of accessibility is that the likelihood that people will apply a particular category to an input is not a function solely of the match between the features of the input and those of the category. Instead, other factors, such as expectancies and need states, can increase the *prior* likelihood that a particular category rather than an alternative will be applied to the input. And, once a particular category is applied to an input, features missing in the input that are part of the category will tend to be filled in.

This consequence of accessibility, however, is not restricted to momentary increases in accessibility from the relatively strategic, stimulus-orienting variables described by Bruner (e.g., instructional sets, stimulus-related goals). It can also result both from momentary increases in accessibility produced by extraneous variables and from chronic accessibility.

In social psychology, a series of studies beginning in the late 1970s demonstrated that simply activating a construct in one task was capable of increasing the accessibility of the construct sufficiently to give it precedence when subjects categorized a target person's behavior in a subsequent, unrelated task (see Higgins, 1981; Higgins & Bargh, 1987; Wyer & Srull, 1981, 1986). For example, in one study (Higgins, Rholes, & Jones, 1977), subjects were initially exposed to one or another set of trait constructs as an incidental aspect of a study on perception. The subjects later participated in an "unrelated" study on reading comprehension, where they were asked to characterize the ambiguous behaviors of a target person portrayed in the essay they read. The study found that the subjects were significantly more likely to use the constructs activated or primed in the perception study than alternative, equally applicable constructs when they later categorized the target person in the second study. Moreover, the subjects' own attitudes toward the target person as measured 2 weeks later were influenced by these contextually primed categorizations.

This basic finding that recent activation increases the likelihood of a construct's being used in subsequent judgments has been replicated in many subsequent studies (e.g., Bargh, Bond, Lombardi, & Tota, 1986; Erdley & D'Agostino, 1988; Fazio, Powell, & Herr, 1983; Herr, 1986; Herr, Sherman, & Fazio, 1983; Higgins, Bargh, & Lombardi, 1985; Higgins & Chaires, 1980; Martin, 1986; Rholes & Pryor, 1982; Sinclair, Mark, & Shotland, 1987; Srull & Wyer, 1979, 1980). Indeed, the results of the Postman and Brown (1952) study, where telling subjects that they had "succeeded" or "failed" influenced how easily they later perceived words related to these constructs, may have been an effect of recent activation rather than of motivation. There is also evidence that frequent activation of a construct increases how long the construct will remain predominant in subsequent categorization (e.g., Higgins, Bargh, & Lombardi, 1985; Lombardi, Higgins, & Bargh, 1987; Srull & Wyer, 1979, 1980).

Other results of these studies suggest that the basic effect of recent and frequent activation—assimilation of subsequent input to the more accessible construct—is more likely to occur if perceivers are not conscious of the priming events when processing the subsequent input than if they are conscious (see Lombardi et al., 1987). Thus, this effect does not require that subjects be aware of (i.e., remember) the primed construct at the point when the construct is to be used in categorization (see Higgins & Chaires, 1980). Indeed, experimental conditions that increase the likelihood of such awareness (e.g., by using highly memorable priming stimuli or actually reminding subjects of the priming events) are more likely to produce a contrast effect on judgment than an assimilation effect (see Herr, 1986; Herr et al., 1983; Lombardi et al., 1987; Martin, 1986; Strack, Schwarz, Bless, Kubler, & Wanke, 1988).[2] And, conversely, experimental conditions that increase the likelihood that subjects' consciousness of a priming event will be suppressed (e.g., when it would be unpleasant to remember a priming event) increases the likelihood that an assimilation effect will be produced (e.g., Martin, 1986).

The importance of recency and frequency of exposure as variables influencing subsequent performance has been recognized for a long time. In the early 19th century, Thomas Brown proposed recency and frequency (along with intensity) as basic conditions under which the general principle of association operates (see Heidbreder, 1933). And in the late 19th century, Edward Lee Thorndike (1898) proposed in his law of exercise that the more recently and the more frequently (as well as the more vigorously) a stimulus–response bond is exercised, the more effectively it is stamped in.

Such learning or practice effects of recent and frequent exposure may underlie certain kinds of priming effects (see Jacoby, 1983; Smith & Branscombe, 1987; Smith, Branscombe, & Bormann, 1988). For example, there are priming effects that appear to be due to procedural learning, where recently or frequently exercising a particular processing procedure (e.g., reading typographically inverted text) increases the likelihood of using that procedure on a subsequent task (e.g., Kolers, 1976; Tulving, Schacter, & Stark, 1982; see Smith & Branscombe, 1987, for a discussion of such effects).

Priming effects from procedural learning, moreover, can involve quite subtle effects of observational learning as well as direct response learning. In one study (Higgins & Chaires, 1980), subjects were shown a series of slides depicting common objects as part of a study purportedly examining long-term memory. Some of the objects would normally be described with a single word (e.g., a banana), whereas other objects would normally be described with a phrase (e.g., a carton containing eggs). In one condition, the experimenter always described the "phrase" slides using an "of" linguistic construction (e.g., "a carton of eggs"). In the other condition, the experimenter described the same slides using an "and" construction (e.g., "a carton and eggs").

After viewing the slides, the subjects performed the Duncker (1945) candle problem, which was presented as a memory interference task to which some subjects were randomly assigned. The difficult part of this problem is to think of using a box filled with thumbtacks as a platform to prevent candle wax from dripping on the table. The results of the priming manipulation were dramatic: Only 20% of the subjects in the "of" condition solved the problem within the 10-minute time period, as compared to 80% of the subjects in the "and" condition. Apparently subjects in the latter condition had learned a procedure for representing "container with contents" stimuli that they used in the subsequent Duncker candle task. This procedure for representing container and contents in a differentiated manner, which subjects had learned from observing the experimenter in the "memory" task, facilitated solving the problem. It should be noted that the subjects were not at all aware of any connection between the two tasks other than the one they had been told, nor were they aware that the "memory" task had influenced their performance on the Duncker task in any way.

Thus, at least some priming effects, and especially those lasting a long time, could be due to procedural learning effects of recent and frequent exposure (see Sherman, 1987; Smith & Branscombe, 1987). (For an example of procedural priming effects on attributional processes, see Fenigstein & Levine, 1984.) But not all priming effects are easily understood in these terms. For example, the accessibility effect found in the Higgins et al. (1977) study is unlikely to have been a procedural learning effect of priming. The priming manipulation involved subjects' orally repeating back a trait word they had received auditorily after performing the central task (naming the background color of a slide), whereas the accessibility effect was measured via subjects' written characterizations of a target person's behavior that they had read about. Thus, the procedures involved in the priming task were different from those in the categorization task. Moreover, the priming effects on subjects' categorizations of the target person's behaviors remained significant even when the particular words produced by subjects in the priming task were excluded from the analysis of their categorizations.

The priming procedures used in various other studies also suggest that procedural learning or strategic processing is not sufficient to explain the full range of accessibility effects (e.g., Bargh & Pietromonaco, 1982; Erdley & D'Agostino, 1988). What else might be involved? Another possibility is that accessibility effects result from the storage and retrieval of specific experiences (see Smith & Branscombe, 1987). In experimental tests of priming effects, for example, the specific experiences associated with priming events themselves could produce the effects observed (see Jacoby & Kelley, 1987; Smith, 1988). By this account, episodic knowledge rather than procedural knowledge is given the leading role. And certainly episodic memory of priming events could produce assimilation effects of priming (Smith, 1988).

One might expect, however, that such episodic learning about the priming events themselves would also be reflected in high recall for the priming events. This in turn suggests a positive relation between people's memory for primed constructs and their use of primed constructs in subsequent categorization. But the Higgins, Bargh, and Lombardi (1985) and Lombardi et al. (1987) studies found no general relation between which primed constructs subjects remembered and which primed constructs they used to categorize the stimulus person. In fact, the classic assimilation effect of priming was only found for subjects who could *not* recall the priming events.

Under certain conditions, one might even expect episodic experiences of priming events to have a contrast effect on categorization rather than an assimilation effect, if these experiences are remembered at the moment of categorization. When a priming event describes a person, as in the Srull and Wyer (1979) and Higgins, Bargh, and Lombardi (1985) paradigms that have been used in many studies, subjects are provided with statements or labels describing people who possess or display a particular trait (e.g., hostility). According to the rules of language comprehension (see, e.g., Huttenlocher & Higgins, 1971), such statements should be interpreted as an instance of a person's possessing or displaying the trait to a greater extent than the average person. If such instances or exemplars are recalled later when subjects are asked to categorize the stimulus person, they may function as a high standard or reference point relative to which the stimulus person's ambiguous or vague behavior is judged. This should produce a contrast effect of the priming events on subjects' categorizations of the stimulus person (see Higgins & Stangor, 1988). Just such contrast effects of priming events on categorization have been found under conditions where subjects are likely to have remembered category instances or exemplars provided by the priming events (e.g., Herr, 1986; Herr et al., 1983; Lombardi et al., 1987; Martin, 1986). On the other hand, when subjects are not provided with or do not remember priming instances (e.g., Bargh et al., 1986; Bargh & Pietromonaco, 1982; Erdley & D'Agostino, 1988; Higgins, Bargh, & Lombardi, 1985; Lombardi et al., 1987), assimilation effects of priming on categorization have been found. It is not clear how a model of accessibility effects based solely on episodic knowledge can account for this pattern of results.

Although a model of accessibility effects based on episodic knowledge does not appear to provide a full account of current findings, it is likely that accessibility and activation of personal experiences do play an important role in many kinds of judgments and decisions. Previous proposals concerning how episodic knowledge may underlie accessibility effects have tended to focus on how memory for the priming events themselves may influence subsequent responses. The impact on subsequent responses from activating episodic knowledge, however, is not restricted to people's personal experiences with the recent priming events themselves. There is research, for example, suggesting that activating people's past life experiences can influence their subsequent behaviors and judgments (see Clark & Isen, 1982; Salancik & Conway, 1975; Schwarz & Clore, 1987; Strack, Schwarz, & Gschneidinger, 1985). And there is also evidence that increasing the availability and accessibility of people's personal experiences with objects influences their subsequent responding to those objects (see Fazio & Zanna, 1981).

In sum, both procedural knowledge and episodic knowledge play a role in accessibility effects. But neither type of knowledge can account for the full range of priming and accessibility effects. Something else is needed. What might this something else be? Before this question is taken up, some additional accessibility effects need to be considered—in particular, the effects of the chronic accessibility of individuals' constructs.

Individual Construct Accessibility: The Case of Chronic Accessibility

As poetically expressed by Kelly (1955), "construct systems can be considered as a kind of scanning pattern which a person continually projects upon his world. As he sweeps back and forth across his perceptual field he picks up blips of meaning" (p. 145). Walter Mischel, a student of Kelly, suggested that individual differences in the subjective meaning of social events may be especially evident in the personal constructs individuals employ, and that these personal constructs may show the greatest resistance to situational presses (Mischel, 1973). More generally, it has been proposed that there are individual differences, including cross-cultural differences, in the theories or viewpoints that people have about human nature and personality (e.g., Kelly, 1955; Sarbin, Taft, & Bailey, 1960; Tagiuri, 1969; Tajfel, 1969).

These early accounts of personal constructs or viewpoints did not specify whether the individual differences involved the *availability* or the *accessibility* of constructs. In discussing individual differences in constructs, Higgins, King, and Mavin (1982) pointed out that there can be both individual differences in the particular kinds of constructs that are present in memory for potential use in processing social input (differences in the kind of stored knowledge that is available for use) and individual differences in the readiness with which available constructs are actually used (differences in the likelihood of using available constructs).

Historically, the effects of temporary category accessibility (e.g., Bruner, 1957b) and personal constructs (e.g., Kelly, 1955) have been treated as completely distinct phenomena. But by distinguishing individual differences in the accessibility of constructs from differences in the availability of constructs, Higgins et al. (1982) proposed a basic conceptual link between the phenomena of temporary category accessibility and personal constructs. First, priming manipulations can be conceptualized as situational factors that temporarily create individual differences in construct accessibility. Second, if frequent priming or activation increases how long a construct will remain accessible or predominant, then long-term individual differences across many situations in the frequency with which different kinds of constructs are activated (as from differences in parental instruction) would be expected to lead to chronic individual differences in construct accessibility. Thus, chronic individual differences in construct accessibility should function like temporary individual differences in construct accessibility.

There is now considerable evidence supporting this chronic-accessibility perspective on personal constructs and knowledge (e.g., Bargh & Pratto, 1986; Bargh & Thein, 1985; Fazio, 1986; Higgins et al., 1982; King & Sorrentino, 1988; Lau, in press; Strauman & Higgins, 1987). For example, in one study (Higgins et al., 1982), subjects' chronically accessible constructs were measured by asking subjects to list the traits of a type of person that they liked, that they disliked, that they sought out, that they avoided, and that they frequently encountered. Chronic accessibility was defined in terms of output primacy—those traits a subject listed first in response to the questions. About 1 week later, subjects participated in an "unrelated" study conducted by a different experimenter. Each subject read an individually tailored essay containing some behavioral descriptions of a target person that moderately exemplified the subject's accessible trait constructs, and other behavioral descriptions that moderately exemplified trait constructs that were not chronically accessible for the subject but were so for some other subject (i.e., a "quasi-yoking" design that controlled across subjects for the content of the accessibility-related and -unrelated descriptions).

On both a measure of subjects' impressions of the target person and a measure of their recall of the behavioral descriptions, the study found that subjects were significantly more likely to exclude information unrelated to their chronically accessible constructs than information that was related to them. These basic effects were also found in another study (Higgins et al., 1982) in which chronic accessibility was defined in terms of the frequency of output to different questions rather than the primacy of output. Moreover, there was evidence from a 2-week delay measure included in this study that the effects persisted or even increased over time.

If chronic accessibility functions like temporary accessibility, as suggested (Higgins et al., 1982), then combining in the same study chronic individual differences in construct accessibility (as measured by the primacy of output measure used in Higgins et al., 1982) and temporary differences in construct accessibility (as produced by a priming manipulation) should yield enhanced effects of construct accessibility. In a direct test of this implication, Bargh et al. (1986) found that, as predicted, the chronic and temporary sources of a construct's accessibility combined additively to increase the likelihood that the construct would be used to interpret behavioral descriptions of a target person.

It should be noted, however, that the Higgins et al. (1982) proposal that chronic and temporary accessibility function similarly does not imply that additive effects of priming and chronic accessibility should always be expected. First, in order for priming to produce an effect, it is necessary that the primed construct both be available in a subject's knowledge system and be perceived as applicable to the input. When a study involves priming the trait constructs of adult subjects, it is reasonable to expect that the trait constructs should be available for everyone. But if a study involves priming trait constructs in children, or involves priming attitudes or opinions that may not be available to all subjects, then an additive effect may not be found. Instead, an interaction effect may be found, because priming should have an additive effect for the chronically accessible subjects (for whom the construct is available) but not for the remaining subjects (for whom the construct is not available to be primed). Indeed, just such an interaction between chronic accessibility and priming of procedural knowledge of a persuasion heuristic (i.e., "Length of message implies strength of message") is reported by Chaiken, Liberman, and Eagly (Chapter 7, this volume; see also Aldrich, Sullivan, & Borgida, in press).

Second, in order for priming to produce a detectable effect, the chronic accessibility of the knowledge prior to priming must not be too high. Otherwise, the addition to the excitation level from priming may not be evident. In the Higgins and Chaires (1980) studies, for example, the chronic accessibility of the "of" procedure for representing "container with contents" stimuli in an undifferentiated manner was probably so high to begin with that any increase in accessibility from the "of" priming was not detectable (i.e., relative to a no-priming condition). Third, the frequent exposure to knowledge-related instances or the long-term goals associated with chronic accessibility may also change the quality of the knowledge over time. To the extent that chronic accessibility influences knowledge availability, one should also not expect simple additive effects with priming.

Bargh and Pratto (1986) used the Stroop color-naming paradigm to test another implication of the proposed similarity between chronic and temporary accessibility—that a chronically accessible construct, like a temporarily accessible construct, should be more ready to be activated by a stimulus input to which it is related. Bargh and Pratto (1986) found that subjects' chronically accessible constructs were indeed at a higher level of activation readiness than their inaccessible constructs, as revealed by greater interference on the Stroop task from the chronically accessible constructs. And in an important test of the proposal that chronic accessibility is likely to be associated with automatic or passive processing (see Bargh, 1984; Higgins & King, 1981), Bargh and Thein (1985) found evidence of the processing efficiency expected with automatic processing for subjects' impressions and recall of a target person's behaviors when the processing involved subjects' chronically accessible constructs.

There is also evidence that chronic knowledge accessibility is an important factor in relation to personal attitudes and opinions. Fazio (1986), for example, reports a series of studies suggesting that the chronic accessibility of object evaluation associations influences the likelihood that people's attitudes about objects will guide their behaviors toward the objects. More recently, Lau (in press) conducted a set of studies using an alternative operationalization of individuals' chronically accessible constructs and found that chronically accessible constructs are relatively stable even over years, and that they guide the processing of information about a wide variety of political objects.

As mentioned earlier, the proposal that chronic and temporary accessibility may function similarly was based on generalizing from more prolonged differences in temporary accessibility due to frequent activation of a construct in a single experimental session, to chronic differences in accessibility from frequent activation across the many natural situations associated with an individual's socialization experiences (Higgins et al., 1982). This analysis suggests that individual differences in chronic accessibility should function like differences in temporary accessibility produced by frequent activation. In an earlier study, Higgins, Bargh, and Lombardi (1985) exposed subjects across a number of trials (in a "scrambled sentences" task) to two different trait constructs that could be used to categorize the same behavior, with one trait being primed more frequently and the other trait being primed more recently. After delays of either 15 seconds or 120 seconds, subjects began another task in which they were asked to categorize the same behavioral description of a target person. When categorizing the target person's behavior, subjects tended to use the more recently activated construct after the brief delay, but the more frequently activated construct after the long delay.

Would the same crossover pattern of results be found if subjects' chronically accessible constructs were substituted for the frequently activated constructs in the design? This question was addressed in a recent study (Bargh, Lombardi, & Higgins, 1988). All subjects were primed by recent exposure to a trait construct that could be used to characterize the behavior of the target person in the subsequent task. The subjects were preselected so that the alternative trait construct for categorizing the behavioral description was a chronically accessible construct for half of the subjects, but was not for the other half. As in our earlier study, the delay between the priming task and the categorization task was either 15 seconds or 120 seconds. The results confirmed our prediction. When the alternative trait construct was chronically accessible for subjects, a crossover pattern was found: Subjects tended to use the recently primed construct after the short delay, but the chronically accessible construct after the long delay. In contrast, no such crossover pattern was obtained among those subjects for whom the alternative trait construct was *not* chronically accessible. This similarity in pattern of results between the Higgins, Bargh, and Lombardi (1985) and Bargh et al. (1988) studies supports our suggestion (Higgins et al., 1982) that chronic accessibility may function like momentary accessibility from frequent activation.

The results of these studies support the proposal that temporary and chronic knowledge accessibility function similarly. And, as stated earlier, it is clear that something in addition to procedural or episodic knowledge underlies accessibility effects. It is time now to consider what that something else might be.

The "Synapse" Model of Knowledge Accessibility and Activation

Higgins and King (1981) suggested an "energy cell" metaphor for construct accessibility, where the energy or action potential of a construct (i.e., the cell) is increased whenever the construct is excited or activated, and the energy slowly dissipates over time. It is assumed in this model that as the energy level of a construct increases, the likelihood of its utilization increases. This metaphor contrasts with a metaphor for construct accessibility suggested by Wyer and Srull (1980). They have proposed a "bin" model, involving a layered storage bin containing constructs in which the construct on top is utilized in processing.

Higgins, Bargh, and Lombardi (1985) have since elaborated the Higgins and King (1981) "energy cell" metaphor into a "synapse" model, in which it is suggested that, as for synapses, the decay over time of the excitation level of a construct following its last activation is slower when the construct has been frequently activated than when it has been activated only once. This model differs from Wyer and Srull's (1980) "bin" model with respect to its interpretation of the effects of frequent activation. According to Wyer and Srull (1980), frequent activation of a construct simply increases the likelihood that, at any point in time, the construct will have been recently activated and thus will be stored on top of the bin where it will be more likely to be used again. In their "bin" model, then, the effects of frequent activation are really due to the effects of recent activation. In the "synapse" model, however, the effects of frequent and recent activation are distinct because of the differences in their decay functions following final activation.

As described earlier, Higgins, Bargh, and Lombardi (1985) tested these alternative conceptualizations of accessibility effects by exposing subjects to two alternative constructs for characterizing subsequent input, one being primed more frequently and the other being primed only once but more recently. Immediately following the last prime, the more recently activated construct would be at its maximum level of excitation, whereas the excitation level of the frequently primed construct would already be below maximum because its final activation occurred earlier. At this point, then, the "synapse" model would predict that the recently primed construct would predominate in categorization. However, because the excitation level of the frequently activated construct was expected to decay more slowly than that of the recently activated construct, it was predicted that with sufficient delay between final priming and the input to be categorized, the construct that was frequently activated would predominate in categorization. In contrast, Wyer and Srull's (1980) "bin" model would predict an advantage for the recently activated construct at both delay periods, because the delay period between final priming and input for categorization was filled with a task that taxed subjects' working memory (i.e., counting backwards by 7's) in such a manner that the recently activated construct would stay on top of the bin. As described earlier, the crossover pattern predicted by the "synapse" model was found.[3]

Applicability and Knowledge Activation

The basic assumption of the "synapse" model is that constructs vary in their levels of excitation prior to stimulus exposure, and that, everything else being equal, the higher the level of excitation of a construct at input, the greater the likelihood that the construct will be activated by exposure to the stimulus.[4] In most studies of accessibility effects, the condition of "everything else being equal" is accomplished by having all subjects exposed to the same target person information. Generally, this has been accomplished in two different ways.

One method, exemplified by the Higgins et al. (1977) study, has been to construct each behavioral description so that its features are (roughly) equal in similarity or overlap to the features of two alternative constructs that could be used to characterize it (e.g., "adventurous/reckless"). That is, each behavioral description is constructed so that two alternative constructs are equally applicable for characterizing it. This method involves exposing all subjects to the same *ambiguous* input. The other method, exemplified by the Srull and Wyer (1979) studies, has been to construct a set of behavioral descriptions that has enough features associated with a particular trait construct (e.g., "hostile") that the construct is applicable to the set, but does not possess enough features associated with the construct that the set requires characterization in terms of the construct. This method involves exposing all subjects to the same *vague* input.

When the former, ambiguous input is used, the effect of increased construct accessibility from priming is typically measured by subjects' choice in categorizing the target person. The prediction is that the target person is more likely to be characterized by the primed trait than by the non-primed trait. When the latter, vague input is used, the effect of increased accessibility is typically measured by subjects' ratings of how much they believe the target person possesses the primed trait. The prediction is that the target person will be rated as possessing the trait to a greater extent when the trait is primed than when it is not primed.

There are some interesting differences between ambiguous and vague input that need to be explored in future research. Vague data only contribute to the excitation level of one construct (e.g., "persistent"). Thus, even if priming one construct (e.g., "persistent") increases the accessibility of a related alternative construct (e.g., "stubborn"), the restricted applicability of the input means that the alternative construct is not competing for activation. In contrast, ambiguous input contributes to the excitation level of alternative constructs (e.g., both "persistent" and "stubborn"). Thus, if priming one construct (e.g., "persistent") increases the accessibility of the related alternative construct (e.g., "stubborn), then with ambiguous data the alternative construct competes for activation. In order for the primed construct to predominate, therefore, it may be necessary for the alternative construct to be inhibited. Thus, priming a construct may produce an increase in accessibility of the alternative construct when the subsequent input is vague, but a decrease when the subsequent input is ambiguous.

More generally, it is critical to control for the *applicability* of the primed construct to the subsequent input. This is because it is the combination of a construct's prior level of excitation and its applicability to the

input that determines the likelihood that the construct will be used in judging the input. It would be extremely rare for a construct to be used to
encode an input when the construct is unrelated to the input. The excitation level of a construct that derives from prior accessibility is usually not
sufficient to reach the threshold of activation required for its subsequent
use. Rather, the additional amount of excitation required to reach activation threshold is typically provided by the match between the features
of the input and the features of the construct (i.e., by the fact that the
construct is applicable to the input). Thus, judgments are typically both
theory-driven (i.e., the prior excitation level of the construct) and data-
driven (i.e., the additional excitation needed for activation that is provided
by the input) (Higgins & Bargh, 1987). Early support for this proposal
was provided in the Higgins et al. (1977) study. The subjects were randomly assigned to four priming conditions: applicable, positive priming
(e.g., "adventurous"); applicable, negative priming (e.g., "reckless"); nonapplicable, positive priming (e.g., "neat"); and nonapplicable, negative
priming (e.g., "disrespectful"). The constructs in the applicable conditions
were denotatively related to the stimulus description, whereas the constructs in the nonapplicable conditions were not. Only the applicable priming influenced subjects' later categorizations of the stimulus person's behaviors.

The Higgins and Chaires (1980) studies (e.g., priming "and") suggest
that it may not always be necessary for all features of the primed knowledge to be applicable to the subsequent input in order to obtain accessibility effects. If applicability does not require all of the features of the primed
knowledge and the input to overlap, then in some cases evaluative applicability might be sufficient to obtain accessibility effects when the response
is evaluative in nature. Some evidence for this possibility has recently been
provided by Martin (1986) and by Sinclair et al. (1987).

The proposal that it is the combination of prior excitation level and
applicability to input that determines the likelihood of a construct being
used in judging the input has a number of implications. First, it implies
that for the same input, increasing the prior excitation level of a construct
should increase the likelihood that the construct will be used to judge the
input. This is basically the effect of construct accessibility. As we have
seen, this effect of prior excitation level will occur as a function of construct-related goals, construct-related expectancies, recent priming, and
frequent priming (including chronic accessibility from long-term frequent
priming). Second, it implies that for the same prior excitation level of a
construct, increasing the applicability of the construct to the input should
increase the likelihood that the construct will be used to judge the input.
Applicability, in turn, can be increased by selecting a construct to prime
whose features are more similar to the input features than those of an
alternative construct, or by selecting an input whose features are more
similar to the primed construct than those of an alternative input.

Thus far, the role of applicability in knowledge activation has received little attention in the literature. If this role is to be considered more fully in future research, the concept of "applicability" needs to be further clarified. "Applicability" does not refer to the relation between the features of a construct and all of the features of an input, but rather to the relation between the construct features and those features of an input that are noticed and receive attention. This is how the parameter of salience can play an important role in knowledge activation. The term "salience" has often been used in the literature to include both the notion of attention focus and the notion of accessibility (e.g., Nisbett & Ross, 1980; Stryker, 1980; Taylor & Fiske, 1978). It is useful, however, to distinguish between variables that influence which information is attended to or focused on and variables that influence the prior excitation level of stored knowledge (see Higgins & Bargh, 1987). In the "synapse" model, the former concerns the salience parameter and the latter concerns the accessibility parameter. When these two parameters are explicitly distinguished, it is possible to consider how accessibility and salience interact to produce knowledge activation (see Sherman, 1987). Salience plays an important role in knowledge activation, because the relative applicability of alternative constructs to an input can vary, depending on which features of the input are currently most salient (e.g., Kruglanski & Ajzen, 1983; Ruble & Feldman, 1976; Trope & Ginossar, 1988; see Higgins & Bargh, 1987, for a review). Momentary contexts, for example, could vary both in the constructs that they prime and in the input features that they make salient, thus setting the stage for complex accessibility–salience interactions.[5]

In regard to salience as a parameter, it should also be noted that the priming event itself may vary in salience. Indeed, by varying the salience of the priming event, it may be possible to manipulate how "intensely" (Thomas Brown; see Heidbreder, 1933) or "vigorously" (Thorndike, 1898) stored knowledge is activated. This is an aspect of priming that has received little theoretical or empirical attention in social cognition (cf. Bargh & Pratto, 1986). Such a manipulation could both increase knowledge accessibility and increase the likelihood that the priming event would be remembered. Thus, a long-lasting effect of priming would be expected, but it could be revealed in either an assimilation effect or a contrast effect, depending on some additional applicability factors to be discussed later.

Just as the concept of applicability does not necessarily refer to all of the input features, it also does not necessarily refer to all of the construct features. Depending on a variety of context variables and the representation of the construct features themselves (e.g., centrality, prominence, or distinctiveness of stored features), some construct features may be more important than others in determining applicability (see Higgins & Chaires, 1980). For example, Herr et al. (1983) suggest that the applicability of their primed extreme-animal exemplars was greater for the animals' size features than for their ferocity features. This greater applicability produced stronger priming effects (in this case, contrast effects from apparently using the primed exemplars as reference points).

It is also important to distinguish the extent to which the features of the stored knowledge and the input overlap, which defines the applicability factor in the "synapse" model of accessibility, from the extent to which the perceiver considers the stored knowledge to be applicable to the data. The latter involves the factor of "perceived applicability." This factor can have independent effects on how information is used (e.g., Ajzen, 1977; Kruglanski, Friedland, & Farkash, 1984; Trope & Ginossar, 1988; see Higgins & Bargh, 1987, for a review). Perceived applicability concerns both the perceived *relevance* of some information for use in a current task and the perceived *appropriateness* of using it. For example, evidence that has been ruled as inadmissible by a trial judge may still be relevant, even though its use has been judged to be inappropriate. If information is perceived as either irrelevant or inappropriate, it will not be consciously used. Indeed, when information is perceived as inappropriate (e.g., intrusive, interfering, or likely to produce a biased response) it is likely to be suppressed, which could produce contrast effects (see Lombardi et al., 1987; Martin, 1986). Conversely, a manipulation that removes subjects' perception that the information is inappropriate, such as a reattribution manipulation, would be expected to yield assimilation effects.

Finally, it should be noted that applicability does not mean consistency. A primed construct whose features are denotatively inconsistent with the input features would have greater applicability to the input than a primed construct whose features are totally unrelated to the input. By being inconsistent, the former construct would necessarily share some feature dimensions and would thus be related to the input. It is true that such inconsistent constructs would not be used to characterize the input, and thus assimilation effects would not be expected. Nevertheless, because they share dimensions with the input, such inconsistent constructs could be used as reference points to judge the input, which could produce contrast effects.

Combinatory Aspects of Knowledge Accessibility

When knowledge is available, the "synapse" model proposes that the various sources of its excitation combine additively (except under certain conditions discussed earlier). As described earlier, the results of the Bargh et al. (1986) study support this proposal in the case of recent and frequent activation as sources of accessibility. More generally, the model proposes that for available knowledge, knowledge-related expectancies and goals combine additively with chronic accessibility and recent and frequent priming to increase the excitation level of the knowledge.

An intriguing hypothesis that follows from this proposal is that different combinations of sources of excitation that yield the same final level of excitation are not distinguishable. That is, analogous to misattribution and excitation transfer effects (see, e.g., Zillman, 1978), people do not know the source of their construct excitation levels. One implication of this hypothesis is that hallucinations may involve cases where the combination of a construct with very high accessibility from multiple sources (e.g., motivation, expectations, frequent activation) but very low applicability to input produces the same experience as the combination of a construct with low accessibility but very high applicability to input (see Higgins & Moretti, 1988). Even in such cases, some contribution from applicability might be necessary, but it could be so minimal that to an outside observer the response to the input would seem totally bizarre.

Another implication of this hypothesis is that recent activation could be experienced as frequent activation. Consistent with this prediction, Gabrielcik and Fazio (1984) found that subliminal priming of the letter T caused subjects to judge that the letter T occurred more frequently in the English language. It is even possible that recent or frequent activation would be experienced as increased construct-related motivation. Such a mechanism could have contributed to the effect described by Carver, Ganellen, Froming, and Chambers (1983), where subjects who had had the construct "hostility" recently primed were more likely to behave aggressively later in a different context (see also Fazio, Chen, McDonel, & Sherman, 1982; Herr, 1986; Neuberg, 1988).

In the original presentation of the "synapse" model, the momentary accessibility effects of priming are described in terms of an increase in the excitation level of a construct stored in general declarative or semantic memory. This is an unnecessarily limited application of the model, because the assumptions and implications of the basic model apply equally to any type of knowledge—procedural, episodic, or general declarative. The increase in accessibility in the case of general declarative knowledge is assumed to involve an increase in the excitation level of an already available construct. But the increase in accessibility in the case of episodic or procedural knowledge may also involve the acquisition of new knowledge, making knowledge available that was not previously available.

Even a brief review of the literature on priming suggests that priming effects can result from increasing the accessibility of procedural knowledge (e.g., Higgins & Chaires, 1980; Kolers, 1976; Smith & Branscombe, 1987), episodic knowledge (e.g., Smith, 1988), or general declarative knowledge (e.g., Bargh & Pietromonaco, 1982; Higgins et al., 1977). Indeed, there are cases where a priming manipulation can function as an active set for processing that influences subsequent judgments independently of any passive accessibility effect (e.g., Ferguson & Wells, 1980). What is perhaps most interesting is that a priming manipulation can simultaneously increase the accessibility of more than one type of knowledge. For example, a priming event can both increase the excitation level of a construct in general declarative memory and make a new instance of the priming event itself available in episodic memory (see also Smith & Branscombe, 1987). It may also be that different sources of accessibility (see Higgins & King, 1981), such as motivation versus recent activation, are likely to increase the accessibility of one type of knowledge more than another (e.g., motivation may increase procedural knowledge accessibility more than episodic knowledge accessibility). The challenge for future theories of priming and accessibility is to predict the information-processing consequences of interactions between the accessibility of different types of knowledge.

Some such interaction may have produced the priming effects found in the Lombardi et al. (1987) studies. As mentioned earlier, in one study assimilation effects of priming were found for subjects who did not recall the priming events, but contrast effects were found for subjects who did recall the events. One interpretation of these findings, discussed previously, is that the subjects who recalled the priming events used the events to form a standard that subsequently functioned as a reference point for judging the stimulus person. The recent and frequent priming events would have contributed differentially to the standard over time as a function of the same accessibility factors in episodic knowledge described for general declarative knowledge. But would not the increased accessibility of the primed constructs in general declarative knowledge have caused an opposite assimilation effect that would compete with this constrast effect? In fact, it could have. The episodic standard, however, would have been functioning actively and thus could have inhibited the passive effect of increased accessibility in general declarative knowledge (see Higgins & King, 1981; Neely, 1977; Posner, 1978; Posner & Warren, 1972).

By this reasoning, one might find that repressing the episodic standard could permit the passive effect of increased accessibility in general declarative knowledge to occur. This should produce an assimilation effect. In fact, this may have been what happened in the second Lombardi et al. (1987) study. The subjects in this study were interrupted after the priming events and were told that the trials were lost and would have to be repeated later. This procedure is likely to have motivated subjects to repress episodic knowledge, either because the priming events were unpleasant to remember or because they were perceived as inapplicable. Consistent with this reasoning, an assimilation effect was found under these conditions (cf. Martin, 1986).

This explanation for the results of these studies is clearly speculative. The main purpose in offering it, however, is to provide an example of the kind of interaction between different types of accessible knowledge that needs to be considered in future theory construction. A variety of different types of interactions are possible. When a construct is primed, the accessibility of both exemplars of the construct stored in general declarative memory (i.e., known category members) and specific instances of the construct stored in episodic memory could be increased and influence subsequent processing. This could set the stage for an interaction between general declarative knowledge and episodic knowledge. Another possibility is that procedures that are activated or made available by one task and are subsequently applied to another task could themselves involve the use of other kinds of knowledge. The procedure may be to make a judgment by using particular types of category exemplars, such as a typical or an extreme exemplar, which would reflect an interaction between procedural knowledge and general declarative knowledge. Or the procedure may be to make a judgment by using personally experienced category instances, which would reflect an interaction between procedural knowledge and episodic knowledge. Future models of knowledge accessibility and activation will need to encompass such interactions among different types of accessible knowledge.

Knowledge Accessibility from Spreading Activation

Another important source of construct accessibility has been mentioned only briefly—increased accessibility of a construct from its relations or connections to other accessible constructs (see Higgins & King, 1981). It is assumed that when a stored construct is activated, other constructs will be automatically activated to the extent that they are closely related to that construct (see Collins & Loftus, 1975). In a Stroop study by Warren (1972), for example, subjects found it more difficult to ignore the meaning of a colored target word (e.g., "tree" printed in red ink) while trying simply to name its color when they had been previously exposed to another word closely related in meaning (e.g., "elm," "oak") than when they had been exposed to a word unrelated in meaning. Apparently the meaning of the target word was activated automatically by the prior activation of the closely related word, and this increased the difficulty of ignoring the target word's meaning.

This effect of increasing the accessibility of a construct by increasing the accessibility of a related construct should not be restricted to object categories, but should hold for social constructs as well. For example, one might expect that activating the construct "fat" would automatically increase the accessibility of "jolly," given the association of these constructs in people's implicit personality theories. If activating one social construct increases the accessibility of related social constructs, one might expect that priming a trait construct would increase the accessibility of other trait constructs to which it is denotatively or connotatively related. There is some evidence that priming of a trait construct increases the likelihood of people's making subsequent judgments that are either connotatively related but denotatively unrelated to the primed construct, or denotatively related but connotatively unrelated to the primed construct (see, e.g., Bargh & Pietromonaco, 1982; Higgins et al., 1977; Sinclair et al., 1987; Srull & Wyer, 1979). In each of these studies, however, the judgments followed the encoding of the target person's behaviors, and thus it is possible that it was the initial encoding that influenced the judgments on these scales, instead of their being a direct effect of priming and spreading activation.

The critical variable determining whether priming of stored knowledge will lead to increased accessibility of related knowledge may be whether the related knowledge currently is or is not in competition with the primed knowledge. In the early 19th century, Johann Friedrich Herbart suggested that every idea has the tendency to maintain itself and to drive out ideas with which it is incompatible. Ideas already in possession of the field regularly repel uncongenial ideas, thrusting them below the threshold of consciousness (see Heidbreder, 1933). The inhibitory effect of ideas in consciousness on other competing ideas has been proposed in many theories since (e.g., Logan, 1980; Milner, 1957; Posner, 1978; Shallice, 1972). It may not be necessary for constructs to be conscious in order for them to inhibit competing constructs; constructs with higher excitation levels may automatically inhibit competing constructs with lower excitation levels. Whether priming a trait construct (e.g., "adventurous") increases or decreases the accessibility of a related trait construct (e.g., "reckless") may depend on whether the two trait constructs are in competition with each other. Perhaps, when priming is followed by a judgment task that places the constructs in competition (e.g., an ambiguous "adventurous/reckless" behavioral description), the alternative construct decreases in accessibility, but when it is followed by a judgment task that does not place the constructs in competition (e.g., an unambiguous but vague "adventurous" behavioral description), the alternative construct increases in accessibility.

This section has described how knowledge accessibility and activation in general produce subjective experiences of social stimuli. In considering the role of knowledge accessibility and activation in producing subjectivity and suffering, the particular domain of self-knowledge is especially important. The next section applies the general model of knowledge accessibility and activation to the case of self-knowledge, in order to address more directly the question raised earlier: How might unconscious processing contribute to people's vulnerability to suffering?

SUFFERING FROM AUTOMATIC ACTIVATION OF SELF-BELIEF PATTERNS

It has been frequently suggested in the literature that the different aspects of people's self-concepts are interrelated in long-term memory; that is, they constitute an integrated cognitive structure (e.g., Epstein, 1973; Kelly, 1955; Lecky, 1961; Rogers, 1951; Sarbin, 1952; Snygg & Combs, 1949; for reviews, see Greenwald & Pratkanis, 1984; Higgins & Bargh, 1987; Markus & Sentis, 1982). If this is the case, then one would expect on the basis of the spreading-activation effect that activation of one self-concept trait would increase the accessibility of other self-concept traits (as revealed in a task where the traits are not in competition). Do self-concept beliefs form such a cognitive structure?

Do Self-Concepts Form a Cognitive Structure?

Many of the consequences that have been attributed to the "fact" that self-concept beliefs form a structure do not require that self-beliefs be structurally interconnected (see Higgins & Bargh, 1987). For example, the "self-referent" effect first described by Rogers, Kuiper, and Kirker (1977)—the finding that material is more easily remembered when it is encoded with reference to self than when it is encoded with reference to some other orientation task—is consistent with self-knowledge's being a cognitive structure, but the memory advantage found does not depend on the self-descriptive traits' being interconnected in memory. The memory advantage should also occur if each self-descriptive trait is completely separate from the others but is highly familiar and emotionally significant (see Greenwald & Pratkanis, 1984), as both familiarity and emotional significance are associated with high accessibility and thus should give the traits a retrieval advantage (see Bower & Gilligan, 1979).

The fact that self-knowledge can have information-processing consequences is also not sufficient evidence for the proposal. For example, it has been demonstrated that self-knowledge is associated with quick decisions, easily retrievable evidence, confident self-prediction, and resistance to contrary evidence (e.g., Bem, 1981; Markus, 1977; Markus, Crane, Bernstein, & Siladi, 1982). But any belief to which a person is committed or in which a person has confidence should have similar properties (see, e.g., Cantril, 1932; Fazio & Zanna, 1981; Howard-Pitney, Borgida, & Omoto, 1986; Kiesler, 1971).

The question is not whether self-concept attributes reflect some kind of cognitive unit. Each attribute must have some independent connection with the self, or at least must be "tagged" as a self-concept attribute. This means that all self-concept attributes have some association with the self in common. In this sense, one might want to argue that such attributes constitute a minimal cognitive unit. But this does not imply that the self-concept attributes themselves are structurally interconnected. Wyer and Gordon (1984) make a similar distinction between a minimal cognitive unit and an organized structure when discussing representations of the attributes of target others. The critical question, then, is whether self-concept attributes are themselves interconnected.

If self-knowledge possesses the same organizational property found for object categories, then exposure to or activation of one self-concept attribute should *automatically* activate other such attributes. If this were so, then individuals' emotional responses to a performance could derive not solely from the affect associated with the performance-related trait, but also from the affect associated with the other traits in their self-structure (see Linville, 1985, for a further discussion of this possibility). Indeed, globality attributions and "overgeneralization" in depression (see Abramson & Martin, 1981; Beck, 1967) could be a consequence of such automatic, uncontrolled spreading among negative self-concept traits.

What kind of evidence would convincingly support the "self as cognitive structure" proposal? Output clustering has been used fruitfully in various social-cognitive studies for examining organization in memory (see Srull, 1984). Clustering, however, is not convincing evidence of automatic activation of one construct by another from pre-established interconnections, because it may reflect an output strategy—an effective tactic for dealing with the current retrieval task at hand—rather than reflecting pretask organization of stored knowledge (see Posner & Warren, 1972). More generally, a task is needed where the effects on performance cannot reflect a deliberate strategy for maximizing performance on the task. Better yet would be a task where maximum performance actually requires avoiding such effects. Then one could demonstrate that the pre-established interconnections influence performance *despite* the performers' active orientation to and strategies for the task.

One such task is Warren's (1972) Stroop test for memory organization of object categories described earlier. The benefit of this technique is that hypothesized effects of constructs' having pre-established interconnections, which is to increase the accessibility of the target word's meaning, is *opposite* to what is required for maximum performance on the task, which is to ignore the meaning of the target word and attend only to its color. Any impact on performance of pre-established interconnections must occur despite performers' deliberate goal to avoid the hypothesized effect of these interconnections.

This technique was used in a set of studies (Higgins, Van Hook, & Dorfman, 1988) to test the proposal that self-concept attributes form a cognitive structure. Subjects were presented with a series of slides of target words printed in different-colored inks and were asked to name the color of each word as quickly as possible. Prior to each slide, subjects were given a memory-load word that they repeated back after naming the color of the target word. The critical experimental manipulation was the relation between the memory-load word, which functioned as a prime, and the target word. In each study there were self-related target traits primed either by other self-related traits or by self-unrelated traits, and object category targets primed either by semantically related categories or by semantically unrelated categories. For both object categories and the self as a category, structural interconnectedness among category attributes themselves should produce slower response times for prime–target pairs.

In the first two studies, self-descriptive traits were defined as being high in both perceived self-applicability and perceived self-relevance (i.e., importance), and non-self-descriptive traits were defined as being low in importance and neither high nor low in self-applicability (similar to the procedure used by Markus, 1977, for identifying schematic and aschematic traits). The object category words were selected from the Battig and Montague (1969) categories.

These studies found clear evidence of structural interconnectedness for the object categories. Replicating Warren's (1972) findings, prime–target pairs involving semantically related objects (e.g., "maple–birch") produced significantly slower response times than pairs involving semantically unrelated objects (e.g., "story–potato"). In contrast, there was no significant difference in response times between prime–target pairs involving self-related traits (i.e., both prime and target were self-descriptive traits) and pairs involving self-unrelated traits (i.e., only one of the traits was self-descriptive). Indeed, in both studies the difference in response times was, if anything, slightly in the wrong direction.

The results of these studies do not support the proposal that self-concept attributes form a cognitive structure. Because it is important whether or not self-concept attributes form a cognitive structure, however, it is worth considering *when* such attributes may form a structure even if they do not always do so. In previous studies, including the two studies just described, the motivational significance of self-concept attributes has been measured by a subject's judging whether a trait on the experimenter-provided list is important to his or her overall self-evaluation. This measure may not be sufficient to tap attributes that are truly motivationally significant. Indeed, without an idiographic measure of self-concept attributes, it is possible that none of a subject's truly significant attributes even appear in the experimenter-provided list.

We have recently devised and tested an idiographic measure of self-concept that taps chronically accessible and personally significant attributes (see, e.g., Higgins, 1987, in press; Higgins, Bond, Klein, & Strauman, 1986; Strauman & Higgins, 1987). This measure, the Selves Questionnaire, first asks respondents to list spontaneously the attributes of the type of person they think they actually are (their "actual self" or self-concept). It then asks them to list the attributes of the type of person that they would ideally like to be (their "ideal/own self"), that they believe it is their duty or obligation to be (their "ought/own self"), that their mother (or father or closest friend) would ideally like them to be (their "ideal/other self"), and that their mother (or father or closest friend) believes it is their duty or obligation to be (their "ought/other self"). These four types of selves represent valued self-standards for the respondent, and are referred to as "self-guides."

After listing the attributes, respondents are asked to rate the extent to which they or the significant other (mother, father, or closest friend) believe that they actually possess or should possess an attribute or the degree to which they or the significant other would like them ideally to possess that attribute. The 4-point rating scale ranges from 1 ("slightly") to 4 ("extremely"). Using these extent ratings and semantic relatedness (as defined by Roget's Thesaurus) as criteria, coders then determine which attributes from a respondent's actual self match or mismatch the attributes listed in each of the self-guides separately.

A self-concept attribute is defined as a "match" when it is synonymous with a self-guide attribute and varies by no more than 1 scale point. It is defined as a "mismatch" when it is the antonym or opposite of an attribute in a self-guide, or is synonymous but varies by 2 or more scale points (e.g., actual/own: "slightly attractive" vs. ideal/own: "extremely attractive"). It is defined as a "nonmatch" when it is unrelated to any of the attributes in a self-guide.

Because the Selves Questionnaire asks respondents to spontaneously list the attributes of their actual self or self-concept, it is likely that those listed are chronically accessible constructs. Moreover, those self-concept attributes that are matches and mismatches are emotionally significant because they are related to the respondent's self-guides. Thus, it is possible that these attributes are structurally interconnected. It is also possible that only the self-concept mismatches, which are evaluatively inconsistent with the respondent's self-guides, would form the basis for structural interconnectedness. In discussing mental representations of target others, Wyer and Gordon (1984) suggest that the attributes most likely to form the basis of interconnectedness among attributes are those that are evaluatively inconsistent with prior expectancies for what the target is like. They suggest that each of these attributes would be problematic and that individuals would attempt to resolve the inconsistency by considering the relation among them as well as between them and the remaining attributes of the category. Applying this suggestion to the case of self-concept attributes, an individual's mismatches, each of which is problematic in relation to some self-guide, should become connected to each other and to the individual's other self-concept attributes. However, self-concept attributes that are not mismatches would not necessarily become connected to each other.

Indeed, this latter possibility could account for why our first two studies found no evidence for self-concept attributes' being interconnected. As in the previous literature, the experimenter-provided list of attributes in both studies contained mostly positive traits, which are generally not mismatching attributes. This method of obtaining self-concept attributes may have minimized the number of mismatching self-concept attributes that appeared as stimuli, thus reducing the likelihood of finding structural interconnections.

The third study, then, was designed to extend the first two studies by having self-related and self-unrelated prime–target pairs that varied in whether the self-descriptive traits were matches, mismatches, or nonmatches. The basic design was a 4×3 within-subjects design: self-relatedness of prime (match, mismatch, or nonmatch self-concept attribute; self-unrelated attribute) × self-relatedness of target (match, mismatch, or non-match self-concept attribute).

If self-concept attributes in general are structurally interconnected, then we should have found more interference (i.e., slower reaction times) when the self-related targets were primed by any other self-related attribute than when they were primed by a self-unrelated attribute. No such effect was found. In contrast, semantically related prime–target object category pairs did produce significantly slower response times than semantically unrelated pairs. Thus, replicating the results of our first two studies, this third study again found evidence of structural interconnectedness for object categories, but not for self-concept attributes *in general*.

However, a significant prime × target interaction was found that was consistent with the hypothesis that mismatch self-concept attributes form the basis for structural interconnectedness. It was hypothesized that "problematic" prime–target pairs, defined as a pair where either the prime or the target is a mismatch self-concept attribute (or both are), would be more likely to be interconnected and thus produce slower response times on the Stroop task than "nonproblematic" pairs, defined as a pair where neither the prime nor the target is a mismatch self-concept attribute. A direct comparison of these conditions revealed, as hypothesized, that the response time (in milliseconds) for problematic pairs ($M = 930$) were significantly slower than the response times for nonproblematic pairs ($M = 883$). Moreover, when the same mismatch self-concept attributes as targets were primed by self-*unrelated* attributes, slower response times were not found ($M = 865$). Thus, it was not simply the content or significance of the mismatch self-concept attributes as individual attributes that produced the self-relatedness effect for problematic pairs.

Across the three studies, then, there was no evidence for general structural interconnectedness among self-concept attributes. Given that the results of previous studies also do not require an interpretation in terms of structure, as discussed earlier, the general question of whether self-concept attributes form a cognitive structure remains open. The results of Study 3, however, suggest that a subset of such attributes may be structurally interconnected, based on connections to mismatch self-concept attributes. The proposal that problematic self-concept attributes form a basis for structure is clearly tentative, but it does seem reasonable from a psychological viewpoint.

Individuals are especially likely to pay attention to and mull over relations involving self-concept attributes that are causing them emotional discomfort or psychological difficulty. Indeed, from the perspective of control theory (see Carver & Scheier, 1981; Miller, Galanter, & Pribram, 1960; Wiener, 1948) or self-discrepancy theory (Higgins, 1987), one would expect individuals to attend to those self-concept attributes that are discrepant from personal standards or expectancies for them in order to reconcile or resolve the evaluative inconsistency. And the more attention these attributes are given, the more likely it is that they will be repeatedly and concurrently stimulated, which should lead to structural interconnectedness (Hebb, 1949; see also Wyer & Gordon, 1984).

As discussed earlier, the presence of structural interconnectedness among self-concept attributes is important, because it has implications for processing beyond the accessibility or significance of individual attributes. In particular, it implies that activation of one self-concept attribute will automatically activate other such attributes. This, in turn, means that an individual's responses to a performance may derive not solely from the attribute related to the performance, but from other attributes connected to this attribute (i.e., overgeneralization and globality). If mismatch self-concept attributes form a basis for structural interconnectedness of self-concept attributes, this should be a vulnerability factor, as people may suffer from feelings associated with self-concept attributes that are automatically activated by other performance-related attributes.

There is considerable evidence that depressed individuals generally possess more mismatches among their self-concept attributes than do nondepressed individuals (see Higgins, 1987). If mismatch self-concept attributes form a basis for structural interconnectedness, whereas match and nonmatch attributes do not, as hypothesized, then the self-concept attributes of depressed individuals should be structurally interconnected to a greater extent than those of nondepressed individuals. This hypothesis was tested in a recent study (Segal, Hood, Shaw, & Higgins, 1988). First, the self-concept attributes of depressed and nondepressed subjects were obtained. One to two weeks later, the subjects were given the Stroop task involving prime–target pairs that were either self-related or self-unrelated attributes, or that were either semantically related or semantically unrelated object categories. Consistent with the results of the studies described above, evidence of structure was found for the object category pairs, but no evidence of overall structure was found for the self-concept attribute pairs of the nondepressed individuals (who had predominantly positive self-concept attributes). As expected, however, evidence of structural interconnectedness *was* found for the self-concept attributes of the depressed individuals. The results of this study support the proposal that problematic self-concept attributes are structurally interconnected. This interconnectedness, by involving the automatic activation of problematic attributes, could be a vulnerability factor for depression—*an unconscious source of suffering.*

The results of this set of studies suggest that problematic self-concept attributes may form a basis for structural interconnections that produce automatic activation of self-concept attributes and emotional problems associated with these attributes. But what is the nature of these emotional problems? Why should self-concept attributes be a source of suffering? Indeed, is it self-concept attributes per se that produce the problem, or is it their relation to self-guide attributes as reflected in mismatches? Let us now consider these basic questions.

The key feature of our (Higgins et al., 1988) third study testing the "self-as-structure" proposal was the distinction it introduced among self-concept attributes—matches, mismatches, and nonmatches. These different types of self-concept attributes are defined in terms of their *relation to* the attributes associated with valued selves or self-guides. From this perspective, it is the relation between self-concept attributes and self-guides that is important, and not the content of self-concept attributes per se. Specifically, it is the psychological situation represented by the structural inter-relation between a self-concept attribute and a self-guide attribute that is critical in determining whether or not there is a "problem." This perspective is now presented more fully (see also Higgins, 1987, in press).

Developmental Roots of the Motivational Significance of Self-Concept Matches and Mismatches

Children between 1½ and 2 years of age become capable of representing the higher-order relation that exists between two other relations (see Case, 1985; Fischer, 1980; Piaget, 1951). As a consequence, they are able to consider the bidirectional relationship between themselves and another person (e.g., their mother) as a relation between two distinct mental objects—self-as-object and other-as-object (see Bertenthal & Fischer, 1978; Harter, 1983; Lewis & Brooks-Gunn, 1979). At this period, then, the following self–other contingency knowledge becomes available to children: "My displaying feature X is associated with response Y of person A, and response Y of person A is associated with my experiencing psychological situation Z." For example, a child can now represent the relation among his or her making a fuss or mess at mealtime; his or her mother frowning, yelling, or leaving; and his or her feeling upset. This self–other contingency knowledge is the early precursor of self-guides.

Another dramatic shift occurs between 4 and 6 years of age in children's available mental representations (see Case, 1985; Fischer, 1980; Piaget, 1932/1965). This shift is traditionally associated with the acquisition of perspective-taking ability (see Higgins, 1981; Shantz, 1983). By becoming capable of coordinating two systems of interrelationships, children can now infer the thoughts, expectations, motives, and intentions of others and evaluate their actions in terms of their relation to some internal standard. A child can now monitor, plan, and evaluate one of his or her features in terms of its relation to the type of feature that the child infers is valued or preferred by another person. The child can now understand that the relation between his or her feature X and response Y of person A is mediated by the relation between feature X and person A's standpoint on feature X. Thus, the child is now able to possess true self-guides.

But children must be motivated to acquire and utilize self-guides. The motivation depends upon the "psychological situation Z" component that is associated with the "response Y of person A" component of the self–other contingency knowledge. Caretaker–child interactions vary in the psychological situations they produce in the child. The basic difference between caretaker–child interactions that involve a positive versus a negative psychological situation for the child is that positive interactions reflect a match between a child's features and those child features valued by the caretaker (as perceived by the child), whereas negative interactions reflect a mismatch. When a match occurs, the caretaker is likely to respond to the child in a manner that places the child in a positive psychological situation (e.g., hugging, holding, reassuring), whereas when a mismatch occurs, the caretaker is likely to respond in a manner that places the child in a negative psychological situation (e.g., punishing, criticizing, withholding).

Children can experience different types of positive and different types of negative psychological situations in their interactions with their caretakers. These reflect the basic types of psychological situations associated with emotional/motivational states that have been described in the psychological literature (see, e.g., Jacobs, 1971; Lazarus, 1968; Mowrer, 1960; Roseman, 1984; Stein & Jewett, 1982). The two basic types of positive psychological situations are the presence of positive outcomes (e.g., a child's mother picking up and hugging the child) and the absence of negative outcomes (e.g., a child's mother removing the child's distress and reassuring the child), and the two basic types of negative psychological situations are the absence of positive outcomes (e.g., love withdrawal as a parental disciplinary technique) and the presence of negative outcomes (e.g., physical punishment as a parental disciplinary technique).

Self-discrepancy theory assumes that children are motivated to approach the positive psychological situations and to avoid the negative psychological situations associated with their caretakers' responses to them. To do so, children must learn to anticipate these responses and discover how their own features influence the likelihood that these responses will occur. They can best accomplish this by learning which of their own features or attributes are valued or preferred by the caretakers. In order to obtain the presence of positive outcomes or avoid the absence of positive outcomes, children attempt to learn what attributes their caretakers would ideally like them to possess, the attributes that their caretakers hope for or wish for—the "ideal self-guide." In order to avoid the presence of negative outcomes or obtain the absence of negative outcomes, children attempt to learn what attributes their caretakers believe they should or ought to possess, the attributes the caretakers believe it is the children's duty or obligation to possess—the "ought self-guide."

As a result of these developments, children acquire ideal or ought self-guides (i.e., self-guides become available). Moreover, in this way the relations between their self-concept attributes (their actual selves) and the attributes in their ideal or ought self-guides acquire motivational/emotional significance. What, then, is the motivational/emotional significance of children and adults possessing actual–ideal and actual–ought discrepancies?

Types of Self-Discrepancies and Kinds of Discomfort

Self-discrepancy theory proposes that it is the relation between and among self-state representations or self-beliefs that produce emotional/motivational vulnerabilities, rather than the content of the self-beliefs per se. In order to distinguish among different types of self-state representations, self-discrepancy theory proposes two psychological parameters—domains of the self and standpoints on the self (see Higgins, 1987, in press). For the purpose of this chapter, the key distinction is among the following three domains of the self: (1) the "actual self," which is your representation of the attributes that someone (yourself or another) believes you actually possess; (2) the "ideal self," which is your representation of someone's hopes, wishes, or aspirations for you; and (3) the "ought self," which is your representation of someone's sense of your duty, obligations, or responsibilities.

The psychological literature has historically distinguished among various facets of the self (for a review, see Higgins, 1987); however, with a few notable exceptions (e.g., James, 1890/1948), there has been little effort to relate different types of self-state representations to different kinds of emotional problems. Self-discrepancy theory proposes that relations between (or among) different types of self-state representations represent different kinds of psychological situations, which in turn are associated with different emotional/motivational states. Although the negative psychological situations are hypothesized to vary as a function of self-guide standpoint (i.e., own standpoint vs. the standpoint of one or more significant others), the two basic negative psychological situations associated with the self-concept vary as a function of self-guide domain, as follows:

1. *Actual/own self versus ideal self.* If a person possesses this discrepancy, the current state of his or her actual attributes, from the person's own standpoint, does not match the ideal self that the person wishes or hopes to attain, or that the person believes some significant other person wishes or hopes he or she would attain. This discrepancy represents the absence of positive outcomes (actual or expected). Given that this kind of negative psychological situation has been associated with sadness, disappointment, dissatisfaction, or dejection-related emotional/motivational problems more generally (see Jacobs, 1971; Lazarus, 1968; Mowrer, 1960; Roseman, 1984; Stein & Jewett, 1982), it is hypothesized that people possessing actual–ideal discrepancies are vulnerable to dejection-related problems.

2. *Actual/own self versus ought self.* If a person possesses this discrepancy, the current state of his or her attributes, from the person's own

standpoint, does not match the state that the person believes it his or her duty or obligation to attain, or believes some significant other person considers to be his or her duty or obligation to attain. Because violation of self- or other-prescribed duties or obligations is associated with self- or other-administered sanctions (i.e., punishment, criticism), this discrepancy represents the other basic kind of negative psychological situation that is associated with negative emotional/motivational states—the presence of negative outcomes (actual or expected). Given that this kind of negative psychological situation has been associated with fear, worry, tension, or agitation-related emotional/motivational problems more generally, it is hypothesized that people possessing actual–ought discrepancies are vulnerable to agitation-related problems.

My colleagues and I have found considerable support for these hypothesized associations in a series of studies. In an initial study (Higgins, Klein, & Strauman, 1985), undergraduates filled out the Selves Questionnaire and a variety of other questionnaires, such as the Beck Depression Inventory (Beck, Ward, Mendelson, Mock, & Erbaugh, 1961) and the Hopkins Symptom Checklist (Derogatis, Lipman, Rickels, Uhlenhuth, & Covi, 1974), that measure various kinds of emotional/motivational problems. Using subjects' responses to the Selves Questionnaire, we calculated the magnitude of a self-discrepancy between a subject's actual/own attributes and the attributes of one of his or her self-guides by summing the number of actual/own attributes that were mismatches with the self-guide attributes and then subtracting the number of matches (for more details about calculating the magnitude of self-discrepancies, see Higgins, 1987).

As predicted, distinct patterns of correlations were found for actual–ideal and actual–ought discrepancies. Partial correlational analyses were performed, in which the contribution of alternative self-discrepancies to the relation between a particular self-discrepancy and a symptom was statistically removed. These analyses revealed that as the magnitude of subjects' actual–ideal discrepancies increased, the intensity and frequency of their suffering from dejection-related symptoms increased (e.g., dissatisfied, lack of pride, feeling blue, feeling no interest in things), and that as the magnitude of subjects' actual–ought discrepancies increased, the intensity and frequency of their suffering from agitation-related symptoms increased (e.g., suddenly scared for no reason, heart pounding or racing, irritability, spells of terror or panic).

In subsequent studies, subjects' chronic discomfort and emotional problems were measured weeks after the subjects' self-discrepancies were measured in order to test the predictive power of self-discrepancy theory. In one study (Strauman & Higgins, 1988, Study 1), a series of factor analyses was performed on the items in the questionnaires used in the initial study (Higgins, Klein, & Strauman, 1985) in order to identify distinct clusters. Two distinct clusters were found, one reflecting a "disappointment/ dissatisfaction" emotional syndrome (e.g., disappointed in oneself; not making full use of one's potential abilities; very satisfied with oneself and one's accomplishments [reversed scoring]), and the other reflecting a "fear/restlessness" emotional syndrome (e.g., feeling afraid to go out of one's house alone; feeling one is or will be punished; feeling so restless one can't sit down). Partial correlational analyses revealed, as predicted, that as the magnitude of subjects' actual–ideal discrepancies increased (specifically, actual/own–ideal/own), their suffering from the "disappointment/dissatisfaction" syndrome increased, and that as the magnitude of subjects' actual–ought discrepancies increased (specifically, actual/own–ought/other), their suffering from the "fear/restlessness" syndrome increased.

A latent-variable analysis was used in another study (Strauman & Higgins, 1988, Study 2) to test the hypothesized relations and at the same time to evaluate the validity of the predicted constructs of mild depression and social anxiety (see Bentler, 1980). The Beck Depression Inventory and the Depression subscale of the Hopkins Symptom Checklist comprised the latent-variable measure for depression; the Interpersonal Sensitivity subscale of the Hopkins instrument, the Fear of Negative Evaluation Scale, and the Social Avoidance and Distress Scale (Watson & Friend, 1969) comprised the latent-variable measure for social anxiety.

The only model to provide an acceptable fit to the sample data $(p > .15)$ was the hypothesized causal structure—the validity of both the depression construct and the social anxiety construct, a relation between actual–ideal discrepancy (specifically, actual/own–ideal/own) and depression that was independent of a relation between actual–ought discrepancy (specifically, actual/own–ought/other) and social anxiety, and vice versa. The results of this study showed, as predicted, that as the magnitude of the subjects' actual–ideal discrepancies increased, their suffering from depression symptoms increased, and as the magnitude of the subjects' actual–ought discrepancies increased, their suffering from social anxiety symptoms increased. The results from this study and the other studies clearly indicate that actual–ideal discrepancies are uniquely associated with (and predictive of) dejection-related problems, and that actual–ought discrepancies are uniquely associated with agitation-related problems.

Self-discrepancy theory proposes that the pattern of attribute relations comprising a self-discrepancy constitutes an available cognitive structure—and not just any cognitive structure, but a cognitive structure representing a negative psychological situation that is associated with a distinctive emotional/motivational state (see Higgins, 1987, in press). Thus, the theory predicts that priming a self-discrepancy should activate the negative psychological situation it represents, thereby producing the emotional/motivational state associated with that negative psychological situation. Moreover, the theory predicts that activating any part of the self-discrepancy structure should be sufficient to activate the whole discrepancy. The next section reviews the evidence for these predictions.

Activation of Self-Discrepancies as a Source of Suffering

Self-discrepancy theory proposes that the interrelations among attributes constituting a discrepancy between the actual self and a self-guide represents, as a whole, a negative psychological situation that functions as available knowledge. As for any available knowledge, then, the likelihood that a self-discrepancy will be activated, thus producing an emotional/motivational episode, depends both on its prior level of accessibility and its applicability to a stimulus event. Thus, the theory predicts that the emotional/motivational state associated with a particular negative psychological situation is more likely to occur when an individual possesses the self-discrepancy representing that negative psychological situation (i.e., the self-discrepancy is available and therefore has a chronic accessibility greater than zero), and the individual is exposed to an event to which the negative psychological situation is applicable.

This prediction was tested in a study by Higgins et al. (1986). On the basis of their responses to the Selves Questionnaire weeks before, undergraduates whose possession of an actual–ideal discrepancy or an actual–ought discrepancy varied were selected for the experiment. In the experiment, the subjects were asked to imagine either a positive event in which performance matched a common standard (e.g., receiving a grade of A in a course) or a negative event in which performance failed to match a common standard (e.g., receiving a grade of D in a course that was necessary for obtaining an important job). According to self-discrepancy theory, the emotional/motivational state associated with the "absence of positive outcomes" psychological situation (feeling sad, discouraged, dissatisfied, slowed down) should have occurred more readily in those subjects who possessed a high magnitude of actual–ideal discrepancy and imagined a negative event, since this negative psychological situation would be both available/accessible to these subjects and applicable to the stimulus event. Similarly, the emotional/motivational state associated with the "presence of negative outcomes" psychological situation (feeling afraid, desperate, agitated) should have occurred more readily in those subjects who possessed a high magnitude of actual–ought discrepancy and imagined a negative event.

In order to measure change in emotional/motivational state, subjects' mood and writing speed were measured both before and after they engaged in imagining the positive or negative event. To measure change in mood, the contribution to subjects' postmanipulation mood from their premanipulation mood was statistically removed. To measure change in writing behavior, subjects' percentage increase in writing speed was calculated, and the contribution of subjects' premanipulation mood was again statistically removed.

The results of the study were consistent with these predictions. The partial correlational analyses on the mood "change" measures are shown in Table 3.1, where the contribution to the relation between one type of

TABLE 3.1. Partial Correlations between Types of Self-Discrepancies and Types
of Postmanipulation Mood in the Positive Event and Negative Event Conditions

| | Guided-imagery manipulation task | | | |
| | Positive event | | Negative event | |
Type of self-discrepancy	Dejection emotions	Agitation emotions	Dejection emotions	Agitation emotions
Actual–ideal	.17	.13	.39***	−.33**
Actual–ought	.05	.26*	−.04	.46***

Note. Partial correlations shown have premanipulation mood and the alternative type of self-discrepancy partialed out of each.
* $p<.10.$
** $p<.05.$
*** $p<.01.$

self-discrepancy and one kind of mood from their common association
with the other type of self-discrepancy was statistically removed. As Table
3.1 shows, increases in dejection-related mood were only associated with
magnitude of actual–ideal discrepancy and exposure to a negative stimulus
event, and increases in agitation-related mood were most strongly associated with magnitude of actual–ought discrepancy and exposure to a negative stimulus event. The same basic pattern of results was found for the
measure of writing speed (e.g., a decrease in writing speed was associated
with higher actual–ideal discrepancies and a negative stimulus event only).

If self-discrepancies are cognitive structures, then it should also be
possible to activate an entire self-discrepancy by activating only one of its
parts. Activation of a self-guide that is part of a discrepancy, for example,
should be sufficient to activate the whole discrepancy and induce its associated emotional problem. And this should occur even for people who possess more than one type of self-discrepancy. Indeed, self-discrepancy theory would predict that when people have more than one type of discrepancy
available, whichever discrepancy is more accessible should predominate.
Thus, if one discrepancy is primed and another discrepancy is not, only
the former should be activated and produce the emotional problems associated with it.

These predictions were tested in another study (Higgins et al., 1986).
Prior to the experiment, two groups of subjects were selected on the basis
of their responses to the Selves Questionnaire. One group possessed both
actual–ideal and actual–ought discrepancies, whereas the other group possessed neither type of discrepancy. In the experimental session held 4–6
weeks later, subjects were randomly assigned to describing either the kind
of person that they and their parents would ideally like them to be, the
attributes that they hoped they would have (the ideal-priming condition);
or the kind of person that they and their parents believed they ought to

TABLE 3.2.   Mean Change in Dejection-Related Emotions and Agitation-Related Emotions as a Function of Level of Self-Concept Discrepancies and Type of Priming

Self-concept discrepancies	Ideal priming		Ought priming	
	Dejection	Agitation	Dejection	Agitation
High actual–ideal and actual–ought discrepancies	3.2	−0.8	0.9	5.1
Low actual–ideal and actual–ought discrepancies	−1.2	0.9	0.3	−2.6

Note. Each emotion was measured on a 6-point scale ranging from "not at all" to "a great deal," and there were eight dejection emotions and eight agitation emotions. The more positive the number, the greater the increase in discomfort.

be, the attributes that they believed it was their duty or obligation to have (the ought-priming condition). Subjects filled out a mood questionnaire measuring dejection-related and agitation-related emotions both before and after the priming manipulation.

As shown in Table 3.2, the results of the study confirmed the predictions. When subjects had self-discrepancies available to be activated, priming increased discomfort. Moreover, the kind of discomfort suffered by these subjects depended on which type of self-discrepancy was primed—an increase in dejection-related emotions when the ideal self-guide was primed, and an increase in agitation-related emotions when the ought self-guide was primed.

The results of this study indicate that suffering can be induced by simply priming one part of a self-discrepancy. This supports the proposal that self-discrepancies are cognitive structures that can be automatically activated to produce emotional problems. It is possible, however, that such effects only occur when people are thinking about themselves in motivational terms, such as their hopes or duties. But if self-discrepancies are truly cognitive structures and, moreover, have bidirectional links between actual-self attributes and self-guide attributes, it may be sufficient to activate a single attribute in the structure to produce an emotional/motivational state. Indeed, if a mismatch between an actual-self attribute and a self-guide attribute constitutes a cognitive structure, then activating even a self-guide attribute should activate the negative psychological situation represented by the discrepancy. If so, then suffering should be produced automatically, even though the prime, the self-guide attribute, is itself a positive attribute. Moreover, it should not be necessary for the self-guide attribute to be primed in a self-relevant task. These predictions were tested in a series of studies (see Strauman, in press; Strauman & Higgins, 1987).

These studies used a covert, idiographic priming technique to activate self-guide attributes in a supposedly non-self-relevant task investigating the "psychological effects of thinking about other people." Subjects were given phrases of the form, "An X person is _____" (where X would be a trait adjective such as "friendly" or "intelligent"), and were asked to complete each sentence as quickly as possible. For each sentence, each subjects' total verbalization time and skin conductance response amplitude were recorded. Subjects' dejection-related and agitation-related emotions were also measured at the beginning and end of the session.

In the first two studies, the subjects were preselected on the basis of their responses to the Selves Questionnaire to be high in either actual–ideal discrepancy or actual–ought discrepancy. Both studies found that priming subjects' self-guide attributes produced a dejection syndrome in subjects with an actual–ideal discrepancy—a greater increase in dejection-related emotions than in agitation-related emotions, a decrease in standardized skin conductance response amplitudes, and a decrease in total verbalization time. In contrast, it produced an agitation syndrome in subjects with an actual–ought discrepancy—a greater increase in agitation-related emotions than in dejection-related emotions, an increase in standardized skin conductance response amplitudes, and an increase in total verbalization time.

In Study 1 it was also possible to examine the effect on subjects' verbalizations and response amplitudes of priming their ideal and ought self-guide attributes, regardless of whether their predominant self-discrepancy was actual–ideal or actual–ought. If discrepancies between the actual self and a self-guide are at the root of people's vulnerabilities, as self-discrepancy theory proposes, then directly activating a particular type of discrepancy should temporarily produce a specific kind of syndrome, regardless of an individual's major vulnerability. The results of Study 1 supported this prediction. Priming subjects' ideal self-guide attributes generally decreased both subjects' total verbalization times and their standardized skin conductance response amplitudes, whereas priming subjects' ought self-guide attributes generally increased both.

Thus, it is not simply that certain kinds of people are predisposed both to possess predominantly a certain type of self-discrepancy and to respond in a particular way when their self-guide attributes are activated. Together with the second study in Higgins et al. (1986), these results indicate that when people possess more than one kind of self-discrepancy, even if one of the discrepancies is greater in magnitude, their emotional/motivational response to the activation of a self-guide attribute will vary, depending on which type of self-discrepancy has been primed.

In Study 1, the priming of the ideal and ought self-guides involved both mismatching and nonmatching self-guide attributes. According to self-discrepancy theory, it is the mismatching attributes, and not the nonmatching attributes, that represent negative psychological situations. Thus, activation of mismatches, and not nonmatches, should produce discomfort. This hypothesis was tested in Study 2. Subjects were randomly assigned to one of two conditions: (1) a "mismatch" priming condition, where the trait adjectives in the incomplete phrase were attributes in a subject's self-guide, and there was a mismatch between the actual self and a self-guide for each attribute; or (2) a "nonmatch" priming condition, where the trait adjectives were attributes in a subject's self-guide, but the attributes did not appear in the subject's actual self. (There was also a "yoked" priming condition to control for the content of mismatch priming.)

As predicted, the pattern of results reported earlier—a dejection syndrome associated with actual–ideal discrepancy and an agitation syndrome associated with actual–ought discrepancy—was found only when the priming involved mismatches. The discriminant pattern across the different trials from priming ideal mismatches versus ought mismatches was quite striking for both the verbalization times and response amplitudes, as shown in Figures 3.1 and 3.2, respectively. (It was not possible to perform this analysis on the mood scores.) Two types of trials are shown in the figures—subject-related and subject-unrelated. The subject-related trials were those on which mismatch priming occurred. The subject-unrelated trials were those on which subjects received adjective traits that did not appear as responses for any subject on the Selves Questionnaire.

The third study in this series extended the previous research in a major way by studying clinical samples for the first time (Strauman, in press). Samples of clinically diagnosed depressed patients and social-phobic patients, as well as normal undergraduates, were given the Selves Questionnaire at one session and were tested in the "incomplete phase" priming paradigm a few weeks later. Self-discrepancy theory would predict that the depressed patients would possess a higher magnitude of actual–ideal discrepancy than the other samples, and that the social-phobic patients would

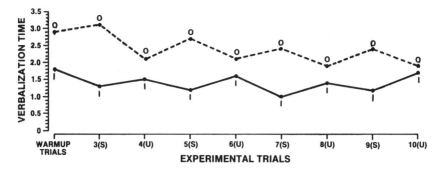

FIGURE 3.1. Verbalization time results across subject-related (S) and subject-unrelated (U) trials for priming of the ideal self-guide (I) versus the ought self-guide (O).

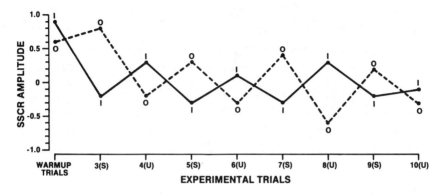

FIGURE 3.2. Standardized skin conductance response (SSCR) amplitude results across subject-related (S) and subject-unrelated (U) trials for priming of the ideal self-guide (I) versus the ought self-guide (O).

possess a higher magnitude of actual–ought discrepancy than the other samples. This prediction was confirmed.

As in Study 2, subjects in each sample were randomly assigned to either mismatch priming or nonmatch priming (or yoked priming). As in Study 1, each subject was primed with both ideal and ought self-guide attributes. There were two major findings. First, the depressed subjects, who had predominantly actual–ideal discrepancies, generally experienced an increase in the dejection syndrome (i.e., mood, verbalization, skin conductance response amplitude), whereas the social-phobic subjects, who had predominantly actual–ought discrepancies, generally experienced an increase in the agitation syndrome. Second, regardless of a subject's predominant type of self-discrepancy and clinical classification, ideal mismatch priming produced the dejection syndrome, and ought mismatch priming produced the agitation syndrome. Nonmatch priming had no effect, as predicted.

These results again provide strong support for the proposal that mismatches between the actual self and a self-guide function as a causal mediator between priming of self-guide attributes and production of discomfort. For clinical patients as well as undergraduates, exposure to a mismatch self-guide attribute, even when the attribute is positive and the focus is on others, can produce suffering automatically. Other results of this study, replicating the results of Study 1, also suggest that people who possess more of a particular type of self-discrepancy are likely to suffer more from the problem associated with that discrepancy, because there will be spreading activation among a greater number of mismatches. This automatic production of syndromes from contextual priming of self-discrepancies is another example of how the interaction between self-structures and context can be an unconscious source of suffering.

CONCLUDING COMMENTS

In this chapter, two types of self-structures have been described as potential sources of subjective experiences and suffering. First, the results of one set of studies have suggested that mismatch attributes form a basis for structural interconnectedness among self-concept attributes (Higgins et al., 1988; Segal et al., 1988). This has been described as a potential vulnerability factor, since people can suffer from feelings associated with contextually unrelated actual-self attributes that are automatically activated by another actual-self attribute that has been contextually activated (e.g., a performance-related attribute). According to the general model of knowledge accessibility and activation, the greater the structural interconnectedness among knowledge attributes, the greater the likelihood of spreading among these attributes. For self-knowledge attributes, then, this suggests that when mismatches are involved, the greater the structural interconnectedness among a person's self-concept attributes, the greater his or her vulnerability to suffering.

This proposal is consistent with Linville's theory that low "self-complexity," which in her model refers to high interrelatedness among self-aspects, is associated with greater vulnerability to suffering. In an impressive set of studies, she has found clear support for this association between interrelatedness of self-aspects and vulnerability to stress-related illness and depression (see Linville, 1985, 1987). The proposal is also consistent with Bargh and Tota's (1988) suggestion that increased structural interconnections between the self and depressed constructs, which arise from frequent activation of self-related depressed constructs during depressive episodes, may contribute to the "spiraling-down" effect in depression.

The second type of self-structure described as a potential source of vulnerability and suffering is the discrepant interrelation between actual-self attributes and self-guide attributes. Various studies have demonstrated that activation of a self-guide, or even just a self-guide attribute, is sufficient to produce suffering. It is suggested that actual-self attributes and self-discrepancies as a whole are automatically activated when self-guide attributes are primed. Following from the knowledge accessibility and activation model, when a person possesses mismatches between the actual self and a self-guide, the greater the structural interconnectedness between a person's self-concept attributes and self-guide attributes, the greater his or her vulnerability to having his or her whole self-discrepancy activated, and thus the greater his or her vulnerability to suffering.

These two sources of suffering from structural interconnectedness of self-concept and self-guide attributes have a common element: mismatches. The mismatches that form the basis of the interconnectedness among the self-concept attributes are themselves composed of the interconnections between self-concept attributes and self-guide attributes. According to this model, then, it is the mismatches that are central to vulnerability. The model proposes that two dimensions of interconnectedness constitute the overall vulnerability: horizontal expansion and vertical expansion. "Horizontal expansion" refers to the spreading activation that occurs either among self-concept attributes or among self-guide attributes when one of them is activated. The extent or breadth of horizontal expansion depends on the centrality of the initially activated attribute. Attributes involved in mismatches between the actual self and a self-guide are assumed generally to have the greatest centrality or interconnectedness, since they form the basis for it. "Vertical expansion" refers to the spreading activation that occurs between self-concept attributes and self-guide attributes. Again, attributes involved in mismatches, and to a lesser degree matches, are assumed to have the greatest vertical expansion. Vertical expansion provides depth of "meaning" or "significance" to an individually activated attribute.

Although they are conceptually distinct, horizontal and vertical expansion typically function in parallel, increasing both the breadth and depth of experience following contextual activation of an individual attribute. Indeed, it is the entire system of interconnections between the self-concept and a particular self-guide that wholistically represents the full-blown psychological situation. And it is the psychological situation as a whole, rather than its component parts, that is experienced phenomenologically. When the psychological situation is negative, this system of interconnections among self-concept and self-guide attributes constitutes an unconscious source of suffering beyond either just self-concept negativity or particular dysfunctional attitudes or irrational beliefs.

Thus from the perspective of the model offered here, the unconscious deserves once again, if not top billing, at least a major role in theories of vulnerability. The role of the unconscious in suffering proposed in this chapter is not the same as the roles described in previous theories of vulnerability. The present model differs from psychodynamic theories in that repression of unpleasant or threatening thoughts (i.e., keeping such thoughts unconscious) is not a critical parameter. And the model differs from cognitive–behavioral theories in that it is not just the automatic (i.e., unconscious) activation of *distinct* negative attitudes or beliefs that is the key vulnerability. Rather, the vulnerability arises from the unitized nature of the self-discrepancy *system*. Because of such unitization, the activation of only a single element in the system, and even a positive element, can automatically activate a pattern of self-beliefs that *as a whole* has negative psychological significance. Although people may be aware of a particular element in the self-system, they are not aware of how this element is interconnected to other elements, both vertically and horizontally, to form a psychologically significant pattern. People are also not aware of how automatic activation of a self-belief pattern from exposure to a single constituent element determines the meaning and importance of social events.

The present chapter proposes that it is this unconscious activation of *psychologically significant patterns* that is a major source of subjectivity and suffering.

ACKNOWLEDGMENTS

Support for the preparation of this chapter and for the studies herein described was provided by Grant MH39429 from the National Institute of Mental Health. I am also grateful to John Bargh, Shelly Chaiken, and Yaacov Trope for their very helpful comments and suggestions.

NOTES

1. The ideas contained in this section were first presented as part of a talk to the Ebbinghaus Empire at the Department of Psychology, University of Toronto, April 1985. I am especially grateful to Endel Tulving for the opportunity to give the talk and receive valuable comments and suggestions.

2. Herr (1986) and Herr et al. (1983) found clear contrast effects when the priming events involved extreme items (e.g., Santa Clause, Dracula) rather than moderate items (e.g., Henry Kissinger, Joe Frazier). Because of the greater novelty and distinctiveness of the extreme primes, it is more likely that they would be better remembered, and thus remain in consciousness, up until the point of judgment than the moderate primes. It is also likely that the procedure used in Martin's (1986) studies, in which contrast effects were found, led to greater subsequent awareness of the priming events by the subjects than is generally the case in priming studies (see Lombardi et al., 1987; Martin, 1986).

3. In a recent paper, Wyer and Srull (1986) have added a couple of new postulates to their original "bin" model that permit the new model to account for this crossover interaction: (1) Given that retrieval of any construct is imperfect, even the most recently activated construct will not necessarily be retrieved first; and (2) when a construct is applicable, a copy of it is used for processing, and following its use the copy is placed back in the bin. Like the "synapse" model, the "bin" model now assumes that frequent activation has processing advantages beyond simply increasing the likelihood that recent activation will have occurred. In their new model, Wyer and Srull's (1986) explanation for recency predominating after a brief delay is that the recently activated construct is more likely to be still in the work space when the categorization task occurs. If this is the case, however, one would also expect that the recently activated construct would be better remembered than the frequently activated construct after the brief delay, and that after the brief delay there would be a positive relation between recall of the recently activated construct and its use in categorization. Neither of these predictions is supported by the results of our studies (see Higgins, Bargh, & Lombardi, 1985; Lombardi et al., 1987). Indeed, recall of the primed constructs is actually associated with the use of the alternative construct (i.e., a contrast effect).

4. The definition of "accessibility" needs to be clarified at this point. In our earlier paper (Higgins & King, 1981), "construct accessibility" was defined as the readiness with which a stored construct is utilized in information processing. This is a useful operational definition, but it is somewhat misleading as a conceptual definition. According to the "synapse" model, "accessibility" refers to the excitation level of stored knowledge. The higher the excitation level of stored knowledge prior to input, the more likely it is that the excitation level of the stored knowledge will reach threshold at input (i.e., the more likely it is that it will be activated at input). However, activation of the stored knowledge at input does not mean that the stored knowledge will necessarily be used at output. A variety of factors determine the use of stored knowledge at output in addition to whether the knowledge has been activated (i.e., in addition to whether it is available in working memory). Thus, strictly speaking, "accessibility" refers to the readiness of stored knowledge to be used, rather than the readiness with which it is used. Everything else being equal, of course, the readiness with which stored knowledge is used increases as its readiness to be used increases.

5. Higgins and King (1981) may also have contributed to some confusion of terminology by proposing that one source of the accessibility of a construct may be its "salience" in memory. We only wished to suggest that the inherent and relational qualities of construct features stored in memory may contribute to the relative likelihood of one versus another construct being activated and used. The term "salience," although useful metaphorically, was an unfortunate choice, because the structural and process variables underlying such an accessibility effect would not involve focus of attention. Indeed, focus of attention would be more likely to be a consequence of such variables. This source of accessibility might be referred to as "inherent and relational features of stored constructs."

REFERENCES

Abramson, L. Y., & Martin, D. J. (1981). Depression and the causal inference process. In J. H. Harvey, W. Ickes, & R. F. Kidd (Eds.), *New directions in attribution research* (Vol. 3, pp. 117–168). Hillsdale, NJ: Erlbaum.

Ajzen, I. (1977). Intuitive theories of events and the effects of base rate information on prediction. *Journal of Personality and Social Psychology, 35,* 303–314.

Aldrich, J. H., Sullivan, J. L., & Borgida, E. (in press). Foreign affairs and issue voting in presidential elections: Are candidates "waltzing before a blind audience"? *American Political Science Review.*

Bargh, J. A. (1984). Automatic and conscious processing of social information. In R. S. Wyer, Jr., & T. K. Srull (Eds.), *Handbook of social cognition* (Vol. 3, pp. 1–43). Hillsdale, NJ: Erlbaum.

Bargh, J. A., Bond, R. N., Lombardi, W. J., & Tota, M. E. (1986). The additive nature of chronic and temporary sources of construct accessibility. *Journal of Personality and Social Psychology, 50,* 869–878.

Bargh, J. A., Lombardi, W. J., & Higgins, E. T. (1988). Automaticity of chronically accessible constructs in person × situation effects on person perception: It's just a matter of time. *Journal of Personality and Social Psychology, 55,* 599–605.

Bargh, J. A., & Pietromonaco, P. (1982). Automatic information processing and social perception: The influence of trait information presented outside of conscious awareness on impression formation. *Journal of Personality and Social Psychology, 43,* 437–449.

Bargh, J. A., & Pratto, F. (1986). Individual construct accessibility and perceptual selection. *Journal of Experimental Social Psychology, 22,* 293–311.

Bargh, J. A., & Thein, R. D. (1985). Individual construct accessibility, person memory, and the recall–judgment link: The case of information overload. *Journal of Personality and Social Psychology, 49,* 1129–1146.

Bargh, J. A., & Tota, M. E. (1988). Context-dependent automatic processing in depression: Accessibility of negative constructs with regard to self but not others. *Journal of Personality and Social Psychology, 54,* 925–939.

Battig, W. F., & Montague, W. E. (1969). Category norms for verbal items in 56 categories: A replication and extension of the Connecticut Category Norms. *Journal of Experimental Psychology Monograph, 80* (3, Pt. 2).

Beck, A. T. (1967). *Depression: Clinical, experimental, and theoretical aspects.* New York: Harper & Row.

Beck, A. T., Rush, A. J., Shaw, B. F., & Emery, G. (1979). *Cognitive therapy of depression.* New York: Guilford Press.

Beck, A. T., Ward, C. H., Mendelson, M., Mock, J., & Erbaugh, J. (1961). An inventory for measuring depression. *Archives of General Psychiatry, 4,* 561–571.

Bem, S. L. (1981). Gender schema theory: A cognitive account of sex typing. *Psychological Review, 88,* 354–364.

Bentler, P. M. (1980). Multivariate analysis with latent variables: Causal modeling. *Annual Review of Psychology, 31,* 419–456.

Bertenthal, B. I., & Fischer, K. W. (1978). Development of self-recognition in the infant. *Developmental Psychology, 14,* 44–50.

Bower, G. H., & Gilligan, S. G. (1979). Remembering information related to one's self. *Journal of Research in Personality, 13,* 420–461.

Bruner, J. S. (1957a). Going beyond the information given. In H. Gruber et al. (Eds.), *Contemporary approaches to cognition.* Cambridge, MA: Harvard University Press.

Bruner, J. S. (1957b). On perceptual readiness. *Psychological Review, 64,* 123–152.

Cantril, H. (1932). General and specific attitudes. *Psychological Monographs, 192.*

Carver, C. S., Ganellen, R. J., Froming, W. J., & Chambers, W. (1983). Modeling: An analysis in terms of category accessibility. *Journal of Experimental Social Psychology, 19,* 403–421.

Carver, C. S., & Scheier, M. F. (1981). *Attention and self-regulation: A control-theory approach to human behavior.* New York: Springer-Verlag.

Case, R. (1985). *Intellectual development: Birth to adulthood.* New York: Academic Press.

Clark, M. S., & Isen, A. M. (1982). Toward understanding the relationship between feeling states and social behavior. In A. Hastorf & A. M. Isen (Eds.), *Cognitive and social psychology* (pp. 73–108). Amsterdam: Elsevier/North-Holland.

Collins, A. M., & Loftus, E. F. (1975). A spreading-activation theory of semantic processing. *Psychological Review, 82,* 407–428.

Derogatis, L. R., Lipman, R. S., Rickels, K., Uhlenhuth, E. H., & Covi, L. (1974). The Hopkins Symptom Checklist (HSCL): A self-report symptom inventory. *Behavioral Science, 19,* 1–15.

Duncker, K. (1945). On problem solving. *Psychological Monographs, 58* (5, Whole No. 270).

Ellis, A. (1973). *Humanistic psychotherapy: The rational–emotive approach.* New York: McGraw-Hill.

Epstein, S. (1973). The self-concept revisited, or a theory of a theory. *American Psychologist, 28,* 404–416.

Erdley, C. A., & D'Agostino, P. R. (1988). Cognitive and affective components of automatic priming affects. *Journal of Personality and Social Psychology, 54,* 741–747.

Fazio, R. H. (1986). How do attitudes guide behavior? In R. M. Sorrentino & E. T. Higgins (Eds.), *Handbook of motivation and cognition: Foundations of social behavior* (pp. 204–243). New York: Guilford Press.

Fazio, R. H., Chen, J., McDonel, E. C., & Sherman, S. J. (1982). Attitude accessibility, attitude–behavior consistency, and the strength of the object–evaluation association. *Journal of Experimental Social Psychology, 18,* 339–357.

Fazio, R. H., Powell, M. C., & Herr, P. M. (1983). Toward a process model of the attitude–behavior relation: Accessing one's attitude upon mere observation of the attitude object. *Journal of Personality and Social Psychology, 44,* 723–735.

Fazio, R. H., & Zanna, M. P. (1981). Direct experience and attitude–behavior consistency. In L. Berkowitz (Ed.), *Advances in experimental social psychology* (Vol. 14, pp. 161–202). New York: Academic Press.

Fenigstein, A., & Levine, M. P. (1984). Self-attention, concept activation, and the causal self. *Journal of Experimental Social Psychology. 20,* 231–245.

Ferguson, T. J., & Wells, G. L. (1980). Priming of mediators in causal attribution. *Journal of Personality and Social Psychology, 38,* 461–470.

Fischer, K. W. (1980). A theory of cognitive development: The control and construction of hierarchies of skills. *Psychological Review, 87,* 477–531.

Freud, S. (1952). *A general introduction to psychoanalysis.* New York: Washington Square Press. (Original work published 1920)

Gabrielcik, A., & Fazio, R. H. (1984). Priming and frequency estimation: A strict test of the availability heuristic. *Personality and Social Psychology Bulletin, 10,* 85–89.

Glanzer, M. (1972). Storage mechanisms in recall. In G. H. Bower (Ed.), *The psychology of learning and motivation: Advances in research and theory* (Vol. 5). New York: Academic Press.

Greenwald, A. G., & Pratkanis, A. R. (1984). The self. In R. S. Wyer, Jr., & T. K. Srull (Eds.), *Handbook of social cognition* (Vol. 3, pp. 129–178). Hillsdale, NJ: Erlbaum.

Harter, S. (1983). Developmental perspectives on the self-system. In E. M. Hetherington (Vol. Ed.), *Handbook of child psychology (4th ed.): Vol. 4. Socialization, personality, and social development* (pp. 275–385). New York: Wiley.

Hebb, D. O. (1949). *The organization of behavior.* New York: Wiley.

Heidbreder, E. (1933). *Seven psychologies.* New York: Appleton-Century-Crofts.

Herr, P. M. (1986). Consequences of priming: Judgment and behavior. *Journal of Personality and Social Psychology, 51,* 1106–1115.

Herr, P. M., Sherman, S. J., & Fazio, R. H. (1983). On the consequences of priming: Assimilation and contrast efforts. *Journal of Experimental Social Psychology, 19*, 323–340.
Higgins, E. T. (1981). Role-taking and social judgment: Alternative developmental
   perspectives and processes. In J. H. Flavell & L. Ross (Eds.), *Social cognitive
   development: Frontiers and possible futures* (pp. 119–153). Cambridge, England: Cambridge University Press.
Higgins, E. T. (1987). Self-discrepancy: A theory relating self and affect. *Psychological Review, 94*, 319–340.
Higgins, E. T. (in press). Self-discrepancy theory: What patterns of self-beliefs cause
   people to suffer? In L. Berkowitz (Ed.), *Advances in experimental social psychology* (Vol. 20), New York: Academic Press.
Higgins, E. T., & Bargh, J. A. (1987). Social cognition and social perception. *Annual Review of Psychology, 38*, 369–425.
Higgins, E. T., Bargh, J. A., & Lombardi, W. (1985). The nature of priming effects
   on categorization. *Journal of Experimental Psychology: Learning, Memory,
   and Cognition, 11*, 59–69.
Higgins, E. T., Bond, R. N., Klein, R., & Strauman, T. (1986). Self-discrepancies
   and emotional vulnerability: How magnitude, accessibility, and type of discrepancy influence affect. *Journal of Personality and Social Psychology, 51*,
   5–15.
Higgins, E. T., & Chaires, W. M. (1980). Accessibility of interrelational constructs: Implications for stimulus encoding and creativity. *Journal of Experimental Social Psychology, 16*, 348–361.
Higgins, E. T., & King, G. (1981). Accessibility of social constructs: Information
   processing consequences of individual and contextual variability. In N. Cantor
   & J. Kihlstrom (Eds.), *Personality, cognition and social interaction* (pp. 69–
   122). Hillsdale, NJ: Erlbaum.
Higgins, E. T., King, G. A., & Mavin, G. H. (1982). Individual construct accessi-
   bility and subjective impressions and recall. *Journal of Personality and Social
   Psychology, 43*, 35–47.
Higgins, E. T., Klein, R., & Strauman, T. (1985). Self-concept discrepancy theory:
   A psychological model for distinguishing among different aspects of depres-
   sion and anxiety. *Social Cognition, 3*, 51–76.
Higgins, E. T., Klein, R., & Strauman, T. (1987). Self-discrepancies: Distinguishing
   among self-states, self-state conflicts, and emotional vulnerabilities. In K. M.
   Yardley & T. M. Honess (Eds.), *Self and identity: Psychosocial perspectives*
   (pp. 173–186). New York: Wiley.
Higgins, E. T., & Moretti, M. M. (1988). Standard utilization and the social-
   evaluative process: Vulnerability to types of aberrant beliefs. In T. F. Olt-
   manns & B. A. Maher (Eds.), *Delusional beliefs: Theoretical and empirical
   perspectives* (pp. 110–137). New York: Wiley.
Higgins, E. T., Rholes, W. S., & Jones, C. R. (1977). Category accessibility and
   impression formation. *Journal of Experimental Social Psychology, 13*, 141–
   154.
Higgins, E. T., & Stangor, C. (1988). A "change-of-standard" perspective on the
   relation among context, judgment, and memory. *Journal of Personality and
   Social Psychology, 54*, 181–192.

Higgins, E. T., Van Hook, E., & Dorfman, D. (1988). Do self attributes form a cognitive structure? *Social Cognition, 6,* 177–206.

Howard-Pitney, B., Borgida, E., & Omoto, A. M. (1986). Personal involvement: An examination of processing differences. *Social Cognition, 4,* 39–57.

Huttenlocher, J., & Higgins, E. T. (1971). Adjectives, comparatives, and syllogisms. *Psychological Review, 78,* 487–504.

Jacobs, D. (1971). Moods–emotion–affect: The nature of and manipulation of affective states with particular reference to positive affective states and emotional illness. In A. Jacobs & L. B. Sachs (Eds.), *The psychology of private events.* New York: Academic Press.

Jacoby, L. L. (1983). Remembering the data: Analyzing interactive processes in readings. *Journal of Verbal Learning and Verbal Behavior, 22,* 485–508.

Jacoby, L. L., & Kelley, C. M. (1987). Unconscious influences of memory for a prior event. *Personality and Social Psychology Bulletin, 13,* 314–336.

James W. (1948). *The principles of psychology (2 vols.).* New York: World. (Original work published 1890)

Jung, C. G. (1956). Symbols of Transformation (R. F. C. Hull, Trans.). In H. C. Read, M. Fordham, & G. Adler (Eds.), *The collected works of C. G. Jung* (Vol. 5, pp. 1–557). New York: Pantheon. (Original work published 1952; revised edition of *The Psychology of the Unconscious,* 1912).

Kelly, G. A. (1955). *The psychology of personal constructs.* New York: Morton.

Kiesler, C. A. (1971). *The psychology of commitment: Experiments linking behavior to belief.* New York: Academic Press.

King, G. A., & Sorrentino, R. M. (1988). Uncertainty orientation and the relation between individual accessible constructs and person memory. *Social Cognition, 6,* 128–149.

Kolers, P. A. (1976). Reading a year later. *Journal of Experimental Psychology: Human Learning and Memory, 2,* 554–565.

Kruglanski, A. W., & Ajzen, I. (1983). Bias and error in human judgment. *European Journal of Social Psychology, 13,* 1–44.

Kruglanski, A. W., Friedland, N., & Farkash, E. (1984). Layperson's sensitivity to statistical information: the case of high perceived applicability. *Journal of Personality and Social Psychology, 46,* 503–518.

Lau, R. R. (in press). Construct accessibility and electoral choice. *Political Behavior.*

Lazarus, A. A. (1968). Learning theory and the treatment of depression. *Behaviour Research and Therapy, 6,* 83–89.

Lecky, P. (1961). *Self-consistency: A theory of personality.* New York: Shoe String Press.

Lewis, M., & Brooks-Gunn, J. (1979). *Social cognition and the acquisition of self.* New York: Plenum.

Liebling, B. A., & Shaver, P. (1973). Evaluation, self-awareness, and task performance. *Journal of Experimental Social Psychology, 9,* 297–306.

Linville, P. W. (1985). Self-complexity and affective extremity: Don't put all of your eggs in one cognitive basket. *Social Cognition, 3,* 94–120.

Linville, P. W. (1987). Self-complexity as a cognitive buffer against stress-related illness and depression. *Journal of Personality and Social Psychology, 52,* 663–676.

Logan, G. D. (1980). Attention and automaticity in Stroop and priming tasks: Theory and data. *Cognitive Psychology, 12,* 523–553.

Lombardi, W. J., Higgins, E. T., & Bargh, J. A. (1987). The role of consciousness in priming effects on categorization. *Personality and Social Psychology Bulletin, 13,* 411–429.

Markus, H. (1977). Self-schemata and processing information about the self. *Journal of Personality and Social Psychology, 35,* 63–78.

Markus, H., Crane, M., Bernstein, S., & Siladi, M. (1982). Self-schemas and gender. *Journal of Personality and Social Psychology, 42,* 38–50.

Markus, H., & Sentis, K. (1982). The self in social information processing. In J. Suls (Ed.), *Psychological perspectives on the self* (Vol. 1, pp. 41–70). Hillsdale, NJ: Erlbaum.

Martin, L. L. (1986). Set/reset: Use and disuse of concepts in impression formation. *Journal of Personality and Social Psychology, 51,* 493–504.

Miller, G. A., Galanter, E., & Pribram, K. H. (1960). *Plans and the structure of behavior.* New York: Holt, Rinehart & Winston.

Milner, P. M. (1957). The cell assembly: Mark II. *Psychological Review, 64,* 242–252.

Mischel, W. (1973). Toward a cognitive social learning reconceptualization of personality. *Psychological Review, 80,* 252–283.

Mowrer, O. H. (1960). *Learning theory and behavior.* New York: Wiley.

Neely, J. H. (1977). Semantic priming and retrieval from lexical memory: Roles of inhibitionless spreading activation and limited-capacity attention. *Journal of Experimental Psychology: General, 106,* 226–254.

Neuberg, S. L. (1988). Behavior implications of information presented outside of conscious awareness: The effect of subliminal presentation of trait information on behavior in the Prisoner's Dilemma game. *Social Cognition, 6,* 207–230.

Nisbett, R. E., & Ross, L. D. (1980). *Human inference: Strategies and shortcomings of informal judgment* (Century Series in Psychology). Englewood Cliffs, NJ: Prentice-Hall.

Piaget, J. (1951). *Play, dreams and imitation in childhood.* New York: Norton.

Piaget, J. (1965). *The moral judgment of the child.* New York: Free Press. (Original work published in English 1932)

Posner, M. I. (1978). *Chronometric explorations of the mind.* Hillsdale, NJ: Erlbaum.

Posner, M. I., & Warren, R. E. (1972). Traces, concepts, and conscious constructions. In A. W. Melton & E. Martin (Eds.), *Coding processes in human memory.* Washington, DC: V. H. Winston.

Postman, L., & Brown, D. R. (1952). The perceptual consequences of success and failure. *Journal of Abnormal and Social Psychology, 47,* 213–221.

Proshansky, H., & Murphy, G. (1942). The effects of reward and punishment on perception. *Journal of Psychology, 13,* 295–305.

Rholes, W. S., & Pryor, J. B. (1982). Cognitive accessibility and causal attributions. *Personality and Social Psychology Bulletin, 8,* 719–727.

Rogers, C. (1951). *Client-centered therapy: Its current practice, implications, and theory.* Boston: Houghton Mifflin.

Rogers, T. B. (1977). Self-reference in memory: Recognition of personality items. *Journal of Research in Personality, 11,* 295–305.

Rogers, T. B., Kuiper, N. A., & Kirker, W. S. (1977). Self-reference and the encoding of personal information. *Journal of Personality and Social Psychology, 35,* 677–688.

Roseman, I. J. (1984). Cognitive determinants of emotion: A structural theory. *Review of Personality and Social Psychology, 5,* 11–36.

Ruble, D. N., & Feldman, N. S. (1976). Order of consensus, distinctiveness, and consistency information and causal attributions. *Journal of Personality and Social Psychology, 34,* 930–937.

Salancik, G. R., & Conway, M. (1975). Attitude inferences from salient and relevant cognitive content about behavior. *Journal of Personality and Social Psychology, 32,* 829–840.

Sarbin, T. R. (1952). A preface to a psychological analysis of the self. *Psychological Review, 59,* 11–22.

Sarbin, T. R., Taft, R., & Bailey, D. E. (1960). *Clinical inference and cognitive theory.* New York: Holt, Rinehart & Winston.

Scheier, M. F., & Carver, C. S. (1983). Two sides of the self: One for you and one for me. In J. Suls & A. G. Greenwald (Eds.), *Psychological perspectives on the self.* Hillsdale, NJ: Erlbaum.

Schwarz, N., & Clore, G. L. (1987). How do I feel about it? The informative function of affective states. In K. Fiedler & J. Forgas (Eds.), *Affect, cognition and social behavior* (pp. 44–62). Toronto: C. J. Hogrefe.

Segal, Z. V., Hood, J. E., Shaw, B. F., & Higgins, E. T. (1988). A structural analysis of the self-schema construct in major depression. *Cognitive Therapy and Research, 12,* 471–485.

Shallice, T. (1972). Dual functions of consciousness. *Psychological Review, 79,* 383–393.

Shantz, C. U. (1983). Social cognition. In J. H. Flavell & E. M. Markman (Vol. Eds.), *Handbook of child psychology* (4th ed.): *Vol. 3. Cognitive development* (pp. 495–555). New York: Wiley.

Sherman, S. J. (1987). Cognitive processes in the formation, change, and expression of attitudes. In M. P. Zanna, J. M. Olson, & C. P. Herman (Eds.), *Social influence: The Ontario Symposium* (Vol. 5, pp. 75–106). Hillsdale, NJ: Erlbaum.

Shiffrin, R. M., & Schneider, W. (1977). Controlled and automatic human information processing: II. Perceptual learning, automatic attending, and a general theory. *Psychological Review, 84,* 127–190.

Sinclair, R. C., Mark, M. M., & Shotland, R. L. (1987). Construct accessibility and generalizability across response categories. *Personality and Social Psychology Bulletin, 13,* 239–252.

Smith, E. R. (1988). Category accessibility effects in a simulated exemplar-based memory. *Journal of Experimental Social Psychology, 24,* 448–463.

Smith, E. R., & Branscombe, N. R. (1987). Procedurally mediated social inferences: The case of category accessibility affects. *Journal of Experimental Social Psychology, 23,* 361–382.

Smith, E. R., Branscombe, N. R., & Borman, C. (1988). Generality of the affects of practice on social judgment tasks. *Journal of Personality and Social Psychology, 54,* 385–395.

Snygg, D., & Combs, A. W. (1949). *Individual behavior.* New York: Harper & Row.

Srull, T. K. (1984). Methodological techniques for the study of person memory and social cognition. In R. S. Wyer, Jr., & T. K. Srull (Eds.), *Handbook of social cognition* (Vol. 2, pp. 1–72). Hillsdale, NJ: Erlbaum.

Srull, T. K., & Wyer, R. S., Jr. (1979). The role of category accessibility in the interpretation of information about persons: Some determinants and implications. *Journal of Personality and Social Psychology, 37,* 1660–1672.

Srull, T. K., & Wyer, R. S., Jr. (1980). Category accessibility and social perception: Some implications for the study of person memory and interpersonal judgments. *Journal of Personality and Social Psychology, 38,* 841–856.

Stein, N. L., & Jewett, J. L. (1982). A conceptual analysis of the meaning of negative emotions: Implications for a theory of development. In C. E. Izard (Ed.), *Measuring emotions in infants and children* (pp. 401–443). New York: Cambridge University Press.

Strack, F., Schwarz, N., Bless, H., Kubler, A., & Wanke, M. (1988). *Remembering the priming events: Episodic cues may determine assimilation vs. contrast effects.* Unpublished manuscript, University of Mannheim.

Strack, F., Schwarz, N., & Gschneidinger, E. (1985). Happiness and reminiscing: The role of time perspective, affect, and mode of thinking. *Journal of Personality and Social Psychology, 49,* 1460–1469.

Strauman, T. J. (in press). Self-discrepancies in clinical depression and social phobia: Cognitive structures that underlie affective disorders? *Journal of Abnormal Psychology.*

Strauman, T., & Higgins, E. T. (1987). Automatic activation of self-discrepancies and emotional syndromes: When cognitive structures influence affect. *Journal of Personality and Social Psychology, 53,* 1004–1014.

Strauman, T. J., & Higgins, E. T. (1988). Self-discrepancies as predictors of vulnerability to distinct syndromes of chronic emotional distress. *Journal of Personality, 56,* 685–707.

Stryker, S. (1980). *Symbolic interactionism.* Mendo Park, CA: Benjamin/Cummings.

Tagiuri, R. (1969). Person perception. In G. Lindzey & E. Aronson (Eds.), *Handbook of social psychology* (2nd ed., Vol. 3, pp. 395–449). Reading, MA: Addison-Wesley.

Tajfel, H. (1969). Social and cultural factors in perception. In G. Lindzey & E. Aronson (Eds.), *Handbook of social psychology* (2nd ed., Vol. 3). Reading, MA: Addison–Wesley.

Taylor, S. E., & Fiske, S. T. (1978). Salience, attention, and attribution: Top of the head phenomena. In L. Berkowitz (Ed.), *Advances in experimental social psychology* (Vol. 11, pp. 249–288). New York: Academic Press.

Thorndike, E. L. (1898). Animal intelligence: An experimental study of the associative processes in animals. *Psychological Review, 5,* Monograph Supplement, 2, No. 8).

Trope, Y., & Ginossar, Z. (1988). On the use of statistical and nonstatistical knowledge: A problem-solving approach. In D. Bar-Tal & A. W. Kruglanski (Eds.), *The social psychology of knowledge* (pp. 209–230). New York: Cambridge University Press.

Tulving, E., Schacter, D. L., & Stark, H. A. (1982). Priming effects in word-fragment completion are independent of recognition memory. *Journal of Experimental Psychology: Learning, Memory, and Cognition, 8,* 336–342.

Warren, R. E. (1972). Stimulus encoding and memory. *Journal of Experimental Psychology, 94,* 90–100.

Watson, D., & Friend, R. (1969). Measurement of social-evaluative anxiety. *Journal of Consulting and Clinical Psychology, 33,* 448–457.

Wertheimer, M. (1923). Untersuchunger zur Lehre von der Gestalt: II. *Psychologische Forschung, 4,* 301–350.

Wiener, N. (1948). *Cybernetics: Control and communication in the animal and the machine.* Cambridge, MA: MIT Press.

Wyer, R. S., Jr., & Gordon, S. E. (1984). The cognitive representation of social information. In R. S. Wyer, Jr., & T. K. Srull (Eds.), *Handbook of social cognition* (Vol. 2, pp. 73–150). Hillsdale, NJ: Erlbaum.

Wyer, R. S., Jr., & Srull, T. K. (1980). The processing of social stimulus information: A conceptual integration. In R. Hastie, E. B. Ebbesen, T. M. Ostrom, R. S. Wyer, D. L. Hamilton, & D. E. Carlston (Eds.), *Person memory: The cognitive basis of social perception* (pp. 227–300). Hillsdale, NJ: Erlbaum.

Wyer, R. S., Jr., & Srull, T. K. (1981). Category accessibility: Some theoretical and empirical issues concerning the processing of social stimulus information. In E. T. Higgins, C. P. Herman, & M. P. Zanna (Eds.), *Social cognition: The Ontario Symposium* (Vol. 1, pp. 161–197). Hillsdale, NJ: Erlbaum.

Wyer, R. S., Jr., & Srull, T. K. (1986). Human cognition in its social context. *Psychological Review, 93,* 322–359.

Zillmann, D. (1978). Attribution and misattribution of excitatory reactions. In J. H. Harvey, W. J. Ickes, & R. F. Kidd (Eds.), *New directions in attribution research* (Vol. 2, pp. 335–368). Hillsdale, NJ: Erlbaum.

4

Affect and Automaticity

ALICE M. ISEN
Cornell University

GREGORY ANDRADE DIAMOND
University of Michigan

This chapter addresses some aspects of the intersection between two lines of psychological inquiry: the study of affect and of automatic cognitive processing. In recent years there has been a growing interest in both of these topics. Although affect has been a topic of general interest from time to time in the past, most experimental work on the topic has been undertaken more recently. Similarly, the concept of automaticity, while rooted in early discussions of volition, traces its modern introduction to the mid-1970s (e.g., Posner & Snyder, 1975a; Schneider & Shiffrin, 1977; Shiffrin & Schneider, 1977). This chapter focuses on aspects of these two lines of recent investigation, in the hope that consideration of the two topics together will help us to learn more about both affective and cognitive processes.

The concept of automaticity has been useful in cognitive psychology for understanding two kinds of phenomena: (1) cognitive processing that seems to occur without awareness and without effort, as, for example, when people drive the usual route to work in the morning without attending to each turn or realizing that they are making the movements that allow them to arrive at their destinations; and (2) cognitive processing that captures attention—seemingly irresistibly—even while one is doing something else, as, for example when a person hears a knock on the door while reading, or hears his or her name in a nearby conversation even though participating in a different conversation (Moray, 1959). The phenomena to which the concept has been applied can involve either perceptual or meaning-based processes and, some authors believe, both innate and learned responses (Glass, Holyoak, & Santa, 1979; but see Lachman, Lachman, & Butterfield, 1979; Schneider & Shiffrin, 1977; and Shiffrin & Schneider, 1977, for the view that most if not all of these processes involve familiarity and "overlearning").[1] In this chapter, we explore the implications that research on automaticity may have for our understanding of affect, and the implications that research on affect may have for theories of automaticity.

The role of affect in automatic processing, and the extent to which affect is processed automatically, have only begun to receive explicit attention within the topic of automaticity. There is now a fast-growing literature on automaticity applied to social judgment, categorization, and other cognitive processes underlying social phenomena—as attested to by the presence of this volume. To the extent that such judgments or categorizations involve evaluation or attitude, they may be considered to involve affect, at least in part.

There are at least two ways in which to conceptualize affect. Affect may be viewed as a quality—valence—assigned to a stimulus. For example, stimuli can be rated with regard to their degree of goodness or badness, attractiveness or unattractiveness, pleasantness or unpleasantness (Osgood, Suci, & Tannenbaum, 1957). Research on automaticity and affect from this perspective might examine how attitudes are formed, as in the research on effects of "mere exposure" (Zajonc, 1968), or might examine how they gain access to consciousness, as in the work of Fazio, Sanbonmatsu, Powell, and Kardes (1986) on attitude accessibility. One might also examine whether the objects of different kinds of attitudes— strong or weak, positive or negative—are affected differentially by automatic processing. Affect may also be viewed as a feeling state that people experience, such as happiness or sadness.[2] Research on automaticity and feeling states might address how automatically such states come into being, how automatically they influence cognitive processing, whether they increase or decrease the ability to process information attentively, and whether the qualitative character of feeling states affects how they interact with automatic processes.

Most existing research relevant to affect and automaticity has focused on valences. Perhaps this is because valences, like size, color, and other characteristics of stimuli, lend themselves more readily to being processed as features than do feeling states, which characterize a person's subjective experience as a whole. Some researchers have explicitly adopted the language of automaticity in their research. Some of the questions they have investigated include whether valences are activated (come to mind) automatically upon the presentation of stimulus objects (e.g., Fazio et al., 1986), and whether affective stimuli are visually processed automatically (e.g., Hansen & Hansen, 1988). Other recent research, while not explicitly using the language of automaticity, may nevertheless be relevant, addressing such topics as some factors that contribute to the perception of valence information about objects (Zajonc, 1968), how valence information is perceived (Zajonc, 1980), or whether valence information may sometimes be blocked from consciousness (as in the "New Look" research; see Erdelyi, 1974, 1985). The processes studied in this research, though not specifically discussed as automatic, may seem to be automatic because they appear to occur without effort or intention.[3]

While there is a great deal of research on such topics that indirectly addresses the intersection of affect and automaticity—in fact, too much to be included in this review—work explicitly investigating the automatic processing of affect, or affect's influence on the operation of automatic processes, is less extensive. Later, we briefly discuss some of this work that deals directly with automaticity and valence, and then we discuss the intersection of automaticity and feeling states. First, however, we need to consider the concept of automaticity in a bit more detail.

DEFINING AUTOMATIC PROCESSING

Let us start with a brief discussion of the ways in which automatic processing is understood and might be understood. Several authors in this volume have provided comprehensive summaries and analyses of the ways in which automatic processes can be defined and distinguished from attentive or controlled processes in useful ways. We only briefly refer to those definitions and analyses here, in order to set the stage for offering some possible extensions or alternative conceptualizations of the phenomena as they interact with affect.

For example, the term "automatic" implies that the processing or response to a stimulus requires neither attention nor effort and therefore does not consume cognitive capacity, which is thought to be limited. Because automatic processes do not take up limited processing capacity, it is said that they can be handled in parallel with other cognitive processing that does require capacity. The ability to deal with material in this way is known as "parallel processing," and it is contrasted with "serial processing," in which material can only be processed after other capacity-consuming activity is put aside. Thus, material that is processed automatically may be processed more rapidly and earlier than other material. In the usual definition of automaticity, an automatic response cannot be blocked from occurring whenever the stimuli eliciting it are present—reminiscent of a "reflex"—and thus it is described as "irresistible." However, an alternative view is that what accounts for this sense of primacy or irresistibility is that the material is processed in parallel with another task, which results in its being processed sooner. Moreover, once such a stimulus is identified, it may seem to interrupt other activity and take primacy. Another way of looking at this phenomenon is that, once identified, this overlearned, familiar material is more interesting or seems more important to the person, with the result that she switches attention to it from the task on which she was previously working. Thus, the automatically processed material may appear to have interrupted the other task and taken primacy (but only part of that sequence of events, the identification of the familiar stimulus, may actually have been automatic). In one sense, the entire process may be seen as irresistible and automatic, but automaticity theorists are now beginning to emphasize that automatic and attentive processes may occur together to produce various phenomena (e.g., Shiffrin, 1988).

This way of viewing the process, then, can account for what might otherwise seem a contradiction—the fact that automatically processed material is thought to be handled without taking capacity, yet is also said to demand attention. Although it is true that people may change their focus of attention to the newly noticed stimulus situation after an automatic process has occurred, this may result from a different process subsequent to the automatic one by which the familiar item was noticed. Moreover, such a shift in attention may not always happen, but rather may depend on the goals, requirements, and plans of the person in the particular situation. The point is that the *process* by which a familiar stimulus is noticed at the same time that attention is directed elsewhere is automatic (requires no cognitive capacity). But what happens subsequently (the change of focus) may be another matter. If one takes this view, however, it remains to be seen whether certain aspects of the customary definition of automatic processing, such as irresistibility, can be maintained. However, the sense of irresistibility may result from other aspects of the process (e.g., parallel processing and choices based on interestingness).

The view of cognitive processes as irresistible or completely dependent on the stimuli presented, and not subject to active participation by the person, is compatible with a particular historical view of mental functioning. More recent conceptualizations of cognition, tending to be more complex, allow for an active role of the person in interpreting stimuli and constructing cognitions rather than simply receiving them (see, e.g., Jenkins, 1974; Neisser, 1967, 1976). It may be that both types of processes can occur, but that the latter is more typical of how people think, with the former reserved for a limited set of stimuli (say, very simple or very familiar ones) or circumstances (say, ones in which capacity is limited or in which the person is not interested in expending capacity on the task).

If this is true, then even if affect (or some other stimulus) were processed automatically, it might not mean that such stimuli were truly irresistible because of their nature and would always *have to be* processed in that way. Rather, when stimuli are processed automatically, it may be a result of their nature in combination with the other demands of the situation and the person's goals, plans, strategies, and perhaps even prior decisions to allow that kind of processing to occur, or "set."[4] A question of interest might then become "Under what conditions are particular stimuli or, say, particular affective experiences likely to be processed automatically?"

As noted, cognitive functions that are "automatic" are sometimes depicted as "data-driven" or "bottom-up" (i.e., based entirely on the stimuli presented, with little or no active cognitive mediation required or possible), and consequent behavior is seen as largely under the control of environmental factors and as involuntary. This aspect of the definition appears to be open to revision, however, as experiments increasingly are showing that meaning and interpretation do play a role in cognitive processing that otherwise fits the definition of "automatic," and that automatic responses can be interrupted or modified. For example, Johnston and Heinz (1978) found that familiar passages were more difficult to ignore than unfamiliar ones in a shadowing task. This is often interpreted as showing that the meaning of the automatically processed material played a role in the process. Similarly, Treisman (1964) found that people noticed that an unattended message had the same meaning as the attended message, and that bilingual subjects noticed that the two messages were the same even when they were presented in two different languages (and therefore were perceptually distinct). Thus, the meaning of the unattended (automatically processed) message had been identified by subjects, and it would be difficult to argue that interpretation or inference of meaning did not occur in this "automatic" process. It should be noted that some automaticity theorists might disagree with our stating here that meaning necessarily involved interpretation and was a constructive inferential process.[5]

Another example of the treatment of meaning in the automaticity literature is available in the "Stroop effect," the name given to the finding that the time to name the color of ink in which a word is printed is lengthened if the word itself names a different color (Stroop, 1935). This finding has traditionally been taken to show that word meaning is processed automatically and is difficult to resist. However, more recent work indicates that response competition, rather than impaired identification of the ink color, may be more responsible for this effect (e.g., Egeth, Blecker, & Kamlet, 1969; Flowers & Stoup, 1977; Hock & Egeth, 1970). Moreover, recent studies suggest that it is the subject's *intent* to name colors that is responsible for this effect, by priming color-name responses, because neutral words produce less interference than color words, and the requirement of emitting other kinds of words as well as color names also produces interference with ink-color naming (Shiffrin, 1988). That is, in a study in which subjects had to give digit names as well as color names, the printed names of the digits interfered with naming the color of the ink in which they were printed as much as did the printed names of colors (Neumann, 1984; cited in Shiffrin, 1988). This means that the subject's goal or intent played a role in the process; but intention surely cannot be automatic.

Shiffrin (1988) suggests, consequently, that it may not be that the entire process involved in phenomena thought to be automatic (such as the Stroop effect) is actually automatic; but that tasks may be accomplished by mixtures of both automatic and attentive processes. This idea is similar to that suggested above in describing how automatically processed material may appear to interrupt ongoing tasks and "take precedence."

Similarly, in a study of the facilitating and interfering effects of high-probability and low-probability primes (i.e., primes that were usually correct and those that were usually incorrect, respectively), Posner and Snyder (1975b) found evidence that both automatic and attentive processes can be involved in the effects of primes. Those authors found that both high-probability and low-probability primes facilitated responding when they were correct, but that only high-probability primes interfered with correct responding when they were incorrect; low-probability incorrect primes could be ignored and did *not* interfere with correct responding. This suggests that interference due to an incorrect prime involves the allocation of attention to that material (and thus is not necessarily automatic), that it is this allocation of attention that causes interference on account of an incorrect prime, and that people can ignore primes that they do not think are useful. Finally, regarding whether automatic processing can be interrupted compatibly with such results, most authors today accept the notion that the influence of automatic processing can be modified, either directly or indirectly (Bargh, Chapter 1, this volume; Logan, Chapter 2, this volume; Shiffrin, 1988).

Other aspects of the usual definition of automatic processes include their being unintentional and outside of awareness. These qualities, too, are difficult to confirm, since work in cognitive psychology has pointed out that studies purporting to establish lack of awareness typically study recall, but inability to recall does not necessarily mean that the stimulus did not enter consciousness briefly, only to be lost because of inadequate encoding or other factors associated with recall. Moreover, recent work has emphasized that phenomena that are automatic often were once conscious and intentionally learned, as, for example, the route to work or even grammar (e.g., Carlson & Dulaney, 1985).

Similar problems arise with the criteria of intentionality and volition. It has been suggested that we cannot allow our subjective awareness of *making* various decisions to lead us to conclude that these decisions are therefore intentional and not automatic. Such self-perceptions may be post facto reconstructions. As Nisbett and Wilson (1977) have reported, people are willing to endorse plausible explanations for their behavior that are objectively incorrect. But this argument works both ways. If introspection is not good evidence for the *active* nature of responses, it is no more valid evidence for their *automatic* nature. Psychologists since James (1890) have realized that the failure to remember consciously making a decision is not good evidence that a decision was not consciously made; people may forget that they have done so.

Several authors now make the important point that it may not be necessary to view automaticity as unitary, requiring or implying *all* of these properties simultaneously, nor to view the automatic–controlled distinction as dichotomous and exhaustive of the alternative modes of processing information that exist. Most reviews now conclude with the notion that not all of the defining criteria that have been used (see Shiffrin & Dumais, 1981, for discussion of 13 possible identifying characteristics) need be considered necessary characteristics for a process to be automatic (e.g., Bargh, Chapter 1, this volume; Shiffrin, 1988; Uleman, Chapter 14, this volume); and many authors now also suggest that the distinction between automatic and attentive processing may not always be a complete or qualitative one. Uleman, for example, has proposed something like a continuum between automatic and controlled processing, suggesting intermediate types of processes that might be called "spontaneous" or "ruminative." Logan (1985) discusses the gradual, continuous development of automaticity in the acquisition of skills. Shiffrin (1988) has introduced the concept of "partial automaticity" and has further noted that in practice automatic and controlled processes usually occur together as a person is trying to accomplish a task, and that therefore it is often difficult to identify automatic processes with certainty. More generally, too, the idea that automaticity depends upon familiarity with the stimulus material and overlearning (very thorough learning) underscores its continuity with other cognitive processes.

As the concept is modified in these ways, however, it will be increasingly important to keep in mind the changed nature of the implications that will follow from a process being identified as "automatic." Authors will need to keep sight of the utility of the concept and its limitations. No longer will material processed automatically be seen as necessarily irresistible or as taking precedence under all circumstances, for example. Rather, emphasis may begin to focus on automaticity as nondeployment of attention, and crucial questions on the topic will center on identifying the circumstances and factors that promote or impair the tendency to process in that way, and the consequences that follow from inattention under different circumstances or with different kinds of material.

Consequently, rather than attempting to select among the defining features to identify crucial ones, the approach that we take in this chapter is to try to understand what is added by the concept of automaticity, what phenomena it helps to illuminate, some of the models or processes that have been proposed for understanding this kind of functioning, what implications this information may have for understanding affect and affect's influence on cognition, and how findings in the affect literature reflect on some of these models and interpretations. Thus, we ask how cognitive psychology has understood and used the concept of automaticity and how this concept relates to basic cognitive processes and models.

AUTOMATICITY IN COGNITIVE PSYCHOLOGY

Given the state of affairs described above, in which the concept of automaticity appears somewhat vague and difficult to define, readers may wonder about the utility of the concept at all. It is important to note, therefore, that despite the problems that have arisen in defining and identifying automatic processes exclusively, many authors (e.g., Shiffrin, 1988) have noted that the concept has been found useful and necessary in all theories of attention (primarily to understand the two kinds of phenomena described at the beginning of this chapter—phenomena in which processing occurs without specific deployment of attention to the task).

Some authors (e.g., see Glass et al., 1979) propose two different kinds of automatic processes, one perceptual and one meaning-based. The former, they suggest, is innate; the latter attributable to overlearning or great familiarity with the stimulus materials. An example of a perceptual automatic phenomenon is apparent in the illustration given earlier of responding to a knock at the door while one is trying to read. Another is what has been called the "pop-out" effect, in which a stimulus from one category embedded in an array of stimuli from another category (e.g., a circle among squares) is effortlessly noticed and seems to "pop out" at the perceiver (e.g., Treisman & Souther, 1985). Schneider and Shiffrin (1977) have reported that for such displays response time is independent of set size, thus confirming the true effortlessness of the process. Examples of automaticity due to overlearning or familiarity include the exercise of well-learned skills such as driving a car or typing; the ability to go to a familiar destination without being aware of executing all of the steps involved; and the ease with which one notices one's name (or some other especially familiar stimulus) in an overheard conversation.

Other authors, however, go further and attribute even apparently perceptual phenomena such as the "pop-out" effect to overlearning and great familarity with the stimulus categories (Schneider & Shiffrin, 1977; Shiffrin, 1988; Shiffrin & Schneider, 1977). Thus, automaticity need not be regarded as a mysterious process, but rather seems to be related to familiarity and overlearning. Overlearning, in turn, seems capable of accounting for both aspects of automatic processing—its ease of processing, and its irresistibility or seeming ability sometimes to capture attention in the midst of other ongoing processing.

As noted earlier, some of the effects attributed to automatic processing may actually result from an influence of the automatic process on *subsequent* cognitive processing. For example, it has been suggested that the sense that the automatic process or stimulus "captures attention" and interrupts may actually result sometimes from a change in focus of attention to the newly noticed stimulus situation after an automatic process has occurred. The findings of Posner and Snyder (1975b), described above, reporting on debilitating effects of incorrect primes as well as facilitating effects of correct primes, suggest still another way in which automaticity may affect subsequent cognitive processing and by which these effects may be limited. Recall that those findings indicated that a high-probability prime (i.e., one that was usually correct) that happened to be incorrect in a given case impaired correct responding in that case, but that a low-probability prime (one that was usually incorrect) that happened to be incorrect in a particular case had no adverse effect. The usual interpretation of this result that has been made is that people can decide to ignore a low-probability prime, and thus it need not interfere with their performance (e.g., Klatsky, 1980). The interference that was observed to result from the incorrect high-probability prime is consequently attributed to subjects' decisions or strategies to rely on the high-probability prime and to allocate attention to it. Thus, although the impaired performance involves an automatic process of priming in some sense, the interference itself actually results from allocation of attention to the usually beneficial stimulus. One question that this raises is whether this allocation of attention results from a decision or strategy regarding the best way to proceed in a particular instance, or whether such decisions might themselves become automatic (overlearned) under some circumstances. However, the main point is that the observed interference results from allocation of attention, not from the mere presence of a prime or the operation of an automatic priming process.

By this point, we can see that strict definitions of automaticity, which posit automatic processing as a kind of cognitive reflex occurring inescapably in the presence of a set of stimuli, may be difficult to maintain. Voluntary allocations of attention can play some role in seemingly "automatic" processing (Posner & Snyder, 1975b), and "automatic" processing of stimulus meanings does appear possible (Johnston & Heinz, 1978; Treisman, 1964). The weakening of the strict formulation of theories of automaticity—by accepting that it may not be a unitary construct, and by suggesting a continuum of automaticity rather than a firm dichotomy—works toward accommodating these findings. But, as the definition of automaticity stretches, it becomes important to keep in mind the more limited ways in which the concept can be applied.

Moreover, it is not clear that the construct of automaticity *can* (or should) be stretched sufficiently to encompass the findings on the automatic processing of meaning. As noted earlier, automaticity theories can accommodate the processing of rudimentary forms of meaning, involving increasing familiarity with stimulus conditions whereby increasingly subtle distinctions among stimulus patterns can be discerned with practice (and thus take on meaning in the sense of being recognizeable). But some phenomena cannot be accounted for in this way, and there has been some suggestion that cognitively mediated stimulus meanings, as well, can be processed automatically—that is, extracted from stimuli effortlessly and without requiring cognitive capacity, although this has not yet been demonstrated. Logically the proposition that cognitively mediated meanings can be processed automatically may blur the distinction between automatic and attentive processing so greatly, and therefore may restrict the uniqueness and the utility of the concept of automaticity so much, that it may actually undermine the concept of automaticity, even as modified. Thus, in order to preserve a useful meaning for the concept of automaticity, it may be preferable to suggest that the apparently automatic apprehension of meaning does not truly qualify as automatic, at least pending evidence regarding whether cognitive capacity is required for such processing.

This distinction has relevance for the application of the construct of automaticity to affect, because as we discuss below, an important influence of affect on memory seems to be mediated through meaning, rather than via affect's simple stimulus features (which would seem to be more amenable to automatic processing). This distinction has important implications for the ways in which affect can be expected to influence memory, for example, and therefore seems a useful distinction to maintain, at least for the present time.

APPLYING THEORIES OF AUTOMATICITY TO AFFECT

We have mentioned that automatic processes and the behavior to which they lead are thought to be under the control of external stimuli. The question being discussed then was whether cognitive mediation was involved. But another question also arises in this context, and that is whether internal sources of stimulation can also function "automatically" or lead to automatic processing. We all know from experience that it is also possible for internal factors such as pain or hunger (and possibly, as we shall discuss, affective states) to come to mind involuntarily and without apparent effort. Such processes are generally considered "feeling" rather than "thinking" in the cognitive literature, however, and on that basis are usually excluded from treatment as automatic cognitive processes (e.g., Glass et al., 1979, p. 187). In this chapter, however, we are trying to see what can be learned from thinking about feelings as having characteristics and effects similar to those of stimuli that are processed automatically, or as influencing the cognitive system in the way that automatic cognitive processes do. Thus, we focus now on automaticity in the affective domain.

In recent years there has been much research investigating the cognitive effects of feelings; these efforts have suggested not only that certain parallels exist in the cognitive and feeling domains, but also that our understanding of both areas may be enhanced by consideration of them in the context of one another. Isen and Hastorf (1982), for example, point out that our understanding of affect can be increased by knowledge of its cognitive impact. At the same time, however, the understanding of cognition is enhanced if models of cognition include those situations, topics, and events about which people frequently think—affective ones.

Automatic processing may seem especially applicable to affect, because much affective experience seems to resemble the two types of phenomena mentioned above as requiring the concept of automaticity in order to be understood: Feelings often seem to occur without a specific effort to achieve them or without awareness of the process (like driving to work), and they seem irresistible. In fact, several lines of research suggest that affect can sometimes have qualities that make it seem like a product of automatic processing.

Considering affect as valence, as already noted, a few authors have suggested that social judgments, inferences about people, and other components of attitudes or contributors to feelings about people can become automated or can function like automatic processes (e.g., Smith & Lerner, 1986). To the extent that such demonstrations involve affect—some do and some do not—these data are relevant to the topic of affect and automaticity.

Although there is a great deal of research on affect as valence that indirectly addresses the intersection of affect and automaticity, as we have already noted, work explicitly investigating affect and automaticity is less extensive. Two recent papers, those by Fazio et al. (1986) and by Hansen and Hansen (1988), set out specifically to address the automaticity of the processing of affective stimuli. Both present findings consistent with theories of automaticity, but in each case it is not clear that the findings demonstrate that the processing of valences is necessarily automatic.

Fazio and colleagues, using a priming paradigm in which subjects were asked to judge the "goodness" or "badness" of stimuli, found that presenting subjects with strongly valenced nouns facilitated (speeded up) their judgments that the succeeding adjective was of the same valence, but inhibited (slowed down) judgments that those adjectives were of the opposite valence. The authors interpret their results as indicating that strongly held attitudes are automatically activated, and they conclude, "[Strongly valenced] attitudes can indeed be activated from memory automatically upon observation of the attitude object. Such activation appears to be spontaneous and inescapable" (Fazio et al., 1986, p. 236).

Although it may be true that the process involved was an automatic one, this is not entirely clear from the study presented, because the procedure employed may have prompted subjects to look for valence information in the priming stimuli as well as in the stimuli about which they were to make judgments. If so, then an attentional process, instead of or in addition to an automatic one, may have contributed to the effect observed. That is, the procedure involved asking subjects to judge and report the "goodness" or "badness" of the adjective presented, and this task may have focused subjects' attention on the affective aspects of the nouns (attitude objects) with which they were presented at the beginning of the following trial. Fazio et al.'s assumption is that the affective value of the presented noun activated (automatically) the attitude; however (as was described in conjunction with work on the Stroop effect, above), it may have been the task requirement of making an affective judgment, which is a nonautomatic process, that brought valence to mind or caused subjects to attend to valence, and influenced subsequent reaction time to similarly or differently valenced words. Consequently, while it remains possible that the process by which affect was activated was automatic, it also seems possible that the effects observed were actually dependent, at least in part, on such attentional processes. It may also be that not just affect, but any aspect of the stimuli made salient or primed by the task, would appear to be automatically activated under those conditions. In order to demonstrate that a process is automatic, it would seem necessary to show that it occurs even under circumstances where attentional processes do not also potentially contribute to the effects.

Similarly, results reported by Hansen and Hansen (1988), using the "pop-out" visual detection paradigm, do not unambiguously demonstrate the automatic perception of affect. Those authors attempted to examine whether happy and angry faces were automatically identified in arrays of dissimilar faces. They found that angry faces could be identified in an array of happy faces more quickly than happy faces could be identified in an array of angry faces. Furthermore, they reported that the time required to detect happy faces increased with the number of distractors present in the array, whereas the time required to detect angry faces was not affected by this factor. (Imperviousness of response time to number of distractors may be the clearest indicator of automaticity; see Shiffrin, 1988.) These results thus suggest that angry faces are processed in parallel (i.e., automatically), while happy faces are processed serially, and that angry faces are thus perceived automatically.

Hansen and Hansen suggest a number of possible interpretations for this effect, including the possibility that subjects automatically perceived the valence of the stimuli without needing to infer the emotion it represented from the features. (Other possible interpretations suggested include that subjects may focus on one critical feature distinguishing happy from angry faces, such as the angle of the brow; and that emotional faces themselves may form coherent perceptual elements.) However, this conclusion is not clearly established by the experiment presented, because in this study a set of perceptual features distinguished the affectively discrepant element from the others in the array. Thus, since perceptual features could distinguish the target element from the distractors, it is possible that subjects responded (automatically) to perception of those, not to valence per se.[6] In contrast, in order to establish that valence itself was automatically perceived, the stimuli would have to be such that only valence distinguished the target pictures from the others and that no perceptual feature varied systematically with valence. This could be done if liked and disliked examples of some class were presented with multiple exemplars so that no set of perceptual features varied systematically with affect.

Thus, these two lines of investigation suggest creative, sophisticated, and promising ways of studying automaticity and affect. However, at the present time their results appear to fall short of establishing unambiguously that affect is activated or perceived automatically.

Turning to experienced affect's possible automatic influence on cognition, there are some findings suggesting that the process is not primarily automatic. Recent work on the influence of affect on cognition indicates that positive affect can have an impact on cognitive processes involved in memory, decision making, categorization, and problem solving (see Isen, 1987, for review). One important example is available in the literature on the influence of affect on memory. Let us begin with a brief review of this area.

Positive affect at time of attempted recall has been found to serve as an effective retrieval cue for positive material in memory (e.g., Isen, Shalker, Clark, & Karp, 1978; Nasby & Yando, 1982; Teasdale & Fogarty, 1979; Teasdale & Russell, 1983). That is, people who are feeling happy show better recall of positive material than of other kinds of material, and also show better recall of such material than do people in whom positive affect has not been induced. This suggests that a pleasant feeling state can cue material stored in memory as relevant to that state; this in turn suggests that the pleasantness or affect associated with things or ideas is a feature that can be (and often is) used in encoding or remembering them. The results suggest that affect is used as an encoding cue, because the encoding-specificity principle (Tulving & Thomson, 1973) holds that cues are effective in facilitating recall at retrieval only if they were used by the person as a means of encoding the material when it was learned. This encoding theoretically may or may not be automatic, but Tulving (e.g., 1979) emphasizes the importance of the meaning of material to subjects in the context of their plans and strategies, in the process of encoding, under most circumstances (i.e., the non-automatic nature of encoding most of the time).

It should also be noted that in examining the impact of affect on memory, many studies report asymmetrical results of positive and negative affect (see Isen, 1985, 1987, for discussion). That is, whereas positive affect has been found to be an effective retrieval cue for positive material in memory, negative affect such as sadness has frequently been seen to be relatively ineffective, or less effective, in cuing sadness-related material from memory (e.g., Bartlett, Burleson, & Santrock, 1982; Bartlett & Santrock, 1979; Isen et al., 1978; Nasby & Yando, 1982; Natale & Hantas, 1982; Riskind, 1983; Snyder & White, 1982; Teasdale & Fogarty, 1979; Teasdale, Taylor, & Fogarty, 1980). This asymmetry also seems compatible with the suggestion that the impact of affect on cognition is not generally automatic (at least not in the most simple sense of the term), but rather is more complexly mediated or developed.

Some studies have reported that a positive feeling state at time of encoding (learning of material) results in improved recall of positive material, when memory is tested later and the subject is in a neutral affective state (e.g., Bower, Gilligan, & Montiero, 1981; Nasby & Yando, 1982). Some authors note symmetrical effects of happiness and sadness (Bower et al., 1981), but again others report the asymmetry described above (Nasby

& Yando, 1982). This, too, suggests that feelings are used by people in encoding material and therefore influence what is later recalled. Again, the encoding process itself logically could be either strategic and effortful, influenced by meaning and interpretation, or automatic.

What does this mean for the automaticity of affective influence, then? Both of these effects involve the encoding, storage, and/or cuing of affective material on the basis of the content or meaning of the material to the person. That is, material in memory seems to be stored and accessible in terms of its affective meaning to the person. Since the meaning of the material is involved, the process would not appear to be automatic. As we have seen, however, some researchers suggest that seemingly automatic phenomena sometimes do involve a rudimentary sort of meaning. Therefore, although the asymmetry effect is compatible with a nonautomatic effect of feelings on memory, another set of affect-and-memory findings— those on affect as a cue in state-dependent learning—may be more convincing regarding the automatic influence of affect on memory.

State-dependent learning is a phenomenon in which people (or animals) show better recall of material learned and recalled under the same stimulus conditions than they do of material recalled under conditions that are different from those present at time of learning. This is thought to be due to a simple context effect, by which nonconceptual elements of the context or stimulus situation (e.g., color of the walls or temperature of the air) are automatically attached to the to-be-learned material and therefore can serve as a memory aid if they are present when recall is attempted. This effect does not involve meaning, in that the effect is independent of the semantic meaning of the stimuli or way in which the stimuli are thought about. In the state-dependent learning paradigm, recall is assessed as a function of the match between conditions present at time of learning and recall, independent of the meaning of the material learned, and thus the nature or meaning of the material is irrelevant to performance.

In looking at the effectiveness of affect as a cue in state-dependent learning, then, one looks at the ability of a feeling state to cue material— any material, regardless of its affective tone or meaning—that was learned when the person was in that same feeling state earlier. Thus, any effect would be due purely to a match between "stimulus" conditions (affective state viewed only as a surrounding stimulus condition) at time of learning and recall. Consequently, this may be a particularly good way to assess an automatic effect of feelings, because meaning and the cognitive processes associated with dealing with meaningful material are minimally involved in this paradigm.

Interestingly in this context, studies on affect as a state-dependent phenomenon suggest that affect independent of the meaning of the material learned does not have strong and reliable effects on memory. At first, some authors thought that affect might function in this way (e.g., Bower, Montiero, & Gilligan, 1978; Bower et al., 1981), as a simple context cue, as might be predicted by associationistic theories such as spreading activation. Others, however, failed to observe such effects from the first (e.g., Isen et al., 1978; Laird, Wagener, Halal, & Szegda, 1982; Nasby & Yando, 1982); more recently, there have been repeated failures to obtain these effects, even among researchers who previously had considered them robust (e.g., Bower & Mayer, 1985; see also Isen, 1984, 1987, for discussion). The failure of this effect frequently to hold, especially in view of the robust meaning-based effects that feelings have been found to have on memory, suggests that perhaps the strongest effect of feelings is not an automatic one (at least not "automatic" in the most fundamental sense of the term—as a function of exposure alone and without regard to meaning or cognitive mediation), but rather a more complex one.

This does not mean that affect cannot ever have such automatic or stimulus-like, state-dependent learning effects under any circumstances. Indeed, a few studies have occasionally reported such effects as a function of affect (more often of positive affect than of negative). It has been suggested that people usually use meaning as a way to encode and recall memories (e.g., Tulving & Thomson, 1973), but that other avenues for learning may be used under conditions most conducive to them: for example, where material is meaningless; where other demands on attention or meaningful memory are great; or where the stimulus (non-meaning-based) cue is especially strong, focal, or for some other reason easy to use (see Eich & Birnbaum, 1982; Isen, 1984, 1987, for discussion).

Thus, one might expect affect-based state-dependent learning under a relatively limited range of conditions, and more cognitively mediated, meaning-based effects of feelings generally, just as has been found true for automatic and attentive cognitive processing more broadly. Similarly, as has been seen with nonaffective material, there may be different degrees of automaticity, and automatic and attentive effects of feelings may occur together to produce overall effects. Consequently, if affect has automatic effects, they most likely will need to be understood in the same ways that other automatic cognitive effects are being explored. Moreover, people's views of their significance, the implications that follow from them, and their utility will have to be modified in those same ways.

Overlearning, Affect, and Automaticity

Thus, again, it appears appropriate to consider automatic processing as cognitive psychology has considered it, even when discussing automatic effects involving feelings. We therefore return to the more general point that in cognitive psychology most automaticity is considered the result of overlearning or repeated exposure (great familiarity). The possible exception that is offered is of a few peripheral perceptual mechanisms, such as perception of contour, that are thought to be probably innate or acquired shortly after birth without much learning (e.g., Shiffrin, 1988). One point we wish to explore is the idea that affect, in most instances in which it operates seemingly automatically, like cognitions found to operate automatically, may also involve overlearning and very familiar material.[7] It seems reasonable to suggest this for feelings—at least some feelings or some feelings in some situations—because some of our earliest and some of our most common and constant experiences are affective. (There may even be a parallel to the distinction between perceptual and cognitive or meaning-based phenomena that has sometimes been drawn in the cognitive area, in that it may be possible to think of situations such as pain or possibly hunger as perceptual, and more complex feelings or other affects as more cognitively mediated or meaning-based. However, as in the cognitive area, this distinction may be relative and ultimately hard to maintain.) Thus, the same kind of process that makes cognitive material appear to operate automatically, or without effort and irresistibly, may be responsible for the sense that we sometimes have that feelings take no effort to be felt and are irresistible: Perhaps this occurs when they involve very common, well-learned basic complexes of stimuli, anticipated effects, responses, and outcomes.

This way of understanding automatic influences of affect, then, may also enable us to suggest ways of understanding when affects will be experienced and have their effects automatically, effortlessly, and seemingly irresistibly, and when, in contrast, they and their effects will be more meaning-based, or will even be figured out or inferred, as some theories describe (e.g., Schachter & Singer, 1962; Weiner, 1985). This analysis would suggest that more frequent, familiar feelings, especially in familiar situations or contexts, would tend to seem more spontaneous and in fact might show characteristics of automaticity, but that less familiar feelings, or feelings in unfamiliar situations or contexts, might take more effort or require conscious attention in order to occur and exert influence.

The question of how much experience is needed to turn an unfamiliar feeling into a familiar one, of course, remains to be determined—it may take only a few exposures—but the same question remains for all automatic processing. That is, the degree of familiarity, or the number of exposures necessary, for something to become automatic is not known. However, it should be noted that this may be a way in which affective stimuli or events may yet differ from other kinds of stimuli. That is, feelings or affective events, compared with nonaffective cognitive material, may require fewer—or more—occasions of experience in order to acquire the capacity to be processed automatically.

Further, individual affects may differ among themselves in this regard (and these differences may differ for individuals). For example, generally, positive affect may be found to become automatic more easily than nonaffective material, whereas sadness may take more exposure. And this may be true for most individuals but not for all (e.g., based on biochemical factors or perhaps frequency of affective experiences of various kinds).

Chunking

Another kind of process that may contribute to automatization, especially of the type involving performance of well-learned tasks such as driving the route to work (described at the beginning of the chapter), is something akin to "chunking." Chunking has been explicitly related to the concept of automaticity, in part because it relates to cognitive capacity and is a means by which cognitive capacity appears to be increased (or not diminished by tasks). The chunking of material in a memory task, for example, involves the organization of the items that are to be recalled into larger units, so that a large number of items becomes more manageable or can be dealt with more efficiently.

Miller (1956), in his classic article on cognitive capacity (capacity limits in short-term memory), called attention to the fact that the upper limit in performance on memory-span tasks is about the same, regardless of the size of the units being recalled (e.g., words vs. letters). To illustrate, the digit string 149217761812 may be too long to recall; however, if recoded into the three familiar dates, 1492, 1776, and 1812, it will be quite a bit more manageable. Thus, Miller's paper suggested that recoding information into chunks (individual items learned and stored as a group) may help people overcome capacity limits, and that information stored in larger units may consequently seem to require less capacity.

Thus, material that is chunked will take less capacity and may therefore seem to be processed "automatically." This may be the means by which complex behavior sequences such as driving to work come to be regarded as automatic: Their components may be chunked into larger units. Some cognitive psychologists (e.g., Anderson, 1983) suggest chunking as the mechanism for that process and relate it to hierarchical organization. Gleitman (1988), for example, points out that when a process is chunked and the substeps have become automatic, a higher-level decision to carry out the task calls forth all of the substeps, without each one being recalled, considered, and decided upon separately. He relates this process to skill development and to the functioning of experts, both of which are generally discussed under the topic of automatic processing. There may be a rote component to this process in some cases, but there is also a grouping of the steps into a larger unit that then unfolds with the decision to perform the action. Anderson (1983) relates the process to compilation of what are called "production rules" or cognitive operations that are similar to covert stimulus–response links.

Some have suggested that this process involves simple "chaining" of stimulus–response sequences, but others disagree with the behavioristic interpretation of these events as resulting from such chains of the stimulus–response bonds making up the components of the action. They argue instead for the creation of a hierarchical structure as described above, pointing out that in some skilled actions such as piano playing, the speed of the actions is too fast for individual messages to be going from fingers to brain and brain to fingers, as would be required if the substeps were merely "chained" to one another. Thus, the bonds must not be individual any longer (Lashley, 1951, as cited in Gleitman, 1988). In this view, a learned program results in a change in the size (or nature) of the units themselves and allows the successive movements to occur without interpolated monitoring. This kind of automatization is essential to expert performance of any kind—in reading, in scientific reasoning—because the learner must come to do in one stroke what at first required many, in order to be free to solve new problems.

It is possible to see this process as distinct from rote repetition, and therefore possibly to consider automaticity based on chunking as different from that based on repetition. Both kinds may exist. (This would account for errors that *are* based on rote repetition, such as beginning the well-learned trip to work when one comes to the first turn, even on a day when one is actually headed somewhere else.) It remains to be seen whether this distinction will be useful.

Nonetheless, it is also apparent that even such a process of chunking is one that is related to overlearning and requires familiarity with the material or event. It should be noted, though, as pointed out by Smith and Lerner's (1986) experiments, that an important component in the phenomena under discussion may be process rather than content—that automatization of a complex process requires repetition of the process (repeated exposure to or familiarity with a given process), not necessarily rote repetition of or experience with the very same content or material.

However, even if simple and complex stimuli share the same basic mechanism, this analysis alerts us to the fact that we might expect automatization not only of very simple stimuli, but also of very complex stimuli. Thus, there may yet be some distinctions to be observed within those processes that are automatic.

Positive Affect and Cognitive Organization

The foregoing discussion of automaticity via chunking relates to recent research showing that positive affect facilitates the very kinds of processes of seeing relationships among ideas that may allow creation of larger units. Thus, positive affect may be involved in promoting chunking or processes similar to chunking.

In a program of research on a related topic, Isen and her students have reported results compatible with the suggestion that positive affect may promote chunking or integration of material. Several studies have shown that under conditions of positive affect people relate ideas to one another more broadly and flexibly, sometimes solving problems more efficiently in that way. For example, Isen, Johnson, Mertz, and Robinson (1985) found that people in whom positive affect had been induced gave a broader range of first associates to neutral stimulus words than did control subjects. This suggests that the pool of associates to a given item is broader under conditions of positive affect. In another series of studies, Isen, Daubman, and Nowicki (1987) showed that people in a positive-affect condition, compared with control subjects, used more remote associates to solve a problem considered reflective of creativity and performed better on a task generally thought to require ingenuity. This too suggests that, under conditions of positive affect, material not usually related to a given set of items is brought into juxtaposition with those items and the task. In addition, Isen and Daubman (1984) found that people in whom positive affect had been induced tended to categorize more stimuli together, using either a rating task or a sorting task. In these studies, fringe exemplars of categories (e.g., "elevator" in the category "vehicle") were given higher ratings as members of the category in a goodness-of-exemplar task like that used by Rosch (1975). That is, items were characterized as more closely related to categories to which, under neutral conditions, they are seen as only remotely related.

All of these effects indicate greater flexibility in thinking about material and a tendency to see ways of grouping ideas together. Since chunking involves a change in categorization, classification, or grouping of material, the process facilitated by positive affect may relate to chunking. In fact, Smith and Lerner (1986) have suggested that the process of treating an ambiguous stimulus as a member of a given category may be mediated by increased efficiency of procedures for classifying stimuli, as a function of automatization. It may be, then, that this effect of positive feelings is also related to the kind of automatization that we have been discussing.

Smith and Lerner (1986) discuss the importance of this kind of phenomenon for social judgment processes. In this context, recent results extending the earlier work on affect and categorization to categorization of types of people are of interest (Isen, Niedenthal, & Cantor, 1988). In one study it was found, similarly, that people in whom positive affect had been induced rated weak exemplars of positive categories of people to be more like members of those categories (e.g., "bartender" as an example of the category "nurturant people"). That is, people in the positive-affect condition were more able to see ways in which categories of people (e.g., bartenders) could be seen as fitting into positive superordinate categories (e.g., "nurturant people"). This process may be important for processes of social categorization and judgment, in that people who are feeling happy may include in positive categories groups of people not typically included in those categories. It should be noted that the effect held only for positive categories, but not for negative; for example, "genius" was not seen as a better example of the category "unstable people" by positive-affect subjects. This suggests that the effect was not attributable to simple response bias or across-the-board changes in inclusion or judgment criteria. It also suggests that the effect of positive feelings is to broaden the social categorization process in the positive direction but not as readily in the negative; this has important implications for the social effects involved.

In another series of studies, Isen and colleagues found that people in whom positive affect had been induced tended more than controls to use heuristics in problem solving (Isen, Means, Patrick, & Nowicki, 1982) and to use a simplified, efficient strategy in decision making (Isen & Means, 1983). In regard to these studies, it should be noted that in one case the process of simplification resulted in improved performance (Isen & Means, 1983), but in another it resulted in impaired performance (Isen et al., 1982). This is not unlike the situation that has been observed for automatic processing: It allows freedom to think about other things, but it can lead to errors. It seems plausible, thus, that positive affect itself may promote these aspects of automatic processing, but much work on this remains to be done.

Consequences of Viewing Automatic Effects of Affect as Stemming from Overlearning (Familiarity)

Now let us consider what may be gained from attributing effects of feelings that appear to be automatic to a process such as overlearning. First, adopting the same approach as has been taken in cognitive psychology suggests several ways to determine whether affect actually operates automatically, taking no capacity (attention). For example, techniques investigating whether set size influences reaction time would be prompted by such an approach. Second, viewing automatic effects involving feelings as resulting from overlearning or great familiarity with those feelings lays out some limits on the effects that may be expected in most situations. Third, it provides some guideposts for understanding when affect may operate automatically and what kinds of feeling states may do so. When the effects of affect are understood in this way, one does not have to maintain that feelings in general are (or are not) generated automatically, are maintained automatically, and/or have effects automatically; rather, one is led to inquire about the circumstances under which affect takes capacity versus when it occurs and/or has effects automatically, or promotes automatic processing.

For example, this analysis suggests that a person's most typically experienced feeling state may more readily be felt in parallel with ongoing cognitive activity and without necessarily disrupting that activity (although disruption is possible, as discussed earlier, depending on the circumstances). Less common affects may have to be processed more attentively. Further, this proposal is compatible with results discussed above, suggesting that positive affect, in contrast with negative feeling states, may tend to influence the cognitive system more readily (e.g., see Isen, 1985, 1987,

and in press, for discussion of the asymmetry between positive and negative affect in effects on memory and cognitive organization) and to be
more likely to become automatized more readily.

This analysis, conceptualizing automatic affect as reflecting an overlearned process involving affect, would also suggest that, even if some feelings seem to arise or have effects automatically now, they may have been
learned and thus may be amenable to unlearning and change. One could
start with the idea that automatic affect would be like any other overlearned process—like any habit—and that the same things that make habits useful or efficient or difficult to change would apply to common affective reactions. This would not reduce all affective experience to the status
of habits, just as all thoughts or cognitive processes would not be equivalent to the common ones that can operate automatically, without attention. There would still be room for noble, sublime, and subtle feelings and
for complex constructive feelings, just as there is room in the cognitive
area for complex, effortful thoughts. But it would suggest that to the extent that affect can have an influence automatically—without attention or
intention and seemingly irresistibly—it can be understood as a deeply ingrained, overlearned habit, or as a process of chunking and organizing the
situation. Thus, such seemingly irresistible feelings might be addressed in
much the same way that other overlearned processes are understood, or in
the way that other broad constructs or conceptualizations are refined (differentiated or "unpacked").

We are reminded of the way in which little boys have often been
taught to keep from crying by substituting anger for sadness: "When
something bad happens, don't get sad; get mad." Thus, people may be
able to regulate their feelings, through their focus and through changing
what they learn in given situations. Similarly, they may be able to change
the impact of certain kinds of feelings, again by directing thoughts along
certain lines. In this way, problem emotions, even though they feel automatic and uncontrollable, may be alterable. This does not mean that unwanted affective reactions will be easy to change (old habits die hard), but
it does suggest that change may be possible and that the very sense of
inevitability may be misleading.

This analysis also points out that because we find that affect can have
an automatic impact, this does not mean that affect *must* always have
automatic effects, or that it is in the *nature* of affect to be automatic. Not
only may affects differ in this regard, but also the requirements of situations may influence whether stimuli are processed automatically, or whether
automatic processes have effects or not. For example, some affects may
tend more than others to be automatic. For most people, positive affect is
probably a frequent, overlearned event, and thus happiness may generally
tend more than other affects to be automatic. But there also may be individual differences in this regard. People who have a lot of experience with
positive affect may find that positive feelings can be induced or perceived
and influence their thought processes without effort and without inter-

rupting ongoing cognitive tasks; by contrast, those who are less accustomed to happy feelings may find it harder to generate good feelings or may have to work at doing so more effortfully. In contrast, people who are especially well practiced at feeling anger may find anger an easily induced companion. As has been suggested elsewhere (Isen, 1985), depressed persons may have greater cognitive facility with sad thoughts than with other thoughts, relative to other people, and they may also tend to have more facility in inducing sad mood apparently effortlessly and irresistibly. Likewise, any of these possibilities may interact with situations and their particular cognitive and affective requirements, goals, possibilities, cues, associated ideas, and so forth.

In fact, as we have seen from our discussion of chunking, it may be that demands of the situation play an important role in whether at least that type of automatic process occurs. That is, in complex or demanding situations, people may be more inclined to chunk (automate) processing, either because of the special need to use capacity efficiently or because the rich context affords opportunities to see connections among stimuli and group them.

This suggests some interesting and complex implications for the interaction between types of affect and demandingness of the context in promoting automatic responding. For example, the foregoing analysis suggests that for most people, positive affect, being more familiar and overlearned, should be more readily processed automatically—it should influence thought and behavior more readily than other states, and should do so without apparent effort and seemingly irresistibly. However, negative affect situations, being less familiar, should be more demanding of attention and cognitive capacity. At first it might seem that this very complexity and drain on capacity might encourage automatization of cognitive processes in the situation. We do seem to see something like this, with people appearing not to think through the situation as well and appearing to rely on more "automatic" processing when demands are great and cognitive capacity is overwhelmed. This may also be related to the principle that arousal facilitates the dominant response, "arousal" being related in this instance to overload of the cognitive system.

Another way of thinking about the situation, however, is to realize that automatization cannot always occur just because it would be nice to be able to process automatically. In the situation described above, a person may decide not to deploy attention to a task because the demands of another task are too great, but the neglected task may not be sufficiently familiar to be processed automatically. Thus, there may be complex situations that drain capacity but that do not involve automatization of responding, because the conditions necessary for automaticity are not present. If that view is taken, then the kinds of behavior and cognitive processing that are observed when people's cognitive capacity is overloaded would be seen simply as the results of the overload and insufficient capacity to perform the task, not of automatization.

However, it is still possible that automatic processes can be triggered in complex situations by the use of strategies that enable them. In this circumstance, we would expect that since there is little basis for chunking or automatization, yet great need for such processing, negative-affect situations might call forth reliance on well-learned rules that are not specifically related to negative affect, but that yet might make processing seem automatic in those situations. However, it might be possible to distinguish these two types of "automatic" processes, or it might be that the latter process is not automatic at all. For example, recall the study described earlier by Posner and Snyder (1975b), in which it was found that high-probability primes interfered with performance when they were incorrect but that low-probability primes did not. It was proposed that this effect was due to subjects' reliance on high-probability primes (possibly attributable to a decision to rely on them). It may be that in cognitively complex, demanding situations, people are more likely to adopt such processing strategies that lower the cognitive load and give rise to effects that appear automatic. This would be in keeping with the idea discussed above, that performance often involves mixtures of automatic and attentive processing. Whether or not such processing differs from other processing that seems automatic remains to be investigated. This means that a productive line of research might be found in investigating the circumstances under which affect or the various specific affective states have automatic effects and the kinds of changes that make this less or more possible.

MODELS OF COGNITION AND AFFECT

We have come to the suggestion that automaticity might be understood as processing without attention, especially on the basis of overlearning or great familiarity with the material to be processed, and possibly also chunking or grouping of this material. There is another sense in which the term "automatic" is often used, not so much technically and explicitly in current cognitive psychology as tacitly and by connotation among people. As mentioned at the beginning of this chapter, the idea of processes that are "automatic" conjures up the idea of something irresistible and relates to a model of cognitive processes in which goals, intent, expectation, and interpretation typically are considered unlikely to play a major role in causing cognition or behavior. We have noted this in our discussion of the influence of affect on memory, in considering the prediction of a state-dependent effect of feelings. The older dichotomy between mechanistic, behavioristic, and associationistic theories on the one hand, and organismic, purposive, and cognitive or constructivist theories on the other, comes to mind (Anderson & Bower, 1972; Bartlett, 1932; Isen & Hastorf, 1982; Jenkins, 1974; Neisser, 1976).

As we have seen, however, discussions of "automatic" processes in the current cognitive literature do not center on this particular set of distinctions. The process of automatization and the operation of automatic processes are now increasingly seen as products of normal cognitive processes such as overlearning. Thus, automaticization may be seen as a gradual process, and automaticity itself as continuous with other kinds of processing, rather than discrete (e.g., Uleman, Chapter 14, this volume); the influence of automatic processes increasingly can be viewed as subject to modification and intervention rather than as inevitable and irresistible. Moreover, the occurrence of seemingly automatic processes may sometimes be the result of earlier decisions to deploy attention elsewhere. Thus, as we have noted, the definition of the concept of automaticity will depend, in part, on the use to which it is to be put. Finally, the fact that certain processes or parts of processes can become so overlearned as to proceed without monitoring under certain circumstances is not taken as a model for all of cognition, nor as evidence that such is the fundamental nature of thought.

Nonetheless, remnants of the older dichotomy remain, and because of the connotation of the word "automatic" in our language usage, it is difficult to resist thinking of "automatic" processes as different in kind from more controlled or conscious or attentive processes—as machine-like, separate from the person, and not able to be controlled. However, it also seems that the word that is used to represent the opposite "pole" or type of processing may play a role in this phenomenon. For example, contrasting "automatic" with "controlled" seems to imply that automatic processes cannot be controlled; contrasting it with "conscious" implies that automatic processes belong to our "unconscious minds" (and to some people this signals a mysterious, irrational phenomenon, such as Freud's concept of an unconscious area of the mind that is inaccessible to conscious mediation regardless of the circumstances). On the other hand, contrasting automatic with "attentive" provides what now appears to be a more accurate sense of the word as simply not requiring attention.

Nowhere is this issue more important than in the domain of affect, because there may be a tendency from the start to think of affect as mysterious, especially demanding, and especially irresistible. Thus, when the topic of the automatic processing of affect is raised, the connotative sense of the term "automatic" may fuel the view that affect or affective material is something apart—different in kind from more normal material—and something that cannot be figured or calculated in understanding the determinants of thought and behavior. Similarly, it may be thought that normal cognitive processes at work in automatic processing have little relevance to the understanding of automatically generated affect or its impact.

In contrast, we view affect as a factor that is similar in fundamental ways to other factors that influence thought and behavior. Although affect may have parameters that distinguish it from other factors, and these must be determined (and affects may differ among themselves in these parameters as well), nonetheless the basic process by which it has influence may be fundamentally the same as that of any other factor influencing the cognitive system. This does not mean that affective material will have precisely the same effect as other material, just as all affects do not have the same influence. (Nor is every kind of nonaffective material equivalent in impact; some are more important, more demanding, more influential in determining thought and action than others.) What it does mean is that affect can influence the cognitive system through the same processes by which other factors do so, and in understandable ways that are compatible with the ways in which other factors have influence. Similarly, the operation of normal cognitive processes applied to phenomena such as automaticity may have much to tell us about our affective experiences and their influence on us. The current view of automatic processes, emphasizing their continuity with attentive processes, is compatible with this goal for our understanding of affective processes and their influence on cognition and behavior.

ACKNOWLEDGMENT

Preparation of this chapter was supported in part by Grant No. 8406352 from the National Science Foundation to Alice M. Isen. The authors wish to thank Keith Williams for his comments on an earlier draft of the manuscript.

NOTES

1. "Overlearning" is defined as learning to a very high criterion level.

2. We present this distinction between valences and feeling states solely for its heuristic value; a full consideration of the relationship between these constructs is beyond the scope of this chapter.

3. However, the phenomena addressed in "New Look" research differ in an important way from automatic processing as it is conceived in the cognitive literature. The "New Look" literature deals with "unconscious processing," but primarily from the perspective of psychoanalytic theory, where unconscious, irresistible processes such as "perceptual defense" and related phenomena are assumed to operate at substantial cost to the capacity of the conscious cognitive and other life systems. In particular, in the psychoanalytic tradition it is thought that keeping unconscious material from awareness requires expenditure of capacity. This is in contradistinction with the modern cognitive concept of automaticity, which is thought to free up capacity.

4. It should be noted that Posner (1978) points out that "set" is not considered an automatic process.

5. Some might agree that "meaning" was processed automatically in the experiments by Johnston and Heinz (1978) and Treisman (1964), but might deny that this required that any active or inferential process took place. For example, they might accept the automatic processing of meaning only insofar as that entails a perceiver's increasing familiarity with stimulus patterns (which, by virtue of being

increasingly distinguishable by the perceiver, are more "meaningful"). This perceptually based, nonconstructive conceptualization of meaning may be useful in explaining some experimental results, but we do not think that it can account, for example, for the fact that the bilingual subjects in the work reported by Treisman (1964) could recognize perceptually distinct messages as synonymous. This ability would seem to require some cognitive interpretation or transformation of the perceived material.

Other researchers suggest, however, that meaning in the more complex sense in which it is normally used can be processed automatically. Bargh (Chapter 1, this volume), for example, argues that the semantic meaning of words can be processed automatically, without awareness or intention. We are not convinced, however, that it has been demonstrated that such processing does not require cognitive capacity, a crucial element in the definition of automaticity. To establish that cognitive capacity is not required, it should be demonstrated that semantic meaning can be processed without being subject to an effect of set size, for example.

6. The asymmetrical effect observed in detection of this feature—that it resulted in automatic detection of one form ("anger") but not the other ("happiness")—is not unusual in studies of the pop-out effect, and is described by Treisman and Souther (1985) as relating to differential effects of "marked" and "unmarked" forms of features.

7. As in the analogous situation in cognition, there may be innate affect of a rudimentary type (or, some might argue, of a complete type). However, the question of innate affect—including its similarity to adult or developed affect, its relative importance in affective life, and so on—is beyond the scope of this chapter.

REFERENCES

Anderson, J. R. (1983). *The architecture of cognition.* Cambridge, MA: Harvard University Press.

Anderson, J. R., & Bower, G. H. (1972). *Human associative memory.* Hillsdale, NJ: Erlbaum.

Bartlett, F. (1932). *Remembering: A study in experimental and social psychology.* Cambridge, England: Cambridge University Press.

Bartlett, J. C., Burleson, G., & Santrock, J. W. (1982). Emotional mood and memory in young children. *Journal of Experimental Child Psychology, 34,* 59–76.

Bartlett, J. C., & Santrock, J. W. (1979). Affect-dependent episodic memory in young children. *Child Development, 50,* 513–518.

Bower, G. H., Gilligan, S. G., & Montiero, K. P. (1981). Selectivity of learning caused by affective states. *Journal of Experimental Psychology: General, 110,* 451–473.

Bower, G. H., & Mayer, J. (1985). Failure to replicate mood-dependent retrieval. *Bulletin of the Psychonomic Society, 23,* 39–42.

Bower, G. H., Montiero, K. P., & Gilligan, S. G. (1978). Emotional mood as a context for learning and recall. *Journal of Verbal Learning and Verbal Behavior, 17,* 573–585.

Carlson, R. A., & Dulaney, D. E. (1985). Conscious attention and abstraction in concept learning. *Journal of Experimental Psychology: Learning, Memory, and Cognition, 11,* 45–58.

Erdelyi, M. H. (1974). A new look at the New Look: Perceptual defense and vigilance. *Psychological Review, 81,* 1–25.

Erdelyi, M. H. (1985). *Psychoanalysis: Freud's cognitive psychology.* San Francisco: W. H. Freeman.

Egeth, H. E., Blecker, D., & Kamlet, A. (1969). Verbal interference in a perceptual comparison task. *Perception and Psychophysics, 6,* 655–656.

Eich, J. E., & Birnbaum, I. M. (1982). Repetition, cueing and state-dependent memory. *Memory and Cognition, 10,* 103–114.

Fazio, R., Sanbonmatsu, D. M., Powell, M. C., & Kardes, F. R. (1986). On the automatic activation of attitudes. *Journal of Personality and Social Psychology, 50,* 229–238.

Flowers, J. H., & Stoup, C. M. (1977). Selective attention between words, shapes, and colors in speeded classification and vocalization tasks. *Memory and Cognition, 5,* 299–307.

Glass, A. L., Holyoak, K. J., & Santa, J. L. (1979). *Cognition.* Reading, MA: Addison-Wesley.

Gleitman, H. (1988). *Psychology.* New York: Norton.

Hansen, C. H., & Hansen, R. D. (1988). Finding the face in the crowd: An anger superiority effect. *Journal of Personality and Social Psychology, 54,* 917–924.

Hock, H. W., & Egeth, H. E. (1970). Verbal interference with encoding in a perceptual classification task. *Journal of Experimental Psychology, 83,* 299–303.

Isen, A. M. (1984). Toward understanding the role of affect in cognition. In R. Wyer & T. Srull (Eds.), *Handbook of social cognition* (pp. 179–236). Hillsdale, NJ: Erlbaum.

Isen, A. M. (1985). The asymmetry of happiness and sadness in effects on memory in normal college students. *Journal of Experimental Psychology: General, 114,* 388–391.

Isen, A. M. (1987). Positive affect, cognitive processes, and social behavior. In L. Berkowitz (Ed.), *Advances in experimental social psychology* (Vol. 20, pp. 203–253). New York: Academic Press.

Isen, A. M. (in press). The influence of positive and negative affect on cognitive organization: Some implications for development. In N. Stein, B. Leventhal, & T. Trabasso (Eds.), *Psychological and biological processes in the development of emotion.* Hillsdale, NJ: Erlbaum.

Isen, A. M., & Daubman, K. A. (1984). The influence of affect on categorization. *Journal of Personality and Social Psychology, 47,* 1206–1217.

Isen, A. M., Daubman, K. A., & Nowicki, G. P. (1987). Positive affect facilitates creative problem solving. *Journal of Personality and Social Psychology, 52,* 1122–1131.

Isen, A. M., & Hastorf, A. H. (1982). Some perspectives on cognitive social psychology. In A. H. Hastorf & A. M. Isen (Eds.), *Cognitive social psychology* (pp. 1–31). New York: Elsevier.

Isen, A. M., Johnson, M. M. S., Mertz, E., & Robinson, G. (1985). The influence of positive affect on the unusualness of word associations. *Journal of Personality and Social Psychology, 48,* 1413–1426.

Isen, A. M., & Means, B. (1983). The influence of positive affect on decision-making strategy. *Social Cognition, 2,* 18–31.

Isen, A. M., Means, B., Patrick, R., & Nowicki, G. (1982). Some factors influencing decision-making strategy and risk-taking. In M. S. Clark & S. T. Fiske (Eds.), *Affect and cognition: The 17th Annual Carnegie Symposium on Cognition* (pp. 243–261). Hillsdale, NJ: Erlbaum.

Isen, A. M., Niedenthal, P., & Cantor, N. (1988). *An influence of positive affect on social categorization.* Unpublished manuscript.

Isen, A. M., Shalker, T., Clark, M., & Karp, L. (1978). Affect, accessibility of material in memory and behavior: A cognitive loop? *Journal of Personality and Social Psychology, 36,* 1–12.

James, W. (1890). *The principles of psychology* (2 vols.). New York: Henry Holt.

Jenkins, J. J. (1974). Remember that old theory of memory? Well forget it! *American Psychologist, 29,* 785–795.

Johnston, W. A., & Heinz, S. P. (1978). The flexibility and capacity demands of attention. *Journal of Experimental Psychology: General, 107,* 420–435.

Klatsky, R. (1980). *Human memory: Structures and processes.* San Francisco: W. H. Freeman.

Lachman, R., Lachman, J. L., & Butterfield, E. C. (1979). *Cognitive psychology and information processing: An introduction.* Hillsdale, NJ: Erlbaum.

Laird, J. D., Wagener, J. J., Halal, M., & Szegda, M. (1982). Remembering what you feel: The effects of emotion on memory. *Journal of Personality and Social Psychology, 42,* 646–657.

Logan, G. D. (1985). Skill and automaticity: Relations, implications, and future directions. *Canadian Journal of Psychology, 39,* 367–386.

Miller, G. (1956). The magical number seven, plus or minus two: Some limits on our capacity for processing information. *Psychological Review, 63,* 81–97.

Moray, N. (1959). Attention in dichotic listening: Affective cues and the influence of instructions. *Quarterly Journal of Experimental Psychology, 11,* 56–60.

Nasby, W., & Yando, R. (1982). Selective encoding and retrieval of affectively valent information. *Journal of Personality and Social Psychology, 43,* 1244–1255.

Natale, M., & Hantas, M. (1982). Effects of temporary mood states on memory about the self. *Journal of Personality and Social Psychology, 42,* 927–934.

Neisser, U. (1967). *Cognitive psychology.* Englewood Cliffs, NJ: Prentice-Hall.

Neisser, U. (1976). *Cognition and reality.* San Francisco: W. H. Freeman.

Neumann, O. (1984). Automatic processing: A review of recent findings and a plea for an old theory. In W. Princz & A. F. Sanders (Eds.), *Cognition and motor processes.* Berlin: Springer Verlag.

Nisbett, R. E., & Wilson, T. D. (1977). Telling more than we can know: Verbal reports on mental processes. *Psychological Review, 84,* 231–259.

Osgood, C. E., Suci, G. J., & Tannenbaum, P. H. (1957). *The measurement of meaning.* Urbana: University of Illinois Press.

Posner, M. I. (1978). *Chronometric explorations of mind.* Hillsdale, NJ: Erlbaum.

Posner, M. I., & Snyder, C. R. R. (1975a). Attention and cognitive control. In R. L. Solso (Ed.), *Information processing and cognition: The Loyola Symposium.* Hillsdale, NJ: Erlbaum.

Posner, M. I., & Snyder, C. R. R. (1975b). Facilitation and inhibition in the processing of signals. In P. M. A. Rabbitt & S. Dornic (Eds.), *Attention and performance V* (pp. 669–682). London: Academic Press.

Riskind, J. H. (1983). Nonverbal expressions and the accessibility of life experience memories: A congruence hypothesis. *Social Cognition, 2,* 62–86.

Rosch, E. (1975). Cognitive representations of semantic categories. *Journal of Experimental Psychology: General, 104,* 192–233.

Schachter, S., & Singer, J. E. (1962). Cognitive, social, and physiological determinants of emotional state. *Psychological Review, 69,* 379–399.

Schneider, W., & Shiffrin, R. M. (1977). Controlled and automatic human information processing: I. Detection, search, and attention. *Psychological Review, 84,* 1–66.

Shiffrin, R. M. (1988). Attention. In R. C. Atkinson, R. J. Herrnstein, G. Lindzey, & R. D. Luce (Eds.), *Stevens' handbook of experimental psychology* (2nd ed., pp. 739–811). New York: Wiley.

Shiffrin, R. M., & Dumais, S. T. (1981). The development of automatism. In J. R. Anderson (Ed.), *Cognitive skills and their acquisition* (pp. 111–140). Hillsdale, NJ: Erlbaum.

Shiffrin, R. M., & Schneider, W. (1977). Controlled and automatic human information processing: II. Perceptual learning, automatic attending, and a general theory. *Psychological Review, 84,* 127–190.

Smith, E. R. (1984). A model for social inference processes. *Psychological Review, 91,* 392–413.

Smith, E., & Lerner, M. (1986). Development of automatism of social judgments. *Journal of Personality and Social Psychology, 50,* 246–259.

Snyder, M., & White, E. (1982). Moods and memories: Elation, depression, and remembering the events of one's life. *Journal of Personality, 50,* 149–167.

Stroop, J. R. (1935). Studies of interference in serial verbal reactions. *Journal of Experimental Psychology, 18,* 643–662.

Teasdale, J. D., & Fogarty, S. J. (1979). Differential effects of induced mood on retrieval of pleasant and unpleasant events from episodic memory. *Journal of Abnormal Psychology, 88,* 248–257.

Teasdale, J. D., & Russell, M. L. (1983). Differential aspects of induced mood on the recall of positive, negative and neutral words. *British Journal of Clinical Psychology, 22,* 163–171.

Teasdale, J. D., Taylor, R., & Fogarty, S. J. (1980). Effects of induced elation–depression on the accessibility of memories of happy and unhappy experiences. *Behaviour Research and Therapy, 18,* 339–346.

Treisman, A. M. (1964). Verbal cues, language, and meaning in selective attention. *American Journal of Psychology, 77,* 215–216.

Treisman, A. M., & Souther, J. (1985). Search asymmetry: A diagnostic for preattentive processing of separable features. *Journal of Experimental Psychology: General, 114,* 285–309.

Tulving, E. (1979). Relation between encoding specificity and levels of processing. In L. S. Cermak & F. I. M. Craik (Eds.), *Levels of processing in human memory.* Hillsdale, NJ: Erlbaum.

Tulving, E., & Thomson, D. M. (1973). Encoding specificity and retrieval processes in episodic memory. *Psychological Review, 80,* 352–373.

Weiner, B. (1985). *Human motivation.* New York: Springer-Verlag.

Zajonc, R. B. (1968). The attitudinal effects of mere exposure. *Journal of Personality and Social Psychology Monograph Supplement, 9*(2, Pt. 2), 1–27.

Zajonc, R. B. (1980). Feeling and thinking: Preferences need no inferences. *American Psychologist, 35,* 151–175.

PART II

UNINTENDED AND UNATTENDED THOUGHT IN DAILY LIFE

5

Spontaneous Trait Inference

LEONARD S. NEWMAN
JAMES S. ULEMAN
New York University

Lily is, for instance, entertaining ladies and I come in with my filthy plaster cast, in sweat socks; I am wearing a red velvet dressing gown which I bought at Sulka's in Paris in a mood of celebration when Frances said she wanted a divorce. In addition I have on a red wool hunting cap. And I wipe my nose and mustache on my fingers and then shake hands with the guests, saying, "I'm Mr. Henderson, how do you do?" And I go to Lily and shake her hand, too, as if she were merely another lady guest, a stranger like the rest. And I say, "How do you do?" I imagine the ladies are telling themselves, "He doesn't know her. In his mind he's still married to the first. Isn't that awful?" This imaginary fidelity thrills them.

—Saul Bellow (1958, p. 9)

The impressions we form of others depend on many things, including how they look, what they do, and even what they don't do (as in the passage above from Saul Bellow's *Henderson the Rain King*). These impressions are captured in images, feelings, and words. Among the most common words in person impressions are those representing traits. Sometimes these traits occur to us spontaneously as we observe others, and sometimes we only find the traits as we try to describe our impressions to others. Of course, we may also set out to evaluate people on particular traits, because we are interested in them as potential employees or students or competitors or lovers, or because a social psychologist has asked us to form an impression of them. But such intentional trait inferences do not concern us here.

This chapter is about spontaneous trait inferences. "Spontaneous inferences" are, by definition, inferences that we make without the intention to do so.[1] Our research demonstrates that they exist. It also shows that we are often unaware that we have made them. That seems to be Henderson's belief in the passage above. The ladies are thrilled and delighted because they have inferred his "fidelity" to his first wife, though they are unaware of their inference and can only comment, "Isn't that awful?" that he fails to recognize his current wife. They are secretly and nonconsciously thrilled at what a faithful fellow he is, but mistake this for pity and talk of him as forgetful rather than faithful. Of course, this is all in Henderson's imagination (in Bellow's imagination), and he is amused by it because, as we learn in the next line, "they are all wrong . . . it was done on purpose." But maybe Henderson is wrong. How can he know what the ladies think but do not discuss? More important, how can we know what people think but do not say, especially if they are not aware of it themselves?

One possibility is that conscious and nonconscious thoughts about an event may serve as effective retrieval cues and help in remembering it later on. The principle of encoding specificity holds that "specific encoding operations performed on what is perceived determine what is stored, and what is stored determines what retrieval cues are effective in providing access to what is stored" (Tulving & Thomson, 1973, p. 369). Research that supports this principle demonstrates that explicitly presented words that provide the context for to-be-remembered words are more effective retrieval cues than strong semantic associates are (see Tulving, 1983, Ch. 11, for a review). Winter and Uleman (1984) extended these demonstrations to inferred, implicit (rather than explicit) context words. They asked subjects to read and remember sentences (e.g., "The secretary solves the mystery halfway through the book") known to imply traits ("clever"), without asking for trait inferences. The implicit traits were more effective cues than strong semantic associates of sentence words ("typewriter," "detective") in subsequent tests of cued recall. Moreover, subjects were unaware of making trait inferences at encoding, or of using them preferentially as cues for recall. These results are analogous to "faithful" bringing Henderson to the ladies' minds, or "mischievous" and "irreverent" reminding us of Henderson, even though we may have had no such conscious thoughts on meeting Henderson.

Two subsequent studies (Uleman, Newman, & Winter, 1987; Winter, Uleman, & Cunniff, 1985) have provided more convincing demonstrations that trait inferences can be unintended and nonconscious. Subjects read the same kind of sentences as "distractors" in a study of "memory for digits." On each trial, they read a digit series aloud, then read a "distractor" sentence and repeated it, and then recalled the digits. After all trials and an intervening task, there was a surprise cued-recall test of memory for the sentences. Again, trait-cued recall exceeded semantic-cued recall and free recall, indicating that traits had been inferred at sentence encoding. In these studies, subjects' thoughts about the last sentence were probed immediately after they read it; again, there was no relationship between awareness of trait or personality inferences and traits' effectiveness in cued recall.

Preliminary evidence on several other characteristics of spontaneous trait inferences, besides their occurrence without intentions to infer traits or awareness of having done so, is worth mentioning briefly. First, the inferences people make seem to depend partly on their characteristic ways of thinking about others. High- and low-authoritarianism subjects differ in the inferences they make from the same behaviors (Uleman, Winborne, Winter, & Shechter, 1986). Second, these inferences are not automatic in the sense of not requiring cognitive capacity for their occurrence (Uleman et al., 1987), even though earlier results had suggested they might be automatic (Winter et al., 1985). Third, some processing goals make trait inferences more likely, even though they do not call for them explicitly—goals such as forming an impression of the person (Bassili & Smith, 1986) or judging the action or actor against other social standards (Moskowitz & Uleman, 1987). Such intentional trait inferences augment spontaneous ones. Fourth, other processing goals, such as attending to isolated features of the stimuli (e.g., particular letters or sounds), sharply reduce spontaneous trait inferences (Moskowitz & Uleman, 1987). And fifth, subjects infer the gists of the action ("reading" in the example above) just as readily and spontaneously as they infer the actors' traits (Moskowitz & Uleman, 1987; Uleman et al., 1987; Winter et al., 1985).

Rather than reviewing these findings in more detail (for that, see Uleman, 1987), we have three other goals in this chapter. First, we briefly review the range of theoretical views in social psychology on the nature of trait inference processes, to make this range explicit and suggest where spontaneous trait inferences may be found within it. Our second goal is to explore when spontaneous trait inferences are most likely to occur. The sentences used in the studies noted above were deliberately designed to imply traits. But this was done intuitively and empirically, without clear theoretical guidance. What kinds of traits are most easily inferred, and what kinds of actions imply traits strongly enough for them to occur spontaneously? To begin to answer this question, we must examine the meanings of "trait." Our third goal is to suggest how spontaneous trait inferences may affect other social phenomena or play a role in them. What difference might they make? The answer to this takes us on a speculative tour of several well-known research programs.

TRAIT INFERENCE PROCESSES IN SOCIAL PSYCHOLOGY

Over the last 20 years or so, attribution theory perspectives have guided most research on when and how people reach conclusions about others' personality characteristics. Jones and Davis' theory of correspondent inference (1965) and Kelley's ANOVA-model (1967) have been particularly influential. The former describes the processes involved in the attribution of dispositional properties to people from their intentional or voluntary behavior. The latter describes how people arrive at causal explanations in general, with the most common causes assumed to be persons, entities, and the environment. As entities are often other persons, Kelley's work is to a large extent also an analysis of the process of inferring that another person's behavior reflects some stable property.

One result of the impact of these theorists' seminal papers—Kelley's work in particular—has been that dispositional properties in general and traits in particular have come to be redefined as *personal causes.* Indeed, Kelley stated that "all judgments of the type 'Property X characterizes Entity Y' are viewed as causal attributions" (1973, p. 107). Trait concepts certainly can be invoked as causal attributions, but as Higgins, Strauman, and Klein (1986) point out (see also Eiser, 1983, and Reeder, 1985), most of the literature on person perception now seems to assume that all dispositional inferences are causal attributions.

A recent review of research on the extent of causal thinking in everyday life is a good case in point. Weiner (1985) notes that "research participants may be thinking about causal attributions, *or trait descriptions,* yet not exhibit or verbalize these thoughts. After all, causal communications *and trait labels* can have far-reaching interpersonal consequences" (p. 75, emphasis added). Clearly, the assumption here is that trait inference is a specific type of causal attribution. Weiner's review concludes that attributional activity is triggered by unexpected events and experiences of failure. As the incidence of attributional activity is thereby limited, so too by implication is the extent of trait inference.

The variables discussed by Weiner do indeed seem to increase attributional activity, including, of course, personal attributions. In addition, expectation of future interaction with a target person has been shown to increase attributional activity (Harvey, Yarkin, Lightner, & Town, 1980) and dispositional inference in particular (Berscheid, Graziano, Monson, & Dermer, 1976; Feldman & Ruble, 1981; Miller, Norman, & Wright, 1978). But to conclude that these are *necessary* conditions for trait inference seems to conflict with the view of early person perception researchers (such as Asch and Heider) that the extraction of dispositional information from the behavior of others is ubiquitous in everyday psychological functioning. This conflict concerns at least two important issues. The first is whether dispositions are always properly thought of as causes, and this depends on what one means by "cause" and "disposition." The second issue is how effortful (or conscious, explicit, intentional, controlled, etc.) the process of inferring dispositions (and causes, if they are the same) is. Our view, in brief, is that some dispositions are causes but others are not, and that there are inference processes that are intentional and effortful, and inference processes that are not. Spontaneous inferences are not intentional.

Some dispositions can clearly be said to cause behavior under almost any conditions (e.g., compulsions and obsessions, appetites and addictions). Other dispositions distinguish their owners by merely enabling behaviors, without requiring them (e.g., intelligence, talent, and immorality). Related dispositions may limit or disable behavioral capacities (e.g., stupidity, ineptness, and moral integrity—which may, of course, also require behaviors under other conditions). Reeder and Brewer (1979) discuss the "hierarchically restrictive schema" of such enabling and limiting dispositions. Other dispositions may be merely descriptive of characteristic behaviors (e.g., friendly, reactionary, or informal) without implying causality. That is, people may be characterized as friendly because they have performed friendly behaviors, without implying that their friendliness caused the behavior; similarly, today's weather may be characterized as sunny because the sun is shining, without implying that sunniness caused the sun to shine, or the stock market may be characterized as bullish because average prices increased, without believing that there is something called "bullishness" that caused the increase. This is discussed further below.

The second issue concerns how effortful or intentional dispositional inferences are. Attribution theorists are not alone in positing that inferring traits from behavior requires special motivating circumstances. Wyer and Srull's (1986) model of social cognition posits a limited-capacity "goal specification box" that stores immediate processing objectives along with information on how to attain them. Unless a task objective is explicitly represented there, it has no effect on the encoding, organization, storage, or retrieval of information. As a result, "behaviors will typically not be spontaneously encoded in terms of trait (attribute) concepts unless a specific processing objective requires it" (p. 328). Carlston and Skowronski (1986, footnote 2), working with Wyer and Carlston's (1979) associative network model of social cognition, assert that under "real-world" conditions people are overloaded with information and have no incentive to carefully process all of the behavioral information they are exposed to. Therefore, people will not infer traits unless they intend to do so.

However, not all social psychologists view trait inferences as effortful, deliberate, and therefore exceptional operations. As Higgins et al. (1986) note (see also Reeder & Brewer, 1979; Trope, 1986), some earlier process must first allow us to represent incoming stimulus information in terms of attribution-relevant categories (e.g., friendly behavior). This is termed the "identification" stage in their model of social evaluation, and they argue that once behavior is identified as being of a particular type, a trait "interpretation" may be based simply on the relation of the behavior to a relevant standard. The actual process of causal reasoning may not be necessary to classify a given behavior in trait-like terms. It should be pointed out, however, that it is unclear whether or not these models allow for the classification of *people* (as opposed to *behaviors*) in terms of traits without some explicit causal attribution process.

Read (1987) presents a model of causal reasoning (based in part on

Schank & Abelson's [1977] script theory) in which such reasoning is essential to the comprehension of any event and requires no special motivating conditions. The model distinguishes between implicit and explicit causal reasoning: The latter refers to the active process frequently studied by attribution researchers (e.g., Weiner, 1985), whereas the former is based on extensive pre-existing knowledge structures and is central to social information processing. Without such implicit processes, "people would simply fail to understand what was going on" (Read, 1987, p. 289). Though the model currently de-emphasizes understanding in terms of traits in favor of teleological causes, it acknowledges that a detailed, well-articulated store of trait knowledge is also necessary to comprehend events. Furthermore, the point is made that Kelley's model in particular is incapable of explaining how people arrive at concrete, content-specific attributions (e.g., "clumsy") as opposed to more abstract person and situation attributions. In fact, such concrete explanations are easier to arrive at than the abstract causal explanations that serve as output in Kelley's model.

Smith and Miller (1983) provided a demonstration of this latter point by using a reaction time measure to explore the distinction between causal attributions and trait inferences. They set out to test whether trait inference is part of a two-stage process, with identification of the actor or situation as the causal locus in the first stage, followed by a trait inference as the second stage. Their data suggested that this is not the case. Subjects read a series of sentences describing trait-relevant behaviors, each followed by one of five questions. Judgments about whether a given trait characterized the subjects of the sentences were not significantly slower than judgments about their gender, and were significantly faster than the slowest judgment of all: person–cause and situation–cause questions. As judgments that take longer to arrive at cannot plausibly mediate judgments that take less time, Smith and Miller concluded that trait inferences may "be made during comprehension, or at least can be readily inferred" (1983, p. 502).

From this perspective, one could infer aggressiveness from aggressive behavior without generating ANOVA-cube information from scratch or searching through other possible causes. One might be able to infer that such behavior is nonconsensual and nondistinctive, on the basis of some schematic, content-specific representation of that behavior, rather than vice versa. Brown and Fish (1983; see also Garvey & Caramazza, 1974) present intriguing data suggesting that causal schemata are even implicit in English verbs that describe interactions (mental or behavioral) between two people. Subjects presented with impoverished sentences of the form "A criticizes B" or "X likes Y" are almost unanimous in how they attribute causality—in these cases, to A and Y. The direction of the attribution can be predicted on the basis of the class of verb involved, and is also predictable from the common derivational adjective of the verb involved when one exists. In the examples presented here, subjects seem to assume that A and Y are "critical" and "likable," respectively, rather than that B and X are "criticizable" and "likeful." (For another perspective on these findings, see Fiedler & Semin, 1988.)

Finally, McArthur and Baron's (1983) ecological theory of social perception specifies that certain dispositional properties (the "structural invariants" of people) are directly perceived without the necessity of intervening inferential processes. In a series of studies, McArthur and her colleagues (Berry & McArthur, 1985; McArthur & Apatow, 1983–1984) have shown that adults with babyish facial appearances are perceived as more childlike (e.g., less strong and domineering) than others whose appearance is more mature. More recently, this research has been successfully extended to the perception of adults with childlike voices (Montepare & McArthur, 1987). Though McArthur and Baron intend their theory to apply specifically to the type of live, dynamic stimulus displays that are uncommon in social-cognition research, and though their subjects are usually asked to form impressions of the target people (so that the impressions are not spontaneous), their work provides additional evidence that forming impressions of others can be a natural, relatively effortless part of social perception.

Even in the attribution literature, evidence is accumulating that a process of causal reasoning may not be necessary for inferences about personality. Johnson, Jemmott, and Pettigrew (1984), using the quiz-game paradigm of Ross, Amabile, and Steinmetz (1977), found that subjects' assessments of the causal determinants of behavior did not match their ratings of the questioner and contestant on dispositional variables (e.g., intelligence). Though they replicated the "fundamental attribution error" (Ross, 1977)—the extraction of dispositional information from behavior without regard to its context—judgments of intelligence could not be accounted for by a misperception of situational forces, as these judgments were not significantly affected by the degree of awareness of situational constraints on the target persons' behavior. Subsequent research by Johnson (1986) has further supported the idea of "separation and independence of causal attributions and dispositional inferences" (p. 60). He found that subjects based personality inferences on such incidents as winning a sweepstakes or sitting in a seat later determined to be lucky, despite their stated recognition that luck determined these outcomes. Reeder and his colleagues (Reeder & Fulks, 1980; Reeder & Spores, 1983) have also found differences between causal attributions and trait inferences that would seem to follow from them, and they have concluded that it is possible that "dispositional inferences are made rather readily as 'snap judgments,' while causal attribution may involve more elaborate information processing and may be based, in part, on a prior dispositional judgment" (Reeder & Fulks, 1981, p. 45). Apparently, the fundamental attribution error cannot be accounted for by a misperception of causal forces, but rather stems from some more immediate process (Jones, 1979).

This point has been made rather forcefully in series of studies by Gilbert and his colleagues (Gilbert & Jones, 1986; Gilbert, Krull, & Pelham, 1987; Gilbert, Pelham, & Krull, 1988). Gilbert (Chapter 6, this volume) suggests that the social inference process can be broken down into a "characterization" stage (what we would call "dispositional inference") followed by "correction" (adjustment for situational influences on behavior). Whereas the latter process requires conscious effort, characterization proceeds relatively automatically (but see Uleman, Chapter 14, this volume). To illustrate, Gilbert et al. (1988) asked their subjects to rate the dispositional anxiety of a clearly nervous woman they observed on film engaging in a conversation. Whereas control subjects rated the woman as relatively less dispositionally anxious when they learned that she had been discussing anxiety-provoking matters, subjects who were required to work at rehearsing words while watching the film failed to take into account the nature of the topics being discussed by the target, despite being well aware of what they were. Apparently, all subjects rather effortlessly made inferences about the target woman's personality, but only those with sufficient cognitive resources available followed up by taking into account the nature of the situation she was in.

Thus there is a growing body of evidence suggesting that (1) dispositional and causal inferences may be either spontaneous, implicit, effortless, automatic, and so on (if we may gloss over potentially important differences among these terms, for present purposes) *or* intentional, explicit, effortful, controlled, deliberative, and the like; and (2) dispositional inferences are not always causal inferences (and vice versa, of course). Note that our brief survey might seem to suggest when the two are distinct, dispositions are inferred spontaneously and causes intentionally; however, this is clearly untrue, as some dispositional inferences require great effort and are subject to explicit consideration and reconsideration. We should not mistake these two distinctions for each other. Dispositions and causes are overlapping content sets; the other distinction(s) describes processes that generate this content.

Bearing this in mind, let us examine the content of trait inferences more closely.

SPONTANEOUS TRAIT INFERENCE: WHAT IS AND WHAT IS NOT INFERRED

Although our data and some of the work reviewed above indicate that personality characteristics can be inferred spontaneously, we have been less clear about which of these characteristics can be so inferred. Clearly, there are limits to the types of conclusions that are effortlessly drawn from observing behavior. To explore these, we must digress briefly to discuss the meaning of the terms "trait" and "disposition."

Psychologists' Conceptions of Traits

Although traits have been at the center of controversy since Mischel's (1968) famous monograph, the exact nature of the target of this controversy has been unclear (Alston, 1975). In fact, there have historically been at least three distinct approaches to the trait concept (Buss & Craik, 1984; Zuroff, 1986). The first one, generally associated with Gordon Allport, is that traits are real entities corresponding to neurophysiological structures. From this perspective, then, traits are traceable to systems of neurons and so provide explanations for behavior. A second position is that traits describe a tendency to perform certain acts in certain situations; this has been called the "dispositional" view of traits (Zuroff, 1986). As Alston (1975) puts it, "a dispositional concept 'embodies' an S-R [situation–response] regularity, differing from a mere report of that regularity only by way of also embodying the claim that there is something more or less stable in X's constitution that is responsible for the regularity (but without specifying what that is)" (p. 20). Traits as dispositions do not refer to specific causal entities, nor do they necessarily imply the frequent occurrence of related behaviors; they "are neither reports of observed or observable states of affairs, nor yet reports of unobserved or unobservable states of affairs" (Ryle, 1949, p. 125). They are hypothetical propositions with situational specifications. Though they do have predictive utility, if the relevant situations never occur, dispositions will never manifest themselves (Buss & Craik, 1984).

The third approach, now associated primarily with Buss and Craik's (1983, 1984) "act frequency approach," is that traits are simply summary statements about observed behavior. To say that "Mary is arrogant" means only that over some period of time Mary has frequently engaged in prototypically arrogant acts. Act *trends* are crucial; single acts, by definition, cannot serve as an appropriate indicator of a trait. Buss and Craik note that Jones and Davis's (1965) work on correspondent inferences contrasts with their view that "a single act is an inadequate basis for dispositional inference" (1983, p. 120), because in that line of research observers are typically asked to infer a trait on the basis of a single instance of behavior (but see Jones & McGillis, 1976, p. 393). As in the dispositional view, traits in the act frequency approach do not have any separate existence and therefore do not offer causal explanations, though on "actuarial grounds" they can serve as a basis for prediction. Buss and Craik emphasize that "This position contrasts markedly with any use of dispositional statements to explain or account for observed manifestations (e.g., 'She issued the command *because* she is dominant')" (1983, pp. 107–108).

Buss and Craik's act frequency conception of traits suggests a fruitful approach to personality research, but it is not always clear whether their rules for trait inference are prescriptive rules for the professional psychologist or are meant to describe the process by which lay perceivers assign trait labels. This is especially apparent in their discussion of Jones and Davis's work. Clearly, Jones and Davis were interested in how trait inferences might be made by laypeople rather than by psychologists. Though their model describes rational baseline principles that are followed imperfectly (hence spontaneous trait inferences; see also Gilbert, Chapter 6, this volume), it attempts to provide a picture of how people might go about inferring dispositions with the suboptimal information that real social interaction generally provides. On the other hand, Buss and Craik's approach serves chiefly to describe an optimal procedure for formal personality assessment by psychologists using trait constructs, given their definition of traits.

However, for a comprehensive account of how laypeople conceive of traits, we must consider the following: First of all, in actuality, people sometimes *do* use trait terms as causal constructs. We would not find it strange to hear someone report that Mary's behavior occurred "because she is dominant." We would probably also not be surprised to discover that our friend's causal account was formed on the basis of a single act; in the context of Tversky and Kahneman's (1971) research demonstrating that we often interpret small samples of observations as if they were quite representative, it would be even more surprising if this were never the case. Finally, the assumption that our trait impressions of others are only based on summaries of individuals' displays of various behaviors over time is hard to reconcile with evidence that people have great difficulty with the covariation estimates that would be necessary to accurately associate people with types of behavior (Nisbett & Ross, 1980; but cf. Epstein & Teraspulsky, 1986).

What traits have meant to psychologists and what they mean to the layperson are related but distinct issues. To learn more about what traits are likely to be spontaneously inferred and when this will occur, we must explicitly consider what traits seem to mean in everyday usage.

Lay Conceptions of Traits

Though the layperson has often been portrayed as a trait theorist (e.g., Nisbett, 1980), trait concepts obviously correspond to only one of the ways in which we categorize ourselves and others. Cantor and Mischel (1979) point out that we also rely on categories pertaining to physical appearance, gender, race, and occupation. Their research demonstrated the use of behavioral *types* as units of everyday categoriation (e.g., "social activist," "comic joker"); traits are said to be organized around these categories. Anderson and Klatzky (1987) argue that such social stereotype categories are actually more natural and efficient than trait categories, and they even suggest that some trait terms may have themselves evolved from labels representing social stereotypes (e.g., "brainy" from "brain," "bullying" from "bully").

However, even Walter Mischel, who criticizes the scientific value of broad trait concepts as explanations for behavior, emphasizes the "importance of the layman's everyday use of trait categories" (1973, p. 263). For example, Jeffery and Mischel (1979) showed that when subjects were asked to organize behavioral information to predict future behavior, the most common approach was to organize the information in terms of traits rather than situations. Fiske and Cox (1979) found that trait terms were the most common category of information offered when adult subjects' instructions were to write descriptions "so that someone else would know what it's like to be around this person." This was especially true when subjects described people they knew well.

Eiser (1983) notes that of the 18,000 person-descriptive terms Allport and Odbert (1936) found in a standard English dictionary, 4,504 seemed to describe stable attributes of individuals. Since it is reasonable to assume that most individual differences that a society's members perceive as significant eventually become encoded into their language (Goldberg, 1981), the referents of these terms are themselves worthy of study. But what do laypeople mean when they characterize an individual with one of these labels?

Stability

In the developmental literature, one finds an abundance of research explicitly assessing subjects' belief in the temporal stability of personality characteristics. For example, Rotenberg (1982) had 5- to 9-year-old children label actors as either "mean" or "kind" after hearing about relevant behavior, and then asked them to characterize the same actors after 1 of 6 days had gone by. Age-related increases in "character constancy" were found: Older children tended to assert that the actors would remain the same. On the other hand, although it is usually assumed that adults' trait labels refer to stable qualities, there is little direct supporting evidence. An exception is a recent study by Chaplin, John, and Goldberg (1988). Chaplin et al. found that subjects' ratings of the trait prototypicality of descriptive terms was best predicted by their ratings of the temporal stability implied by those terms. (See also Greenberg, Saxe, & Bar-Tal, 1978, on the *relative* perceived stability of various traits.)

Other indirect evidence supports the assumption that adults are strong believers in character constancy. Wimer and Kelley (1982) factor-analyzed ratings of a wide range of causal attributions. Possible trait causes of various behaviors (e.g., ability, compulsiveness) were seen as temporally stable, loading highly on their Enduring versus Transient factor. Hayden and Mischel (1976) found that people presented with behaviors that clearly clashed with previous trait impressions would either try to interpret the behaviors so as to confirm previous trait impressions or dismiss them as being due to transient, situational pressures. In other words, "underlying consistency at the trait level" (p. 131) was assumed. Indeed, one of the reasons why behavior inconsistent with a previous trait impression is relatively well remembered (Hastie & Kumar, 1979) is that we actively try to reconcile this behavior with the previous impression (Crocker, Hannah, & Weber, 1983). The tendency to do this both reflects and encourages the belief in trait stability.

Predictive Utility

As one might intuitively expect, belief in traits' stability is accompanied by an appreciation of their predictive value. Rotenberg (1982) found that character constancy correlated with the degree to which his younger subjects predicted that actors would engage in trait-consistent behavior, and almost all of his third-grade subjects predicted behavior in line with their previous trait judgments (see also Rholes & Ruble, 1984). Similar results have been reported in the adult literature. Reeder and Spores (1983) found that fictional characters most likely to be judged immoral by college students on the basis of their sexual behavior were also judged to be more likely to engage in other immoral behaviors such as lying or stealing. Traits are thus understood to imply some degree of cross-situational stability.

But once inferred, are traits seen as expressing themselves in a cross-situationally rigid fashion? It has been suggested that once a person labels another with a trait term, predictions of future behavior are completely unaffected by situational context (Nisbett, 1980). To some degree, insensitivity to situational variability is perhaps inherent in the linguistic nature of trait terms (Semin & Greenslade, 1985). However, intuition and evidence suggest that this insensitivity is limited. Zuroff (1982) found that his subjects stored not only trait information about their friends' behavior, but also situational information and person × situation interactions. Epstein and Teraspulsky's (1986) subjects did not perceive unreasonably high correlations among various behavioral referents of traits, and when estimating these relationships, they reported relying on situational as well as trait categories for doing so. Allen and Smith (1980) showed that college students were more likely to endorse interactional explanations of human behavior than either trait or situational explanations, and Wimer and Kelley (1982) found that trait causes of the behaviors they studied loaded negatively on a factor that seemed to reflect to what extent causes were seen as necessary for the occurrence of behavior.

Therefore, though trait concepts are seen by the lay perceiver as having predictive value, they are not seen as necessary causes of behavior. A more recent illustration of this point was provided by Sande, Goethals, and Radloff (1988), who found that people often see others and (especially) themselves as possessing opposing pairs of traits (e.g., "serious" and "carefree"). Such reports clearly imply a recognition of variability and flexibility across situations.

Traits as Causes

This brings us to the question of whether laypeople generally even see traits themselves as causal constructs. Because psychologists usually see trait inferences as the result of a causal attribution process, they tend to think of traits as stable personal causes and assume that lay psychologists also see them that way. But Fletcher (1984) notes that causal accounts using traits as explanatory concepts may contain circular logic. For example, if we know that a man is aggressive because he hits people, to assert that he hits people because he is aggressive somehow seems less than enlightening. Fletcher therefore makes a distinction between what he calls "behavioral" and "mental" dispositions. The former encompass what we usually think of as personality traits ("talkative," "aggressive," "punctual," etc.). They refer to regularity with regard to specific types of behavior, but do not explain them. The latter, on the other hand, are more clearly located "in the head." They include beliefs, attitudes (knowledge structures), abilities, and various affect-related traits (uncontrollable internal qualities). This analysis is almost identical to Alston's (1975) distinction between "T-concepts" and "purposive–cognitive concepts." Alston called the latter (which correspond to Fletcher's mental dispositions) "causal concepts," and the former (which are like Fletcher's behavioral dispositions) "dispositional concepts" in the sense described in the section above.

This distinction is intuitively appealing, and also highlights the danger of treating personal dispositions as a homogenous class (Ross & Fletcher, 1985). In fact, in addition to attitudes, beliefs, and abilities, Ryle (1949) presents a whole catalogue of "behavioral tendencies" that could be considered dispositional—habits, tastes, interests, bents, hobbies, occupations, addictions, ambitions, missions, loyalties, and devotions (pp. 132–133). Furthermore, some indirect evidence from a study by Miller, Smith, and Uleman (1981) supports the utility of the distinction. Their subjects were provided with some standard attributional scales for rating a number of friendly and unfriendly behaviors. Though responses were dutifully provided, a subsequent comparison of subjects' "causal attributions" with various other measures indicated that their attributional thought regarding these prototypical behavior dispositions was not well represented by the internal–external causal dimension assumed to underlie the attributional measures. These results indicate that people do not think of friendliness or unfriendliness as internal causes, and suggest that the same might be true for other common trait terms.

As both Alston and Fletcher emphasize, a basic contrast between their two classes of dispositions concerns how they relate to observable behaviors. Though T-concepts and behavioral dispositions are by definition directly associated with prototypical behaviors, purposive–cognitive and mental concepts require a more complex theory to translate into behavior. Saying that one is "sociable" means that one is inclined to seek the company of others. However, one can "need social contact" without ever engaging in sociable behaviors. And how such mental dispositions as "insecurity" or "anal retentiveness" map onto behavior is even less clear. In our research, we have focused for the most part on inferences about personality characteristics best classified as behavioral dispositions (see Winter & Uleman, 1984, Table 1; Winter et al., 1985, Table 1). It is not clear whether mental dispositions can be spontaneously inferred, though with sufficient practice and expertise, it may be possible. However, for the time being, we assume that trait concepts appearing to fit the definition of behavioral dispositions/T-concepts function as optimal, middle levels of personality categorization (but see Hampson, John, & Goldberg, 1986). That is, this level may be the ideal one for most possible observational goals, and so most likely to be inferred spontaneously from behavior.

It should be acknowledged, finally, that many dispositional concepts straddle the fence: "Excitability" and "introversion" imply cognitive–affective factors as well as predictable behaviors (Fletcher, 1984). In other cases, the same trait term may refer to both a mental and a behavioral disposition (or even a "state"—see Chaplin et al., 1988). When used in one sense, "crazy" is of the former type, and negative in valence; it implies unobserved factors that cause maladaptive or socially unacceptable behavior. However, the same term can be used in a positive way to describe someone who consistently behaves in exciting, unpredictable ways. In the latter case, "crazy" is simply a description of the type of behavior that one can expect from a person, and functions as a behavioral disposition. It should also be noted that people in everyday conversation *will* tell us that someone "won't shut up because he is talkative." Behavioral dispositions used in this way serve as "proximal causes" (Ross & Fletcher, 1985). One can explain rude behavior in terms of the person's rudeness, but this trait may then be attributed to the person's upbringing, which can be attributed to his or her parents' personalities, which may be a function of *their* upbringings, and so on. Once again, these deeper levels of causal analysis are more likely with greater perceiver practice and effort.

Conclusions

Though traits are not the only way to classify or think about people, they are important categories for social understanding. They are seen by lay perceivers as stable attributes and reasonably predictive of future behavior, but there is no expectation that they will be rigidly expressed—traits are not seen as necessary causes of behavior. Nor are they necessarily causal constructs at all. The lay perceiver seems to be agnostic with regard to their causal status. Finally, traits are not simply summaries of behavior; they can be inferred from even single instances of behavior.

It seems, then, that the lay understanding of traits corresponds closely to the second psychologists' view described above, the dispositional view.

A recent conceptual analysis by Eiser (1983) leads to a conclusion similar to ours. Are people "looking for *causes* of the actor's behavior within the actor's personality? This is far too narrow a view of the bases of predictability that can be implicit in such interpersonal descriptions" (p. 105). Trait descriptions, Eiser goes on to say, "are special kinds of descriptions in that they assume and predict high consistency and low distinctiveness— but not in that they refer to a logically separable, unobservable (internal cause)" (pp. 103–104).

This conclusion leaves us with something of a paradox. On the one hand, the evidence indicates that our conception of traits is not particularly rigid or mechanical. Traits are not expected to express themselves in every situation, and are not seen as necessary causes of behavior. But on the other hand, other research indicates that we seem to effortlessly extract some trait meanings from behavior. This state of affairs is perhaps best illustrated by the Johnson et al. (1984) study discussed above. Their subjects made inferences about a stable disposition even when they "should have known better"—that is, even when they understood the constraints of the situation. The present review of the layperson's understanding of traits suggests that while in general we all "know better" about the causes of behavior, spontaneous trait inferences occur anyway.

The Behavior–Trait Link

Although there is a multitude of interesting ways of differentiating among traits (see especially Buss & Craik, 1983), most recent treatments focus on the behavior–trait link—that is, the ease with which a given trait can be confirmed or instantiated by observed behavior. Confirmability is of particular interest to us, as it seems to be directly related to limits on the spontaneity of trait inference.

Reeder and Brewer (1979; see also Reeder, 1985) have presented perhaps the best-developed model of the implicit links between dispositions and the behaviors they imply. Several "implicational schemata" are described. For example, some dispositions are associated with a fairly wide range of relevant behaviors; though people differ in their average standing on these dispositions, there is a great deal of intraindividual variability. Such dispositions, primarily "personality characteristics that have no clear skill component" (Reeder & Brewer, 1979, p. 70)—for example, traits such as "friendly"—are related to behavior with a "partially restrictive schema." Behavior is partially but not totally restricted by one's standing on some dispositional continuum. On the other hand, other attributes are inferred with a "hierarchically restrictive schema," in which dispositional levels at the upper extreme of a continuum are not restricted while those at lower levels are. Moral and ability attributes are the best examples. In order to turn in a stellar performance of some sort, one must have the ability to do so, but a poor or mediocre performance is less diagnostic;

anyone can have a bad day. Similarly, moral people are not expected to engage in dishonest behavior, whereas even the most detestable person can occasionally be expected to do something virtuous. One implication of this model is that less normative (e.g., "brilliant") and more undesirable (e.g., "selfish") traits are easier to instantiate. Similar predictions were made by Jones and Davis (1965).

Rothbart and Park (1986) assessed the relationship between behavioral evidence and trait inferences for a wide range of trait concepts. Subjects gave answers to the question, "How many confirming behaviors would a person have to engage in before you would consider this trait to be an accurate description of that person?" Confirmability correlated most strongly with subjective favorability of the trait. More favorable traits ("honest," "faithful") required more occasions for instantiation than unfavorable traits ("hostile," "humorless"), and were also easier to disconfirm. However, there was no relationship between confirmability and the judged frequency of a trait once favorability was partialed out, and high-ability traits (a class of mental dispositions) did not display the "easy to confirm–hard to disconfirm" pattern suggested by Reeder and Brewer and other attribution theorists. Funder and Dobroth (1987; see also Funder & Colvin, 1988), using a similar procedure, derived a "visibility" index from the set of rating dimensions used by Rothbart and Park. Traits relating to extraversion were judged by subjects to be the most visible, and these traits were also the ones that yielded the most interjudge agreement when applied to people known by the subjects.

Another factor some have noted as a moderator of the behavior–trait link is "category breadth" (Hampson et al. 1986). Broader, less concrete traits are associated with a relatively large and diverse set of behaviors with looser boundaries, whereas more concrete traits are more clearly linked with prototypical behaviors. Pryor, McDaniel, and Kott-Russo (1986) make a similar point, though they call this dimension "abstractness," which they define as "the generality of behavioral descriptions" (p. 315). Pryor et al., using both speeded classifications and recall tasks, found that subjects classified behaviors more easily in terms of concrete ("uses money wisely") than abstract ("practical") schemata. It should be pointed out, however, that Rothbart and Park's data show that in the set of traits they studied, neither of the measures that arguably resemble abstractness (ease of imagining confirming–disconfirming behaviors) correlated with the confirmability measure, though this may have been due to a restricted range of concepts; few if any of the trait terms they examined were as concrete as "spends money wisely." A separate issue, of course, is the level at which behaviors are generally classified in everyday interaction. "Keith Larsen clips coupons from the paper" (one of Pryor et al.'s stimulus sentences) may be classified more easily in terms of "spends money wisely" than "practicality," but could probably be classified even more easily in terms of the more concrete "uses scissors." But we doubt that one would spontaneously encode this behavior at such a concrete level. As stated above, the evidence for the importance of trait concepts implicates them as the most typical level of behavior and person classification.

Spontaneous Trait Inference and Confirmability

Allen and Ebbesen (1981) reported results indicating that target actors' standings on abstract traits—in this case, defined as those less likely to "be confirmed by watching a person engage in a single behavior" (p. 129)— needed to be computed from stored behavioral information, whereas less abstract traits seemed to be rather quickly judged on the basis of some "stored global representation" of the behavior (the nature of which they left unspecified). From our perspective, these results suggest that some traits will be more likely to be spontaneously inferred than others—specifically, those traits scoring low on Rothbart and Park's (1986) "number to confirm" measure, which Allen and Ebbesen's measure of abstractness closely resembles.

A post hoc analysis of data from a recent study of ours (Uleman et al. 1987) provides tentative support for this hypothesis. The paradigm was similar to that described by Winter et al. (1985). Subjects read behavorial exemplars of traits while working on digit recall tasks of varying difficulty, and then performed a surprise cued-recall task. Of the 16 traits we used, 13 could either be found on Rothbart and Park's list or were synonyms of traits they studied. The amount of sentence recall cued by each trait correlated $-.46$ with the "number of instances to confirm" measure, meaning that trait-cued recall was highest for those traits that required relatively few behaviors to confirm. If one considers only the conditions where there appeared to be enough available cognitive capacity for trait inferences to occur, then the correlation was .51 ($p < .05$). Research designed to more directly examine the relationship between spontaneous inference and various trait dimensions (confirmability, visibility) and other characteristics (the mental–behavioral distinction, relevance to extraversion) is currently being planned.

WHAT MIGHT SPONTANEOUS TRAIT INFERENCES AFFECT?

All of the research on spontaneous trait inferences to date concerns the conditions under which they occur, particularly in terms of people's goals and concurrent cognitive load (see "Trait Inference Processes in Social Psychology," above). Is there any evidence that spontaneous trait inferences affect social behaviors or judgments? Specifically, (1) can spontaneous trait inferences have effects on conscious decisions and behavior that are undetected and unintentional? Or (2) are they merely the results of a hypothetical processing stage, and either lost without any practical effect if there is no relevant conscious processing goal, or taken as input for conscious decision processes where they are critically examined anyway? If (2) is the case, why do they matter, since the cognitive output should be the same with or without them? If (1) is the case, isn't there at least some indirect evidence of them in research on other phenomena?

Of course, we are most interested in the possibility that (1) is the case—that spontaneous trait inferences can have undetected and unintentional effects on social judgments and behavior. But we know of no research that directly tests or demonstrates this. So in this section, we offer some clues we think can be found in other research programs—indications that spontaneous trait inferences may have a heretofore unrecognized role in social judgments and behavior. Because the research we describe was not designed with spontaneous trait inferences in mind, it is important to remember that any evidence is indirect and that the interpretations are speculative. In several cases, we can only describe phenomena that may involve spontaneous inferences, describe how the evidence is not inconsistent with that idea, and encourage future research that will look at this issue directly.

Spontaneous Trait Inferences about the Self

Self-perception undoubtedly depends on a variety of processes, including conscious expectancies and intentions, and biased retrieval from memory. Most self-perception studies offer no evidence regarding a possible role for spontaneous inferences. But Fazio, Effrein, and Falender (1981) have provided evidence that is at least consistent with unintended and nonconscious inferences about the self. They induced self-perceptions of introversion or extraversion by interviewing 42 subjects with biasing questions (e.g., "What things do you dislike about loud parties?" or "What would you do if you wanted to liven things up at a party?", respectively) developed by Snyder and Swann (1978). Immediately after the interview, subjects described themselves on 10 bipolar trait scales related to introversion–extraversion and then interacted with a confederate for 10 minutes. As expected, their responses to the interview questions were biased, as were their subsequent self-descriptions. And this bias carried over to their interaction with the confederate in a waiting room. The biased interview apparently induced changes in self-perceptions, which changed both conscious self-descriptions and behavior.

To what extent were these changes in self-perceptions intentional and conscious? Unfortunately, subjects were not questioned about this, so we have no direct evidence. It is possible, for example, that subjects were surprised by some of their own answers, and engaged in conscious self-reflection and reassessment during the interview. It is also possible that the interview's effects on subsequent interactions did not depend on any revision in self-perceptions, conscious or not (both possibilities noted by R. H. Fazio, personal communication, Dec. 2, 1987). However, the most interesting and plausible possibility for us is that subjects did revise their self-perceptions in response to the interview, were unaware of doing so, and were then affected by these revisions in their interview behavior.

If one adopts the working hypothesis that the interview prompted spontaneous revisions in self-perceptions (unintended and nonconscious, by definition), the next issue is whether these revisions affected interactions with the confederate directly. Or did their effects depend on self-perceptions becoming conscious and explicit in the self-description task? Two kinds of evidence indicate that their effects did *not* depend on revisions becoming explicit. First, Fazio et al. (1981) reported that "partialling out self-description scores reduces the correlation between interview responses and later behavior from .497 to a still statistically significant .398 ($p <$ .02)" (p. 239). In other words, the conscious self-descriptions did not capture much of the assumed self-perception revision engendered by the biased interview; moreover, they apparently did not have to, for that revision to affect behavior. This finding is also consistent with our supposition that the revision was not conscious. Second, the order of self-descriptions and interactions was counterbalanced; some subjects interacted with the confederate before the self-description task, so it could not have affected the interaction. There was no significant order effect on either self-descriptions or interactions (pp. 237–238).

Thus, the biased interviews' effects on interactions with the confederate were not mediated by or dependent on the self-description task, performed intentionally and consciously. Spontaneously revised self-perceptions during the biased interview offer one possible explanation of these effects that merits investigation.

One of the most interesting self-perception phenomena is the perseverance of a newly acquired self-concept after the evidence for it has been discredited. Ross, Lepper, and Hubbard, (1975) and Lepper, Ross, and Lau (1986) have employed materials that seem ideal for triggering spontaneous self-descriptions (of ability to detect genuine suicide notes and of math aptitude, respectively). Unfortunately, the relevant self-descriptions were elicited from subjects explicitly, so we do not know whether they would have occurred spontaneously, or whether spontaneous self-descriptions would show such strong perseverance effects.

However, there is evidence that belief perseverance occurs in part because people spontaneously generate explanations for their beliefs. Anderson (1983, Experiment 2) asked subjects to "discover relationships between personal characteristics and behavioral outcomes" in information about firefighter trainees' risk preferences and their subsequent job success. Immediately after subjects estimated the strength of the relationship, three self-reports of their thoughts were obtained and scored for causal thinking.

More causal thinking was associated with greater subsequent belief perseverance in the face of information discrediting. It is unlikely that these causal thoughts have to be explicit for perseverance to occur, because Experiment 1 did not elicit them explicitly and yet obtained the same perseverance effects. More recently, Anderson, New, and Speer (1985) showed that individual difference in the implicit availability of causal thoughts is an important mediator of belief perseverance. What is not clear is whether the instruction to "discover relationships" is necessary for spontaneous causal thoughts to occur. Whether it is or not, discovering relationships does not require causally explaining them. This seems to occur spontaneously.

Self-Fulfilling Prophecies and Spontaneous Trait Inferences

Do self-fulfilling prophecies require conscious goals and beliefs, and does behavioral disconfirmation require an intentional cost–benefit analysis? Miller and Turnbull's (1986) choice of terms in discussing these processes suggests a fairly high degree of awareness and intentional analyses of social situations, even though they never address this issue directly. For example, "Which prophecy effect will emerge depends on both how *perceivers react to their expectancies* and how targets react to the behavior of perceivers" (p. 243, italics added). Among "the many factors that probably moderate the [perceiver's] expectancy–behavior link are (a) the perceiver's *interaction goals* . . . and (b) the perceiver's *belief in the target's modifiability*" (p. 239, italics added). Furthermore, when "the costs associated with disconfirmation are greater than those associated with confirmation, targets can be expected to be *reluctant to challenge* the perceiver's false expectancy. When the balance of costs and rewards are reversed, targets can be expected to *attempt disavowal*" (p. 243, italics added).

The same is true of Darley and Fazio's (1980) model of social interactions that produce self-fulfilling prophecies (see also Deaux & Major, 1987). Four of its six components are described in terms that seem to imply conscious characterizations of someone's behavior, though again the question is never explicitly addressed and the implication may be unintended. These six components are "(a) a perceiver's formation of an *expectancy* about a target person, (b) his or her behavior congruent with the expectancy, (c) the target's *interpretation* of this behavior, (d) the target's response, (e) the perceiver's *interpretation* of the response, and (f) the target's *interpretation* of his or her own response" (p. 867, italics added). Similarly, in discussing their elegant demonstration of compensatory strategies that produce behavioral disconfirmation, Ickes, Patterson, Rajecki, and Tanford (1982) "assumed that compensation occurs when the perceiver (1) *views* the target's anticipated behavior as undesirable, but (2) *believes* that it is modifiable via the norm of reciprocity, and (3) *is aware of* and *willing* and able to display a contrasting pattern of behavior that, if reciprocated by the target, would render the target's behavior more desirable" (p. 163, italics added).

We do not mean to imply that these theorists believe that these processes depend on intentionally formulated and conscious goals, expectancies, interpretations, and so on. Most would probably not take such a restrictive view. But their terms seem either to suggest this or to ignore the issue. Most of the research on these phenomena has provided subjects with explicit expectancies and sometimes explicit goals. And to the extent that conscious, intentional reasoning produces more firmly held expectancies, their effects are probably stronger (Swann & Ely, 1984). However, it is also possible that expectancies are often neither conscious nor intentional, yet have reliable effects. For example, Word, Zanna, and Cooper (1974) showed that white interviewers distanced themselves from black interviewees, and that interviewees who were treated in this way created a worse impression. Assuming that the white interviewers' interaction expectations were only implicit and their distancing behavior was unintentional, this suggests several important questions for future research. Which, if any, of the steps in self-fulfilling prophecies require conscious expectations or interpretations? Which steps require verbal mediation of any kind, conscious or nonconscious (cf. Friedman, 1967)? And are there differences between the effects of nonconscious rather than conscious expectancies, besides the obvious one that effects of nonconscious expectancies are less subject to self-correction?

Stereotype Confirmation and Spontaneous Trait Inferences

Slusher and Anderson (1987) showed that people may maintain their stereotypes by confusing self-generated imaginary evidence with actual confirmatory evidence. In their first experiment, subjects read sentences about occupational groups in particular settings (e.g., lawyers playing basketball in a local park) and described their images of the scenes. These images often included stereotypic traits (e.g., aggressive) when the context was relevant to the trait, but not otherwise. In Experiment 2, they read such sentences carefully for a subsequent memory test and imagined the scenes without describing them. The sentences contained roles, situations, and sometimes traits. Then they estimated the frequency with which traits were actually paired with occupational roles. Consistent with the imaginal confirmation hypothesis, they overestimated the frequency of actual pairings, apparently confusing the actual with the imaginary.

The relevance of spontaneous trait inferences to this phenomenon is obvious and important. The procedure was very similar to ours. Subjects read sentences that implied traits, under both a memory set as in Winter and Uleman (1984) and an "image set." And this combined set led to inferred traits that subjects confused with traits that were explicitly presented in other sentences. Apparently subjects were unaware of these inferences, or were unable to take them into account in judging actual frequencies. This similarity of spontaneous trait inferences to imaginal stereotype confirmation strongly suggests that the latter could be a special case of the former. What is not clear from available evidence is whether this effect depends on intentional imaging. Or might imaginal confirmation occur spontaneously? The literature on spontaneous trait inference suggests that it would, but this should be investigated directly.

There is another process that has been implicated in stereotype maintenance and that may also occur spontaneously, though there is not yet evidence directly relevant to this. Darley and Gross (1983) have shown that people can infer tentative trait expectancies or hypotheses without being willing to report them as impressions, and that these hypotheses can then influence the processing of subsequent nondiagnostic information so that it is interpreted as confirmatory. They asked subjects to help them test a "teachers' evaluation form" by using it to rate a white fourth-grade child on several academic variables, including abilities in liberal arts, reading and mathematics, and work habits. Half the subjects saw only a 6-minute film of Hannah playing in her neighborhood. The "negative-expectancy" version of this film was shot in a poor urban setting, and the "positive-expectancy" version was filmed in a prosperous suburban neighborhood. The other half of the subjects saw an additional 12-minute film of Hannah performing 25 achievement test problems with mixed success. The expectancy films had no effect on the ratings of those who did not see the performance film. But those who saw the performance film, which was the same for all subjects, rated her higher when their expectancy film was positive and lower when it was negative.

Darley and Gross suggest that sometimes "expectancies function as hypotheses, and the task of evaluating an individual for whom one has an expectancy is a hypothesis-testing process. Expectancy confirmation . . . occurs as the end product of an active process in which perceivers examine the labeled individual's behavior for evidence relevant to their hypothesis" (p. 28). Only subjects who saw the performance film found evidence to confirm their hypotheses, even though the film was entirely uninformative.

One might suppose that this process of hypothesis formation and confirmation is deliberate and conscious; subjects did have instructions and intentions to form an impression of Hannah. However, additional findings suggest that subjects were unaware that they had derived hypotheses from the two expectancy films. Manipulation checks at the end of the study showed that all subjects correctly identified Hannah's socioeconomic status, but they also indicated that it was "not useful" in rating her. Furthermore, those who did not see the performance film showed no expectancy effects in rating Hannah, even though elaborate and apparently effective steps were taken to eliminate demand characteristics and make it easy to anonymously rate her on the basis of tentative stereotypic hypotheses. Subjects could have "guessed," but they did not. Perhaps they were deliberately awaiting further "evidence," as Darley and Gross suggest. Or perhaps they were even unaware of having hypotheses at this point. Whenever they became aware of having hypotheses to test, they seemed to be unaware of their source.

The occurrence of spontaneous trait inferences raises the possibility of spontaneous trait hypotheses, which could then bias the processing of subsequent information to produce hypothesis confirmation. Such a possibility seems even more insidious than the one Darley and Gross describe, because it would occur without awareness of even the initial hypothesis. People's awareness of their initial hypotheses and their sources is an important topic for future research, particularly as it applies to stereotyping.

Vividness Effects and Spontaneous Inferences

Shedler and Manis (1986) examined relations among the vividness of stimuli, memory for those stimuli, and their impact on subsequent judgments. They predicted that more vivid stimuli would be better remembered and thereby influence judgments more, demonstrating the importance of the availability heuristic (Tversky & Kahneman, 1973) in mediating vividness effects. More vivid stimuli were better remembered and more important in judgments in their two studies, but path analyses showed that judgments were not mediated by memory differences.

In seeking a plausible explanation for these surprising results, Shedler and Manis suggested that "vivid information may have a disproportionate influence on human judgment because it evokes a rich associative network, which (in turn) is readily available when judgments are made" (1986, p. 35). That is, spontaneous elaborations may have occurred at encoding, particularly for vivid stimuli. These elaborations may have included information more relevant to making subsequent judgments than the stimuli themselves, and the elaborations rather than the stimuli may have been used to make judgments.

Shedler and Manis's tasks (and those of others they cited) seemed to involve not only spontaneous trait-like inferences, but also spontaneous elaborations relevant to frequency judgments and logical reasoning tasks. This suggests that such spontaneous elaborations may include using well-learned schemata that can facilitate subsequent social reasoning (e.g., Crockett, 1982).

Intentional Thought and Spontaneous Inferences

One might think that spontaneous inferences strongly affect the stream of thought and behavior because they enter it uninvited and unnoticed. On the other hand, they may be easily ignored for the same reasons and be without any effects whatever. That is, intentional thought may easily disrupt or override spontaneous inferences, so their effects may be fleeting and unstable. Several lines of research suggest this.

Hazlewood and Olson (1986) had subjects interact with and then rate a confederate, after they had seen the confederate act impolitely on videotape as part of a study of "impression formation and acquaintanceship." Before the interaction (which subjects did not anticipate), they were also casually given covariation information designed to indicate that the rude behavior was unique to the confederate or was a common response to the question she was asked. Half the subjects were then asked for explicit causal attributions for the rude behavior: Was it caused by something about her, or something about the question she was asked? Then they interacted with and rated her. Subjects who had *not* been asked for explicit causal attributions showed consistent effects of the covariation information on both their subsequent interactions with the confederate and their ratings of her. But those who had answered the causal attribution questions showed no such effects, on several behavioral and impression rating measures. Hazlewood and Olson note that causal and dispositional attributions are not the same thing (see above) and argue convincingly that "the explicit attribution question interfered with the effects of covariation information on some measures, presumably by introducing uncertainty about the actual cause of the stimulus event" (1986, p. 289).

Subjects in this study knew it concerned impression formation, and their initial inferences about the confederate were not spontaneous. Even so, they were apparently disrupted by causal attribution questions. This suggests that explicit reconsideration of initial as-yet-unexpressed impressions may disrupt them, if the reconsideration calls for a different perspective or set of considerations. We would predict that spontaneous impressions are at least as easily disrupted.

Apparently similar effects have been noted in the area of attitude–behavior consistency by Wilson (1985; Wilson & Dunn, 1986): Analyzing the reasons for feelings, rather than simply focusing on those feelings, reduces the consistency. Of course, this is but one aspect of a large and complex literature (e.g., Quattrone, 1985). A detailed examination of the possible role of spontaneous inferences in affecting consistencies between "cognition" and behavior is beyond the scope of this chapter. But recognizing a possible role for spontaneous inferences in these phenomena, and investigating them directly with recently developed techniques, may help clarify the conditions under which consistency will and will not occur.

SPONTANEOUS TRAIT INFERENCE: CAVEATS

Though the evidence presented here indicates that the extent to which we can control the interpretation and encoding of others' behavior in dispositional terms has been overestimated, one should keep in mind Ross's (1981) observation that "trait theorists are made and not born" (p. 28). The young American adults participating in our studies seemed to extract trait meaning naturally and effortlessly from our experimental stimuli. However, though spontaneous processes are surely universal, the *content* of such processes is a function of developmental level and cultural assumptions about the underlying causes of behavior.

As suggested by Rotenberg's (1982) study discussed above, there is some disagreement as to whether children younger than 7–8 years of age even understand the concept of the stable disposition (Shantz, 1983). Rholes and Ruble (1984) found that 5- to 6-year-olds did not base their predictions of other children's behavior on those children's past behaviors. For example, they were as likely to predict that a boy who had previously refused to share his lunch with a friend would behave generously as they were to predict the opposite. Older children (9- to 10-year-olds), on the other hand, almost always predicted trait-consistent behavior. These findings held up even when subjects were led to overtly label the actors' previous behaviors with appropriate trait terms. Young children's apparent lack of use of the trait information for prediction implies that they expect less consistency in others' behavior and do not understand trait terms to apply to stable, abiding characteristics of people. Rholes and Ruble's findings dovetail with other research showing that children of this age are much less likely to describe themselves and others in central or dispositional terms than are older children and adults (Livesley & Bromley, 1973; Peevers & Secord, 1973), and are less likely to describe recently witnessed behavioral episodes in such terms (Flapan, 1968). Thus, it is doubtful that young children spontaneously infer traits.

This suggests that our research has captured only one point on a developmental continuum. Sears (1986) notes that social psychology's reliance on college students as subjects may bias substantive conclusions. For example, relative to adults, adolescents do not have a very strong sense of self-definition. Perhaps by studying late adolescents we have overestimated the spontaneity of trait inference, for a preoccupation with defining attributes of the self might lead to such constructs' being more cognitively accessible (Higgins & King, 1981) and thus likely to "capture" witnessed behavior. There are no data relevant to this question. However, some evidence suggests that relative to children in late childhood/early adolescence, late adolescents are actually *less* likely to infer a stable disposition from behavior. Josephson (1977) tested subjects over a wide age range with a procedure similar to that of Rholes and Ruble (1984), and found that the tendency to generalize from past to future behavior peaked at about 11 years of age and declined thereafter. Barenboim (1981) found that starting at 12 years of age, the proportion of unqualified trait constructs used in free descriptions of others began to decline, and Block and Funder (1986) discovered that though the fundamental attribution error has been described as a social information-processing liability, the degree to which young adolescents were prone to overattribute behavior to dispositions correlated positively with social competence, good emotional adjustment,

and high self-esteem. In sum, preadolescents seem to be particularly ortho-
dox trait theorists. On the other hand, studies of the naive psychology of
undergraduates show that they appreciate situational influences on behavior and person × situation interactions (Allen & Smith, 1980; Epstein &
Teraspulsky, 1986; Zuroff, 1982). These findings suggest that the spontaneity of trait inference among preadolescents may be even greater than
among college students.

The developmental changes described here have been documented almost exclusively with North American and British subjects. That cross-
cultural consistency can be assumed is implicit in accounts of attributional
phenomena that are based on perceptual processes (e.g., the fundamental
attribution error and the actor–observer effect; Jones, 1979; Jones & Nisbett, 1971). Such explanations seem to leave little room for variability due
to cultural factors. Ross (1981), however, suggests that something about
Western culture and ideology may bias people toward a view that individuals take primacy over situations and are ultimately responsible for what
happens to them. Miller (1984) provides support for this idea. Whereas
her American subjects showed developmental increases in references to stable
dispositions when explaining others' behavior, an opposite pattern was
found for Hindus: References to situational factors increased with age.
Different "cultural conceptions of the person," Miller suggests, can lead
to differences in what is likely to be inferred from observed behavior. Once
again, though spontaneous processes and their nature are universal, their
content is not.

Finally, intracultural variability should be acknowledged. Some traits
are more likely to be inferred by some people than others. Individual differences in long-term construct accessibility (Higgins & King, 1981; Higgins, King, & Marvin, 1982) have been shown to determine the readiness
with which one will interpret behavior and encode it into memory in terms
of a particular trait construct. Higgins et al. (1982; see also Bargh, Bond,
Lombardi, & Tota, 1986) demonstrated that when a trait term appeared
frequently and early in a person's free descriptions of others, that trait
played a greater role in his or her impressions of a target person described
in ambiguous terms that included information moderately related to this
accessible trait. Uleman et al. (1986) found that high- and low-authoritarianism subjects reliably differed in their spontaneous interpretations of
various behaviors (see above). And Bargh and Thein (1985) further demonstrated that people need fewer attentional resources to process stimuli
relevant to their accessible constructs.

Therefore, though we have argued for the spontaneous use of trait
constructs in everyday social understanding, there are individual differences in the likelihood of behavior being classified as an exemplar of a
particular trait. This is an especially important consideration, for most behaviors are probably diagnostic of more than one trait (Borkeneau, 1986;
Reeder & Brewer, 1979). In other words, behaviors can be prototypical of

many or no traits—and, arguably, the former is the rule. Reeder and Brewer's (1979) model suggests that a behavior will be classified with respect to the trait for which it is the most prototypical, and that this will be followed by spreading of activation to related trait concepts. Future research should explore whether this is true of spontaneous trait inferences.

CONCLUSION

To some extent, then, our impressions of others are out of control. The ladies Lily is entertaining in *Henderson the Rain King* jump to spontaneous conclusions about Henderson's fidelity, though they might have stopped at simply characterizing his behavior. Or they might have gone on to explain it not in terms of Henderson's traits, but in terms of circumstances and social roles. People explaining their own behavior often do that (Jones & Nisbett, 1971), and that is what poor Henderson later does. But his interpretation of his wife's behavior, though qualified, is predictable:

> Because when I was brought home from the hospital in this same bloody heavy cast, I heard her saying on the telephone, "It was just another one of his accidents. He has them all the time but oh, he's so strong. He's unkillable." Unkillable! How do you like that! It made me very bitter. . . . I put an antagonistic interpretation on it, even though I knew better. (Below, 1958, pp. 9–10)

We all know better, but our inferences about behavior may not always reflect this knowledge.

ACKNOWLEDGMENTS

Preparation of this chapter was faciliated by National Institute of Mental Health Grant No. BSR 1 R01 MH43959 to the second author (J.U.) We are grateful to Craig Anderson, Russ Fazio, Dan Gilbert, Doug Hazlewood, Mel Manis, Randy Osborne, and Felicia Pratto for their generous comments and suggestions on all or part of this chapter. The views expressed in it are ours, however, and not necessarily theirs.

NOTES

1. They might be called "unintended inferences," except that this implies a preference for avoiding them, as if they were anticipated or controllable, as in "I didn't mean to do it; it was unintended." Thus, "unintended" is too specific a term. "Not intended" is more accurate but awkward.

REFERENCES

Allen, B. P., & Smith, G. F. (1980). Traits, situations, and their interaction as alternative "causes" of behavior. *Journal of Social Psychology, 111*, 99–104.

Allen, R. B., & Ebbesen, E. B. (1981). Cognitive processes in person perception: Retrieval of personality trait and behavioral information. *Journal of Experimental Social Psychology, 17*, 119–141.

Allport, G. W., & Odbert, H. S. (1936). Trait names: A psycholexical study. *Psychological Monographs: General and Applied, 47*(1, Whole No. 211).

Alston, W. P. (1975). Traits, consistency, and conceptual alternatives for personality theory. *Journal of the Theory of Social Behavior, 5*, 17–47.

Andersen, S. M., & Klatzky, R. L. (1987). Traits and social stereotypes: Levels of categorization in person perception. *Journal of Personality and Social Psychology, 53*, 235–246.

Anderson, C. A. (1982). Inoculation and counterexplanation: Debiasing techniques in the perseverance of social theories. *Social Cognition, 1*, 126–139.

Anderson, C. A. (1983). Abstract and concrete data in the perseverance of social theories: When weak data lead to unshakable beliefs. *Journal of Experimental Social Psychology, 19*, 93–108.

Anderson, C. A., New, B. L., & Speer, J. R. (1985). Argument availability as a mediator of social theory perseverance. *Social Cognition, 3*, 235–249.

Barenboim, C. (1981). The development of person perception from childhood to adolescence: From behavioral comparisons to psychological constructs to psychological comparisons. *Child Development, 52*, 129–144.

Bargh, J. A., Bond, R. N., Lombardi, W. L., & Tota, M. E. (1986). The additive nature of chronic and temporary sources of construct accessibility. *Journal of Personality and Social Psychology, 50*, 869–878.

Bargh, J. A., & Thein, R. D. (1985). Individual construct accessibility, person memory, and recall–judgment link: The case of information overload. *Journal of Personality and Social Psychology, 49*, 1129–1146.

Bassili, J. N., & Smith, M. C. (1986). On the spontaneity of trait attribution: Converging evidence for the role of cognitive strategy. *Journal of Personality and Social Psychology, 50*, 239–245.

Bellow, S. (1958). *Henderson the rain king.* New York: Avon.

Berry, D. S., & McArthur, L. Z. (1985). Some components and consequences of a babyface. *Journal of Personality and Social Psychology, 48*, 312–323.

Berscheid, E., Graziano, W., Monson, T., & Dermer, M. (1976). Outcome dependency: Attention, attribution, and attraction. *Journal of Personality and Social Psychology, 34*, 978–989.

Block, J., & Funder, D. C. (1986). Social roles and social perception: Individual differences in attribution and error. *Journal of Personality and Social Psychology, 51*, 1200–1207.

Borkeneau, P. (1986). Toward an understanding of trait interrelations: Acts as instances for several traits. *Journal of Personality and Social Psychology, 51*, 371–381.

Brown, R., & Fish, D. (1983). The psychological causality implicit in language. *Cognition, 14*, 237–273.

Buss, D. M., & Craik, K. H. (1983). The act frequency approach to personality. *Psychological Review, 90,* 105–126.

Buss, D. M., & Craik, K. H. (1984). Acts, dispositions, and personality. In B. A. Maher & W. B. Maher (Eds.), *Progress in experimental personality research* (Vol. 13, pp. 241–301). New York: Academic Press.

Cantor, N., & Mischel, W. (1979). Prototypes in person perception. In L. Berkowitz (Ed.), *Advances in experimental social psychology* (Vol. 12, pp. 3–52). New York: Academic Press.

Carlston, D. E., & Skowronski, J. J. (1986). Trait memory and behavior memory: The effects of alternative pathways on impression judgment response times. *Journal of Personality and Social Psychology, 50,* 5–13.

Chaplin, W. F., John, O. P., & Goldberg, L. R. (1988). Conceptions of states and traits: Dimensional attributes with ideals as prototypes. *Journal of Personality and Social Psychology, 54,* 541–557.

Crocker, J., Hannah, D. B., & Weber R. (1983). Person memory and causal attributions. *Journal of Personality and Social Psychology, 44,* 55–66.

Crockett, W. H. (1982). Balance, agreement, and positivity in the cognition of small social structures. In L. Berkowitz (Ed.), *Advances in experimental social psychology* (Vol. 15, pp. 1–57). New York: Academic Press.

Darley, J. M., & Fazio, R. H. (1980). Expectancy confirmation processes arising in the social interaction sequence. *American Psychologist, 35,* 867–881.

Darley, J. M., & Gross, P. H. (1983). A hypothesis-confirming bias in labeling effects. *Journal of Personality and Social Psychology, 44,* 20–33.

Deaux, K., & Major, B. (1987). Putting gender into context: An interactive model of gender-related behavior. *Psychological Review, 94,* 369–389.

Eiser, J. R. (1983). Attribution theory and social cognition. In J. Jaspers, F. Fincham, & M. Hewstone (Eds.), *Attribution theory and research: Conceptual, developmental, and social dimensions* (pp. 91–113). London: Academic Press.

Epstein, S., & Teraspulsky, L. (1986). Perception of cross-situational consistency. *Journal of Personality and Social Psychology, 50,* 1152–1160.

Fazio, R. H., Effrein, E. A., & Falender, V. J. (1981). Self-perceptions following social interaction. *Journal of Personality and Social Psychology, 41,* 232–242.

Feldman, N. S., & Ruble, D. N. (1981). The development of person perception: Cognitive and social factors. In S. M. Kassin & F. K. Gibbons (Eds.), *Developmental social psychology* (pp. 191–206). New York: Oxford University Press.

Fiedler, K., & Semin, G. R. (1988). On the causal information conveyed by different interpersonal verbs: The role of implicit sentence context. *Social Cognition, 6,* 21–39.

Fiske, S. T., & Cox, M. G. (1979). Person concepts: The effect of target familiarity and descriptive purpose on the process of describing others. *Journal of Personality, 47,* 136–161.

Flapan, D. (1968). *Children's understanding of social interaction.* New York: Teachers College Press.

Fletcher, G. J. O. (1984). Psychology and common sense. *American Psychologist, 39,* 203–213.

Friedman, N. (1967). *The social nature of psychological research: The psychological experiment as a social interaction.* New York: Basic Books.

Funder, D. C., & Colvin, C. R. (1988). Friends and strangers: Acquaintanceship, agreement, and the accuracy of personality judgment. *Journal of Personality and Social Psychology, 55,* 149–158.

Funder, D. C., & Dobroth, K. M. (1987). Differences between traits: Properties associated with interjudge agreement. *Journal of Personality and Social Psychology, 52,* 409–418.

Garvey, C., & Caramazza, A. (1974). Implicit causality in verbs. *Linguistic Inquiry, 5,* 459–464.

Gilbert, D. T., & Jones, E. E. (1986). Perceiver-induced constraint: Interpretations of self-generated reality. *Journal of Personality and Social Psychology, 50,* 269–280.

Gilbert, D. T., Krull, D. S., & Pelham, B. W. (1987). *Of thoughts unspoken: Social inference and the self regulation of behavior.* Unpublished manuscript, University of Texas at Austin.

Gilbert, D. T., Pelham, B. W., & Krull, D. S. (1988). On cognitive busyness: When person perceivers meet persons perceived. *Journal of Personality and Social Psychology, 54,* 733–740.

Goldberg, L. R. (1981). Language and individual differences: The search for universals in personality lexicons. In L. Wheeler (Ed.), *Review of personality and social psychology* (Vol. 2, pp. 141–165). Beverly Hills, CA: Sage.

Greenberg, M. S., Saxe, L., & Bar-Tal, D. (1978). Perceived stability of trait labels. *Personality and Social Psychology Bulletin, 4,* 59–62.

Hampson, S. E., John, O. P., & Goldberg, L. R. (1986). Category breadth and hierarchical structure in personality: Studies of asymmetries in judgments of trait implications. *Journal of Personality and Social Psychology, 51,* 37–54.

Harvey, J. H., Yarkin, K. L., Lightner, J. M., & Town, J. P. (1980). Unsolicited interpretation and recall of interpersonal events. *Journal of Personality and Social Psychology, 38,* 551–568.

Hastie, R., & Kumar, P. A. (1979). Person memory: Personality traits as organizing principles in memory for behavior. *Journal of Personality and Social Psychology, 37,* 25–38.

Hayden, T., & Mischel, W. (1976). Maintaining trait consistency in the resolution of behavioral inconsistency: The wolf in sheep's clothing? *Journal of Personality, 13,* 141–154.

Hazlewood, J. D., & Olson, J. M. (1986). Covariation information, causal questioning, and interpersonal behavior. *Journal of Experimental Social Psychology, 22,* 276–291.

Higgins, E. T., & King, G. A. (1981). Accessibility of social constructs: Information processing consequences of individual and contextual variability. In N. Cantor & J. Kihlstrom (Eds.), *Personality, cognition, and social interaction* (pp. 69–121). Hillsdale, NJ: Erlbaum.

Higgins, E. T., King, G. A., & Marvin, G. H. (1982). Individual construct accessibility and subjective impressions and recall. *Journal of Personality and Social Psychology, 43,* 35–47.

Higgins, E. T., Strauman, T., & Klein, R. (1986). Standards and the process of self-evaluation: Multiple affects from multiple stages. In R. M. Sorrentino & E. T. Higgins (Eds.), *Handbook of motivation and cognition* (pp. 23–63). New York: Guilford Press.

Ickes, W., Patterson, M. L., Rajecki, D. W., & Tanford, S. (1982). Behavioral and

cognitive consequences of reciprocal versus compensatory responses to prein-
teraction expectancies. *Social Cognition, 1,* 160–190.

Jeffery, K. M., & Mischel, W. (1979). Effects of purpose on organization and
recall of information in person perception. *Journal of Personality 47,* 397–
419.

Johnson, J. T. (1986). The knowledge of what might have been: Affective and
attributional consequences of near outcomes. *Personality and Social Psychology Bulletin, 12,* 51–62.

Johnson, J. T., Jemmott, J. B., III, & Pettigrew, T. F. (1984). Causal attribution
and dispositional inference: Evidence of inconsistent judgments. *Journal of
Experimental Social Psychology, 20,* 567–585.

Jones, E. E. (1979). The rocky road from acts to dispositions. *American Psychologist, 34,* 107–117.

Jones, E. E., & Davis, K. E. (1965). From acts to dispositions: The attribution
process in person perception. In L. Berkowitz (Ed.), *Advances in experimental
social psychology* (Vol. 2, pp. 219–266). New York: Academic Press.

Jones, E. E., & McGillis, D. (1976). Correspondent inferences and the attribution
cube: A comparative reappraisal. In J. H. Harvey, W. J. Ickes, & R. F. Kidd
(Eds), *New directions in attribution research* (Vol. 1, pp. 389–420). Hillsdale,
NJ: Erlbaum.

Jones, E. E., & Nisbett, R. E. (1971). The actor and the observer: Divergent perceptions of the causes of behavior. In E. E. Jones, D. E. Kanouse, H. H.
Kelley, R. E. Nisbett, S. Valins, & B. Weiner (Eds.), *Attribution: Perceiving
the causes of behavior* (pp. 79–94). Morristown, NJ: General Learning Press.

Josephson, J. (1977). *The child's use of situational and personal information in
predicting the behavior of another.* Unpublished doctoral dissertation, Stan-
ford University.

Kelley, H. H. (1967). Attribution theory in social psychology. In D. Levine (Ed.),
Nebraska Symposium on Motivation (Vol. 15, pp. 192–238). Lincoln: University of Nebraska Press.

Kelley, H. H. (1973). The processes of causal attribution. *American Psychologist,
28,* 107–128.

Lepper, M. R., Ross, L., & Lau, R. R. (1986). Persistence of inaccurate beliefs
about the self: Perseverance effects in the classroom. *Journal of Personality
and Social Psychology, 50,* 482–491.

Livesley, W., & Bromley, D. (1973). *Person perception in childhood and adolescence.* Chichester, England: Wiley.

McArthur, L. Z., & Apatow, K. (1983–1984). Impressions of baby-faced adults.
Social Cognition, 2, 315–342.

McArthur, L. Z., & Baron, R. M. (1983). Toward an ecological theory of social
perception. *Psychological Review, 90,* 215–238.

Miller, D. T., Norman, S. A., & Wright, E. (1978). Distortion in person perception
as a consequence of the need for effective control. *Journal of Personality and
Social Psychology, 36,* 598–607.

Miller, D. T., & Turnbull, W. (1986). Expectancies and interpersonal processes.
Annual Review of Psychology, 37, 233–256.

Miller, F. D., Smith, E. R., & Uleman, J. S. (1981). Measurement and interpretation of situational and dispositional attributions. *Journal of Experimental Social Psychology, 17,* 80–95.

Miller, J. G. (1984). Culture and the development of everyday social explanation. *Journal of Personality and Social Psychology, 46,* 961–978.

Mischel, W. (1968). *Personality and assessment.* New York: Wiley.

Mischel, W. (1973). Toward a cognitive social learning reconceptualization of personality. *Psychological Review, 80,* 252–283.

Montepare, J. M., & McArthur, L. Z. (1987). Perceptions of adults with childlike voices in two cultures. *Journal of Experimental Social Psychology, 23,* 331–349.

Moskowitz, G. B., & Uleman, J. S. (1987, August). *The facilitation and inhibition of spontaneous trait inferences.* Paper presented at the annual convention of the American Psychological Association, New York.

Nisbett, R. E. (1980). The trait construct in lay and professional psychology. In L. Festinger (Ed.), *Retrospections on social psychology* (pp. 109–130). New York: Oxford University Press.

Nisbett, R. E., & Ross, L. (1980). *Human inference: Strategies and shortcomings of social judgment.* Englewood Cliffs, NJ: Prentice-Hall.

Peevers, B. H., & Secord, P. F. (1973). Developmental changes in attribution of descriptive concepts to persons. *Journal of Personality and Social Psychology, 27,* 120–128.

Pryor, J. B., McDaniel, M. A., & Kott-Russo, T. (1986). The influence of level of schema abstractness upon the processing of social information. *Journal of Experimental Social Psychology, 22,* 312–327.

Quattrone, G. A. (1985). On the congruity between internal states and action. *Psychological Bulletin, 98,* 3–40.

Read, S. J. (1987). Constructing causal scenarios: A knowledge structure approach to causal reasoning. *Journal of Personality and Social Psychology, 52,* 288–302.

Reeder, G. D. (1985). Implicit relations between dispositions and behaviors: Effects on dispositional attribution. In J. H. Harvey & G. Weary (Eds.), *Attribution: Basic issues and application* (pp. 87–116). New York: Academic Press.

Reeder, G. D., & Brewer, M. B. (1979). A schematic model of dispositional attribution in interpersonal perception. *Psychological Review, 86,* 61–79.

Reeder, G. D., & Fulks, J. L. (1980). When actions speak louder than words: Implicational schemata and the attribution of ability. *Journal of Experimental Social Psychology, 16,* 33–46.

Reeder, G. D., & Spores, J. M. (1983). The attribution of morality. *Journal of Personality and Social Psychology, 44,* 736–745.

Rholes, W. S., & Ruble, D. N. (1984). Children's understanding of dispositional characteristics of others. *Child Development, 55,* 550–560.

Ross, L. D. (1977). The intuitive psychologist and his shortcomings. In L. Berkowitz (Ed.), *Advances in experimental social psychology* (Vol. 10, pp. 173–220). New York: Academic Press.

Ross, L. D. (1981). The "intuitive scientist" formulation and its developmental implications. In J. H. Flavell & L. D. Ross (Eds.), *Social cognitive development* (pp. 1–42). Cambridge, England: Cambridge University Press.

Ross, L. D., Amabile, T. M., & Steinmetz, J. L. (1977). Social roles, social control, and biases in social perception. *Journal of Personality and Social Psychology, 35,* 485–494.

Ross, L. D., Lepper, M. R., & Hubbard, M. (1975). Perseverance in self-perception and social perception: Biased attributional processes in the debriefing paradigm. *Journal of Personality and Social Psychology, 32*, 880–892.

Ross, M., & Fletcher, G. J. O. (1985). Attribution and social perception. In G. Lindzey & E. Aronson (Eds.), *Handbook of social psychology* (Vol. 2, pp. 73–122). New York: Random House.

Rotenberg, K. J. (1982). Development of character constancy of self and other. *Child Development, 53*, 505–515.

Rothbart, M., & Park, B. (1986). On the confirmability and disconfirmability of trait concepts. *Journal of Personality and Social Psychology, 50*, 131–142.

Ryle, G. (1949). *The concept of mind.* New York: Barnes & Noble.

Sande, G. N., Goethals, G. R., & Radloff, C. E. (1988). Perceiving one's own traits and others': The multifaceted self. *Journal of Personality and Social Psychology, 54*, 13–20.

Schank, R. C., & Abelson, R. P. (1977). *Scripts, plans, goals and understanding: An inquiry into human knowledge structures.* Hillsdale, NJ: Erlbaum.

Sears, D. O. (1986). College sophomores in the laboratory: Influences of a narrow data base on social psychology's view of human nature. *Journal of Personality and Social Psychology, 51*, 515–530.

Semin, G. R., & Greenslade, L. (1985). Differential contributions of linguistic factors to memory-based ratings: Systematizing the systematic distortion hypothesis. *Journal of Personality and Social Psychology, 49*, 1713–1723.

Shantz, C. U. (1983). Social cognition. In J. H. Flavell & E. M. Markman (Vol. Eds.), *Handbook of child psychology* (4th ed.): *Vol. 3. Cognitive development* (pp. 495–555). New York: Wiley.

Shedler, J., & Manis, M. (1986). Can the availability heuristic explain vividness effects? *Journal of Personality and Social Psychology, 51*, 26–36.

Slusher, M. P., & Anderson, C. A. (1987). When reality monitoring fails: The role of imagination in stereotype maintenance. *Journal of Personality and Social Psychology, 52*, 653–662.

Smith, E. R., & Miller, F. D. (1983). Mediation among attributional inferences and comprehension processes: Initial findings and a general method. *Journal of Personality and Social Psychology, 44*, 492–505.

Snyder, M., & Swann, W. B., Jr. (1978). Hypothesis testing processes in social interaction. *Journal of Personality and Social Psychology, 36*, 1202–1212.

Swann, W. B., Jr., & Ely, R. J. (1984). A battle of wills: Self-verification versus behavioral confirmation. *Journal of Personality and Social Psychology, 46*, 1287–1302.

Trope, Y. (1986). Identification and inferential processes in dispositional attribution. *Psychological Review, 93*, 239–257.

Tulving, E. E. (1983). *Elements of episodic memory.* New York: Oxford University Press.

Tulving, E. E., & Thomson, D. M. (1973). Encoding specificity and retrieval processes in episodic memory. *Psychological Bulletin, 30*, 352–373.

Tversky, A., & Kahneman, D. (1971). Belief in the law of small numbers. *Psychological Bulletin, 76*, 105–110.

Tversky, A., & Kahneman, D. (1973). Availability: A heuristic for judging frequency and probability. *Cognitive Psychology, 5*, 207–232.

Uleman, J. S. (1987). Consciousness and control: The case of spontaneous trait inferences. *Personality and Social Psychology Bulletin, 13*, 337–354.

Uleman, J. S., Newman, L. S., & Winter, L. (1987). *Making spontaneous trait inferences uses some cognitive capacity at encoding.* Unpublished manuscript, New York University.

Uleman, J. S., Winborne, W. C., Winter, L., & Shechter, D. (1986). Personality differences in spontaneous personality inferences at encoding. *Journal of Personality and Social Psychology, 51,* 396–403.

Weiner, B. (1985). "Spontaneous" causal thinking. *Psychological Bulletin, 97,* 74–84.

Wilson, T. D. (1985). Strangers to ourselves: The origins and accuracy of beliefs about one's own mental states. In J. H. Harvey & G. Weary (Eds.), *Attribution: Basic issues and applications* (pp. 9–36). New York: Academic Press.

Wilson, T. D., & Dunn, D. S. (1986). Effects of introspection on attitude–behavior consistency: Analyzing reasons versus focusing on feelings. *Journal of Experimental Social Psychology, 22,* 249–263.

Wimer, S., & Kelley, H. H. (1982). An investigation of the dimensions of causal attribution. *Journal of Personality and Social Psychology, 43,* 1142–1162.

Winter, L., & Uleman, J. S. (1984). When are social judgments made? Evidence for the spontaneousness of trait inferences. *Journal of Personality and Social Psychology, 47,* 237–252.

Winter, L., Uleman, J. S., & Cunniff, C. (1985). How automatic are social judgments? *Journal of Personality and Social Psychology, 49,* 904–917.

Word, C. O., Zanna, M. P., & Cooper, J. (1974). The nonverbal mediation of self-fulfilling prophecies in interracial interaction. *Journal of Experimental Social Psychology, 10,* 109–120.

Wyer, R. S., Jr., & Carlston, D. E. (1979). *Social cognition, inference, and attribution.* Hillsdale, NJ: Erlbaum.

Wyer, R. S., Jr., & Srull, T. K. (1986). Human cognition in its social context. *Psychological Review, 93,* 322–359.

Zuroff, D. C. (1982). Person, situation, and person-by-situation interaction components in person perception. *Journal of Personality, 50,* 1–14.

Zuroff, D. C. (1986). Was Gordon Allport a trait theorist? *Journal of Personality and Social Psychology, 51,* 993–1000.

6

Thinking Lightly about Others: Automatic Components of the Social Inference Process

DANIEL T. GILBERT

University of Texas at Austin

We cannot avoid referring to psychic activities and the laws that govern them . . . [but] we might run the risk of losing our hold of established facts and of not adhering steadily to a method founded on clear well-recognized principals [sic].

—Herman von Helmholtz (1910/1925, p. 1)

With this caveat, the hard-nosed Helmholtz grudgingly took his first steps into the realm of mentalism, where he dwelled for a mere 35 pages before returning once more to the safe and familiar world of optical physiology and established facts. But during his brief foray, Helmholtz described a concept that would anger, excite, and inspire mentalists for a century to come: the *umbewusster Schluss,* or unconscious inference.[1]

By insisting that unconscious inferential activity is a prerequisite of simple visual perception, Helmholtz offered a proposition with far-reaching implications: Human beings engage in involuntary mental activities of which they can never be aware, and these activities are the necessary antecedents of conscious experience. By and large, Helmholtz limited his claim to visual perception, but most modern theorists would agree that the construction of precepts, cathedrals, and omelettes all require the occurrence of unconscious inferential operations. Helmholtz presaged many current thinkers not only by postulating the existence of such operations, but also by describing their general features.

According to Helmholtz, unconscious inferential processes are unique in that (1) they are triggered by the environment rather than by volition (their products "are urged on our consciousness, so to speak, as if an external power had constrained us, over which our will has no control"); (2) they are obscured from conscious awareness (they "never once can be elevated to the plane of conscious judgments," and thus their product "strikes our consciousness as a foreign and overpowering force of nature"); (3) they are routine and computational, rather than insightful or creative (they "lack the purifying and scrutinizing work of conscious thinking"); and (4) they are relatively impervious to conscious control or disruption (their products are "irresistible" and "impossible to get rid of," and "the effect of them cannot be overcome"; Helmholtz, 1910/1925, pp. 26–27). Today, Helmholtz's *umbewusster Schluss* would be recognized as the product of an automatic process, and although theorists have extended and refined the criteria for such processes, Helmholtz's suggestions have a surprisingly modern ring.

So what has social psychology to learn from this champion of the brass instrument? After all, Helmholtz is commonly remembered as the Sergeant Joe Friday of psychophysics, a devotee of hard facts and a critic of soft thinking, a pragmatic Teuton who surely would have scoffed at the study of person impressions and social judgments. Witness his prize example of unconscious inference:

> An actor who cleverly portrays an old man is for us an old man there on the stage, so long as we let the immediate impression sway us, and do not forcibly recall that the programme states that the person moving about there is the young actor with whom we are acquainted . . . and the deep-seated conviction that all this is only show and play does not hinder our emotions at all . . . (Helmholtz, 1910/1925, p. 28)

Clearly, Helmholtz was a catholic thinker who saw his ideas at work all around him, and his point here about social inference is really quite profound. Helmholtz argued that reading a person is, like reading a word, a largely involuntary and unconscious enterprise. Features of the actor's behavior (e.g., facial expression, speech, dress, demeanor) are unconsciously analyzed by the perceiver, and an inference about the actor's inner state pops into the perceiver's consciousness. "This person is happy and that one is cruel," we conclude on a daily basis, and yet we are hard pressed to explain just how such conclusions are achieved. Furthermore, and most important to the concerns of this chapter, we draw such conclusions even when we know they are wrong. As Helmholtz (1910/1925, p. 28) warned, "the tendency to abide by the false conclusions persists in spite of the better insight into the matter based on conscious deliberation."

OF STRAW MEN AND MANNEQUINS

It is probably fair to say that Helmholtz's ideas about the social inference process have exerted no impact whatsoever on social psychology. Rather, social psychology's cognitive landscape has been dominated by a pantheon of attributional theories (i.e., theories about how ordinary perceivers determine the causes of behavior), the most influential of which have been those of Jones and Davis (1965), Kelley (1967), and Bem (1972). For all their differences, these theories do share two general features.

First, each theory turns on Heider's (1958) distinction between "dispositional" and "situational" causation. Heider's fundamental insight was that perceivers consider behavior to be the joint product of the actor's enduring internal character traits and of vagrant external forces. Furthermore, Heider specified that to the extent that one of these causal agents is clearly effective, the status of the other must be indeterminate. Thus, for example, behavior executed in response to strong situational forces (e.g., a bribe or a threat) should be seen by ordinary perceivers as relatively uninformative with regard to the actor's character.

The second feature common to the attributional theories lies in what they neither claim nor do (nor claim they do). None is offered as a theory of mental events so much as a theory of mental logic; that is, each describes a set of rules or *procedures* by which an intelligent system (e.g., a person or a machine) might determine the causes of observed behaviors, but none attempts to describe the *processes* by which these procedures are executed. None specifies what actually happens when an attribution is made—which chutes drop open, which bells go "ding," which lights wink on and off.

Instead, these theories hang their inferential garments on a mannequin. They describe a dispassionate and rational perceiver who, after some deliberation, chooses either situational or dispositional explanations of behavior according to a well-explicated set of decision rules. This rational deliberator is not, of course, offered as a model of real psychological processes, but as a dummy—a device whose purpose is to display the wares that attributional theories have to sell. As Jones and McGillis (1976, p. 404) note, attribution theory "does not summarize phenomenal experience," but rather "presents a logical calculus in terms of which accurate inferences *could* be drawn by an alert perceiver" (italics added).

Attributional theories, then, do not tell us how social inferences are made any more than Euclid's axioms tell us how young kickball players bisect lines when carving up a play yard. And this deficit does not invalidate the attributional theories any more than it invalidates geometry; rather, it suggests that attributional theories provide an incomplete picture of the world and that a more complete picture is needed—one that includes the attributional theories in its canvas, but one that goes beyond their procedural concerns and addresses the issues of mental process. So what *do* we know about the process of social inference? Two things.

Becoming Unaware

Although attributional theories are not designed to elucidate psychological processes, this has not stopped some from trying to make them do the very work for which they are so poorly suited. Interestingly, though, by using attributional theories as straw men (i.e., by taking them to task for assumptions they do not really make), theorists have begun to develop a new and useful perspective on attributional issues.

Langer (1978) quite colorfully articulated a widespread discontent when she urged attribution theorists to "rethink the role of thought in social interaction." She pointed out that social inference is not always a conscious and deliberate act; rather, it is often the province of mindless automata. Attributional theories (according to Langer) have been too quick to assume that perceivers engage conscious processes in order to achieve their causal conclusions. This clarion call was widely appreciated, and if Langer did not quite set the stage for a psychology of unconscious social inference, she at least rented the theatre. The same might be said of those who abandoned the notion of inference altogether and adopted instead the so-called "ecological" or "Gibsonian" perspective (e.g., Kassin & Baron, 1985; McArthur & Baron, 1983; Newtson, 1980). These theorists, too, advocated a view of "social knowing" as something other than a conscious decision-making process.

While all of this was happening, experimental psychology was itself becoming unaware. Almost a century earlier, William James (1890, p. 163) had dismissed the unconscious as "the sovereign means for believing what one likes in psychology," and, indeed, the supernatural flavor of Freud's *Umbewusst* made the concept generally unpalatable to the emerging scientific discipline (cf. Erdelyi, 1985). However, when theorists such as LaBerge and Samuels (1974), Posner and Snyder (1975), Shiffrin and Schneider (1977), and Hasher and Zacks (1979) began to explicate the parameters of automatic, "off-line" processes in a computer-based vernacular, the ghost somehow fled the machine. All of this is to say that there has, in recent years, been a discernible shift in the wind: The role of awareness and control in the social inference process has been appropriately questioned, and the role of unconscious and unintentional processes has been approved for exploration. And this is the first thing we know.

Unwarping the Woof

By questioning the role of awareness in social inference, theorists have essentially asked at what place or level the social inference process occurs. But a process unfolds over time as well as in a conceptual place, and as such, it can often be decomposed into meaningful constituent events or chains of successive subprocesses. When we see big things happen, we should suspect that many little things are happening in a very particular order.

We are beginning to see that social inference is in fact just such a consortium of successive subprocesses. Quattrone (1982), for example, has shown that perceivers do not (as the attributional mannequin insists) make either–or decisions about situational or dispositional causation; rather, perceivers *first* draw dispositional inferences about others and *then* correct these inferences with information about the situational forces that may have coerced the other's action.Thus, perceivers do not ponder, "Did Arthur take the money because he is dishonest [dispositional causation], or because his friends pressured him to do so [situational causation]?" Rather, perceivers of such behavior first draw a dispositional inference ("Arthur is dishonest") and then correct this inference with information about the situational constraints on the actor ("But given that his friends pressured him to take the money, I guess he isn't *really* dishonest"). Causal attributions are the net result of a chain of events, and this is the second thing we know.

ONE-THIRD LESS EFFORT THAN REGULAR THINKING

Attributional theories have outlined the procedures by which the causal determinants of behavior may be appreciated, but have been silent with regard to the processes by which these procedures are enacted. However, two leads appear promising. First, the social inference process seems to be a chain of sequential subprocesses: *Characterization* (or dispositional inference) is followed by *correction* (or situational adjustment). Second, at least some of these subprocesses may be relatively effortless and unconscious. But which ones?

For the past few years, Doug Krull, Brett Pelham, and I have been trying to make a dent in just this sort of question: In what ways do the two major components of the social inference process (characterization and correction) qualitatively differ? That is, what *kinds* of processes are they? What must happen for them to unfold? What do they require and how are they controlled? A preliminary answer to these sorts of questions lies in Helmholtz's story of the young actor who portrays an old man. In that story, a perceiver is immediately taken by the actor's persona; the perceiver characterizes the "old man" on the stage in dispositional terms, and only later corrects this erroneous characterization by "forcibly recalling" that the old man is in fact a young actor.

A hypothesis is lurking just beneath the surface of this story: Could it be that characterization is a relatively automatic process that requires little effort or attention, whereas correction is a deliberate form of conscious reasoning that happens slowly and effortfully, if at all? Perhaps when we see others act, we draw dispositional inferences from their actions—even if we "know" that these actions are coerced and therefore inappropriate grounds for such inferences. And perhaps it is only *after* we have drawn these erroneous, but effortless, inferences of disposition that we are afforded an opportunity to correct them through the labor of reason.

What specific sorts of predictions might fall out of such a broad hypothesis? One hallmark of automatic processes is that they require scant "resources" (i.e., effort, attention, energy, consciousness, calories—choose one), and thus are not disrupted by concurrent processing demands; the automatic processes that enable depth perception do not desist, for example, when the individual is concurrently called upon to alphabetize some words, recite poetry, or play the piano. On the other hand, nonautomatic processes require significant resources and are therefore mutually debilitating; alphabetizing words and reciting poetry are, for most of us, activities done quite well alone but quite poorly in tandem.[2]

If characterization is a relatively automatic process, then it should be relatively impervious to disruption. Perceivers who find themselves short on cognitive resources should nonetheless be able to draw dispositional inferences from the behavior of others. However, because correction is not an automatic process, such perceivers should be *unable* to correct their characterizations with information about the situational constraints that conditioned the actor's behavior. As a result, these perceivers should be particularly likely to accept internal, dispositional accounts of others' externally caused behavior.

The "Sexual Fantasies" Experiment

We (Gilbert, Pelham, & Krull, 1988) sought to test this notion. In one experiment, subjects watched a videotape of a young woman (the target) engaged in conversation with a stranger. Subjects were not allowed to hear the conversation (concern for the target's privacy was offered as a rationale), but they were told what sorts of topics the woman and her strange partner had been assigned to discuss. In all conditions of the experiment, the target appeared generally anxious and distressed: She bit her nails, twirled her hair, tapped her fingers, and shifted in her chair from cheek to cheek.

Some subjects were led to believe that an external force had caused the target's apparent distress. These subjects were told that the woman had been asked to discuss with her strange partner several anxiety-provoking topics (e.g., her sexual fantasies). Clearly, a normal person could be expected to shift and tap in such a situation, and thus the target's anxious behavior should have told subjects in this "anxious-topics" condition relatively little about the target's dispositional anxiety level (i.e., her tendency to behave anxiously across situations). Other subjects were told a different story: Subjects in the "bland-topics" condition were told that the target was discussing with her strange partner several mundane topics (e.g., world travel). In this case, the target's behavioral anxiety should have been taken as a telling sign of character, and subjects should have confidently labeled the target as dispositionally anxious.

In other words, all subjects should have drawn dispositional inferences about the target ("She appears to be an anxious sort"). However, subjects in the anxious-topics condition should have then used the situational-constraint information (i.e., information about the topics) to correct these inferences ("But she was discussing some awfully anxiety-provoking topics, so maybe she is a *less* anxious person than she appears to be") and subjects in the bland-topics condition should have used the same information to correct their inferences ("Given that those topics were as bland as oatmeal, I bet she's actually a *more* anxious person than she appeared to be"). And that is, of course, just what subjects did. Subjects in the bland-topics condition considered the woman much more dispositionally anxious than did subjects in the anxious-topics condition.

More interesting were the judgments of a second set of subjects who were asked to do everything the first set did and one thing more. This new set of subjects was asked to rehearse some words while watching the film. We assumed that rehearsing words would usurp the subjects' cognitive resources, thus disabling the relatively effortful or controlled (but not the relatively effortless or automatic) component of the social inference process. The simple prediction was that these cognitively busy subjects would draw dispositional inferences from the target's anxious behavior, but would fail to correct these dispositional characterizations, because such a correction would require resources that the rehearsal task had already usurped. Thus, cognitively busy subjects should have concluded that the target was dispositionally anxious, *regardless* of the topics she was ostensibly discussing.

The reader will, I hope, have serious objections. After all, cognitively busy subjects were asked to rehearse some words while watching the film and then failed to use information about the topics that the woman was discussing. Isn't it entirely possible that these subjects were too busy rehearsing the words even to *notice* the topics? Perhaps they didn't *use* the situational constraint information simply because they didn't *have* it—and all this talk of resources and Helmholtz be damned!

In order to eliminate this possibility, we had subjects rehearse a very special set of words: the topics themselves. We made subjects cognitively busy by asking them to rehearse and memorize the situational-constraint information, and our prediction was that those subjects who were asked to rehearse and memorize the situational-constraint information would in fact be the least likely to use it. As Figure 6.1 shows, this is exactly what happened. When subjects were asked how dispositionally anxious they thought the target was, the judgments of cognitively busy subjects were

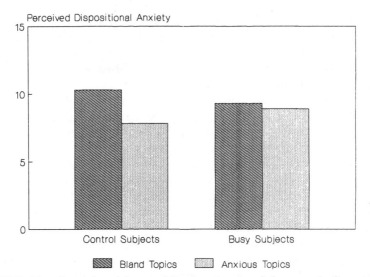

FIGURE 6.1. Control and busy subjects' estimates of the target's dispositional anxiety level. Adapted from "On Cognitive Busyness: When Person Perceivers Meet Persons Perceived" by D. T. Gilbert, B. W. Pelham, and D. S. Krull, 1988, *Journal of Personality and Social Psychology, 54,* p. 735. Copyright 1988 by the American Psychological Association. Adapted by permission.

virtually unaffected by the type of topic (anxious or bland) the target had ostensibly discussed—despite the fact that busy subjects had rehearsed this very information. Indeed, when subjects were finally asked to recall the discussion topics, busy subjects remembered them significantly *better* than did control subjects.

The "Preoccupied Listener" Experiment

These data are consistent with our hypothesis that the social inference process has both a relatively automatic and a relatively controlled component. Characterization appears to be less susceptible to disruption than correction, and thus, cognitively busy perceivers draw dispositional inferences from behaviors that are, in fact, situationally induced. Several experiments confirm and extend this conclusion. For example, in another experiment, we (Gilbert, Pelham, & Krull, 1988) asked subjects first to listen to a confederate (the reader) give either a pro- or an antiabortion speech, and then to estimate the reader's attitude toward abortion. Our subjects were told that the reader had been assigned to defend a particular position and that he had had no choice with regard to the position he defended (cf. Jones & Harris, 1967).

Some of our subjects merely heard the speech, and, as we expected, these subjects corrected their characterizations and concluded that the reader was only slightly pro- or antiabortion in the respective experimental conditions. However, a second set of subjects was given a "mental preoccupier." These subjects were also asked to listen to the speech, but in addition they were told that later they too would be assigned to give a speech on some political topic.

One might expect that these preoccupied subjects would be particularly sensitive to the constraints on the reader's behavior (given that they themselves would soon be experiencing similar constraints), and would therefore refrain from drawing dispositional inferences about the reader. Our prediction, however, was that these subjects would consciously ruminate about the upcoming speech-writing event. This preoccupation should have cost the subjects resources, thus disabling the relatively controlled (but not the relatively automatic) component of the social inference process. Thus, we expected these subjects to fail to correct their characterizations of the reader, and, as Figure 6.2 shows, they failed quite well.

The "Don't Look Now" Experiment

In both of the foregoing experiments, we decreased the cognitive resources that subjects could devote to social inference by giving them something extra to do. It occurred to us, however, that resources could also be decreased by giving subjects something extra *not* to do. As several theorists

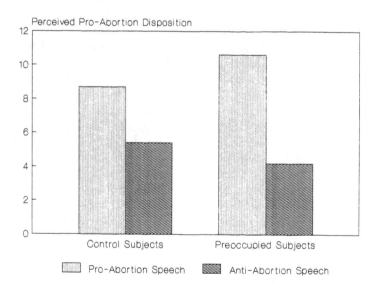

FIGURE 6.2. Control and preoccupied (busy) subjects' estimates of the speaker's attitude toward abortion. Adapted from "On Cognitive Busyness: When Person Perceivers Meet Persons Perceived" by D. T. Gilbert, B. W. Pelham, and D. S. Krull, 1988, *Journal of Personality and Social Psychology, 54,* p. 737. Copyright 1988 by the American Psychological Association. Adapted by permission.

have argued, the active inhibition of behavior is a form of cognitive work (Gray, 1975; Pennebaker & Chew, 1985; Wegner, Schneider, Carter, & White, 1987), and if our suggestions regarding the relative automaticity of the two inferential subprocesses were correct, then subjects who attempted to inhibit their actions should fail to adjust their dispositional inferences about others.

We (Gilbert, Krull, & Pelham, 1988) conducted an experiment that was in one sense similar to the "sexual fantasies" experiment described above. In this experiment, a woman (the target) appeared sad and depressed during a clinical interview; some subjects were told that she was answering sadness-inducing questions (e.g., "Describe a time when your parents made you feel unloved") and other subjects were told that the woman was answering happiness-inducing questions (e.g., "What is your fondest childhood memory?"). The obvious prediction was that all subjects would characterize the woman as dispositionally sad, but that subjects in the "sad-questions" condition would then correct that characterization ("She isn't as sad as she looks"), as would subjects in the "happy-questions" condition ("She's even sadder than she looks"). And, this was what they did.

However, the experimental procedure contained two noteworthy oddities. First, during the film, a one-syllable noun (e.g., "tree," "chair," "sky") would appear at the bottom of the screen, move upward toward the center of the screen, and then suddenly disappear. This oddity happened 38 times in the course of the 5-minute clinical interview. Subjects were forewarned that the words would appear and disappear (the rationale being that they were relevant to some other condition of the experiment), and they were told that they should feel free to ignore the words. The second oddity was that all subjects were told that their eye movements were being tracked and recorded by a "parafoveal optiscope," and that this was being done so that the experimenter could determine which parts of the target's face the subjects had spent the most time watching. Subjects were told not to worry about the presence of the eye-tracking device.

Why these oddities? Because a new group of subjects was not to be let off as easily as the controls. This new group of "self-regulating" subjects was given the same social inference task, but was additionally told that they should under no circumstances look at the disappearing words, because if they did, they would cause the parafoveal optiscope to "lose its alignment." Thus, whereas control subjects were told that they *need* not look at the disappearing words, self-regulating subjects were told that they *must* not look at the disappearing words. As the reader may suspect, these self-regulating subjects failed to correct their characterizations of the target. Figure 6.3 shows that self-regulating subjects considered the target to be just as dispositionally sad when she ostensibly answered sadness-inducing questions as when she ostensibly answered happiness-inducing questions. And although self-regulating subjects did not use the situational-

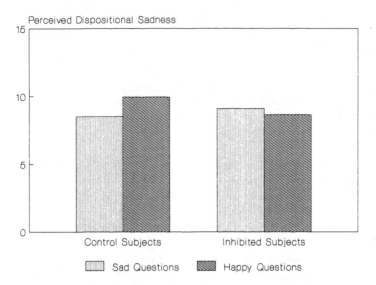

FIGURE 6.3. Control and self-regulating (busy) subjects' estimates of the inter-viewee's dispositional sadness. Adapted from *Of Thoughts Unspoken: Social In-ference and the Self-Regulation of Behavior* by D. T. Gilbert, D. S. Krull, and B. W. Pelham, 1988, *Journal of Personality and Social Psychology, 55,* p. 688. Copyright 1988 by the American Psychological Association. Adapted by permis-sion.

constraint information to adjust their inferences, they remembered that information quite well (just as well, in fact, as did control subjects).

The "Mr. Smile and Mr. Sneer" Experiment

In each of the experiments discussed so far, subjects were given some ar-tificial task to do or to refrain from doing, and we became curious about the natural conditions that might produce the effects we were finding with such regularity. It occurred to us that in the real world, perceivers often are cognitively busy because they are putting a dull edge on the truth. As every philanderer knows, telling a lie requires a great deal more effort and attention than does telling the truth, and thus we reasoned that an act of deception should be enough to change the inferences that deceptive per-ceivers draw about others.

Although people may rarely tell egregious lies, even a routine social interaction can include polite falsehoods, pointed omissions, and sanitized truths. It is, for example, commonplace for people to act nicely toward those whom they do not really like, and we (Gilbert et al., 1988) at-tempted to model this phenomenon in our laboratory. Two female subjects met a handsome male confederate in a waiting room. Sometimes the con-federate played the role of "Mr. Smile": He offered the subjects some gum, smiled and fawned, made polite inquiries about classes and friends, and so forth. At other times, the confederate played the role of "Mr. Sneer." He offered the subjects a lickerish grin and a few choice words, and then ignored them quite thoroughly—all of this simply to lead the subjects to like or dislike the confederate. (And they did.)

Next, one subject was asked to play the role of interviewer and another the role of observer, while the confederate played the role of interviewee. We asked the interviewer to interrogate the confederate with regard to his attitudes on several political issues, but explained (with appropriate rationale) that he would be constrained to read only the conservative answers that we had prepared. In addition, interviewers were asked to use nonverbal means to ingratiate the confederate as they interviewed him. They were asked to smile, lean forward, nod—anything to communicate liking for the confederate. Observers (who were fully informed of the interviewer's ingratiation instructions) were simply asked to watch this charade unfold.

Thus, interviewers heard a confederate read several politically conservative statements and, in addition, expressed positive feelings for the confederate via their nonverbal behavior. Of course, those subjects who interviewed Mr. Smile were expressing their true feelings, but those who interviewed Mr. Sneer were forced to do some effortful dissembling. Finally, all subjects estimated the confederate's true political attitudes. Our prediction was that interviewers would consider Mr. Sneer more politically conservative than Mr. Smile—simply because those who interviewed Mr.

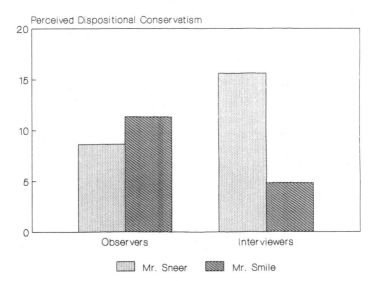

FIGURE 6.4.   Interviewers' and observers' estimates of the confederate's political orientation. Adapted from *Of Thoughts Unspoken: Social Inference and the Self-Regulation of Behavior* by D. T. Gilbert, D. S. Krull, and B. W. Pelham, 1988, *Journal of Personality and Social Psychology, 55*, p. 690. Copyright 1988 by the American Psychological Association. Adapted by permission.

Sneer should have been making a conscious effort to disguise their true feelings and to express false ones. This effortful task should have rendered Mr. Sneer's interrogator unable to correct the conservative characterization she made.

Of course, it is entirely possible that nasty people are simply considered more politically conservative than are nice people, and that our predictions would be borne out for this rather uninteresting reason. (We chose to have the confederate read conservative statements because we suspected that our Texan subjects would, if anything, more readily equate nastiness with liberalism.) But a moment's reflection should convince the reader that the presence of observers controlled for this possibility. We predicted that interviewers would consider Mr. Sneer to be more conservative than Mr. Smile, but that observers (who liked or disliked the confederate just as much as the interviewers did, but who were not required to ingratiate him) would consider Mr. Sneer and Mr. Smile equally conservative. As Figure 6.4 shows, this is just what we found. (The apparent reversal for observers was not statistically significant.)

SOME BEHAVIORS ARE MORE EQUAL THAN OTHERS

These experiments tell a short story: Characterization is relatively unaffected by concurrent processing demands, but correction is readily impaired by tasks as varied as ingratiating a lout, not moving one's eyeballs, memorizing some words, and thinking about the future. (Just for the record, intense squinting and chanting a phone number seem to have similar effects.) These experiments, in conjunction with other recent evidence (e.g., Uleman, 1987; Winter & Uleman, 1984; Winter, Uleman, & Cunniff, 1985) provide strong support for our contention that people are easily swayed by "immediate impressions," and must perform conscious work to "forcibly" correct these impressions when they are wrong.

By decomposing the social inference process, we have been able to make a first stab at describing some features of its component processes; we have identified, so to speak, various bells that go "ding" and have learned how much work each dinging requires. Thus, it did not strike us as overly optimistic to expect that we might learn something more by taking the first of these processes (characterization) further to pieces.

Up to this point, we had considered drawing dispositional inferences from behavior to be a relatively fuel-efficient process. But all behaviors are not equally easy to analyze, and it occurred to us that fewer resources might be required to draw dispositional inferences from nonverbal than from verbal behavior. This hypothesis seemed plausible for several reasons. First, nonverbal behavior is structurally simpler than is verbal behavior: Whereas a sentence is like a motion picture that requires the cognitive integration of discrete elements over time, a gesture or expression is like a still photograph that may be apprehended in a single optical gulp. Second, at both the ontogenetic and phylogenetic levels, people have greater experience in drawing inferences from nonverbal than from verbal behavior: Babies, cats, and primitives can decipher a coo but not a codex. Thus we hypothesized that although characterization is in general a relatively automatic process, characterizations from nonverbal behavior may be *more* automatic than characterizations from verbal behavior.

The "Hungry Chameleon" Experiment

Our initial investigation of this hypothesis turned on the fact that job seekers are often needy enough to overstate their qualifications by claiming to possess whatever attributes the prospective employer suggests are appropriate. We (Gilbert & Krull, 1988) created films of two job interviews: In one film an interviewer told an applicant that the job of laboratory coordinator required someone who was quite extraverted, and the applicant quickly claimed to be an extravert ("Boy, do I love crowds!"). In the other film the interviewer explained that an introvert was needed to fill the job of library researcher, and the applicant promptly claimed to be that introvert ("Boy, do I love closets!").

The most important feature of these films was that the applicants dif-

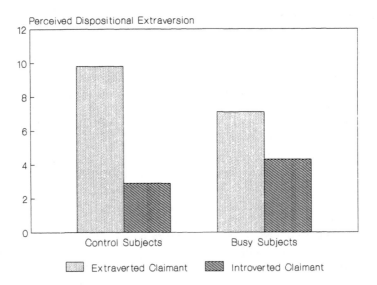

FIGURE 6.5. Control and busy subjects' estimates of the job applicant's dispositional extraversion. Adapted from "Seeing Less and Knowing More: The Benefits of Perceptual Ignorance" by D. T. Gilbert and D. S. Krull, 1988, *Journal of Personality and Social Psychology, 54,* p. 196. Copyright 1988 by the American Psychological Association. Adapted by permission.

fered in the verbal claims they made, but they did *not* differ in the nonverbal behavior they displayed. That is, the applicants claimed extraversion and introversion, respectively, but both displayed the same neutral tone of voice, facial expressions, postures, and so on. (The same confederate acted in both films, and ratings of acoustically degraded tapes confirmed that his nonverbal behavior was indeed constant.) In addition, the films contained an oddity: Every few seconds, a roman letter would appear and then rapidly disappear at some location on the screen. Control subjects watched the film with the goal of diagnosing the applicant's true personality and were told to ignore the flashing letters. Cognitively busy subjects were given the same goal of personality diagnosis, but were additionally required to press a button whenever one of three particular letters appeared on the screen.

As Figure 6.5 shows, the personality judgments of control subjects were strongly influenced by the applicants' claims, but the judgments of cognitively busy subjects were not. (The apparent differences for busy subjects were not statistically significant.) Interestingly, busy subjects *remembered* the applicant's verbal claims just as well as control subjects did, but these subjects apparently did not draw dispositional inferences from the verbal behaviors they heard and remembered.

The "Silly Faces" Experiment

The "hungry chameleon" experiment suggests that concurrent processing demands can, under some circumstances, impair the characterization process itself: Busy subjects were apparently able to draw dispositional inferences from the applicant's nonverbal behavior, but not from his verbal behavior. Of course, a rigorous test of this hypothesis would require the orthogonal manipulation of verbal and nonverbal behavior, and in another experiment, we (Gilbert & Krull, 1988) did just that.

In this experiment we utilized "conflictual behavior"; that is, we used behavior whose verbal component suggested one thing about the speaker's character, but whose nonverbal component suggested precisely the opposite. Subjects were recruited as members of a studio audience in the (wholly bogus) "Texas Television Journalism Project." Upon arriving at the laboratory, subjects were told that a journalism major would be playing the role of newscaster and that he would read aloud a political editorial that he neither wrote nor necessarily endorsed. Subjects then heard a confederate read one of two editorials (either a pro- or an antiabortion editorial) with a severe lack of vocal enthusiasm. Thus, when the confederate read a proabortion editorial, his well-reasoned words suggested a proabortion attitude, while his torpid delivery suggested that he actually believed quite the opposite. Afterwards, subjects were asked to estimate the newscaster's true attitude toward abortion.

Control subjects did just what we expected they would do: They drew dispositional inferences from the newscaster's behavior and (given that the newscaster had been constrained to read a particular editorial) corrected those inferences moderately. These subjects concluded that to some extent the newscaster personally approved the editorial he had read, and this finding mirrors the well-documented tendency for subjects to overemphasize verbal behaviors (even highly constrained verbal behaviors) in their attributions (Jones, 1979; Ross, 1977; see especially Jones, Worchel, Goethals, & Grumet, 1971; Schneider & Miller, 1975).

A second set of subjects was given another task to perform concurrently. These subjects were told that real newscasters must quickly learn to tune out distractions in the studio and that, in addition to making a judgment about the newscaster's true attitude toward abortion, the subject would also be asked to provide such a distraction. Cognitively busy subjects were asked to distract the newscaster by making him "crack up" as he read his editorial: They were instructed to stick out their tongues, scrunch up their noses, roll their eyes, and make altogether silly faces at the newscaster (whom they could not see, but who presumably could see them on camera).

Although subjects performed this task with apparent ease (and with more than a hint of glee), the job of making silly faces had a profound effect on their judgments about the newscaster. As Figure 6.6 shows, busy subjects did not draw dispositional inferences from the newscaster's verbal claims; rather, they drew dispositional inferences from the newscaster's

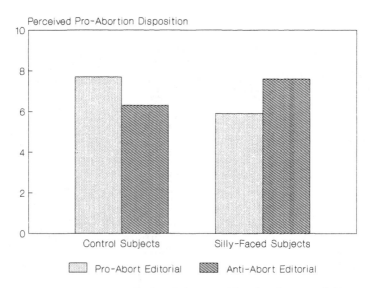

FIGURE 6.6. Control and silly-faced (busy) subjects' estimates of the newscaster's attitude toward abortion. Adapted "Seeing Less and Knowing More: The Benefits of Perceptual Ignorance" by D. T. Gilbert and D. S. Krull, 1988, *Journal of Personality and Social Psychology, 54,* p. 200. Copyright 1988 by the American Psychological Association. Adapted by permission.

nonverbal behavior, and concluded that an unenthusiastic reader of a proabortion editorial was, in fact, personally antiabortion. These results are consistent with the notion that the characterization of nonverbal behavior is easier than the characterization of verbal behavior.

Is it possible, though, that busy subjects made these judgments simply because they did not *hear* the newscaster's words? In a word, no. First, at the end of the experiment, each of the busy subjects correctly reported the position of the editorial; second, both busy and control subjects were equally persuaded by the verbal claims of the particular newscaster they heard. Thus, for example, those busy subjects who heard a newscaster read a proabortion editorial judged the newscaster to be antiabortion, but the subjects themselves became proabortion—which would be quite a trick had they not been able to hear the editorial in the first place. (It is worth noting that the effects shown in Figure 6.6 were replicated in a less colorful but more highly controlled experiment [Gilbert & Krull, 1988], in which busy subjects were asked to do mental arithmetic rather than to make silly faces.)

THE STUPID TAILORS OF TELEOLOGY

We have, then, a picture of an inferential system that (with relative ease) draws characterological inferences from the human actions it observes and (with relative effort) corrects those inferences when necessary. The logic employed by each of these subprocesses is spelled out in some detail by attributional theories, but the operational parameters of the processes themselves are only now being revealed. Knowing how fragile or resource-dependent these processes are is but a first and small step toward a fuller understanding of their operation.

Yet, even in its current underdeveloped phase, this picture has implications that range from the practical to the esoteric. On the practical side, it tells us something about how person perceivers who are actively engaged in social interaction (and who are thus cognitively busy) may come to construe their worlds; on the esoteric side, it suggests some particular perspectives on the architecture of mind. I have discussed the practical sorts of implications elsewhere (e.g., Gilbert & Krull, 1988; Gilbert, Krull, & Pelham, 1988; Gilbert, Pelham, & Krull 1988), and thus will squander the remainder of the reader's attention on this more esoteric question: How is the inferential system designed to employ conscious attention, and why is it designed this way?

The Design of Inferential Systems

Blaise Pascal, the 17th-century philosopher and mathematician, argued that "the most powerful cause of error is the war existing between the senses and reason. . . . These two sources of truth, reason and the senses, besides being both wanting in sincerity, deceive each other in turn" (1670/ 1908, p,. 27). In other words, errors of understanding result from the improper combination of knowledge that is *given to* consciousness by the senses and knowledge that is *produced by* consciousness through reason— a view quite compatible with the work presented here. Subjects in our studies often drew erroneous conclusions about others because the subjects were too busy to apply a conscious correction to the character inferences they had automatically generated.

But underlying Pascal's proposition (as well as Helmholtz's and mine) is one of the most vexing and intriguing assumptions in the history of epistemology—namely, that we have knowledge to whose conception we did not contribute and whose birth we neither attended nor condoned. And if we have within our minds bits of knowledge that are the obvious products of reasoning, but that were not consciously or intentionally produced through reasoning, then only one conclusion seems plausible: Someone or something else did the reasoning for us.

Indeed, consciousness may well be an inferential mechanism whose work is preceded by the work of many unconscious mechanisms that can deliver their inferential products to consciousness, but about whose identities and interworkings consciousness knows nothing. This picture of consciousness as only one machine among many seems necessary not only to a scientific epistemology, but to the explanation of phenomena in neuropathology (Gazzaniga, 1985), artificial intelligence (Minsky, 1985), and psycholinguistics (Fodor, 1983). It is, in fact, one of the few theoretical assumptions to span so many diverse areas of inquiry and to be embraced by so many otherwise disparate thinkers.[3]

If a mind is a society of separate systems, then it must avoid chaos by dint of its internal organization. Thus, when we adopt a multiple-systems view of mind, we must immediately ask how these systems are organized with respect to one another. The work described earlier is consistent with a view of consciousness as a limited-capacity mechanism that does not itself perform tedious and routine analyses (e.g., the sorts of analyses that turn behavioral observations into dispositional inferences), but merely checks and corrects the outputs of other "upstream" or "off-line" systems. Thus, one (but *only* one) of the duties of consciousness is to act like the inspector in a garment factory: It does not make a product, but it checks to make sure a product is perfect. If an imperfection is found, it institutes a remedy.

To understand why an inferential system should employ consciousness in such a post hoc manner, it may be useful to indulge the metaphor a bit longer and examine an imaginary garment factory. The primary constraint on the design of this factory is that the little tailors who sew the clothes are simpletons and dullards. They can only be taught to make one size of each garment, and so, when called upon to make a pair of men's trousers, these tailors always make a modal product (e.g., size 34). This is usually not a problem because the modal product will, by definition, fit most customers. But on occasion there will be a Triton among the minnows who requires something in a size 52, and when this happens, the smart inspector must alter the size 34 pants that the stupid tailors have made.

There are obvious problems with this sort of system. For example, because there are many important things that cannot be done by the dim little tailors, the alteration of trousers becomes but one of the smart inspector's many responsibilities. The inspector must also check the quality of the work on shirts and socks, deal with breakdowns of the conveyor belt, communicate with other factories in the area, and so forth. In fact, the inspector is often too busy to alter (or alter properly) the products manufactured by the little tailors, and thus from time to time a portly or puny customer will end up wearing erroneous trousers.

Given these sorts of problems, why should the factory be so organized? Why, for example, should it always manufacture trousers in size 34 only to alter them, rather than simply manufacturing them in the right size to begin with? For the same reason why most real men buy off-the-rack trousers: Custom tailoring takes too long and is too damned expensive. By producing a common trouser, the factory can make trousers quickly and cheaply. And when something other than a size 34 is required, the inspector can always alter the trousers to fit. It is true that on occasion the inspector will fail to do the appropriate alterations and that some customers will therefore go away clad in tents or bound in tourniquets, but on balance (and this is what counts) the factory can turn out an absolutely greater number of trousers that fit *perfectly* than can the custom tailor. And, on average, each pair costs less.

The garment metaphor is wearing thin, but its point should by now be clear. Mental systems (at least those that inhabit viable organisms) must quickly produce the best inferences they can for the least investment. It seems reasonable to assume that our characterizations of others are *usually* correct, at least in a pragmatic sense: Just as tables often appear flat because they have the property of flatness, people often appear kind because they have the property of kindness. If we accept that dispositional inferences are, in fact, the size 34 trousers of social perception, then we can understand why a system would utilize several stupid tailors to make such inferences and just one smart inspector to correct them. The system can automatically produce, at little cost, an inference that is right more often than wrong. If some corrections are required, the system can tuck a little here and hem a little there—but in any event, this way of doing things gets inferences to consciousness quickly and cheaply. Such a mind, it seems, does not manufacture its conclusions about others so much as it tailors them.

The Evolution of Inferential Systems

At the outset of this section, I have asked why any organism should employ a two-step inference-making system, and I have speculated that this way of doing business has certain benefits—namely, that inferences can be made quickly and cheaply. Now I would like to argue that this "one step forward, half step backward" system is awkward, overly complicated, aesthetically displeasing, and prone to severe errors of undercorrection; in short, it is *not* the best way to design an inferential system from scratch.

One of the dangers of teleology is that when we ask *why* organisms are designed as they are, we may forget that organisms, unlike computers, are not designed at all. Biological systems are made to serve no premeditated purpose, but are instead randomly implemented and then continuously modified by their own effects. In addition, whereas human engineers have the luxury of interconnecting any number of otherwise useless parts, nature can only make modifications to parts that are already capable of functioning on their own. Complicated natural systems can evolve only from subcomponents that have established their own worth; as a result, natural systems often look like Rube Goldberg machines—jury-rigged amalgams of new parts appended to old. The human brain itself is essentially a reptilian weenie wrapped in neocortical bun.

The two-step inference system that I have described may be similarly construed: Unconscious characterizers may be primitive mechanisms to which conscious correctors are (in evolutionary time) relatively new addenda. We can easily imagine a simple organism that understands the world by attributing properties or propensities to things that behave. Such an organism would need only remember how the things in its world act and assume that such things will generally act as they have in the past. Of course, such dispositional inferences are among the least penetrating sorts of causal conclusions, and an organism that could not transcend them would make plenty of mistakes: It would imbue raindrops with fallingness, lightning with hurtability, politicians with conviction—but (and this is what counts) it would probably be able to feed and copulate without much ado.

Thus, when we ask *why* the human inferential system is designed as it is, we must keep in mind that it isn't. Rather, it is haphazardly evolved with the constraint that each subcomponent must prove itself viable before new features can be tested. The two-step inference maker may not be the best way to engineer a sophisticated information-processing device. But it may be the *only* way to turn an amoeba into one.

A SHORT CONCLUSION

In the quotation that opens this chapter, Helmholtz warned us against analyses of mental life. Yet he did not do so because he thought that such analyses were inevitably wrong, but because he thought that no one ever acknowledged them when they were right.

> We know by experience that people very seldom come to any agreement about abstract questions of this nature. The keenest thinkers, philosophers like Kant for instance, have long ago analyzed these relations correctly and demonstrated them, and yet there is no permanent and general agreement about them among educated people. . . . [These are] questions that always have been, and perhaps always will be, subjects of debate . . . (Helmholtz, 1910/1925, p. 2)

Certainly the problems of consciousness and cognition, intention and awareness, attribution and action, will be with us for a long, long time. But we are beginning to question some basic assumptions about these matters and, as such, are well on our way to a better understanding of both the problems and their solutions. We must hope that we will recognize the truth when we rediscover it.

ACKNOWLEDGMENTS

The writing of this chapter and the research reported herein were supported by National Science Foundation Grant No. BNS-8605443. I thank Bill Swann, Brett Pelham, and Dough Krull for their helpful comments and suggestions.

NOTES

1. There has been some controversy regarding the appropriate translation of this term, but "unconscious inference" and "unconscious conclusion" are its most popular English equivalents. The German *Schluss* literally means "termination" or "ending," and Helmholtz probably meant "ending" or "end product" in the sense that a proposition is the syllogistic end product of its premises. It should also be noted that, much to William James's delight, Helmholtz ultimately disavowed both the term and the concept it represented. So much for brief forays.

2. Currently, the term "automatic" means so many things that it threatens to mean nothing at all (Bargh, Chapter 1, this volume). Shiffrin and Schneider (1977) contrast "automatic" with "controlled" processes, implying that the ability of consciousness to guide or alter a process is the benchmark of that process's automaticity. Hasher and Zacks (1979), on the other hand, find "effortful" to be a better antonym for "automatic," implying that the resource requirements of a process determine the legitimacy of its claim to automaticity. The criteria offered by these and other theorists are generally variations on these dual notions of capacity and control, which may themselves be two faces of the same coin (e.g., a resource may be that which is required to institute control).

This terminological fog may lift when psychology achieves a comprehensive model of mind. In the meantime, I use the term "automatic" to mean something like "capable of proceeding on the basis of scant resources or with limited conscious assistance." This definition departs from others in that it does not preclude the possibilities (a) that an automatic process may require a jump-start (i.e., the initial activation of a process may require conscious control) or (b) that an automatic process may be controll*able* (e.g., control of the process may be possible even if it is unnecessary).

3. Although this assumption would, at various points in history, have warranted charges of felonious homunculism, today's information-processing vernacular enables such possibilities to be entertained without a hint of circularity or paradox (see Dennett, 1978, pp. 109–126; Erdelyi, 1974).

REFERENCES

Bem, D. J. (1972). Self-perception theory. In L. Berkowitz (Ed.), *Advances in experimental social psychology* (Vol. 6, pp. 1–62). New York: Academic Press.

Dennett, D. C. (1978). *Brainstorms: Philosophical essays on mind and psychology.* Cambridge, MA: MIT Press.

Erdelyi, M. H. (1974). A new look at the New Look: Perceptual defense and vigilance. *Psychological Review, 81,* 1–25.

Erdelyi, M. H. (1985). *Psychoanalysis: Freud's cognitive psychology.* San Francisco: W. H. Freeman.

Fodor, J. A. (1983). *The modularity of mind.* Cambridge, MA: MIT Press.

Gazzaniga, M. S. (1985). *The social brain.* New York: Basic Books.

Gilbert, D. T., & Krull, D. S. (1988). Seeing less and knowing more: The benefits of perceptual ignorance. *Journal of Personality and Social Psychology, 54,* 193–202.

Gilbert, D. T., Krull, D. S., & Pelham, B. W. (1988). Of thoughts unspoken: Social inference and the self-regulation of behavior. *Journal of Personality and Social Psychology, 55,* 685–694.

Gilbert, D. T., Pelham, B. W., & Krull, D. S. (1988). On cognitive busyness: When person perceivers meet persons perceived. *Journal of Personality and Social Psychology, 54,* 733–740.

Gray, J. A. (1975). *Elements of a two-process theory of learning.* New York: Academic Press.

Hasher, L., & Zacks, R. T. (1979). Automatic and effortful processes in memory. *Journal of Experimental Psychology: General, 108,* 356–388.

Heider, F. (1958). *The psychology of interpersonal relations.* New York: Wiley.

Helmholtz, H. von. (1925). *Treatise on psychological optics* (3rd ed., Vol. 3, J. P. C. Southall, Trans.). Menasha, WI: Banta. (Original 3rd ed. published 1910)

James, W. (1890). *The principles of psychology* (Vol. 1). New York: Holt.

Jones, E. E. (1979). The rocky road from acts to dispositions. *American Psychologist, 34,* 107–117.

Jones, E. E., & Davis, K. E. (1965). From acts to dispositions: The attribution process in person perception. In L. Berkowitz (Ed.), *Advances in experimental social psychology* (Vol. 2, pp. 219–266). New York: Academic Press.

Jones, E. E., & Harris, V. A. (1967). The attribution of attitudes. *Journal of Experimental Social Psychology, 3,* 1–24.

Jones, E. E., & McGillis, D. (1976). Correspondent inferences and the attribution cube: A comparative reappraisal. In J. H. Harvey, W. J. Ickes, & R. F. Kidd (Eds.), *New directions in attribution research* (Vol. 1, pp. 389–420). Hillsdale, NJ: Erlbaum.

Jones, E. E., Worchel, S., Goethals, G. R., & Grumet, J. F. (1971). Prior expectancy and behavioral extremity as determinants of attitude attribution. *Journal of Experimental Social Psychology, 7,* 59–80.

Kassin, S. M., & Baron, R. M. (1985). Basic determinants of attribution and social perception. In J. Harvey & G. Weary (Eds.), *Attribution: Basic issues and applications* (pp. 37–64). New York: Academic Press.

Kelley, H. H. (1967). Attribution theory in social psychology. In D. Levine (Ed.), *Nebraska Symposium on Motivation* (Vol. 15, pp. 192–238). Lincoln: University of Nebraska Press.

LaBerge, E. J., & Samuels, S. J. (1974). Toward a theory of automatic information processing in reading. *Cognitive Psychology, 6,* 293–323.

Langer, E. J. (1978). Rethinking the role of thought in social interaction. In J. H. Harvey, W. J. Ickes, & R. F. Kidd (Eds.), *New directions in attribution research* (Vol. 2, pp. 35–58). Hillsdale, NJ: Erlbaum.

McArthur, L. Z., & Baron, R. M. (1983). Toward an ecological theory of social perception. *Psychological Review, 90,* 215–238.

Minsky, M. (1985). *The society of mind.* New York: Simon & Schuster.

Newtson, D. (1980). An interactionist perspective on social knowing. *Personality and Social Psychology Bulletin, 6,* 520–531.

Pascal, B. (1908). *Pensées* (W. F. Trotter, Trans.). New York: Dutton. (Original work published 1670)

Pennebaker, J. W., & Chew, C. H. (1985). Behavioral inhibition and electrodermal activity during deception. *Journal of Personality and Social Psychology, 49,* 1427–1433.

Posner, M. I., & Snyder, C. R. R. (1975). Attention and cognitive control. In R. L. Solso (Ed.), *Information processing and cognition: The Loyola Symposium* (pp. 55–85). Hillsdale, NJ: Erlbaum.

Quattrone, G. A. (1982). Overattribution and unit formation: When behavior engulfs the person. *Journal of Personality and Social Psychology, 42,* 593–607.

Ross, L. (1977). The intuitive psychologist and his shortcomings. In L. Berkowitz (Ed.), *Advances in experimental social psychology* (Vol. 10, pp. 173–220). New York: Academic Press.

Schneider, D. J., & Miller, R. (1975). The effects of enthusiasm and quality of arguments on attitude attribution. *Journal of Personality, 43,* 693–708.

Shiffrin, R. M., & Schneider, W. (1977). Controlled and automatic human information processing: II. Perceptual learning, automatic attending, and a general theory. *Psychological Review, 84,* 127–190.

Uleman, J. S. (1987). Consciousness and control: The case of spontaneous trait inferences. *Personality and Social Psychology Bulletin, 13,* 337–354.

Wegner, D. M., Schneider, D. J., Carter, S. R., & White, T. L. (1987). Paradoxical effects of thought suppression. *Journal of Personality and Social Psychology, 53,* 5–13.

Winter, L., & Uleman, J. S. (1984). When are social judgments made? Evidence for the spontaneousness of trait inferences. *Journal of Personality and Social Psychology, 47,* 237–252.

Winter, L., Uleman, J. S., & Cunniff, C. (1985). How automatic are social judgments? *Journal of Personality and Social Psychology, 49,* 904–917.

7

Heuristic and Systematic Information Processing within and beyond the Persuasion Context

SHELLY CHAIKEN
AKIVA LIBERMAN
New York University

ALICE H. EAGLY
Purdue University

The distinction between "heuristic" and "systematic" information processing has been central to the development of a theory of persuasion that we call the "heuristic–systematic model" (HSM; see also Chaiken, 1978, 1980, 1982, 1987). Because we believe that the ideas embodied in this model are applicable beyond the persuasion context, it is important to describe the model's two processing modes in general terms.

At the most generic level, we conceive of systematic processing as a comprehensive, analytic orientation in which perceivers access and scrutinize all informational input for its relevance and importance to their judgment task, and integrate all useful information in forming their judgments. Obviously, systematic processing can vary in its extensiveness. For purposes of theory development, however, our model often treats systematic processing more prototypically. To wit, (prototypal) systematic processing refers to the upper end of a data-seeking/analysis/integration continuum and, as such, is assumed to require more than marginal levels of effort and cognitive capacity. Because of these assumptions, our model further assumes that people must be motivated to process systematically and that this mode is adversely affected by situational variables and individual differences that constrain people's capacities for in-depth information processing (e.g., time pressures, lack of domain-specific expertise). Our definition of systematic processing may suggest to some readers that we regard this mode as ubiquitously open-minded and unbiased. Not so. Systematic processing can be unbiased or biased, depending upon motivational factors (e.g., processing goals) and cognitive factors (e.g., the accessibility of knowledge structures that influence perceivers' interpretation and evaluation of information).

We conceive of heuristic processing as a more limited processing mode that demands much less cognitive effort and capacity than systematic processing. When processing heuristically, people focus on that subset of available information that enables them to use simple inferential rules, schemata, or cognitive heuristics to formulate their judgments and decisions. Because heuristic processing entails minimal amounts of data collection and analysis, it might be construed as anchoring the low end of a systematic-processing continuum. Yet, because we regard heuristic processing as more exclusively theory-driven than systematic processing and assume that the two modes can co-occur, our model's mode-of-processing distinction is not merely a quantitative one.

The rules or heuristics that define heuristic processing are learned knowledge structures that may be used either self-consciously or non-self-consciously by social perceivers. Although the model has focused on persuasion heuristics such as "Experts' statements can be trusted," we believe that other sorts of declarative and procedural knowledge structures also serve as simple heuristics in social judgment settings. Examples of these include social stereotypes (e.g., "Attractive people are sociable") and implicit beliefs about the causes of events and behavior (e.g., "People's actions reflect their attitudes").

Our model's effort and capacity assumptions are relevant to a central concern of this volume—the distinction between "controlled" and "automatic" processes. Although we do tend to regard systematic processing as generally controlled and intentional, the status of heuristic processing is less clear. We believe that perceivers sometimes use heuristics in a highly deliberate, self-conscious fashion, but at other times they may use heuristics more spontaneously, with relatively little awareness of having done so. Thus, heuristic processing can be controlled and intentional, but at times it may achieve some—though not all—of the criteria that have been used to define an automatic process (lack of intention, lack of awareness, involuntariness, noninterference with other ongoing mental processes; Bargh, 1984; Posner & Snyder, 1975; Shiffrin & Schneider, 1977). However, we concur with a growing opinion that a strict automatic-controlled dichotomy is too restrictive to capture many phenomena of interest, including heuristic processing, because the criteria that connote automaticity often occur independently (Bargh, Chapter 1, this volume; Logan & Cowan, 1984; Shiffrin, in press; Uleman, Chapter 14, this volume). Because little evidence currently exists concerning the minimal degree of attention, effort, or intention necessary for heuristic processing, we feel it premature to make detailed predictions about the degree of automaticity that heuristic processing may attain (see Sherman, 1987, for an interesting discussion of this issue). Nonetheless, we do believe that people may often be relatively unaware of or, at the least, may underestimate the extent to which simple rules, schemata, or heuristics influence their social judgments and behavior.

In this chapter, we offer a detailed discussion of the HSM as we have applied it to date—that is, to persuasion settings in which people are motivated to attain valid attitudes. Afterward, we argue that the core ideas of the model are applicable beyond this one persuasion context. First, we show that the model can be extended to incorporate multiple motivational orientations, and that this multiple-motive version of the model can provide a useful framework for studying a broader range of social influence settings in which people's attitude judgments are focal. Second, we argue that a generic version of our extended model can also provide a broad framework for studying a variety of other social judgments, such as those investigated in traditional impression formation, stereotyping, attribution, and decision-making tasks.

THE HEURISTIC–SYSTEMATIC MODEL OF PERSUASION

The description of the HSM we offer here is compatible with earlier expositions (Chaiken, 1978, 1980, 1982, 1987; Chaiken & Eagly, 1983; Eagly & Chaiken, 1984). Here, however, we articulate the model more completely than we have in past papers—by more fully explicating its assumptions and their implications, and by discussing in detail several principles and hypotheses that have received less attention previously.

An Important (and Limiting) Motivational Assumption

The HSM was explicitly developed to apply to persuasion settings in which the individual's dominant motivational concern could be assumed to be *the desire to form or to hold valid, accurate attitudes*—that is, to attain attitudes that are perceived to be congruent with relevant facts (see Katz, 1960; Kelman, 1961; Smith, Bruner, & White, 1956). Because of this functional assumption, the HSM assumes that the primary processing goal of message recipients is to assess the validity of the persuasive messages they encounter. Moreover, the model assumes that *both* heuristic and systematic processing occur in the service of this goal.

The assumption that people desire to maximize the validity of their attitudes clearly limits our model's current range of applicability. As presently formulated, for example, the HSM is not necessarily applicable to influence settings in which people are more concerned with establishing or maintaining relationships with social influence agents (see Kelman, 1961; Smith et al., 1956). Later, we argue that our mode-of-processing distinction *can* be applied to settings in which such alternative motives operate. For now, we wish to stress that the current version of the HSM is limited to validity-seeking persuasion contexts, and to note that the decision to limit the model in this way reflected two considerations. First, we desired to align the HSM with other cognitive theories of attitudes, most of which explicitly or implicitly assume that people in persuasion settings are motivated to attain valid attitudes (see Chaiken & Stangor, 1987; Eagly & Chaiken, 1984). Second, we wished to differentiate the HSM from theories sharing its view that persuasion is not invariably the outcome of extensive processing of persuasive argumentation, but postulating underlying motives and/or psychological mechanisms that are quite different from the validity-seeking motive and cognitive heuristics featured in the HSM (e.g., reactance, identification, classical conditioning; see Chaiken, 1987; Eagly & Chaiken, 1984).[1]

Definitions, Assumptions, and Their Implications

Two of the HSM's assumptions have already been noted. We assume that recipients' primary processing goal is to assess the validity of persuasive messages, and that both heuristic and systematic processing serve this objective.

Two Concurrent Modes of Judging Message Validity

Our model assumes that systematic and heuristic processing may co-occur. This is not to say that both modes *always* occur, only that the two modes *can* proceed concurrently. The implications of this assumption are discussed in subsequent sections of this chapter.

For the validity-seeking persuasion context, we use more specific definitions of heuristic and systematic processing than the generic definitions introduced earlier. When engaged in systematic processing, people judge the validity of a message's advocated position by scrutinizing all relevant information (especially persuasive argumentation) and by thinking about this information in relation to other knowledge they may possess about the object or issue discussed in the message. Two aspects of our conceptualization should be emphasized. First, although systematic processing connotes extensive processing of message- and issue-relevant information, it does not designate the *particular* processing mechanisms (e.g., comprehension of persuasive arguments, cognitive responding) or integration rules (e.g., weighted averaging) that may mediate people's attitude judgments.[2] Second, although systematic processing can be characterized as methodical, the systematic information processor is not necessarily processing message- and issue-relevant data impartially (see subsequent sections of this chapter).

In contrast to the systematic mode, heuristic processing is more exclusively theory-driven because recipients utilize minimal informational input in conjunction with simple (declarative or procedural) knowledge structures to determine message validity quickly and efficiently. More specifically, when processing heuristically, message recipients use simple decision rules such as "Experts' statements can be trusted" and "Consensus implies correctness" to judge the validity of persuasive messages. As a consequence, they may agree more with expert communicators, with messages that most other persons appear to endorse, and so on, without having fully absorbed the semantic content of persuasive argumentation.

The cornerstone of heuristic processing is the idea that specific rules, schemata, or heuristics can mediate people's attitude (or other social) judgments. We use the term "heuristic cue" to refer to any variable whose judgmental impact is hypothesized to be mediated by a simple decision rule. In validity-seeking persuasion contexts, these rules or "persuasion heuristics" associate particular levels of the heuristic cue (e.g., high source expertise, high consensus) with a high probability that the position advocated in the message is valid, and other levels (e.g., low source expertise, low consensus) with a low probability that the message's position is valid.

Some of the heuristic cues (and their associated persuasion heuristics) that have been successfully examined from the HSM perspective include source expertise ("Experts' statements can be trusted"), source likability ("People generally agree with people they like"), message length ("Length implies strength"), and consensus information ("Consensus implies correctness"; see Axsom, Yates, & Chaiken, 1987; Chaiken, 1980, 1987; Chaiken et al., 1988; Chaiken & Eagly, 1983; Liberman, de La Hoz, & Chaiken, 1988; Maheswaran & Chaiken, 1988; Ratneshwar & Chaiken, 1986; Wood, Kallgren, & Preisler, 1985).[3]

Knowledge Accessibility and Heuristic Processing

We assume that the heuristics postulated by the HSM are learned knowledge structures. That is, we assume that people have abstracted persuasion heuristics such as "Experts' statements can be trusted" and "Length implies strength" on the basis of their past experiences and observations or via direct instruction from socialization agents (or both). Moreover, we assume that these heuristics are represented in memory much as other knowledge structures are assumed to be (see Higgins, Chapter 3, this volume; Smith, 1984). Several principles governing heuristic processing follow from these assumptions.

Like other declarative and procedural knowledge structures, persuasion heuristics can impact on people's attitude judgments only to the extent that they are cognitively available (i.e., stored in memory for potential use; Higgins, King, & Mavin, 1982). Clearly, for a cue such as communicator likability to be processed heuristically, recipients must have learned and stored in memory the liking–agreement heuristic ("People generally agree with people they like"). Of course, recipients might agree with likable, attractive sources for other reasons (e.g., to establish rapport; Chaiken, 1986; Kelman, 1961). Yet, from the perspective of the single-motive HSM, they would not be regarded as having processed this cue heuristically (see note 3).

Heuristic processing depends also on whether cognitively available heuristics are activated or accessed from memory. Clearly, one prerequisite for activation is that the setting contains cues that can be processed heuristically. In the absence of consensus-related cues, for example, the consensus heuristic would not be activated. Another determinant of activation is the individual's processing goals; the goal of assessing message validity should itself increase the likelihood that relevant heuristics are activated. Moreover, any factor that enhances the importance of this processing goal should increase the accessibility of relevant persuasion heuristics (Bruner, 1957; Higgins, Chapter 3, this volume). When recipients do not have this goal, it is more likely that knowledge structures relevant to alternate goals would become accessible.

The accessibility principle is important, because it implies that (1) situational factors that influence the temporary accessibility of persuasion heuristics and (2) individual differences in the chronic accessibility of such heuristics should (all else being equal) influence the persuasive impact of heuristic cues. For example, manipulating the salience or vividness of heuristic cues should increase their persuasive impact, because such manipulations should increase the likelihood that these cues' associated persuasion heuristics will be activated. Findings consistent with this logic have been obtained by Pallak (1983), who manipulated the vividness of communicator physical attractiveness (via photographs), and by Chaiken and Eagly (1983), who varied the salience of communicator likability (via communication modality). Regarding individual differences, people lower in need for cognition (NFC; Cacioppo & Petty, 1982; Cohen, 1957) may use cognitive heuristics more frequently than those higher in NFC (Chaiken et al., 1988). Since frequency of use leads to chronic differences in construct accessibility (Higgins, Chapter 3, this volume), one can infer that persuasion heuristics may be more chronically accessible among low-NFC persons. Consistent with this logic, low NFC (vs. high-NFC) subjects are more influenced by heuristic cues in persuasion settings (Axsom et al., 1987; Chaiken et al., 1988). Finally, we have investigated the joint effect of temporary and chronic sources of accessibility on the persuasive impact of heuristic cues in several priming studies. In one study, for example, subjects classified as chronic users of the length–strength rule agreed more with a message that ostensibly contained many (vs. few) arguments, especially after exposure to a task that primed this heuristic. In contrast, chronic nonusers of this rule were no more persuaded by the long message than by the short one, regardless of whether the length–strength heuristic had or had not been primed (Chaiken et al., 1988; see also Chaiken, 1987).

There is a third aspect to persuasion heuristics that the concepts of construct availability and accessibility do not fully capture. Persuasion heuristics vary not only in their availability and accessibility; they also vary in their strength or perceived reliability (see Higgins, in press). A person whose past experience with likable and unlikable persons has yielded many confirmations and few disconfirmations of the liking–agreement rule should perceive a stronger association between the concepts of liking and interpersonal agreement than a person whose experience has yielded proportionately more disconfirmations (see Stotland & Canon, 1972). Because the former person should attribute greater reliability to the liking–agreement heuristic, he or she may be more likely to use it in relevant persuasion settings, and hence more likely to express agreement with likable (vs. unlikable) communicators.

In addition to the fact that the same heuristic may be perceived as more reliable by some persons than by others, some persuasion heuristics may be perceived as more reliable than other heuristics by most people. For example, unpublished data of ours suggests that college students attribute greater reliability to the expertise heuristic than to the liking–agreement heuristic. All else being equal, then, we might expect expertise manipulations to exert generally larger effects on persuasion than communicator likability or attractiveness manipulations.

Because the persuasive impact of heuristic cues increases with the perceived reliability of the heuristics associated with these cues, factors that influence rule reliability should exert a corresponding effect on the persuasive impact of relevant heuristic cues. Support for this conjecture was obtained among low-NFC subjects who participated in a study that manipulated the reliability of the liking–agreement heuristic and a persuasive communicator's likability. Compared with control subjects, high-reliability subjects manifested a greater tendency and low-reliability subjects manifested a lesser tendency to agree more with the likable (vs. unlikable) communicator's message (see Chaiken, 1987).

Effort and Capacity Assumptions

Because systematic and heuristic processing differ in the extensiveness of processing they entail, the HSM assumes (1) that systematic processing is more effortful than heuristic processing; and (2) that systematic processing both demands and consumes cognitive capacity, whereas heuristic processing makes relatively few capacity demands. The first of these assumptions is important, because it is grist for the additional assumption that message recipients must be motivated to engage in systematic processing. The second assumption is equally important, because it implies that even when motivation for systematic processing is high, this processing mode—to a far greater extent than heuristic processing—may be constrained by factors that limit people's abilities to engage in detailed information processing.

The assumption that message recipients must be motivated to engage in systematic processing has been supported in numerous studies (for reviews, see Chaiken, 1987; Chaiken & Stangor, 1987; Petty & Cacioppo, 1986). In this research, subjects who received messages on topics of high (vs. low) personal relevance, or who were led to believe that their attitude judgments had important (vs. unimportant) consequences, or who were given sole (vs. shared) responsibility for message evaluation have been regarded as motivated to engage in systematic processing. Consistent with this view, these subjects engaged in greater amounts of systematic processing, as indexed by their heightened sensitivity to message content manipulations (e.g., argument quality, valence of argumentation) and their higher scores on measures such as reading time, argument recall, and the number of message- and issue-relevant cognitions generated on thought-listing tasks (e.g., Axsom et al., 1987; Chaiken, 1980; Leippe & Elkin, 1987; Maheswaran & Chaiken, 1988; Petty & Cacioppo, 1984; Petty, Harkins, & Williams, 1980; Weldon & Gargano, 1985). Supporting the assumption that systematic processing also requires ability, studies that have measured or manipulated subjects' capacities for systematic processing have produced similar findings (for reviews, see Chaiken, 1987; Chaiken & Stangor, 1987; Petty & Cacioppo, 1986). For example, subjects who lack knowledge about the message topic or who must process under severe time constraints or whose moods drain their resources show less sensitivity to manipulations of message content and score lower on measures of systematic processing than do subjects who are more expert about the message topic or who receive ample time for processing or whose moods do not drain their resources (Liberman et al., 1988; Mackie & Worth, in press; Wood et al., 1985; Worth & Mackie, 1987; see also Alba & Hutchinson, 1987).

Systematic Processing and the Impact of Heuristic Cues

Heuristic processing is presumed to require much less effort and cognitive capacity than systematic processing.[4] Thus, so long as heuristic processing is feasible (e.g., the setting contains heuristic cues; see earlier discussion), people should engage in this processing mode even when they are unmotivated or unable to engage in more than negligible amounts of systematic processing. As a consequence, the persuasive impact of heuristic cues should be maximal in such situations. In contrast, heuristic cues will often exert much less persuasive impact when recipients are highly motivated *and* able to process systematically. In these settings, heuristic and systematic processing are assumed to co-occur. Nevertheless, systematic processing should provide recipients with additional evidence regarding message validity, and some of this information may contradict the validity of persuasion heuris-

tics. As a result, the persuasive impact of heuristic cues will often be attenuated. For example, although experts' messages will often induce greater
persuasion than nonexperts' messages because recipients apply the expertise heuristic, careful scrutiny of the semantic content of persuasive argumentation may provide information contradicting this rule of thumb (e.g.,
the expert's message is weak while the nonexpert's message is strong; Petty,
Cacioppo, & Goldman, 1981). Thus, when recipients process systematically, a heuristic cue such as source expertise may not exert a detectable
persuasive impact (especially in laboratory experiments that feature explicit contradictions between message content and heuristic cues).

This *attenuation hypothesis* has been demonstrated in numerous studies using a variety of heuristic cues (e.g., source expertise, likability, and
physical attractiveness; message length and number of persuasive arguments; and audience reactions and consensus information). Specifically, this
research has shown that heuristic cues exert a significantly greater persuasive impact when motivation *or* ability for systematic processing is low
than when motivation *and* ability are high (e.g., Axsom et al., 1987; Chaiken, 1980; Maheswaran & Chaiken, 1988; Petty & Cacioppo, 1984; Petty,
Cacioppo, & Goldman, 1981; Ratneshwar & Chaiken, 1986; Wood et
al., 1985; Worth & Mackie, 1987).

Importantly, the attenuation hypothesis is only one of several hypotheses that follow from the HSM's assumption that heuristic and systematic processing can co-occur. For example, the *bias hypothesis* asserts
that heuristic processing can bias systematic processing, and the *additivity
hypothesis* asserts that heuristic and systematic processing can exert additive effects on people's attitude judgments. In subsequent sections of this
chapter we will discuss these additional hypotheses, contrast their predictions with the prediction of the attenuation hypothesis that systematic processing diminishes the persuasive impact of heuristic cues, and discuss the
circumstances under which each of these various hypotheses is most likely
to apply.

Efficiency and the Principle of Sufficiency

We assume, as others have, that people prefer less effortful to more effortful modes of information processing. This assumption does not imply that
we view people as lazy or "mindless" (cf. Langer, 1978). Instead, we agree
with Simon (1976; Simon & Stedry, 1969) and others (Mischel, 1979;
Taylor & Fiske, 1978) that people are economy-minded souls who wish
to satisfy their goal-related needs in the most efficient ways possible. The
goal of validity-seeking message recipients is to assess the validity of a
message's advocated position (in order to satisfy their underlying motivation to hold accurate attitudes), and both heuristic and systematic processing *can* serve this goal. But in the interest of efficiency, message recipients
may be inclined to avoid systematic processing because of its effortful nature.

Although validity-seeking recipients prefer to minimize effort expenditure, their foremost motivational concern is to attain valid attitudes. People cannot know with complete certainty that their attitudes (or other judgments) are correct, but they can hope to achieve some reasonable or sufficient level of confidence. The "sufficiency principle" embodies the idea that efficient information processors must strike a balance between minimizing their processing efforts and maximizing their judgmental confidence. In general, it asserts that people will exert whatever level of effort is required to attain a sufficient degree of confidence that they have satisfactorily accomplished their processing goals. In validity-seeking persuasion settings, the principle asserts that recipients will invest whatever amount of effort is required to attain a sufficiently confident assessment of the validity of a message's advocated position.

To understand the sufficiency principle better, imagine a judgmental confidence continuum and a point (somewhere) along this continuum that represents the person's sufficiency threshold (i.e., criterion point of sufficient confidence). Confidence levels to the left of this point are perceived as insufficient, and levels to the right as more than sufficient. The sufficiency principle holds that people will exert whatever effort is required to attain their sufficiency threshold. Importantly, what constitutes sufficient confidence for one person may be insufficient (or more than sufficient) for another; and what is deemed sufficient in one situation may be considered insufficient (or more than sufficient) in another setting. In other words, sufficiency thresholds vary as a function of individual difference and situational factors.

Attaining Confidence through Systematic Processing

The sufficiency principle implies that if a less effortful mode of processing does not afford a sufficiently confident judgment, a more effortful mode will be invoked. It therefore suggests that validity-seeking message recipients will engage in greater amounts of systematic processing when heuristic processing cannot occur, or, more importantly, when heuristic processing confers insufficient judgmental confidence.

The latter hypothesis was tested in a study that manipulated the congruency of consensus information and message content (Maheswaran & Chaiken, 1988).[5] Subjects learned either that a majority or a minority of consumers liked a new product, the "XT-100" answering machine, and read a message describing this product as either superior or inferior to two competing brands. Thus, the valence of consensus information and message content was either congruent (e.g., both positive) or incongruent (e.g., positive consensus/negative message). Finally, we also manipulated motivation for systematic processing by telling subjects that the study and their responses were either very important or "preliminary" and unimportant.

We hypothesized that incongruency would increase systematic processing among subjects not otherwise disposed to do so—that is, among low-task-importance subjects. The rationale was this: Heuristic processing of the positive (negative) consensus cue should produce positive (negative) evaluations of the XT-100. However, even the barest attention to the message was expected to reveal its congruency–incongruency with the consensus cue. In the congruent conditions, low-importance subjects' minimal systematic processing should confirm the validity of the consensus heuristic. Because these subjects' confidence in their heuristic-based product evaluations should be high (and their motivation for systematic processing low), there would be little reason for them to pay much additional attention to the message. In the incongruent conditions, however, marginal processing of the message should undermine subjects' confidence in their heuristic-based product evaluations. To attain sufficient confidence, we reasoned that these subjects would step up their systematic-processing efforts.[6] Theoretically, incongruency should also increase systematic processing among high-task-importance subjects. We felt that this effect would be undetectable, however, given the high overall amount of systematic processing expected of these subjects.

The results of the experiment confirmed our predictions. As expected, high-importance subjects engaged in a great deal of systematic processing, as indexed by the large number of product-related cognitions they generated on a thought-listing task. Consistent with this, message valence but not consensus information exerted a significant impact on these subjects' product attitudes, and the only significant predictor of these attitudes was the valence of subjects' product-related cognitions. Overall, low-importance subjects did less systematic processing than high-importance subjects. As predicted, however, this difference was due to low-importance subjects in the study's congruent conditions. When incongruent information was received, low-importance subjects did just as much systematic processing as high-importance subjects. Consistent with this mixed pattern of systematic processing, low-importance subjects' product attitudes were best predicted by the valence of their product-related cognitions in the study's incongruent conditions and by the valence of their consensus-related cognitions in the congruent conditions.

Understanding Motivation for Systematic Processing

A large amount of research relevant to the HSM has investigated situational and individual-difference variables (e.g., personal relevance) that are hypothesized to affect motivation for systematic processing. As reviewed earlier, this research supports the hypothesis that systematic processing often requires motivation (see "Effort and Capacity Assumptions"). Whereas this empirical fact has been treated axiomatically by most researchers (e.g., Petty & Cacioppo, 1986), the HSM addresses the issue of *why* certain variables motivate systematic processing.

The motivating effect of variables such as personal relevance and task importance can be understood from the perspective of the HSM's sufficiency principle. Such factors presumably influence processing effort *because* they affect recipients' sufficiency thresholds. Consider the variable of personal relevance (also known as "issue involvement" or "outcome-relevant involvement"; see Chaiken & Stangor, 1987; Johnson & Eagly, in press; Petty & Cacioppo, 1986). Its motivating effect on systematic processing can be understood by assuming that increased personal relevance enhances recipients' desires to attain valid attitudes. Because they should therefore aspire to attain greater confidence in their assessment of message validity, their sufficiency thresholds should be higher on the judgmental confidence continuum. Because the likelihood that recipients will attain their sufficiency thresholds via heuristic processing decreases as these thresholds increase, recipients who encounter personally relevant messages should generally exhibit heightened levels of systematic processing.

The argument is similar for other motivational variables. For example, consider individual differences in NFC. High-NFC subjects have been shown to engage in more systematic processing than low-NFC subjects (e.g., Cacioppo, Petty, & Morris, 1983). This effect on systematic processing can be understood by assuming that higher-NFC persons generally desire to achieve greater levels of judgmental confidence. As a consequence, the sufficiency thresholds of high-NFC persons would be higher on the judgmental confidence continuum than those of low-NFC persons.[7]

Ability Issues and Attaining Confidence through Heuristics

We have discussed two main hypotheses derived from the sufficiency principle. First, when the less effortful heuristic-processing mode yields insufficient judgmental confidence, or, more obviously, when heuristic processing cannot occur, people are more likely to expend the effort required to engage in systematic processing. Second (and corollary to the first hypothesis), because higher sufficiency thresholds decrease the probability that heuristic processing will confer sufficient confidence, motivational factors that increase sufficiency thresholds typically will increase the magnitude of systematic processing. These hypotheses are conditional, however, because they entail several assumptions that may not always be met.

Most obviously, our hypotheses presume that people have the *ability* to process systematically. As such, they should prove valid only when situational or individual-difference factors (e.g., time pressure, lack of knowledge) do not severely constrain systematic processing. For example, the hypothesis that personal relevance increases systematic processing should be true only when ability for this processing mode is intact. Unfortunately, the limitations of motivational hypotheses such as this one have not been explored, because relevant research has used materials and procedures that ensure high capacity for systematic processing (see Chaiken, 1987, p. 11).

Less obviously, our hypotheses also presume that people believe that they *can* increase judgmental confidence through systematic processing. If this belief were not held, there would be little advantage to systematic processing. In previous papers, we have glossed over differences in such self-efficacy beliefs by making the unqualified assumption that systematic processing is a more reliable means of judging message validity than relying on simple decision rules (e.g., Chaiken, 1987, p. 8). In retrospect, this assumption is too sweeping, although there are reasons to consider it generally applicable. For example, research indicates that attitudes based on direct experience are held with more confidence than those based on indirect experience (Fazio & Zanna, 1981). Since attitudes formed primarily by systematic processing can be likened to attitudes based on direct experience, whereas those formed via heuristic processing can be likened to attitudes based on indirect experience, it follows that systematic processing often *will* yield greater judgmental confidence than heuristic processing. Indeed, this analogy partially underlies the HSM's (substantiated) hypothesis that systematic processing often confers greater attitude persistence and attitude–behavior consistency than heuristic processing (Cacioppo, Petty, Kao, & Rodriguez, 1986; Chaiken, 1980, Experiment 1; Chaiken & Eagly, 1983, Experiment 2; Pallak, Murroni, & Koch, 1983; Petty, Cacioppo, & Schumann, 1983; for more detailed discussion of this hypothesis and its contingencies, see Chaiken, 1978, 1980, 1987; Chaiken & Stangor, 1987).

Motivational Impact of Ability Deficits

Although systematic processing may often confer greater judgmental confidence, and although people may often believe this to be the case, there are clear exceptions. Most obviously, when ability for systematic processing is constrained, the potential for this mode to actually enhance confidence is severely compromised. Moreover, it is unlikely that people are oblivious to such constraints. For this reason, factors that impair ability for systematic processing probably also reduce people's beliefs that this mode can enhance their judgmental confidence. As a consequence, ability-impairing variables probably undermine people's *motivation* for systematic processing, as well as their capacity for systematic processing. A novice about economics may attend little to debates on the federal deficit, because he or she realizes that even the most compulsive attention will not afford a confident opinion on this topic.

Importantly, though, the motivational impact of ability-impairing variables has a different source than the motivational impact of variables such as personal relevance, task importance, or need for cognition. We have argued that the latter variables affect systematic processing via their impact on sufficiency thresholds, the level of judgmental confidence people aspire to attain. In contrast, the effect of ability-impairing variables on motivation for systematic processing is mediated by self-efficacy beliefs, people's beliefs that systematic processing can increase judgmental confidence.

Heuristic Processing in High-Stakes Settings

What happens when people's sufficiency thresholds are high, but they doubt the efficacy of systematic processing or, for other reasons, cannot process systematically (see Chaiken, 1980, Experiment 2; McCroskey, 1969)? One obvious possibility is that a less-than-desired degree of judgmental confidence will have to suffice. To illustrate, imagine a study manipulating personal relevance, argument quality, and message comprehensibility. Previous research has shown that argument quality exerts a greater persuasive impact when personal relevance is high *or* when ability for systematic processing is not impaired (e.g., Petty & Cacioppo, 1979, 1984; Wood et al., 1985; Worth & Mackie, 1987). Our three-factor study would extend this research in several important ways. It would presumably demonstrate that (1) personal relevance enhances systematic processing *primarily* when ability for such processing is high (i.e., high-comprehensibility conditions), and (2) ability enhances systematic processing *primarily* when people are motivated to enhance their judgmental confidence (i.e., conditions of high personal relevance). Moreover, the study should also reveal differences in attitudinal confidence. In particular, confidence should be lowest among high-relevance/low-comprehensibility subjects, for their ability for systematic processing is impaired but their sufficiency thresholds are high.

In this hypothetical study, high-relevance/low-comprehensibility subjects have no opportunity to seek out information *other* than message content that may enhance their judgmental confidence—at least not within the laboratory setting. But what if heuristic cues were available to them? We have cited research indicating that personal relevance *attenuates* the persuasive impact of heuristic cues when ability for systematic processing is high (e.g., Axsom et al., 1987; Chaiken, 1980; Petty & Cacioppo, 1984; Petty, Cacioppo, & Goldman, 1981). If ability for systematic processing were constrained, would this attenuation effect still be observed? We think not. In fact, in these settings we would predict the opposite—that heightened personal relevance (task importance, etc) should *enhance* the persuasive impact of heuristic cues.

There are two reasons why this *enhancement hypothesis* should be true. First, as discussed earlier in this chapter, enhancing the accessibility of persuasion heuristics increases the persuasive impact of their associated heuristic cues. And any factor that enhances the importance of the goal of assessing message validity should increase the accessibility of heuristics relevant to accomplishing this goal. Since personal relevance is probably one of these factors, it follows that this variable should increase the persuasive impact of heuristic cues. Second, because personal relevance raises people's sufficiency thresholds, they may scrutinize persuasion settings more carefully in order to ferret out cues that might be diagnostic of message validity. In other words, people may be more likely to notice (and use) heuristic cues when they encounter messages of high personal relevance.[8]

We are arguing, then, that motivational variables such as personal relevance do not influence only the magnitude of systematic processing. These variables should also enhance the likelihood of heuristic processing, because they increase the cognitive accessibility of relevant persuasion heuristics and/or increase the vigilance with which people search (the setting or their memories) for relevant heuristic cues. Yet the fact that these variables enhance the liklihood of heuristic processing does not imply that they will *always* increase the persuasive impact of heuristic cues. As we have pointed out, when motivation *and ability* for systematic processing are high, the persuasive impact of heuristic cues is often attenuated. In contrast, the enhancing effect of motivational variables on the persuasive impact of heuristic cues should be most detectable in *low-ability* situations, where systematic processing is not, or is not perceived to be, a feasible means of assessing message validity.

Although this enhancement hypothesis requires explicit testing, Sorrentino, Bobocel, Gitta, Olson, and Hewitt (1987) reported data congenial to it. These authors examined the effects of personal relevance and source expertise (and argument quality) on the attitudes of uncertainty-oriented and certainty-oriented subjects. The former subjects yielded data consistent with previous research on personal relevance (e.g., Chaiken, 1980, Experiment 2; Petty, Cacioppo, & Goldman, 1981): Source expertise influenced their attitudes less when personal relevance was higher (and argument quality influenced them more). In contrast, certainty-oriented subjects were *more* influenced by source expertise when personal relevance was high (and were less influenced by argument quality). If we assume that certainty-oriented subjects were disinclined to process systematically because they doubted its efficacy—an assumption compatible with Sorrentino et al.'s conceptualization of this personality variable—these results are consistent with the hypothesis that motivational variables *can* (under specifiable circumstances) enhance the persuasive impact of heuristic cues.

Our discussion of ability issues underscores our belief that the use of heuristics is more ubiquitous than existing persuasion research suggests. Although previous research suggests that heuristic processing exerts a detectable persuasive impact mainly when motivation for systematic processing is low, most of this research has been conducted in high-ability settings. In contrast, heuristic processing probably exerts a stronger persuasive impact in low-ability settings. Moreover, we would argue that capacity for systematic processing is often lower in real-world settings than in the modal laboratory persuasion study (Chaiken & Stangor, 1987; Eagly & Chaiken, 1984). Outside the laboratory, people encounter innumerable messages virtually every day via the mass media and their social interactions with others. Given the sheer amount of this information, the capacity to process every message systematically is well-nigh impossible. In addition, the complexity of such information, particularly regarding important social and political issues, may undermine people's beliefs in the (self-)efficacy of systematic processing. For these reasons, people probably turn to simple decision rules on a much more frequent basis than current laboratory research suggests.

Interaction Effects and Biased Systematic Processing

Because systematic processing (in more than negligible amounts) requires effort and capacity, it will not occur in all persuasion settings. Similarly, because heuristic processing depends (at a minimum) on the presence of heuristic cues and the cognitive availability of relevant heuristics, its occurence is also conditional. In situations conducive to both modes, however, the HSM assumes that heuristic and systematic processing can co-occur. The HSM thus allows for the possibility that its two processing modes may influence each other, and hence for the possibility that they may exert interdependent (i.e., interactive) or independent (i.e., additive) effects on people's judgments. In this section, we focus upon interaction effects, especially the hypothesis that heuristic processing may bias systematic processing.

In earlier sections of this chapter, we have touched upon two ways in which heuristic and systematic processing may be viewed as interdependent. First, systematic processing can override the judgmental impact of heuristic processing. Support for this attenuation hypothesis is most likely to be obtained in settings marked by high motivation and, especially, high ability for systematic processing. In these situations, heuristic processing furnishes information relevant to message validity (e.g., the message contains many arguments), but so does systematic processing. In addition, systematic processing may yield information that contradicts the validity of simple persuasion heuristics (e.g., the message contains lots of ridiculous arguments or very few but excellent ones; e.g., Petty & Cacioppo, 1984). For these reasons, the persuasive impact of heuristic cues will often be negligible in persuasion settings characterized by high motivation and high ability for systematic processing.[9]

The second sense in which heuristic and systematic processing affect each other is mediated by sufficiency thresholds. As shown by our XT-100 study, the failure of heuristic processing to confer sufficient judgmental confidence can stimulate systematic processing. When low-importance subjects in that study lacked confidence in their heuristic-based evaluations of the XT-100 (due to incongruency), they stepped up their systematic processing (Maheswaran & Chaiken, 1988). Analogously, the failure of systematic processing to confer sufficient judgmental confidence may stimulate heuristic processing. As we have discussed, rather than settling for uncertainty, recipients may actively search the persuasion setting for heuristic cues, and their memories for relevant heuristics that may afford a more confident attitude judgment (see also Chaiken, 1980, p. 763).

Heuristic Processing May Bias Systematic Processing

The third way in which the HSM's two modes can interact is that heuristic processing may sometimes bias systematic processing. That is, because heuristic cues influence recipients' perceptions of the probable validity of persuasive messages, they may also function to bias recipients' perceptions of message content. Thus, if a message is delivered by an expert, its arguments may be viewed more positively than if the message is delivered by a nonexpert. Similarly, if other persons appear to endorse a message's advocated position, its content may be evaluated and elaborated upon in a more positive manner than if other persons appear to oppose its position.

The conditions under which heuristic cues may bias systematic processing are fairly circumscribed, because message content must be ambiguous enough to be *amenable to differential interpretation* as a function of recipients' processing of heuristic cues. In essence, heuristic cues can be used to disambiguate message content. Since prior knowledge about the message topic can also function to disambiguate message content, heuristics should exert a greater biasing effect when recipients are motivated to process (ambiguous) messages systematically but lack knowledge about the message topic.[10] In these situations, the "bias hypothesis" predicts that heuristic cues will exert a detectable persuasive impact, and, more importantly, that this persuasive impact will be mediated (at least partially) by biased systematic processing.

Findings consistent with this bias hypothesis were reported by Mackie (1987, Experiment 1). She presented subjects with arguments allegedly endorsed by a majority of others and with opposing arguments allegedly endorsed by a minority, and found that subjects agreed more with the majority's position than with the minority's. Suggesting that agreement was mediated by biased systematic processing, subjects recalled more majority than minority arguments and generated more favorable thoughts about the majority's arguments. Because Mackie's subjects probably possessed little knowledge about the message topic (whether the United States should ensure a military balance in the Western Hemisphere), they probably found it an enigmatic task to judge the relative merits of the majority versus the minority arguments on the basis of these arguments alone. As a consequence, their heuristic processing of consensus information led them to perceive the majority's (vs. minority's) arguments as better, and this perception in turn fostered greater attention to (and subsequent memory for) these arguments and more positive elaborations of them.[11]

Notwithstanding Mackie's (1987) results, it is difficult to find much empirical support for the bias hypothesis. Although the hypothesis could be wrong, we feel that the main reason it lacks support is that its preconditions have not been well represented in persuasion studies. Most importantly, the messages used in persuasion research virtually always consist of straightforward and unambiguously strong (and sometimes weak) arguments whose intrinsic validity can be ascertained with ease by the typical college-age subject. If persuasive argumentation were made more ambiguous, we believe that the bias hypothesis would be confirmed. In this regard, it is noteworthy that research showing that cognitive structures such as stereotypes and trait constructs can bias person perception has intentionally used ambiguous stimuli (see Higgins & Bargh, 1987).

Our bias hypothesis raises an apparent paradox. If it is correct, subsequent research using appropriate stimuli should demonstrate that heuristic cues can influence persuasion via their impact on systematic processing. On the surface, this projected result seems inconsistent with one of the HSM's fundamental assertions—that heuristic cues affect persuasion via simple decision rules—and supportive of earlier theoretical perspectives, which assumed that heuristic cues such as source expertise influence persuasion via their impact on people's acceptance of persuasive argumentation (e.g., Fishbein & Ajzen, 1975; McGuire, 1969). In reality, there is no contradiction. The original purpose of the HSM, rather than to deny the validity of these earlier accounts, was to argue for the *additional* (and, at the time, novel) possibility that the persuasive impact of heuristic cues might *often* reflect little more than recipients' use of simple decision rules (Chaiken, 1978, 1980). Moreover, the bias hypothesis refines earlier views of how heuristic cues function, for it argues that recipients' heuristic processing of these cues establishes expectancies about message validity, which then influence recipients' systematic processing of message content. By specifying when the persuasive impact of heuristic cues will be mediated by simple persuasion heuristics versus heuristics plus systematic processing, the HSM provides a rapprochement between older and newer views of how this class of variables affects persuasion.

Sources of Bias Other Than Heuristic Cues

The HSM's bias hypothesis posits a cognitive mechanism—validity expectancies established by recipients' processing of heuristic cues—that can produce biased systematic processing. In addition, systematic processing may be biased by other factors, such as prior knowledge, vested interests, and preferences for or commitments to particular attitudinal positions. In this section, we address these other motivational and cognitive sources of bias and comment on their connection to our model.

The idea that systematic processing might be biased by people's vested interests and attitudinal commitments that stem from important values or reference groups follows from earlier theorizing about "ego-involving" attitudes (e.g., Ostrom & Brock, 1968; Sherif & Hovland, 1961). Nevertheless, this possibility has not been well researched (see Johnson & Eagly, in press). Contemporary studies of persuasion have largely ignored these independent variables, and earlier research typically included either no measures of cognitive processing or measures capable of detecting only limited aspects of selective information processing (e.g., perceived message position—Hovland, Harvey, & Sherif, 1957; see Johnson and Eagly, in press, for a review and discussion of this research and its relation to contemporary research on "involvement"). In a similar vein, the idea that systematic processing might be biased by people's preferences or desires for particular attitudinal positions is suggested by experiments showing that subjects are more persuaded by messages that espouse desirable rather than undesirable conclusions—for example, that unemployment is declining versus rising (Eagly & Chaiken, 1975; see also Eagly & Acksen, 1971; Eagly & Whitehead, 1972; McGuire, 1957, 1969, 1981). Unfortunately, this possibility cannot be evaluated on the basis of existing research, for a variety of methodological reasons (e.g., experimental confounds, lack of direct measures of cognitive processing).

The impact that vested interests, attitudinal commitments, and preferences for particular conclusions have on cognitive processing and judgment can be understood in terms of the underlying motives that these variables represent. In general, all of these variables can be conceptualized under one umbrella motive—the desire to form or to defend particular attitudinal positions. Because the HSM has heretofore assumed only a single motive (achieving valid attitudes), to postulate additional motives constitutes an extension of the model. For this reason, we reserve further discussion of variables related to the defense motive we have postulated until we have presented an extended version of the HSM.

Prior knowledge may at times also bias systematic processing. In contrast to the biasing effects of vested interests and preferred attitude positions, which are motivational, prior knowledge represents a cognitive source of bias insofar as this knowledge may be evaluatively skewed. Such a skewed knowledge base is often likely, since people's beliefs tend to be evaluatively consistent with their attitudes (Feather, 1969, 1971; Fishbein & Ajzen, 1975). Possessing an evaluatively biased store of knowledge may enhance recipients' abilities to rebut counterattitudinal arguments and to generate proattitudinal arguments. If so, more knowledgeable recipients may be less persuaded by counterattitudinal messages but more persuaded by proattitudinal messages in comparison to recipients who lack prior knowledge. Alternatively, prior knowledge may function not to bias systematic processing, but rather to enhance recipients' abilities to process messages systematically and critically, *regardless* of these messages' positions. If so, more knowledgeable recipients may be less persuaded than less knowledgeable recipients by both proattitudinal and counterattitudinal messages.

The impact of prior knowledge on persuasion has been investigated by Wood and her colleagues in research with subjects who differ in their abilities to retrieve attitude-relevant beliefs and behaviors from memory (Wood, 1982; Wood & Kallgren, 1988; Wood et al., 1985). Supporting the hypothesis that domain-specific expertise enhances ability for systematic processing, Wood's high-retrieval (vs. low-retrieval) subjects have generated more message-relevant thoughts in response to her persuasive communications and have been more influenced by variations in argument quality. Regardless of argument quality, however, high-retrieval subjects have also generated more negative thoughts about Wood's messages and have been less persuaded than low-retrieval subjects (e.g., Wood et al., 1985). Does this negativity effect reflect biased systematic processing by high-retrieval subjects, or simply their greater ability to critically evaluate even strongly argued messages?

The bias interpretation is favored by the fact that Wood's subjects received counterattitudinal messages, and the fact that attitude-relevant knowledge tends to be evaluatively consistent with attitudes. Thus, the greater knowledge possessed by high-retrieval (vs. low-retrieval) subjects may have been biased in favor of their prior attitudes—a factor that would enhance the likelihood that they would rebut arguments contained in the counterattitudinal messages they received and generate arguments bolstering their prior attitudes.

Although this bias interpretation is reasonable, there are several reasons why it may be premature. First, its assumption that high-retrieval subjects' knowledge was evaluatively consistent with their prior attitudes was not documented in Wood's research. Such documentation is important, because there exists substantial variation in the degree to which people manifest evaluative–cognitive consistency (e.g., Chaiken & Baldwin, 1981; Rosenberg, 1968). Second, the fact that Wood has statistically controlled for prior attitudes through analysis of covariance procedures somewhat weakens the plausibility of the bias interpretation. That is, to the extent that this technique implicitly controls for the valence of prior knowledge *in addition to* explicitly controlling for the valence of prior attitudes, it is difficult to argue forcefully that *differences* in the former contributed to Wood's negativity findings. For these reasons, high-retrieval subjects' more negative responses to Wood's messages may have been the product of their enhanced abilities to process information critically, rather than the product of biased systematic processing. Further research could test between these interpretations by using proattitudinal messages. If high-retrieval subjects exhibited more negative systematic processing and less persuasion in response to such messages, the heightened-criticality interpretation would be supported. If, however, their systematic processing was more positive and their persuasion greater, the bias interpretation would be supported.

Regardless of how Wood's research is best interpreted, an important point in our view is that prior knowledge per se does not bias systematic processing. Rather, prior beliefs represent a potential source of bias to the extent that their valence is distinctly positive or negative (see also Alba & Hutchinson, 1987). Because prior knowledge is probably most likely to be evaluatively polarized when people's prior attitudes are strongly held, it is probably more accurate to assert that strong prior attitudes may bias systematic processing, and that an evaluatively biased knowledge base may mediate this effect.

Surprisingly, the biasing effects of prior attitudes have received little attention by contemporary cognitively-oriented researchers, even though earlier persuasion researchers often accorded prior attitudes an important theoretical role (e.g., Sherif & Hovland, 1961). Most contemporary studies do not even assess prior attitudes. In these "after-only" experiments, subjects' pre-experimental attitudes typically are assumed to be opposed to the message's advocacy. Moreover, when prior attitudes are assessed, they are rarely represented in the analytic design. In some cases, they are "dismissed" because, consistent with random assignment of subjects to conditions, preliminary analysis reveals that they do not vary across experimental conditions. In other cases, they are used (with postmessage attitudes) to create attitude change scores, but are still not represented as an independent variable in the study's design (see Mackie, 1987, for an exception). Finally, prior attitudes sometimes enter the design as a covariate, as in Wood's (e.g., 1982) research. Although the covariate strategy can yield information regarding the overall (i.e., main) effect of prior attitudes on various dependent measures, it ignores possible interactions between prior attitudes and other independent variables in the study.

To explore whether prior attitudes affect systematic processing (and, if so, when and how), researchers could use regression models in which relevant dependent measures are regressed on prior attitudes and other independent variables and, in subsequent steps, on cross-product terms that represent these variables' interactions. As we have already suggested, prior attitudes may bias systematic processing because attitude-relevant knowledge is evaluatively biased. Another possibility follows from the HSM's hypothesis that heuristic processing can bias systematic processing. If one's prior attitude (in conjunction with a message's position) is conceptualized as a heuristic cue—and its associated heuristic is something like "Messages that espouse agreeable (disagreeable) positions probably are (aren't) valid"— the content of messages that appear proattitudinal may be processed in a more benevolent fashion than the content of messages that appear counterattitudinal (see Liberman et al., 1988; for alternate theoretical perspectives, see Petty & Cacioppo, 1979; Sherif & Hovland, 1961).[12]

Additivity Effects

We have discussed three ways in which the HSM's two modes of processing can be regarded as interdependent. In addition, however, our model's co-occurrence assumption allows for the possibility that heuristic and systematic processing can proceed relatively independently of each other. If so, there should be circumstances under which the two processing modes exert *additive* effects on people's attitude judgments. To illustrate, consider a study manipulating a heuristic cue, source expertise, and a message content variable, argument quality. An inference that the HSM's two modes combined additively to influence attitudes would be warranted if source expertise and argument quality each exerted a main effect on postmessage attitudes; and if regression analyses supported the ideas that the persuasive impact of argument quality was mediated by the valence of message-relevant thought, while the persuasive impact of source expertise was mediated by the expertise heuristic.

Studies that have simultaneously manipulated heuristic cues and message content variables under conditions conducive to systematic processing are numerous, but almost none have yielded support for the additivity hypothesis we have described. Instead, most existing research indicates that when recipients are willing and able to process systematically, message content manipulations exert strong main effects on postmessage attitudes, whereas heuristic cue manipulations exert no significant persuasive impact (alone or in interaction with the message manipulation). In other words, this research overwhelmingly demonstrates the attenuation effect, in which systematic processing overrides the judgmental impact of heuristic processing (see earlier discussion).

Akin to our defense of the HSM's bias hypothesis, we feel that methodological factors have not been congenial to the additivity hypothesis. To see why this is so, let us reconsider the 2×2 study described above and assume that the experimental situation is conducive to systematic processing. Additivity would predict (at the least) that *both* main effects (i.e., source expertise, argument quality) should be significant on subjects' postmessage attitudes. Like previous research, however, this hypothetical study would no doubt yield *only* a main effect for argument quality (strong > weak). Such a design is a poor test of additivity, however, for the chances of its yielding a main effect for expertise are slim. The main reason why this is so is that two of the study's four cells represent clear-cut cases in which message content blatantly *contradicts* the expertise heuristic (i.e., expert/weak arguments, inexpert/strong arguments). Thus, the design is heavily stacked in favor of the attenuation hypothesis and against the additivity hypothesis. Even if the attitudes expressed by subjects in the two noncontradictory cells (expert/strong, inexpert/weak) *did* exhibit additivity—that is, if their attitudes were independently influenced by heuristic and systematic processing—the attenuation effect in the two contradictory cells would make it difficult for the expertise main effect to reach significance. The inclusion of no-heuristic-cue control conditions in such a study should make additive effects in the two noncontradictory cells more detectable. That is, in comparison to a strong-arguments-only condition, expert/strong subjects should exhibit more positive postmessage attitudes; and in comparison to a weak-arguments-only condition, nonexpert/weak subjects should exhibit more negative attitudes. In essense, a fairer test of the HSM's additivity hypothesis necessitates experimental designs that, unlike most previous studies, are not so heavily stacked against it.

BEYOND THE VALIDITY-SEEKING PERSUASION CONTEXT

We have stressed that the HSM's current domain of applicability is limited because it posits only one underlying motivational orientation: the desire to form or to hold valid, accurate attitudes. It is important to realize, however, that most existing work in persuasion has explicitly or implicitly assumed that people are validity seekers (see Eagly & Chaiken, 1984). It might be argued, then, that a single-motive HSM does provide a good account of persuasion as it has been traditionally studied. Yet the fact that most research has emphasized one motive does not mean that others are unimportant. Thus, despite the HSM's utility for validity-seeking contexts and the heavy representation of such contexts in the literature, we offer an extended model that should have even greater value. In particular, our extended model is intended to apply to a variety of social influence settings in which people either *receive* attitude-relevant information from external sources, as in persuasion and some self-perception and group influence paradigms (see Chaiken & Baldwin, 1981; Maass, West, & Cialdini, 1987), or *generate* such information in response to direct or indirect inducements to do so, as in some induced compliance, mere thought, and anticipatory attitude change experiments (see Cialdini & Petty, 1981; Higgins & McCann, 1984; Stroebe & Diehl, 1988; Tetlock, 1983).

Sketch of a Multiple-Motive Model for the Social Influence Domain

The single-motive HSM posits one motive, achieving valid attitudes, and one corresponding processing goal, assessing the validity of persuasive messages (or, more generally, assessing the validity of attitude-relevant information). The first step, then, in building a multiple-motive model is to list other motives that may operate in influence settings and to link these motives to processing goals. At present, we believe that accuracy motivation and two other capacious motives may be adequate to describe the motivational space of most social influence settings (but see note 13).

   We have already discussed one of these additional motives. Specifically, we have argued that the impact of variables such as vested interests and attitudinal commitments and preferences can be conceptualized in terms of "defense motivation," the desire to form or to defend particular attitudinal positions (see "Sources of Bias Other Than Heuristic Cues"). The processing goal of defense-motivated recipients, then, is to confirm the validity of particular attitudinal positions and disconfirm the validity of others. Theorizing about different aspects of the self and their relation to social influence suggests that we should also postulate an "impression motive" (cf. Greenwald & Pratkanis, 1984; Johnson & Eagly, in press, 1988; Leippe & Elkin, 1987; Smith et al., 1956). When *impression motivation* is paramount, people desire to express attitudes that will be socially acceptable to potential evaluators, both real and imagined (see Higgins, 1981; Kel-

man, 1961; Leippe & Elkin, 1987; Smith et al, 1956; Tetlock, 1983, 1985).
The processing goal of impression-motivated individuals, then, is to assess
the social acceptability of alternative attitudinal positions. Impression motivation is likely to be aroused when people anticipate communicating (or
justifying) their attitudes to others (e.g., Tetlock, 1983), especially when
potential evaluators' attributes or social roles cast them as an important
audience (Schlenker, 1982). However, impression–motivation may also be
aroused in other influence situations when interpersonal relationships are
salient to the individual or when the identities of significant others and
groups (and their relevance to the focal attitude topic) are made salient
(see Higgins, 1981; Kelman, 1961; Smith et al., 1956).

The single-motive HSM posits that *both* heuristic and systematic processing serve the accuracy-motivated goal of assessing the validity of attitude-relevant information. Similarly, we posit that both of these modes can
serve the defense-motivated goal of confirming the validity of particular
attitudinal positions, and the impression-motivated goal of assessing the
social acceptability of alternative attitudinal positions. In other words, the
multiple-motive HSM views processing mode and processing goal as orthogonal; heuristic and systematic processing occur in the service of the
individual's processing goal, whatever that goal may be.[13]

The essence of heuristic and systematic processing remains the same,
regardless of perceivers' processing goals. Whereas heuristic processors will
use simple decision rules to accomplish their goals, systematic processors
will accomplish the same by extensively processing available attitude-relevant
information. Although their essence is unchanged, the purpose of heuristic
and systematic processing does shift as a function of processing goal.

Accuracy Motivation

Most familiar, of course, is accuracy-motivated processing. Heuristic perceivers assess the validity of attitude-relevant information using simple rules
such as the expertise heuristic or the consensus heuristic. All else being
equal, they adopt attitudinal positions that square with those of experts,
with the majority opinion, and so forth. In contrast, systematic perceivers
scrutinize *all* attitude-relevant information. Accuracy-motivated systematic
processing may sometimes be biased by cognitive factors such as prior
knowledge (if biased by prior attitudes) and heuristic cues. Nevertheless,
because of its motivational basis, accuracy-motivated systematic processing (and accuracy-motivated heuristic processing) can be characterized as
open-minded.

Defense Motivation

Next, let us consider defense-motivated processing. Defense-motivated perceivers use the same persuasion heuristics that accuracy-motivated perceivers do, but they use them *selectively*. For example, the expertise heuristic

should be used by these persons only to the extent that an expert advocates a position whose validity they desire to confirm or a nonexpert advocates a position they wish to disconfirm. Similarly, the consensus heuristic is more likely to be invoked when it would validate, rather than invalidate, a favored attitudinal position. Defense-motivated systematic processing is also selective. Attitude-relevant information that supports favored positions or opposes nonfavored ones should receive more attention and be more positively interpreted than information that opposes favored positions or supports nonfavored ones. Given its motivational agenda, this type of systematic processing can be characterized as closed-minded.

Impression Motivation

As we have noted, impression motivation may be aroused when the identities of significant audiences (real or imagined) are salient to the individual, when social relationships are important, or when people must communicate their attitudes to potential evaluators. When impression-motivated processing reflects people's intentions to express attitudes that will please or appease potential evaluators, it can be characterized as strategic. Most research suggests that such attitudes reflect accommodations to situational pressures that revert to prior levels when these pressures are removed (e.g., Cialdini, Levy, Herman, Kozlowski, & Petty, 1976; Kelman, 1961; Shechter, 1987; see Cialdini & Petty, 1981, for a review). Yet there is some evidence that attitudes expressed for strategic reasons may eventually become internalized (e.g., Higgins & McCann, 1984; see also Chaiken & Stangor, 1987). For this reason, the issue of whether attitudinal responses that result from strategic impression-motivated processing are dissimulations or genuine should be dealt with empirically rather than by definitional fiat (cf. Kelman, 1961).

Impression-motivated heuristic processing involves the use of simple rules to guide one's selection of a socially acceptable attitudinal position (e.g., "Moderate positions minimize disagreement," "Agreement facilitates liking"), whereas impression-motivated systematic processing connotes that the same task has been accomplished through a more extensive consideration of attitude-relevant information. More concrete descriptions of impression-motivated heuristic and systematic processing require knowledge of particular influence contexts, because what constitutes socially acceptable attitude judgments will vary as a function of potential audiences, their salience, and other situational factors. For example, conformity to others' attitudes may be more acceptable in some situations than in others.

Recent research supports the value of our mode-of-processing distinction in settings that arouse impression motivation (e.g., Leippe & Elkin, 1987; Shechter, 1987; Tetlock, 1983). For example, Tetlock (1983) told subjects that they would be discussing their attitudes on affirmative action, capital punishment, and defense spending with another person whose views were unknown to subjects or were described as liberal or conservative. In the study, subjects listed their thoughts about each issue and then gave their attitudes. The results indicated that subjects who were unaware (vs. aware) of their partner's ideology engaged in more extensive thinking, as indexed by the integrative complexity of their listed thoughts. Moreover, this systematic processing apparently served these subjects' impression-motivated goal of forming a socially acceptable middle-of-the-road attitude, for their thought protocols revealed a mix of pro–con thinking on the issues, and their subsequently expressed attitudes were relatively neutral. In contrast, subjects who were aware of their partner's ideology seemed to use a simple agreement heuristic (see also Tetlock, 1985). They expressed relatively liberal attitude positions when their partner was liberal and conservative views when he was conservative (see also Higgins & McCann, 1984).

Given Tetlock's attitude issues, subjects could easily discern what the liberal–conservative position was on each, and it is this knowledge that no doubt enabled those aware of their partner's ideology to use a simple agreement heuristic. For example, the pro position on defense spending communicates agreement with conservatives. If the study had used less ideologically clear-cut issues, their liberal–conservative positions would have been less apparent. As a consequence, subjects aware of their partner's ideology might have engaged in just as much impression-motivated systematic processing as those who were unaware—with an important difference. The purpose of unaware subjects' processing was to formulate a socially acceptable middle-of-the-road position. In contrast, we would predict that the purpose of aware subjects' extensive processing would be to ascertain the liberal (vs. conservative) position on each discussion issue, so that they could formulate a socially acceptable liberal (vs. conservative) attitudinal response.

Summary and Example Predictions

In essence, the multiple-motive HSM features three underlying motives and three correspondent processing goals, and the assertion that both heuristic and systematic processing occur in the service of these processing goals. These ideas will require refinement, especially in relation to understanding impression-motivated processing and the complexities that may arise when more than one motive and processing goal are important to individuals (see note 13).

The remaining features of our extended model would be virtually identical to the cognitive and motivational aspects outlined in relation to the single-motive model. That is, regardless of which motive and processing goal are operative, the multiple-motive HSM assumes that heuristic and systematic processing may co-occur; that heuristic processing depends upon the cognitive availability, accessibility, and perceived reliability of

relevant judgmental heuristics; that systematic processing is both more effortful and more capacity-limited than heuristic processing; that heuristic
processing can proceed in either a more or less self-conscious manner; and
that effort minimization and the principle of sufficiency are crucial determinants of processing mode.

The bulk of this chapter has detailed the testable implications of the
HSM for settings in which accuracy motivation is paramount. In settings
in which defense motivation or impression motivation is paramount, analogous implications follow from our extended model's parallel set of cognitive—functional assumptions and principles. For example, capacity-lim-
iting factors should constrain defense- or impression-motivated systematic
processing, and, as a consequence, should enhance the judgmental impact
of heuristic processing. Likewise, the level of judgmental confidence that
defense-motivated or impression-motivated recipients aspire to attain should
be increased by motivational factors that enhance defense-motivated recipients' desires to confirm particular attitudinal positions (e.g., making salient vested interests or the attitudes of important reference groups) and
impression-motivated recipients' desires to express socially appropriate attitudes (e.g., making salient potential evaluators' reward or coercive power;
French & Raven, 1959). Therefore, with defense- or impression-motivated
processing, these sorts of motivational variables should (1) increase the
magnitude of systematic processing in situations where ability for such
processing is high, and (2) increase the likelihood of heuristic processing
in situations that constrain ability for systematic processing or in other
ways undermine its feasibility.

A final example illustrates the predictive utility of the sufficiency principle. Consider two recipients, one goaded by accuracy motivation and the
other by defense motivation, who encounter a persuasive message from an
expert or a nonexpert. Regardless of the message's specific position, the
accuracy-motivated recipient should assess message validity using the expertise heuristic. Thus, he or she should agree with the expert's advocated
position (or disagree with the nonexpert's position) without deliberating
much about the message's persuasive arguments (unless, of course, his or
her sufficiency threshold is very high).

In contrast, whether the defense-motivated recipient stops at the heuristic-processing stage depends upon the nature of the message's position.
When the recipient desires to confirm the validity of the message's position, he or she should use the expertise heuristic and eschew systematic
processing in response to the expert communicator, because heuristic processing should confer sufficient judgmental confidence. In response to the
nonexpert, however, he or she would probably manifest defense-motivated
systematic processing, because heuristic processing should undermine the
validity of the recipient's preferred position. The reverse pattern should
obtain when the message's position is one whose validity the recipient desires to disconfirm. In these situations, the defense-motivated recipient would

probably use the expertise heuristic and eschew systematic processing in response to the nonexpert's message, but would probably engage in systematic processing in response to the expert's message.

Relevance of the Multiple-Motive HSM to Other Social Judgment Contexts

Since the single-motive HSM was originally developed to apply to validity-seeking persuasion settings, we geared its vocabulary to this context. In comparison, the language of the multiple-motive HSM is less specialized, given its applicability to a broader range of social influence settings. Nevertheless, in both versions of the model, our vocabulary is pitched to social judgment domains in which people's *attitudes* are focal.

Although the focalized nature of the HSM maximizes its clarity as a theory of the cognitive and functional mechanisms underlying the formation, change, and expression of attitudes, it may obscure its relevance to other kinds of social judgments. Yet we believe that the HSM has utility for the broader domain of social judgment. In particular, we believe that a generic version of the HSM can provide a framework for studying a variety of situations in which people are exposed to information about themselves, other persons, and events, and make decisions or formulate judgments about these entities. We are referring, then, to a variety of social judgments investigated in research on impression formation, stereotyping, attribution, social prediction, and decision making.

A multiple-motive HSM of social judgment and decision making would feature the generic definitions of heuristic and systematic processing offered at the beginning of this chapter, as well as more precise definitions for particular contexts. The specific definitions we have used in relation to the validity-seeking persuasion context exemplify this strategy. Our general model would also postulate the three motives and processing goals discussed in the preceding section, although they too would be more broadly defined. For example, defense motivation would be defined as the desire to form or to defend particular social judgments or decisions, and the processing goal of defense-motivated social perceivers would be described as confirming the validity of particular judgments and disconfirming the validity of others. As these examples illustrate, the vocabulary of our generic HSM would be broad enough to apply to a variety of social judgments and settings. Yet our general model's definitions, assumptions, and principles would be identical to those we have articulated in this chapter.

A Hypothetical Empirical Example

To illustrate the HSM's relevance to nonattitudinal settings, consider the following hypothetical experiment. Subjects are asked to form an impression of a female target after reading a story about a party she attended and seeing her picture. The picture portrays the target as either physically attractive or unattractive, and the story portrays her party behavior as "sociable." However, the story's descriptions of other partygoers' behavior (consensus) and of the target's behavior at other parties (consistency) and social gatherings (distinctiveness) are varied in order to create two versions—one designed to foster an internal attribution for the target's sociability (low consensus, high consistency, low distinctiveness), and one designed to foster an external attribution (high consensus, low consistency, high distinctiveness; see Kelley, 1972).

In this study, story content is analogous to a persuasive message. If this story is carefully processed, subjects should rate the target as being more sociable in the internal-attribution (vs. external-attribution) condition. The target's physical attractiveness is analogous to a persuasion study's heuristic cue, because its impact on subjects' sociability judgments can be mediated by the simple decision rule, "Attractive people are sociable" (see Bassili, 1981). Heuristic processing of the attractiveness cue should thus lead subjects to regard the attractive (vs. unattractive) target as more sociable.

Obviously, a variety of predictions can be generated for this study. For example, perceptions of target sociability may be influenced only by story content or only by the attractiveness cue. Alternatively, story content and attractiveness may exert independent effects on subjects' sociability judgments or might interact to affect these perceptions. According to the HSM, each of these predictions should be confirmed under certain specifiable circumstances. More important, the model possesses the ability to specify what these circumstances should be. For the sake of simplicity, we assume that subjects' processing goal is to form an accurate impression of the target person.[14]

Under what circumstances should we expect to find a strong attractiveness effect on perceived sociability and little, if any, impact due to story content? According to the HSM, this particular result is most likely to occur when subjects engage in minimal to nil levels of systematic processing. Thus, provided that the relevant heuristic, "Attractive people are sociable," is cognitively available to subjects, the judgmental impact of the attractiveness cue should be pronounced (and the impact of story content weak) when situational or individual-difference factors (1) minimize subjects' motivation for systematic processing (e.g., low-task-importance instructions) or, regardless of motivation, (2) constrain subjects' capacities for systematic processing (e.g., time pressures). The effect of the attractiveness cue should be enhanced further by priming manipulations or other treatments that increase either the accessibility or the perceived reliability of the relevant heuristic (see Chaiken et al., 1988; Pallak, 1983).

In contrast, the judgmental impact of story content (i.e., the attributional manipulation) should be more pronounced when situational or individual-difference factors ensure moderate to high ability for systematic processing (e.g., the story is easy to comprehend) and moderate to high motivation to engage in this processing mode (e.g., high-task-importance instructions). Whether physical attractiveness also influences subjects' sociability judgments in these circumstances depends on other factors. For example, this cue should have little influence to the extent that the "Attractive people are sociable" heuristic is unavailable to subjects or low in its perceived reliability or accessibility. Even if this heuristic is available, accessible, and reliable, the judgmental impact of the attractiveness cue may be attenuated due to subjects' systematic processing. This result is somewhat unlikely, however, because our story portrays the target's behavior as sociable. Thus, systematic processing should not yield information blatantly contradicting the "Attractive people are sociable" heuristic.[15]

The hypotheses we have outlined assume that story content is unambiguous. As suggested by the HSM's bias hypothesis, however, if story content were to be made more ambiguous, subjects exposed to the attractive (vs. unattractive) target might "see" more evidence for her sociability. In other words, their heuristic processing of the attractiveness cue would bias their systematic processing.

Compatible Social Judgment Research

Our hypothetical experiment illustrates the potential applicability of a generalized version of the HSM to nonattitudinal social judgment settings. Obviously, its actual worth must be assessed in the same manner in which we and others have assessed the worth of the single-motive HSM in relation to validity-seeking persuasion contexts—through programmatic research. Nevertheless, there are notable commonalities between findings in the recent social judgment literature and the persuasion research we have focused upon in this chapter, and these findings lead us to be optimistic that more explicit tests of our general model will confirm its value as a framework for studying the cognitive and functional mechanisms that underlie social judgment.

Numerous social-cognitive experiments featuring diverse types of social judgments and decisions have yielded findings in accord with one of the HSM's basic assumptions: that people must be motivated to engage in more than minimal levels of systematic processing. These studies have shown that subjects process information more extensively, more critically, and often more complexly when they are made to feel more responsible or accountable for their judgments (e.g., Kruglanski & Freund, 1983; McAllister, Mitchell, & Beach, 1979; Tetlock & Kim, 1987; Wells, Petty, Harkins, Kagehiro, & Harvey, 1977); when they are made to feel more concerned about controlling or predicting events in their social environments (see Pittman & D'Agostino, 1985); or when they are led to make judgments about issues, events, or targets that have important personal consequences (e.g., Berscheid, Graziano, Monson, & Dermer, 1976; Borgida & Howard-Pitney, 1983; Erber & Fiske, 1984; Taylor, 1975). For example, Harkness, DeBono, and Borgida (1985) found that female subjects made more complex judgments of a male target's dating preferences when they expected to date him. Similarly, Kassin and Hochreich (1977) found that subjects were more likely to attribute behaviors to multiple (vs. single) causes when the importance of their attributional task was emphasized by describing it as a "social intelligence test." Although most of these studies have not featured heuristic cues, those that have support the HSM's hypothesis that the judgmental impact of heuristic cues is often attenuated when motivation for systematic processing is high (e.g., Borgida & Howard-Pitney, 1983; Kruglanski & Freund, 1983). Similarly, the few social judgment studies that have varied subjects' capacities for detailed systematic processing have shown that this mode is constrained by capacity-reducing variables (Gabrenya & Arkin, 1979) and that heuristic cues exert a greater judgmental impact when ability for systematic processing is low (e.g., Bodenhausen & Lichtenstein, 1987; Kruglanski & Freund, 1983). For example, Bodenhausen and Lichtenstein (1987) had subjects read information about a criminal trial and make judgments of a non-Hispanic or Hispanic defendant's aggressiveness or guilt. They reasoned that if stereotypes function as simplifying heuristics, they ought to exert a greater influence when perceivers make complex (vs. simple) judgments, because such judgments draw more heavily upon cognitive capacity. Consistent with this reasoning, the defendant's ethnicity had a significantly greater impact on subjects' guiltiness ratings than on their aggressiveness ratings.

Concluding Comments

Although our intention in this section has been to argue that a general multiple-motive HSM has utility as a general cognitive–functional framework for understanding the processes underlying social judgment, we do not wish to imply that our model is necessarily superior to other dual-process perspectives that have recently been developed in social cognition (Brewer, 1988; Fiske, 1982; Fiske & Pavelchak, 1986). Like our own model, these dual-process perspectives, as well as other recent discussions of social judgment and decision making, play upon the idea that social perceivers are flexible information processors who—depending upon a range of factors—can be more or less diligent, more or less efficient, and more or less biased in the way they process and utilize information in their social environments (see Alba & Hutchinson, 1987; Ginossar & Trope, 1987; Higgins & Bargh, 1987; Kruglanski, in press; Payne, 1982). Although we have not thoroughly compared our theoretical perspective to these other formulations, such an analysis would no doubt reveal points of agreement as well as disagreement. But, more importantly, such a comparison would probably also reveal that the various frameworks emphasize different levels of analysis, and therefore different but complementary aspects of the cognitive and functional mechanisms that underlie social judgments and decisions.

ACKNOWLEDGMENTS

Development of the model discussed in this chapter has been facilitated by grants to Shelly Chaiken from the National Science Foundation (No. BNS-8309159) and National Institute of Mental Health (No. RO1 MH43299-01). We thank John Bargh, Doug Hazlewood, Tory Higgins, Beth Meyerowitz, Ratti Ratneshwar, and Wendy Wood for their comments on a draft of this chapter.

NOTES

1. The elaboration likelihood model of persuasion (ELM; Petty & Cacioppo, 1986) posits two routes to persuasion, the "central" route and the "peripheral" route. Although there are similarities between the ELM and HSM, there are also important differences. Most importantly, the ELM's peripheral route refers to family of attitude change theories that specify factors or motives that can produce persuasion without engendering message- and issue-relevant thinking. Thus, the ELM would place heuristic processing in the same category as theories that feature psychological mechanisms quite different from the HSM's cognitive heuristics (see Chaiken & Stangor, 1987). The ELM's central route to persuasion is defined similarly to the HSM's systematic-processing mode. Thus, the central route entails what Petty and Cacioppo (e.g., 1986) have termed "message processing" or "elaboration" of the persuasive issue or the arguments contained in the message. Similarly, we define systematic processing for the persuasion context as scrutinizing all message- and issue-relevant information and thinking about this information in relation to relevant stored knowledge. Finally, the HSM includes a number of assumptions and propositions not shared by the ELM—for example, the idea that heuristic processing depends on the availability, accessibility, and reliability of persuasion heuristics, the model's sufficiency principle, and the idea that systematic and heuristic processing can have additive or interactive effects on persuasion, under specified conditions. These and other assumptions and propositions are developed in detail in the present chapter.

2. The notion of systematic processing is congruent with the explicit or implicit emphasis of most information-processing models of persuasion. Inherent in McGuire's (e.g., 1969) information-processing paradigm and the cognitive response approach (e.g., Greenwald, 1968; Petty, Ostrom, & Brock, 1981), for example, is the idea that people attend to, comprehend, and cognitively elaborate upon persuasive argumentation, and think in some depth about the issue discussed in the persuasive message (see Eagly & Chaiken, 1984, for detailed discussion).

3. Our use of the term "heuristic cue" to refer to variables such as source expertise, source likability, and consensus information conveys our belief that the per-

suasive impact of these variables is *often* mediated by simple decision rules—not a belief that these variables *cannot* affect persuasion via other psychological mechanisms.

4. Our effort assumption does not imply that heuristic processing is "effortless," only that it is less effortful than systematic processing. As noted in the beginning of this chapter, we believe that heuristic processing may sometimes achieve some of the criteria associated with automaticity (e.g., lack of awareness), but at other times may represent a more intentional, controlled process because perceivers may actively search for heuristic cues to guide their attitude (and other) judgments. In the latter case, heuristic processing would indeed require some degree of effort, although presumably less than systematic processing would require (see "Heuristic Processing in High-Stakes Settings").

5. Although numerous studies have manipulated heuristic cues, none (that we know of) has featured a "no-heuristic-cue" control group. Thus, the hypothesis that people engage in greater amounts of systematic processing when heuristic processing cannot occur awaits testing.

6. These predictions regarding the effects of incongruency on systematic processing are compatible with research indicating that expectancy-inconsistent information leads to greater attention and recall, as well as increased causal reasoning (Hastie, 1981, 1984; Hastie & Kumar, 1979). In essence, heuristic cues can create expectancies regarding message content (e.g., an expert's message will be strong), and these expectancies can be either confirmed or disconfirmed by message content (see "Heuristic Processing May Bias Systematic Processing").

7. This interpretation of the motivating effect of NFC on systematic processing does not follow immediately from Cacioppo and Petty's (1982) conceptual definition of this variable as "the tendency for an individual to engage in and enjoy thinking" (p. 116). It is, however, consistent with Cohen's (1957; Cohen, Stotland, & Wolfe, 1955) original conceptualization of the construct as "a need to understand and make reasonable the experiential world" (Cohen et al., 1955, p. 291). Interestingly, if our interpretation of the motivating effect of NFC is correct, it suggests that Cacioppo and Petty's conceptual definition of this construct is more a consequence than the essence of NFC.

8. Standard manipulations of heuristic cues are unlikely to be missed by *any* subject. Thus, to address the hypothesis that motivational variables such as personal relevance enhance the persuasive impact of heuristic cues in low-ability settings, subtler manipulations of heuristic cues would need to be implemented (e.g., vague allusions to source expertise).

9. Whereas our attenuation hypothesis assumes that heuristic processing occurs in high-motivation/high-ability situations but that systematic processing overrides its judgmental impact, it might instead be argued that systematic processing actually *suppresses* heuristic processing. Although we favor the former point of view, we acknowledge the latter possibility as well. However, if heuristic processing ever proceeds fully automatically—a possibility that awaits empirical investigation—it should be noted that there is currently little evidence that controlled processes can suppress automatic ones (see Bargh, Chapter 1, this volume).

10. The bias hypothesis is not inconsistent with the idea that systematic processing often attenuates the judgmental impact of heuristic processing, for the two hypotheses apply to different circumstances. The attenuation hypothesis applies to situations marked by moderate to high motivation and, especially, high ability for systematic processing. In contrast, the bias hypothesis applies to moderate- to high-motivation settings in which recipients can be characterized as lacking the ability to confidently judge the intrinsic validity of persuasive arguments. In addition to the factors we have highlighted—lack of knowledge and, most importantly, ambiguity of message content—this specific ability may also be compromised by situational factors that limit capacity for critical thought (e.g., time pressures, distractions). Thus, so long as such factors do not totally undermine systematic processing (e.g., by reducing comprehension to nil levels), they may also enhance the likelihood that recipients' perceptions and interpretations of argumentation will be biased by heuristic cues.

11. We should acknowledge an alternate, motivational interpretation for Mackie's (1987, Experiment 1) biased-systematic-processing results. Because consensus information described the attitudes of the majority/minority of subjects' peers (i.e., other students at their university), subjects' group identity needs may have fostered a sense of commitment to the majority's position. Instead of our cognitive explanation (i.e., that heuristic processing of consensus information biased the valence of message-relevant thought), then, it might be argued that subjects were motivated to defend the validity of the majority's position, and hence engaged in a processing strategy that allowed them to confirm the validity of the majority's arguments and disconfirm the validity of the minority's arguments (see Mackie, 1987, and our discussion of defense motivation in this chapter).

12. This reasoning does not imply that proattitudinal messages will necessarily produce greater persuasion than counterattitudinal ones. In fact, since proattitudinal messages espouse positions that are, by definition, consistent with recipients' prior attitudes, attitude change will almost invariably be greater when counterattitudinal messages are received (e.g., Hovland & Pritzker, 1957; Mackie, 1987).

13. For simplicity, our discussion of the multiple-motive HSM assumes that only one of its three postulated motives will be paramount in any one social influence setting. Yet, two or even all three of these motives may be equally important to individuals in some settings. Our model will require broadening in order to take such complexities into account. An additional aspect of our model that may require broadening concerns the generality of its motivational system. The virtue of the validity–defense–impression system is that it subsumes a larger number of more discrete motives without being so abstract as to be unwieldy (e.g., defense motivation encompasses motives such as preserving vested interests and defending attitudes to which one is committed). Eventually, however, this system may be supplemented by a more general classification consisting of maintaining outcomes, maintaining relationships, and maintaining values and other important knowledge structures. This more abstract system is probably a truer reflection of the complex motivational dynamics underlying social influence, as evidenced by the fact that it is orthogonal to the validity–defense–impression system. For example, in the interest of maintaining a relationship, one might sometimes be motivated to seek valid, accurate attitudes, sometimes motivated to defend particular attitudinal positions, and sometimes motivated to express socially acceptable attitudes.

14. Research on social judgment and decision making has tended to emphasize accuracy motivation or "truth seeking" (Higgins & Bargh, 1987), relative to other motives, to an even greater extent than has persuasion research. As we have stressed in relation to persuasion, however, the fact that most research has implicitly or explicitly emphasized one motive does not mean that others are unimportant. Although space limitations do not permit a full discussion of how defense motivation and impression motivation may operate in nonattitudinal settings, we believe that these alternate motives do play an important role in real-world judgment and decision contexts and that future research in these areas, as well as in the attitudes area, should devote greater attention to them.

15. Although two of the study's cells describe a sociable, unattractive person, it is doubtful that this configuration would be viewed as contradictory. Since subjects might perceive a greater contradiction between being unsociable and being physically attractive, however, systematic processing might well attenuate the judgmental impact of attractiveness if our hypothetical experiment were to use a story depicting the target's party behavior as unsociable.

REFERENCES

Alba, J. W., & Hutchinson, J. W. (1987). Dimensions of consumer expertise. *Journal of Consumer Research, 13*, 411–454.

Axsom, D., Yates, S. M., & Chaiken, S. (1987). Audience response as a heuristic cue in persuasion. *Journal of Personality and Social Psychology, 53*, 30–40.

Bargh, J. A. (1984). Automatic and conscious processing of social information. In R. S. Wyer, Jr., & T. K. Srull (Eds.), *Handbook of social cognition* (Vol. 3, pp. 1–43). Hillsdale, NJ: Erlbaum.

Bassili, J. N. (1981). The attractiveness stereotype: Goodness or glamour? *Basic and Applied Social Psychology, 2*, 235–252.

Berscheid, E., Graziano, W., Monson, T., & Dermer, M. (1976). Outcome dependency: Attention, attribution, and attraction. *Journal of Personality and Social Psychology, 34*, 978–989.

Bodenhausen, G. V., & Lichtenstein, M. (1987). Social stereotypes and information-processing strategies: The impact of task complexity. *Journal of Personality and Social Psychology, 52*, 871–880.

Borgida, E., & Howard-Pitney, B. (1983). Personal involvement and the robustness of perceptual salience effects. *Journal of Personality and Social Psychology, 45*, 560–570.

Brewer, M. B. (1988). A dual process model of impression formation. In T. K. Srull & R. S. Wyer, Jr. (Eds.), *Advances in social cognition* (Vol. 1, pp. 1–36). Hillsdale, NJ: Erlbaum.

Bruner, J. S. (1957). On perceptual readiness. *Psychological Review, 64*, 123–152.

Cacioppo, J. T., & Petty, R. E. (1982). The need for cognition. *Journal of Personality and Social Psychology, 42*, 116–131.

Cacioppo, J. T., Petty, R. E., Kao, C. F., & Rodriguez, R. (1986). Central and peripheral routes to persuasion: An individual difference perspective. *Journal of Personality and Social Psychology, 51*, 1032–1042.

Cacioppo, J. T., Petty, R. E., & Morris, K. J. (1983). Effects of need for cognition on message evaluation, recall, and persuasion. *Journal of Personality and Social Psychology, 45,* 805–818.

Chaiken, S. (1978). The use of source versus message cues in persuasion: An information processing analysis (Doctoral dissertation, University of Massachusetts–Amherst). *Dissertation Abstracts International, 39,* 438B.

Chaiken, S. (1980). Heuristic versus systematic information processing and the use of source versus message cues in persuasion. *Journal of Personality and Social Psychology, 39,* 752–766.

Chaiken, S. (1982, October). *The heuristic/systematic processing distinction in persuasion.* Paper presented at the meeting of the Society of Experimental Social Psychology, Nashville, IN.

Chaiken, S. (1986). Physical appearance and social influence. In C. P. Herman, M. P. Zanna, & E. T. Higgins (Eds.), *Physical appearance, stigma, and social behavior: The Ontario Symposium* (Vol. 3, pp. 143–177). Hillsdale, NJ: Erlbaum.

Chaiken, S. (1987). The heuristic model of persuasion. In M. P. Zanna, J. M. Olson, & C. P. Herman (Eds.), *Social influence: The Ontario Symposium* (Vol. 5, pp. 3–39). Hillsdale, NJ: Erlbaum.

Chaiken, S., Axsom, D., Yates, S. M., Wilson, D., Hicks, A., & Liberman, A. (1988). *Heuristic processing of persuasive messages: The role of temporary and chronic sources of accessibility.* Unpublished manuscript, New York University.

Chaiken, S., & Baldwin, M. W. (1981). Affective–cognitive consistency and the effect of salient behavioral information on the self-perception of attitudes. *Journal of Personality and Social Psychology, 41,* 1–12.

Chaiken, S., & Eagly, A. H. (1983). Communication modality as a determinant of persuasion: The role of communicator salience. *Journal of Personality and Social Psychology, 45,* 241–256.

Chaiken, S., & Stangor, C. (1987). Attitudes and attitude change. *Annual Review of Psychology, 38,* 575–630.

Cialdini, R. B., Levy, A., Herman, C. P., Kozlowski, L. T., & Petty, R. E. (1976). Elastic shifts of opinion: Determinants of direction and durability. *Journal of Personality and Social Psychology, 34,* 663–672.

Cialdini, R. B., & Petty, R. E. (1981). Anticipatory opinion effects. In R. E. Petty, T. M. Ostrom, & T. C. Brock (Eds.), *Cognitive responses in persuasion* (pp. 217–235). Hillsdale, NJ: Erlbaum.

Cohen, A. R. (1957). Need for cognition and order of communication as determinants of opinion change. In C. I. Hovland (Ed.), *The order of presentation in persuasion* (pp. 79–97). New Haven, CT: Yale University Press.

Cohen, A. R., Stotland, E., & Wolfe, D. M. (1955). An experimental investigation of need for cognition. *Journal of Abnormal and Social Psychology, 51,* 291–294.

Eagly, A. H., & Acksen, B. A. (1971). The effect of expecting to be evaluated on change toward favorable or unfavorable information about oneself. *Sociometry, 34,* 411–422.

Eagly, A. H., & Chaiken, S. (1975). An attribution analysis of the effect of communicator characteristics on opinion change: The case of communicator attractiveness. *Journal of Personality and Social Psychology, 32,* 136–144.

Eagly, A. H., & Chaiken, S. (1984). Cognitive theories of persuasion. In L. Berkowitz (Ed.), *Advances in experimental social psychology* (Vol. 17, pp. 267–359). New York: Academic Press.

Eagly, A. H., & Whitehead, G. I., III. (1972). The effect of choice on receptivity to favorable and unfavorable evaluations of oneself. *Journal of Personality and Social Psychology, 22,* 223–230.

Erber, R., & Fiske, S. T. (1984). Outcome dependency and attention to inconsistent information. *Journal of Personality and Social Psychology, 47,* 709–726.

Fazio, R. H., & Zanna, M. P. (1981). Direct experience and attitude–behavior consistency. In L. Berkowitz (Ed.), *Advances in experimental social psychology* (Vol. 14, pp. 161–202). New York: Academic Press.

Feather, N. T. (1969). Attitude and selective recall. *Journal of Personality and Social Psychology, 12,* 310–319.

Feather, N. T. (1971). Organization and discrepancy in cognitive structures. *Psychological Review, 78,* 355–379.

Fishbein, M., & Ajzen, I. (1975). *Belief, attitude, intention, and behavior: An introduction to theory and research.* Reading, MA: Addison-Wesley.

Fiske, S. T. (1982). Schema-triggered affect: Applications to social perception. In M. S. Clark & S. T. Fiske (Eds.), *Affect and cognition: The 17th Annual Carnegie Symposium on Cognition* (pp. 55–78). Hillsdale, NJ: Erlbaum.

Fiske, S. T., & Pavelchak, M. A. (1986). Category-based versus piecemeal-based affective responses: Developments in schema-triggered affect. In R. M. Sorrentino & E. T. Higgins (Eds.), *Handbook of motivation and cognition* (pp. 167–203). New York: Guilford Press.

French, J. R. P., & Raven, B. T. (1959). The bases of social power. In D. Cartwright (Ed.), *Studies in social power* (pp. 150–167). Ann Arbor: University of Michigan Press.

Gabrenya, W. K., Jr., & Arkin, R. M. (1979). Motivation, heuristics, and the psychology of prediction. *Motivation and Emotion, 3,* 1–17.

Ginossar, Z., & Trope, Y. (1987). Problem solving in judgment under uncertainty. *Journal of Personality and Social Psychology, 52,* 464–476.

Greenwald, A. G. (1968). Cognitive learning, cognitive response to persuasion, and attitude change. In A. G. Greenwald, T. C. Brock, & T. M. Ostrom (Eds.), *Psychological foundations of attitude* (pp. 147–170). New York: Academic Press.

Greenwald, A. G., & Pratkanis, A. R. (1984). The self. In R. S. Wyer, Jr., & T. K. Srull (Eds.), *Handbook of social cognition* (Vol. 3, pp. 129–178). Hillsdale, NJ: Erlbaum.

Harkness, A. R., DeBono, K. G., & Borgida, E. (1985). Personal involvement and strategies for making contingency judgments: A stake in the dating game makes a difference. *Journal of Personality and Social Psychology, 49,* 22–32.

Hastie, R. (1981). Schematic principles in human memory. In E. T. Higgins, C. P. Herman, & M. P. Zanna (Eds.), *Social cognition: The Ontario Symposium* (Vol. 1, pp. 39–88). Hillsdale, NJ: Erlbaum.

Hastie, R. (1984). Causes and effects of causal attribution. *Journal of Personality and Social Psychology, 46,* 44–56.

Hastie, R., & Kumar, P. A. (1979). Person memory: Personality traits as organizing principles in memory for behaviors. *Journal of Personality and Social Psychology, 37,* 25–38.

Higgins, E. T. (in press). Continuities and discontinuities in self-regulatory and self-evaluative processes: A developmental theory relating self and affect. *Journal of Personality.*

Higgins, E. T., & Bargh, J. A. (1987). Social cognition and social perception. *Annual Review of Psychology, 38,* 369–425.

Higgins, E. T., King, G. A., & Mavin, G. H. (1982). Individual construct accessibility and subjective impressions and recall. *Journal of Personality and Social Psychology, 43,* 35–47.

Higgins, E. T., & McCann, C. D. (1984). Social encoding and subsequent attitudes, impressions, and memory: "Context driven" and motivational aspects of processing. *Journal of Personality and Social Psychology, 47,* 26–39.

Hovland, C. I., Harvey, O. J., & Sherif, M. (1957). Assimilation and contrast effects in reactions to communication and attitude change. *Journal of Abnormal and Social Psychology, 55,* 242–252.

Hovland, C. I., & Pritzker, H. A. (1957). Extent of opinion change as a function of amount of change advocated. *Journal of Abnormal and Social Psychology, 54,* 257–261.

Johnson, B., & Eagly, A. H. (in press). The effects of involvement on persuasion: A meta-analysis. *Psychological Bulletin.*

Kassin, S. M., & Hochreich, D. J. (1977). Instructional set: A neglected variable in attribution research? *Personality and Social Psychology Bulletin, 3,* 620–623.

Katz, D. (1960). The functional approach to the study of attitudes. *Public Opinion Quarterly, 24,* 163–204.

Kelley, H. H. (1972). Attribution in social interaction. In E. E. Jones, D. E. Kanouse, H. H. Kelley, R. E. Nisbett, S. Valins, & B. Weiner (Eds.), *Attribution: Perceiving the causes of behavior* (pp. 1–26). Morristown, NJ: General Learning Press.

Kelman, H. C. (1961). Processes of opinion change. *Public Opinion Quarterly, 25,* 57–78.

Kruglanski, A. W. (in press). Motivations for judging and knowing: Implications for causal attribution. In E. T. Higgins & R. M. Sorrentino (Eds.), *Handbook of motivation and cognition* (Vol. 2). New York: Guilford Press.

Kruglanski, A. W., & Freund, T. (1983). The freezing and unfreezing of lay inferences: Effects on impressional primacy, ethnic stereotyping, and numerical anchoring. *Journal of Experimental Social Psychology, 19,* 448–468.

Langer, E. J. (1978). Rethinking the role of thought in social interaction. In J. H. Harvey, W. Ickes, & R. F. Kidd (Eds.), *New directions in attribution research* (Vol. 2, pp. 35–58). Hillsdale, NJ: Erlbaum.

Leippe, M. R., & Elkin, R. A. (1987). When motives clash: Issue involvement and response involvement as determinants of persuasion. *Journal of Personality and Social Psychology, 52,* 269–278.

Liberman, A., de La Hoz, V., & Chaiken, S. (1988, April). *Prior attitudes as heuristic information.* Paper presented at the annual meeting of the Western Psychological Association, Burlingame, CA.

Logan, G. D., & Cowan, W. B. (1984). On the ability to inhibit thought and action: A theory of an act of control. *Psychological Review, 91,* 295–327.

Maass, A., West, S. G., & Cialdini, R. B. (1987). Minority influence and conversion. In C. Hendrick (Ed.), *Group processes: Review of personality and social psychology* (Vol. 8, pp. 55–79). Newbury Park, CA: Sage.

Mackie, D. M. (1987). Systematic and nonsystematic processing of majority and minority persuasive communications. *Journal of Personality and Social Psychology, 53*, 41–52.

Mackie, D. M., & Worth, L. T. (in press). Cognitive deficits and the mediation of positive affect in persuasion. *Journal of Personality and Social Psychology.*

Maheswaran, D., & Chaiken, S. (1988). *Heuristic processing can enhance systematic processing: The effect of consensus information and message valence on persuasion.* Unpublished manuscript, New York University.

McAllister, P. W., Mitchell, T. R., & Beach, L. R. (1979). The contingency model for the selection of decision strategies: An empirical test of the effects of significance, accountability, and reversibility. *Organizational Behavior and Human Performance, 24*, 228–244.

McCroskey, J. C. (1969). A summary of experimental research on the effects of evidence in persuasive communication. *Quarterly Journal of Speech, 55*, 169–176.

McGuire, W. J. (1957). Order of presentation as a factor in "conditioning" persuasiveness. In C. I. Hovland (Ed.), *The order of presentation in persuasion* (pp. 98–114). New Haven, CT: Yale University Press.

McGuire, W. J. (1969). The nature of attitudes and attitude change. In G. Lindzey & E. Aronson (Eds.), *Handbook of social psychology* (2nd ed., Vol. 3, pp. 136–314). Reading, MA: Addison-Wesley.

McGuire, W. J. (1981). The probabilogical model of cognitive structure and attitude change. In R. E. Petty, T. M. Ostrom, & T. C. Brock (Eds.), *Cognitive responses in persuasion* (pp. 219–307). Hillsdale, NJ: Erlbaum.

Mischel, W. (1979). On the interface of cognition–personality: Beyond the person–situation debate. *American Psychologist, 34*, 740–754.

Ostrom, T. M., & Brock, T. C. (1968). A cognitive model of attitudinal involvement. In R. P. Abelson, E. Aronson, W. J. McGuire, T. M. Newcomb, M. J. Rosenberg, & P. H. Tannenbaum (Eds.), *Theories of cognitive consistency: A sourcebook* (pp. 373–383). Chicago: Rand McNally.

Pallak, S. R. (1983). Salience of a communicator's physical attractiveness and persuasion: A heuristic versus systematic processing interpretation. *Social Cognition, 2*, 158–170.

Pallak, S. R., Murroni, E., & Koch, J. (1983). Communicator attractiveness and expertise, emotional versus rational appeals, and persuasion: A heuristic versus systematic processing interpretation. *Social Cognition, 2*, 122–141.

Payne, J. W. (1982). Contingent decision behavior. *Psychological Bulletin, 92*, 382–402.

Petty, R. E., & Cacioppo, J. T. (1979). Issue involvement can increase or decrease persuasion by enhancing message-relevant cognitive responses. *Journal of Personality and Social Psychology, 37*, 1915–1926.

Petty, R. E., & Cacioppo, J. T. (1984). The effects of involvement on responses to argument quantity and quality: Central and peripheral routes to persuasion. *Journal of Personality and Social Psychology, 46*, 69–81.

Petty, R. E., & Cacioppo, J. T. (1986). The elaboration likelihood model of persuasion. In L. Berkowitz (Ed.), *Advances in experimental social psychology* (Vol. 19, pp. 123–205). New York: Academic Press.

Petty, R. E., Cacioppo, J. T., & Goldman, R. (1981). Personal involvement as a determinant of argument-based persuasion. *Journal of Personality and Social Psychology, 41*, 847–855.

Petty, R. E., Cacioppo, J. T., & Schumann, D. (1983). Central and peripheral routes to advertising effectiveness: The moderating role of involvement. *Journal of Consumer Research, 10*, 135–146.

Petty, R. E., Harkins, S. G., & Williams, K. D. (1980). The effects of group diffusion of cognitive effort on attitudes: An information processing view. *Journal of Personality and Social Psychology, 38*, 81–92.

Petty, R. E., Ostrom, T. M., & Brock, T. C. (1981). *Cognitive responses in persuasion.* Hillsdale, NJ: Erlbaum.

Pittman, T. S., & D'Agostino, P. R. (1985). Motivation & attribution: The effects of control deprivation on subsequent information processing. In G. Weary & J. Harvey (Eds.), *Attribution: Basic issues and applications.* (pp. 117–141). New York: Academic Press.

Posner, M. I., & Snyder, C. R. R. (1975). Attention and cognitive control. In R. L. Solso (Ed.), *Information processing and cognition: The Loyola Symposium* (pp. 55–85). Hillsdale, NJ: Erlbaum.

Ratneshwar, S., & Chaiken, S. (1986). When is the expert source more persuasive? A heuristic processing analysis. In T. A. Shimp, S. Sharma, G. John, J. A. Quelch, J. H. Lindgren, Jr., W. Billon, M. P. Gardner, & R. F. Dyer (Eds.), *American Marketing Association Summer Marketing Educator's Conference proceedings* (p. 86). Chicago: American Marketing Association.

Rosenberg, M. J. (1968). Hedonism, inauthenticity and other goads toward expansion of a consistency theory. In R. P. Abelson, E. Aronson, W. J. McGuire, T. M. Newcomb, M. J. Rosenberg, & P. H. Tannenbaum (Eds.), *Theories of cognitive consistency: A sourcebook* (pp. 73–111). Chicago: Rand McNally.

Schlenker, B. R. (1982). Translating actions into attitudes: An identity-analytic approach to the explanation of social conduct. In L. Berkowitz (Ed.), *Advances in experimental social psychology* (Vol. 15, pp. 193–247). New York: Academic Press.

Shechter, D. (1987). *Relational and integrity involvement as determinants of persuasion: The self-monitoring of attitudes.* Unpublished doctoral dissertation, New York University.

Sherif, M., & Hovland, C. I. (1961). *Social judgment: Assimilation and contrast effects in communication and attitude change.* New Haven, CT: Yale University Press.

Sherman, S. J. (1987). Cognitive processes in the formation, change, and expression of attitudes. In M. P. Zanna, J. M. Olson, & C. P. Herman (Eds.), *Social influence: The Ontario Symposium* (Vol. 5, pp. 75–106). Hillsdale, NJ: Erlbaum.

Shiffrin, R. M. (in press). Attention. In R. C. Atkinson, R. J. Herrnstein, G. Lindzey, & R. D. Luce (Eds.), *Stevens' handbook of experimental psychology* (2nd ed.). New York: Wiley.

Shiffrin, R. M., & Schneider, W. (1977). Controlled and automatic human information processing: II. Perceptual learning, automatic attending, and a general theory. *Psychological Review, 84*, 127–190.

Simon, H. A. (1976). *Administrative behavior* (3rd ed.). New York: Free Press.

Simon, H. A., & Stedry, A. C. (1969). Psychology and economics. In G. Lindzey & E. Aronson (Eds.), *Handbook of social psychology* (2nd ed., Vol. 5, pp. 269–314). Hillsdale, NJ: Erlbaum.

Smith, E. R. (1984). A model of social inference processes. *Psychological Review, 91*, 392–413.

Smith, M. B., Bruner, J. S., & White, R. W. (1956). *Opinions and personality.* New York: Wiley.

Sorrentino, R. M., Bobocel, D. R., Gitta, M. Z., Olson, J. M., & Hewitt, E. C. (1987). Uncertainty orientation and persuasion: Individual differences in the effects of personal relevance on social judgments. *Journal of Personality and Social Psychology, 55,* 357–371.

Stotland, E., & Canon, L. K. (1972). *Social psychology: A cognitive approach.* Philadelphia: W. B. Saunders.

Stroebe, W., & Diehl, M. (1988). When social support fails: Supporter character- istics in compliance-induced attitude change. *Personality and Social Psychol- ogy Bulletin, 14,* 136–144.

Taylor, S. E. (1975). On inferring one's own attitudes from one's behavior: Some delimiting conditions. *Journal of Personality and Social Psychology, 31,* 126– 131.

Taylor, S. E., & Fiske, S. T. (1978). Salience, attention, and attribution: Top of the head phenomena. In L. Berkowitz (Ed.), *Advances in experimental social psychology* (Vol. 11, pp. 249–288). New York: Academic Press.

Tetlock, P. E. (1983). Accountability and complexity of thought. *Journal of Per- sonality and Social Psychology, 45,* 74–83.

Tetlock, P. E. (1985). Accountability: The neglected social context of judgment and choice. In B. M. Staw & L. Cummings (Eds.), *Research in organizational behavior* (Vol. 7, pp. 297–322). Greenwich, CT: JAI Press.

Tetlock, P. E., & Kim, J. I. (1987). Accountability and judgment processes in a personality prediction task. *Journal of Personality and Social Psychology, 52,* 700–709.

Weldon, E., & Gargano, G. M. (1985). Cognitive effort in additive task groups: The effects of shared responsibility on the quality of multiattribute judgments. *Organizational Behavior and Human Development, 36,* 348–361.

Wells, G. L., Petty, R. E., Harkins, S. G., Kagehiro, D., & Harvey, J. H. (1977). Anticipated discussion of interpretation eliminates actor–observer differences in the attribution of causality. *Sociometry, 40,* 247–253.

Wood, W. (1982). Retrieval of attitude-relevant information from memory: Effects on susceptibility to persuasion and on intrinsic motivation. *Journal of Person- ality and Social Psychology, 42,* 798–810.

Wood, W., & Kallgren, C. A. (1988). Communicator attributes and persuasion: Recipients' access to attitude-relevant information in memory. *Personality and Social Psychology Bulletin, 14,* 172–182.

Wood, W., Kallgren, C. A., & Preisler, R. M. (1985). Access to attitude-relevant information in memory as a determinant of persuasion: The role of message attributes. *Journal of Experimental Social Psychology, 21,* 73–85.

Worth, L. T., & Mackie, D. M. (1987). The cognitive mediation of positive affect in persuasion. *Social Cognition, 5,* 76–94.

8

Examining the Role of Intent: Toward Understanding Its Role in Stereotyping and Prejudice

SUSAN T. FISKE

University of Massachusetts at Amherst

Recent cognitive social psychology has led to a view of people's interpersonal attention, memory, and inference as predominantly driven by the demands of cognitive economy (Fiske & Taylor, 1984; Markus & Zajonc, 1985; Nisbett & Ross, 1980). Research on the cognitive bases of stereotyping is an especially apt example of this (Ashmore & Del Boca, 1981; Fiske & Neuberg, in press; Hamilton & Trolier, 1986). Its central assumption is that stereotyping is based on categorization, and that when people stereotype, they categorize others in order to simplify the tasks of social cognition and thus to maximize scarce cognitive resources. In effect, stereotypers categorize because it requires too much mental effort to individuate. Cognitive stereotyping research holds that people categorize other people by race, sex, ethnicity, and the like in the same way that they categorize furniture as chairs, tables, couches, and the like. According to this viewpoint, both types of categorization are perfectly natural.

This well-taken perspective creates an all-too-common misinterpretation, however—namely, that the social categorizer cannot easily do otherwise. The cognitive view is too easily misinterpreted to mean that people automatically stereotype others without express intent simply because built-in or overlearned factors make them "wired" to categorize. For example, in reviewing this literature, Jones et al. (1984) note that

> if stereotypes are normal by-products of the inevitable selecting and packaging of data from a complex world, . . . will stigma not always be with

us? Contemporary cognitive approaches to stereotyping . . . [project] a rather weary fatalism. The subprocesses involved in stigmatization are seen as . . . ingrained human proclivities. (p. 300)

In his review, Hamilton (1979) calls the same thing "a rather depressing dilemma" (p. 80). The assumption that cognitive explanations for stereotyping imply a lack of intent also surfaces frequently in the original empirical articles, including those I coauthored: "Race is used as an encoding strategy . . . regardless of whether a perceiver is intentionally trying" (Taylor, Fiske, Etcoff, & Ruderman, 1978, p. 782). Another cognitively oriented empirical article states that "stereotypes operate unconsciously as automatic expectations" (Brown & Geis, 1984, p. 812). That stereotyping is unintentional and perhaps inevitable is a mistaken assumption at worst, and an inadequately examined one at best.

This common misinterpretation is important, because an absence of intent ultimately implies an absence of responsibility for the effects of categorization (cf. Shaver, 1985). It has led me to have the following nightmare: After testifying for the plaintiff in a case of egregious and demonstrable discrimination, a cognitive social psychologist faces the cross-examining attorney. The hostile attorney, who looms taller than Goliath, says, "Tell us, Professor, do people intend to discriminate?" The cognitive social psychologist hedges about not having any hard data with regard to discrimination, being an expert mainly in stereotyping. When pressed, the psychologist admits that stereotypic cognitions are presumed to underlie discriminatory behavior. Pressed still further, the psychologist reluctantly mumbles that, indeed, a common interpretation of the cognitive approach is that people do not stereotype intentionally, whereupon the cross-examining attorney says in a tone of triumph, "No further questions, Your Honor." The plaintiff is led shaking from the courtroom, and the psychologist is left stewing about the misuse of science outside the ivory tower.

This courtroom drama is not merely a fantasy. As the end of this chapter will show, most versions of discrimination law hold that an absence of discriminatory intent releases defendants from responsibility for the discriminatory impact of their actions. Moreover, conservative interpretations of discriminatory intent require that it be conscious—that is, that defendants be aware their actions were based on the other person's social group membership. According to this viewpoint, if alleged discriminators behaved without express intent—for example, because of cognitive factors outside their control—then they need not be responsible for even the most egregiously harmful discrimination. Although it is quite unlikely that cognitive research on stereotyping will directly alter fundamental principles of the law, social science has a history of bearing on discrimination law (*Brown v. Board of Education of Topeka, Kansas*, 1954), and cognitive social psychology has recently been considered as expert testimony in discrimination cases that have reached the Supreme Court (Hopkins v. Price-

Waterhouse, 1985; Price-Waterhouse v. Hopkins, 1988). Hence, there is potential for damage due to misinterpretations of cognitive approaches to stereotyping as necessarily implying a lack of intent on the part of the social categorizer.

This sobering realization has motivated me to examine more closely the all-too-common misinterpretation of cognitive approaches to stereotyping. The necessary first step is to understand what is meant by "intent," in order to synthesize theoretically derived principles that ultimately can be applied to the role of intent in prejudice and stereotyping. Investigating intent is not itself a small task, so this chapter is mostly about intent, and not so much about stereotyping. But possible applications to stereotyping are woven in as a refrain echoing the fundamental goal of the undertaking. Moreover, this conceptualization of intent has informed my own empirical work on motivation and stereotyping (see Fiske & Neuberg, in press, for a review). A broader message reflects the themes of this book: a friendly reminder that explanations of behavior as influenced by built-in or over-learned cognitive factors need not mean that behavior is dominated by such factors.

IS INTENT REALLY NECESSARY?

Before addressing the variety of approaches to intent, one might wonder whether intent is a necessary concept in the context of cognitive stereotyping research. One might suggest, first, that it is totally obvious that people can intentionally control whether or not they stereotype other people. One might ask, second, whether the concept of intent is really necessary here at all.

In regard to the first point that the operation of intent in stereotyping is obvious, the idea that intent can influence stereotyping and individuation is not meant to be counterintuitive; rather, the influence of intent is simply systematized and delineated here. Moreover, the role of intent has *not* so far been obvious in cognitively oriented research on stereotyping. Although the cognitive approach has been misinterpreted as meaning that stereotypic responses are unintentional and inevitable, this possible misinterpretation has not, unfortunately, been confronted thoroughly. Finally, even if the role of intent in stereotyping should be obvious, it has not been empirically demonstrated within a framework informed by past writing on this subject.

To turn to the second point, is intent a necessary concept in the current context? The literature on intent provides a conceptual basis for deciding whether it is reasonable to interpret a person's actions as intentional. This conceptual analysis potentially applies psychological knowledge about stereotyping to legal and organizational settings. To assign legal responsibility for past discrimination, one must know how to decide whether it was intentional or not, for unintentional discrimination is not illegal. To develop an organizational intervention to prevent future discrimination, one must know whether, when, and how people can control their category-based and individuating processes. If the principles of intent are supported empirically, then we may be in a better position to judge accordingly (1) *whether* the stereotyper has a choice; (2) *when* people are most likely to choose to stereotype or not; and (3) *how* intent operates cognitively on stereotyping processes. Finally, all the preceding arguments for the conceptual utility of intent should be complemented by the operational utility of intent, to be tested in future work. The task for the present, then, is to be conceptually clear about what we mean by "intent."

WHETHER, WHEN, AND HOW INTENT OPERATES

It is the business of this main section to define "intent." A preliminary example can preview the more detailed discussion. Suppose one needs to decide whether Jane is discriminating against Hamid, who is Iranian, because of unintentional stereotyping. Informed by psychological inquiry (to be reviewed), one would consider three features of intent. First, intent is defined as existing when a person has *options*—that is, a perceived choice among cognitively available alternatives. One would therefore want to know whether Jane knows how to individuate other people, rather than to stereotype them, and whether she has any choice in applying this individuating process to Hamid as an Iranian. Having options is the minimal condition for exercising intent.

Second, intent typically entails a choice between a more dominant alternative and a weaker alternative. Intent is especially obvious when one makes the *hard choice*, by pursuing the nondominant alternative—that is, doing what one would not otherwise do. If Jane is someone who thinks stereotypically about most people, then if she instead individuates Hamid, one immediately presumes that it must involve some intent on her part. On the other hand, choosing the dominant alternative is intentional also, but it is a less obvious form of intent. If Jane stereotypes Hamid, it does not at first seem so intentional, because she stereotypes everyone. Nevertheless, suppose we have established previously that she knows how to individuate and has some choice in how she thinks about Hamid in particular. Then, even if she exercises her dominant mode of stereotypic thinking in considering Hamid, that is intentional, although in a more subtle sense than if she uncharacteristically individuates him.

Finally, intent is mediated by *motivated attention*. The alternatives on which a person emphatically concentrates the mind determines what the person intends. If she wants to, Jane can allow herself to stereotype Hamid by concentrating on his category membership as an Iranian and all that this implies to her, or she can concentrate on his qualities as a unique individual. Either way, she is implementing her intent to stereotype or individuate him. Each of the three main features of intent—having options, making the hard choice, and paying attention—is elaborated in detail throughout this chapter. The discussion draws on scientific, lay, and legal psychology.

In undertaking this review, I noticed that the investigation of intent has been out of scientific fashion lately. I suspect that this is due in part to mainstream psychology's historical reaction against introspection and in favor of behaviorism. Ironically, even as psychology has returned to cognitive explanations, the spirit with which they are sometimes adopted (by social psychologists at least) has assumed that people have little control, and so the specific investigation of intent seems essentially irrelevant. Nevertheless, a great variety of psychological scholars (and others) have long grappled with issues related to intent, control, volition, will, and the like. This review confines itself to the writings of scientific psychologists, although even there the contributions sprawl across a considerable range of traditions. Despite the variety of approaches, however, virtually all the discussions conceptualize intent similarly in crucial respects. Let the reader beware that this project involves that abstract, nonempirical area at the borderline between philosophy and psychology, although the ultimate goal is empirical accountability.

Having Options

From Early to Modern Conceptions

William James (1890/1981) laid the foundations for many later scientific discussions of intent. He essentially defined "volition" (intent) as a choice between two conflicting courses of thought. Whenever a person has two antagonistic ideas in mind, one of them must be neutralized. If there are two alternatives available, then volition implies giving consent to one over the other. Giving consent then allows action; action is preceded by the idea of the act, according to James. James discussed colorful and enduring examples of conflicts that are resolved by the exercise of intent: staying in a warm bed or getting out into the cold air, joining or avoiding a provoked fight, pocketing one's money or squandering it on one's cupidities, and walking away from or toward a coquette's door. Another relevant conflict, not mentioned by James, might include using or ignoring one's most familiar and comfortable stereotypes.[1]

The role of intent in Edward Tolman's (1925, 1927) purposive behaviorism built on the foundations laid by James. Of course, Tolman was analyzing the intentions of rats running for food in mazes, rather than a person hesitating before a coquette's door. But, like James, Tolman described intent as existing when a task can be performed in more than one way. According to Tolman, intent has meaning when observable behavior changes, for then the organism displays consciousness. The organism is acting to bring about a result not yet present. Thus intent is the behavioral possibility that an organism imputes to a particular environment, or, in other words, perceived options. Tolman invoked intent because he found the repeated trials of strict associationism to be theoretically insufficient for explaining a rat's otherwise arbitrary novel choice in a maze.

In a similar vein, Kurt Lewin found repeated associative trials insufficient to explain people's chosen responses (Deutsch, 1954; Tolman, 1938). As a remedy, the early work of Lewin and his students was a focused defense of intent, purpose, and motivation in the face of imperialistic associationism (Lewin, 1935, 1951). They argued that repeated associations do not by themselves produce behavior; rather, motivation decides the particular cognitive structure that in turn guides behavior.[2]

In Lewin's view, intent essentially causes one to cognize the relevant psychological situation differently. Intent prepares one for a desired behavioral possibility by restructuring the perceived situation. According to Lewin, one creates new "valences," which are the relevant behavioral possibilities in the environment. For example, if one has an important letter to mail, or if one wants a small child to see over the crowds at a parade, the first mailbox takes on a different valence or behavioral pull than it does if one has been warned of possible terrorism by letter bomb. In this framework, intent is most demonstrably a motivation that alters valences, so it determines which of many possible cognitive structures provides the basis for action. Note that intent again arises when one has options, but Lewin in addition highlighted a motivational restructuring mechanism, which was abandoned by subsequent writers.

Writing a quarter century after Lewin, early information-processing theorists inherited the main idea of intent as requiring cognitively available alternatives or options. According to Miller, Galanter, and Pribram (1960), Lewin's work had been the "last serious attempt to make sense of the will" (p. 11), and they cited him extensively. As did Lewin, Miller et al. tackled the translation of cognitive structures into action. They distinguished between an "Image," which is a cognitive structure, and a "Plan," which is the program for action. An Image is accumulated, organized world knowledge, approximately what is now sometimes called "declarative [semantic and episodic] memory." A Plan is any hierarchical process that controls the order in which actions are performed; in a later theoretical incarnation, it is essentially" procedural knowledge" (Anderson, 1982).

Intent, in the view of Miller et al., consists of the "uncompleted parts of a Plan whose execution has already begun" (p. 61). Hence, to explain intent, one need only specify the choice of a Plan. The choice of one Plan implies rejecting other available alternatives, so intent again occurs only when one has options. As before, then, intent is defined by a choice among cognitively available alternative courses of thought and action, only one of which dominates at a given time. This fits with the classical definition of volitional behavior as that which can be inhibited by choice, either through instigations to competing acts or through its own completion (Kimble & Perlmuter, 1970; Logan & Cowan, 1984).

Other information-processing approaches to this problem essentially concur that intent is closely linked to the control of action when multiple options are available. Shallice and Norman in particular view the will as a mechanism for the "direction of action by deliberate conscious control" (Norman & Shallice, 1986, p. 14; Shallice, 1972), which is only possible when one has multiple viable alternatives.

Another contemporary perspective on intent rejects most of the basic information-processing assumptions, while agreeing on intent as choice. Marcel (1983) argues that intent lies at the very basis of human consciousness (cf. Mandler, 1984). Consciousness "is the ability to base intentional categorical action upon a perceptual (or imaginal) experience. . . . Thus we can choose or set up what aspect of an event is to control the *categories* of our behavior, as opposed to those aspects which merely affect the parameters of the act" (pp. 240–241, italics in original). That is, people can choose which direction to follow (category), but not, for example, how quickly to do it (parameter). Intent again arises from choice, but it implies nothing about the nature of the processes executed thereby.

A variety of viewpoints over time thus concur that intent at a minimum requires having cognitively available options. Although not always easy to determine, this is the defining feature of intent. What this definition means for applications to stereotyping is that it becomes crucial to know whether stereotypers have cognitively available alternatives—that is, whether, when, and how they have the option not to employ their stereotypes. In our view, people do have options to stereotype or individuate, as shown by the flexibility with which they use the different options (e.g., Erber & Fiske, 1984; Fiske, Neuberg, Beattie, & Milberg, 1987; Fiske & Pavelchak, 1986; Neuberg & Fiske, 1987; see Fiske & Neuberg, in press, for a review of other people's research).

A Note on Awareness of Options

Having options defines those situations in which it is permissible to speak of another's intent. But what if the person fails to recognize the options? Can we say that a person intends something when the individual is not aware that there is any choice? What if one has options available but does not know it?

The clearest answer is that options must be at least potentially cognitively available to the individual. "Potentially" is an important but tricky term here. Upon reflection, the individual should be able to report that there are possible alternatives. The alternatives may not be consciously considered at the time, but they are cognitively available at some level, so the particular alternative is controllable. For example, suppose one encounters a middle-aged black woman on a suburban street and assumes that she is a housekeeper. One presumably does not consciously consider the inference, but if asked, one has to admit that there are alternative ways to think about this person. If one were to act without thinking, based on this inference, one would certainly be responsible for the stereotypic assumption that underlay the behavior. Suppose, in contrast, that a dramatically deceived white child has been told that all black women are housekeepers. If the child then makes the same inference about the woman on the street, one should not assume the child capable of thinking about her in any other way (pending re-educatiion). Thus, even an "unthinking" choice may be considered intentional, but only when it has the potential to be consciously accessed. Even if one does not explicitly think about a given choice at the time, one nevertheless intends it, in the sense that one has options cognitively available to do otherwise and could potentially reflect on those options.

This view contradicts some common-sense uses of the term "intent," as conscious planning or premeditation ("I didn't intend to say that; it just came out"). But there are many thoughts and activities to which one implicitly assents, although there are alternatives. From the perspective of psychological theory, it is conceptually clearest to consider this implicit assent equivalent to intent, although it may fly in the face of some readers' intuitions.

As an example of the conceptual reason for defining intent in terms of potentially available options, consider different possible degrees of intent as indicated by the accessibility of options. Suppose a person even upon reflection simply cannot consider thinking about the situation differently and cannot imagine how anyone else could do so (An isolated villager who says, "In my culture, all women are considered the property of their husbands or fathers, and I have never heard of anything else," or an unimaginative psychologist who says, "In my experience, psychology articles are always written in prose, and I cannot imagine a person writing one in verse"); it is not reasonable to treat such a blind, core assumption and subsequent actions as intentional.

Suppose, however, that the person has never thought otherwise but admits that one could conceive as a realistic possibility that other options exist (i.e., there may be cultures where women are treated as equal to or more important than men, or one could conceivably imagine writing a journal article in verse rather than prose); then whether options are available is open to debate. One might describe this as the potential availability of options. Applying intent in this instance is controversial from a psychologist's perspective. If I have never considered writing a psychology article in verse, does that mean that my writing one in prose is intentional? Certainly, if asked, I would say I intended prose. Similarly, the villager who treats his wife as subservient presumably would say that this also is intentional, although he has never actively considered alternatives prior to being asked.

Suppose, at a third level, that one has considered alternatives at other times, but not this one. For example, the villager may be aware that people who live in the big city are supposed to treat women as equal to comparable men, and he himself has managed to do so in the city, but not on any occasion in the village. Or a psychologist may have heard of journal articles published in verse and may have at one time considered the idea, but may not ever have done so. The options have clearly been available to the person, so intent unambiguously applies in this instance.

The most obvious form of intent, of course, fits the common-sense notion of intent: The person has actively considered alternatives at this particular time. After elaborating further perspectives on intent, I will return to these issues.

Using the criterion that options be at least potentially available to consciousness raises another issue. The person may not openly acknowledge that options exist. That is, the actor's own report about intent may be suspect, especially when intent would imply responsibility for a harmful act. Because of this problem, intent sometimes must be inferred from behavior and from assumptions about the psychology of a reasonable person. To infer intent, therefore, an observer must concentrate on alternatives that the actor could conceivably have had in mind and that are within the actor's understanding and repertoire (Shaver, 1985, pp. 120–121). The actor may not have actively considered all the options at the moment of choice, but if the person was capable of choosing and enacting each of them, and if on reflection the person would know this, then the person may be considered to have had cognitive options available, and intent applies.

Making the Hard Choice

Early Conceptions of the Hard Choice

Almost invariably, when a person has several options available, one alternative is dominant. One alternative may be dominant because the association is habitual, because a strong impulse or emotion inclines that way, or because the thought is what one would follow by default, without other intervention. The dominant alternative or easy choice is the one that requires less mental effort. For example, James's typical conflicts involve the choice between a strong initial impulse and the wiser, more "difficult" idea. Volition is clearest when a dominant, unacceptable thought conflicts with the "still, small voice" of a wiser one. Although this is not always simple to determine, it is the dominant but unwise thought that one is motivated to "neutralize," in Jamesian terms. If the dominant thought per-

sists, according to James, the corresponding action will follow. His examples of typically dominant choice are the thoughts that precede staying
in bed, getting provoked into a fight, squandering one's money, and knocking
on the coquette's door. Another dominant thought may be one's most accessible stereotypic category.

Competing against the dominant thought is another, weaker thought
that one is motivated to encourage (e.g., getting out of bed, avoiding the
coquette, not using the stereotype). This is the difficult thought, in James's
terms. The tension between dominant thoughts and weaker but preferable
thoughts is central to understanding intent. Intent is most obvious—it most
dramatically occurs—when one chooses the nondominant alternative, thus
making what people commonly call the "hard choice." Nevertheless, if one
demonstrably has options, then whatever choice one makes is intentional;
thus, by definition, the easy choice (the dominant alternative) is also a
form of intent.

The view of intent as most obvious in making the harder choice also
appears in discussions by Tolman: Intent, because it requires change, rests
on choosing between the previously dominant behavior and a novel nondominant alternative. And in particular, according to Tolman, intent most
demonstrably exists when the chosen alternative requires a more differentiated response, which is the heretofore weaker but now preferable one.
Like James, then, Tolman conceptualized intent as especially clear when
one chooses a nondominant but preferred course over a previously dominant one.

Not surprisingly, Lewin made essentially the same point. Lewin emphasized that intent imposes a new direction on what the person would
do otherwise: Intent "arises when the foreseen situation by itself would
lead to . . . actions contrary to the desired action" (1951, p. 149). Intent
most obviously creates valences other than the most usual ones. For example, mailboxes usually have a neutral valence, but the important letter
creates a strong pull from the first mailbox one sees. Intent, in its most
dramatic form, interferes with the otherwise dominant action in the situation.

Automatic and Controlled Processing

Subsequent to these early discussions of the "hard choice," information-
processing psychologists became concerned with how people control otherwise dominant responses. When instructions (giving rise to intentions)
override habitual (dominant) responses, the performance is termed "controlled"; when they do not, performance is termed "automatic." For the
sake of readers who wonder whether an old-fashioned idea such as intent
is really necessary, given the more current discussions of controlled and
automatic processes, a digression on this point is warranted.

First, the very definition of controlled processing implies not equating it with intent. Controlled processing, as commonly defined, entails awareness, intent, and interference with other ongoing processes (e.g., Posner & Snyder, 1975; see Bargh, 1984, for a review). If intent is a criterion for controlled processing, the two ought to be distinguishable. Otherwise, the definition of controlled processing is circular.

Second, intent has not been carefully examined in the literature on controlled processing, although intent plays a major role both operationally and conceptually. Of the three criteria for controlled processing, intent has been treated as an independent variable that invokes control. In contrast, the other two criteria, interference and awareness, have been treated as dependent variables that reveal control. Considering that intent plays such a major role, the research on controlled processing is surprisingly unhelpful on the nature of intent. The typical study merely operationalizes intent as the explicit task instruction (Posner & Snyder, 1975; Schneider & Shiffrin, 1977; Shiffrin & Schneider, 1977).[3]

Third, as just noted, controlled processing by definition requires awareness or conscious processing. In contrast, it is conceptually useful to "tolerate 'unconscious intentions' " (Miller et al., 1960, p. 61, footnote 3). As discussed earlier ("A Note on Awareness of Options"), the critical factor is whether the availability of options is potentially accessible to consciousness, not whether the person has consciously considered all the options originally.

Finally, as Lewin (1951) observed, intent can set in motion *either* controlled and conscious or uncontrolled and unconscious processes.[4] When people choose one alternative over another—that is, when they behave intentionally—the processes that ensue may be controlled or automatic or some combination. For example, a perceiver's intent to respond in a nonstereotypic way can involve both relatively automatic processes (such as attribute averaging) and controlled processes (such as searching for individuating information about the other). And, indeed, the literature on automatic and controlled processing specifically considers such interactions of the two types of process (e.g., Logan, 1980; Neely, 1977; Posner & Snyder, 1975; Schneider & Shiffrin, 1977; Shiffrin & Schneider, 1977). But the point is that intentionality can precede the implementation of automatic, controlled, or combined processes. The occurrence of an intent does not determine the exact nature of the processes that follow. It means that the choice itself is potentially controllable, not that the ensuing processes are controlled.

For all these reasons, intent and controlled processing are by no means redundant, although examining the one may illuminate the other. To return to our main theme, then, in the literature on automatic and controlled processes, intent is clearly viewed as intervening to bring about control when otherwise dominant automatic processing is problematic or counter

to an instruction. Thus, even in the current information-processing research, intent is especially obvious when one picks the nondominant alternative, making what is here called the hard choice.

Paying Attention

Early Perspectives on Paying Attention

As suggested so far, intent is defined as having options, but it is especially
clear when one chooses the nondominant alternative. What, therefore, is
the mechanism for picking the dominant or nondominant alternative? How
does one make the "hard choice"—or fail to make it? One makes the hard
choice essentially by concentrating attention on the weaker but preferable
alternative. James of course put it well:

> Attention with effort is all that any case of volition implies. The essential
> achievement of the will, in short, when it is most "voluntary," is to attend
> to a difficult object and hold it fast before the mind. . . . Sustained in
> this way by a resolute effort of attention, the difficult object erelong be-
> gins to call up its own congeners and associates and ends by changing the
> disposition of the man's consciousness. . . . Though the spontaneous drift
> of thought is all the other way, the attention must be kept strained on
> that one object until at last it grows, so as to maintain itself before the
> mind with ease. This strain of attention is the fundamental act of will.
> (1890/1981, pp. 1166, 1168, original italics omitted)

It is not, however, a simple matter to focus one's attention. James's discussion implies but does not say that motivation is the key; notice the
"resolute effort of attention" that "must be kept strained on that one object." On a common-sense level, the necessity of motivated attention is
clear. Consider how one resists a dominant but nonpreferred alternative,
whether it is staying in bed, joining a fight, squandering money, visiting a
coquette, or not stereotyping. Concentrating on what one must do instead
(i.e., get up, make peace, etc.) allows one to act on the hard choice. A
failure of attention allows one to backslide from the difficult good intention. In stereotyping, concentrated attention on what one actually knows
about the unique individual is the key (Fiske & Neuberg, in press).

Lewin's work is helpful on exactly how attention might be motivated
in the service of intent. His explicit mechanism for intent is the tension
system. He described intent as a "quasi-need" that creates tension until it
is fulfilled. Once one intends to follow a particular choice (the preferred
alternative), one essentially creates a motivational need state. Like actual
needs, this quasi-need (intent) creates valences associated with various features of one's psychological environment. One perceives valences associated with, for example, a forbidden hot fudge sundae either in terms of its
consummatory features (creamy cold ice cream with thick bittersweet hot
fudge), in terms of its health risk (540 calories and 210 milligrams of cholesterol), or perhaps in terms of a consumption-irrelevant sensory meta-

phor (a volcano erupting out of a snow-covered mountain; cf. Mischel, 1974). As another example, when a man encounters an attractive woman, he may think mainly of her face and body and interpret friendly behavior as seductive. Alternatively, he can also concentrate on what she is specifically saying and doing about the task on which they are collaborating. Valences change to reflect the perceived and desired action possibilities associated with objects. Whether coming from an actual need or a quasineed, valences "challenge us to certain activities" (Lewin, 1951, p. 117); in that sense, they are motivating.

Moreover, Lewin linked intent-based valences to attention. Attention can override the default valence—that is, the one that would exist without intent, or the otherwise dominant tendency. Attention allows one to overcome the ordinary valences and substitute those imposed intentionally. Similarly, a failure of attention causes the normally dominant valences to prevail. Hence, motivated attention is the key to exercising intent.

Information-Processing Mechanisms for Intent

Motivation would hardly seem to fit with an information-processing perspective on intent. To determine the possible role of motivation in intent, it is helpful to examine how far the information-processing perspective can go without motivation. Consider, for example, Miller et al.'s view of intent, which shuns Lewinian motivational dynamics, including valences. Miller et al. rejected the need for motivation as a motor for intentional behavior, saying that "once a biological machine starts to run, it keeps running twenty-four hours a day until it dies. The dynamic "motor" that pushes our behavior along its planned grooves . . . is located in the nature of life itself. . . . The stream of thought can never stop flowing" (1960, p. 64). To avoid motivation, Miller et al. embedded behavior in a cybernetic system. Which of the several available Plans (action structures) a person executes is determined by values embedded in the Image (cognitive structure) of the current situation. Although values may sound like valences, they do not operate as valences do. As a Plan is being executed, its actions are tested to see whether they increase the value of the situation. Ordinarily, executing a Plan increases the value of the immediate situation, except when the action is embedded in a larger Plan expected to result in a positive value in the long run (Miller et al., 1960, p. 62). Thus, the choice of a Plan, and hence intent, depends on the value of its expected results. In short, the intent mechanism proposed by Miller et al. is the choice of a Plan or program, which depends on the value associated with its probable outcome.

Other theorists subsequently built on this framework, some arguing that motivation should be reincorporated into it (Kimble & Perlmuter, 1970). However, in fact, their view of motivation does not differ especially from Miller et al.'s concept of choosing a Plan, driven by its expected value. Conceptually, Kimble and Perlmuter define motivation as the "predominating desire of performing the response" (1970, p. 369), but the definition is never operationalized in this spirit. Operationally, their definition of motivation simply involves the instruction to the subject. Certainly, instructions are a likely condition for executing one Plan over another, but not a very traditional or compelling operationalization of motivation.

Although they did not view motivation as necessary, Miller et al. did argue that attention is a determining mechanism for intent. When a Plan is moved into working memory, where it can be easily attended, then it is the currently active intent.

Similarly, according to Shallice and Norman (Shallice, 1972; Norman & Shallice, 1986), the nonmotivational determining mechanism for intent is attention. In their view, the will operates by way of a supervisory attentional system that intervenes to select action in settings that are problematic for automatic activity. Hence, again, attention essentially facilitates intent. The idea is that attention helps to raise the activation of the relevant action structures, which causes them to become the dominant plan or, in other words, the intent. It is interesting that in this respect the mainstream information-processing view is reminiscent of William James's mechanism for the will, in which attention holds fast the difficult idea, which "erelong begins to call up its own congeners and associates." The role of motivation as driving attention, however, is abandoned in this information-processing perspective.

Conscious and Unconscious Intent

If attention is a major mechanism for intent, does this mean that processes must be wholly conscious to be intentional? No, rather the existence of unconscious intents seems highly plausible, for several reasons already discussed ("A Note on Awareness of Options"). Some additional reasons follow from the discussion of intent and attention.

A close examination of work from the information-processing perspective suggests that, just because attention is a major mechanism for its operation, intent need not necessarily be conscious. Recall that intentionality is one of several features (intent, awareness, interference) that distinguish automatic and controlled processes. This implies that intent can occur without awareness (and vice versa), or else intent and awareness would be redundant criteria for control. Moreover, although the relevant literature explicitly addresses the controllability of responses, it makes no uniform assumptions about the necessity for awareness. That is, in discussing controlled processing, some writers discuss the necessity for attention to the nondominant or controlled course of action (Miller et al., Norman & Shallice) or for conscious compliance with instructions (Posner & Snyder, Kimble & Perlmuter). At the same time, they may explicitly allow for unconscious intents (Miller et al.). Thus, sometimes the theorists assume that intent must be conscious, and sometimes they allow unconscious intent.

Reiterating a distinction may clarify this issue. The most obvious form of intent occurs when one makes a conscious choice among alternatives by attending to the nondominant course of action. That obvious form of intent corresponds to what one emphatically means to do, and it operates by motivated attention. The most dramatic form of intent occurs when one makes the hard choice previously described. Such clearly intentional acts include getting out of bed, not squandering one's money, avoiding the coquette's door, and valiantly overcoming one's stereotypes.

On the other hand, intent also occurs when one makes an unconscious or semiconscious choice to follow the dominant course of action, even though potentially perceived alternatives exist. Recall that the defining feature of intent is having cognitively available options. Even when one follows the dominant alternative, this is a form of intent, although admittedly a less obvious one. Intent can correspond to what one does carelessly, recklessly, or by default, although one could certainly do otherwise. Examples of the less obvious types of intentional acts include staying in bed, wasting one's money, not resisting the coquette, and continuing to rely on one's stereotypes. Like the most obvious form of intent, the less obvious form of intent also operates by motivated attention, but in this case it operates by a failure of motivated attention. That is, the less obvious form of intent occurs when one's attention is distracted away from the difficult but wiser idea, away from the nondominant but preferred course of action.[5]

Both forms of intent—making the easy or the hard choice—assume that one is or can be aware of the dominant and nondominant alternatives, as well as of one's ability to control one's attention, and through it, one's actions. Neither type of intent assumes that one need be aware of why one chooses one or the other (cf. Nisbett & Wilson, 1977) or of how the cognitive processes operate.

The distinction between the more and less obvious forms of intent is important. Without it, one is forced to state that when people have options, if they choose one alternative, that is intentional, but if they choose the other, that is not intentional. This amounts to a confusion between the definition of intent and the most obvious form of intent. Such confusion does not make good psychological theory. Hence, because intent is defined as having cognitively available options, both the dominant and nondominant alternatives must be viewed as intentional, even though one is a more obvious form of intent than the other. Logic compels us to include what people most obviously intend, as well as what they can control and therefore also intend.

Summary of Intent as Viewed by Scientific Psychologists

The history of work on intent and related concepts touches some major traditions of cognitive and social psychology. Nor has this discussion exhausted the possibilities; we have much to learn about the intentional control of cognitive and affective processes. Nevertheless, intent has been commonly defined as occurring when people have options—that is, when they have the ability to choose among cognitively available alternatives. This is the single necessary condition for intent.

Intent is especially obvious when one makes the hard choice, by following a previously nondominant alternative. The most dramatic form of intent involves the choice not to follow the dominant alternative. At its most obvious, then, intent involves actively following the previously more difficult alternative. The difficult alternative may be nondominant because another is simpler (less differentiated), because another has stronger prior associations, or because another is more motivationally compelling. On the other hand, intent also occurs when one follows the dominant alternative despite the availability of options. Although a less obvious form of intentional response, it too fits the basic definition.

Finally, intent appears to be mediated by motivated attention; that is, the alternative on which one concentrates the mind—or allows the mind to be concentrated—is the intended one. Concentrating the mind then facilitates enacting the intended alternative. Throughout, potential implications for cognitively oriented explanations of stereotyping have emerged.

INTENT AS VIEWED BY LAY PSYCHOLOGY

Scientific psychologists approach intent with cautious reluctance. In contrast, ordinary people attribute intent all the time, with considerable abandon. Nevertheless, although they are not systematically aware of it, lay psychologists generally agree with scientific psychologists about how to impute intent. Like scientists, laypeople infer intent when actions result from choosing among cognitively available alternatives. Also, when actions involve rejecting the dominant alternative, then intent is especially obvious. To infer intent, perceivers look for actions that reveal the actor's attentional focus on a particular goal. Hence, in crucial respects, lay and scientific psychologies agree. Naive psychology is helpful because it tells us what people consider good evidence for intent, and it gives additional detail about what clues to notice when examining intent. The remainder of this section elaborates on these points, analyzing "the naive psychology of action by making explicit what is not always phenomenally explicit" (Heider, 1958, p. 123).

Fritz Heider (1958) first described the ways in which ordinary people infer intent from the behavior of others. Intent is crucial to understanding purposive action, according to Heider:

> Unless intention ties together the cause–effect relations, we do not have a case of true personal causality. . . . Above all, it is the goal of an action, its source in the intention of a person, that often determines what

the person really is doing, or what really is happening. The situation is quite different, and carries different implications for the future, if something is done to me intentionally or accidentally. It is the difference between a stone accidentally hitting me and a stone aimed at me. (Heider, 1958, pp. 100, 117)

In short, psychologically, "the meaning of an action [is] its intentional significance" (Jones & Davis, 1965, p. 222).

Perceiving That a Person Has Options

Before attributing intent to someone else's actions, perceivers first analyze whether the person "can" perform the action (Heider, 1958). "Can" is equivalent to having options. It is the balance between personal power (ability) and environmental contingencies. Having options requires that the person be able to perform the action or not, given the facilitative and inhibitory contingencies in the environment. We do not infer that a person acts intentionally when the environment constrains his or her action in a manner beyond normal control. For example, we do not infer purposive (in)action when a small person fails to lift a boulder or when a naive driver skids on an icy road or when anyone flinches at a hot stove. Nor do we infer purpose action when a very young child mimics ethnic categories used by all the surrounding adults. In each case, the particular person does not have the power to counteract compelling environmental forces.

To impute "can," then, perceivers judge how the person's ability to act (or not) combines with environmental contingencies. Jones (Jones & Davis, 1965; Jones & McGillis, 1976), who built on Heider's analysis, similarly describes the fundamental conditions for intent.[6] The actor must have ability (capacity to perform the act), as well as behavioral freedom (having a choice without undue physical or social constraints from the environment). Jones also makes explicit the role of knowledge (understanding which actions cause which effects). Note, however, that knowledge does not mean that intent need be conscious: "The actor's intention may or may not be conscious and deliberate, but it is marked by some aspect of desire or volition which comes from the person and is not predetermined by environmental forces" (Jones & Davis, 1965, p. 224). In sum, the difference between the ability of the person and the constraints of the environment allows the inference of what I have called having options—namely, the potential to choose among cognitively available alternatives.

Perceiving That a Person Has Made the Hard Choice

Intent "derives from some consideration of the alternative action possibilities available to but foregone by the actor" (Jones & Davis, 1965, p. 222). When the foregone alternatives would normally be considered the dominant choice—that is, when the person picks the nondominant alternative—then the actor especially reveals intent. People are normally expected to choose what is culturally desirable, unless they belong to a deviant group or have maverick personalities. When people make a choice that is socially undesirable, then they have picked a nondominant alternative and made the hard choice, in our terms. People are also expected to behave consistently with their social category and their personalities. When people make a choice that is atypical for their social category, or atypical for them personally, then also they have made the hard choice. When someone does something unexpected, according to the perceiver's expectations, then the action is perceived as obviously intentional, to countermand all the normally prevailing forces. Choosing the otherwise nondominant alternative is viewed as especially indicative of intent.

Following the dominant alternative is, as noted earlier, a nonobvious form of intent. Accordingly, discussions of lay psychology do not describe it as a time when people necessarily attribute intent. Common-sense psychology is inconsistent about attributing intent to people who make the easy choice. For example, a person who treats an affirmative action appointee as less competent than other colleagues is following a fairly dominant (misguided) assumption; many lay psychologists would probably not attribute intent to that behavior, although it is certainly controllable. On the other hand, a person who estimates driving time by assuming an average speed 5 miles per hour above the speed limit is equally thinking in a fairly normative fashion, but lay psychologists would certainly say that the person intentionally thinks about driving at that speed. Hence, lay psychologists agree with scientific psychologists that following the *non*dominant alternative is obviously intentional, but they are more variable concerning the dominant alternative.

Perceiving the Focus of a Person's Attention

The inference of purposive action requires that the actor be perceived as striving with some effort in the direction of a plausible goal. The "trying" component of purposive action consists of both goal (direction of action) and exertion (effort expended). For example, we do not say that someone staring at a boulder is "trying" to lift it, for that is an unlikely intent, and moreover there is no observable effort (outside of psychokinesis). Nor do we say that the driver in a skid is "trying" to prevent the skid, although this is a likely intent, unless we observe some effort in that direction. Certainly, people may "try" to do such things (or try not to), but we infer whether they are trying by what they do and how hard they do it. If the actions are directed toward some goal and the actions require exertion, then perceivers impute that particular goal and amount of effort, respectively, and therefore the actions show that the person is "trying."

There is little direct evidence about what exactly lay psychologists observe to infer trying. It seems likely, however, that one mechanism by which perceivers infer another person's intention is to observe where and how closely the person's attention is focused. Heider (1958) described the several types of evidence that people use to decide what an actor intends, and each can be interpreted as determining what the actor has in mind (i.e., the focus of attention). Naive psychologists directly observe the following indicators of equifinality: When a particular behavior is thwarted, does the person try other behaviors that would have the same effect? Does the person give up trying when the effect is obtained? Does the person attempt several coordinated behaviors all aimed at the same outcome? Note that all of these factors indicate the alternative on which the other person's attention is concentrated. Although this is indirect evidence of its importance, focused attention seems to be an underlying theme in each of these lay observations. If the perceiver observes behavior patterns consistent with a particular attentional focus, then intent seems more likely.

Perceivers may also obtain evidence of intent by asking the person. Or perceivers may infer intent indirectly, based on their knowledge of the person (is the goal in line with this person's character and usual motives?). Similarly, perceivers may infer intent based on their knowledge of people in general (is the goal in line with typical social desirability?). Through direct observation of goal-directed behavior, through self-report, through prior knowledge of the person, or through knowledge of human nature, perceivers analyze actions for their underlying intents by attempting to discover what the actor has in mind, the actor's attentional focus. For lay psychologists, as for scientific psychologists, attention is a crucial mechanism for intent.

Summary of Lay Psychology and Intent

In sum, naive psychologists tend to agree with scientific psychologists on many features of intent. Choice among cognitively available alternatives—having options—is determined by the two "can" factors (ability and environment). Choosing a presumably nondominant alternative—making the hard choice—allows an especially clear inference of intent. And attention essentially determines which alternative the person follows, so naive and scientific observers both search for the two "trying" factors (a plausible goal and observable effort), as indications of focused attention.

Perceiving Intent in Stereotyping

In order to infer intent, a lay psychologist observing a stereotyper would first want to consider whether the person has options to think in other ways. Presumably, the stereotyper's personal and cultural history would be informative: Has the stereotyper been exposed to alternative ways of thinking about the stereotyped outgroup? Does the stereotyper's culture present alternatives to stereotypic thinking? Does the stereotyper have the cognitive capacity to individuate the other person? Second, the lay perceiver would consider whether stereotyping is the dominant or nondominant alternative. If it is nondominant—for example, if everyone else surrounding the stereotyper is thinking in *non*stereotypic terms—then the stereotyper's mode of thinking should seem especially intentional. If it is dominant—if everyone else is stereotyping too—then lay psychologists would not be so certain of intent, and inferences would be more variable. Finally, the mechanism that the observer would use to infer intent should be considering what the stereotyper apparently has in mind: Does the person seem to have a stereotype-consistent goal in mind? Does the person usually seem to think this way? In short, the lay psychologist would operate much as a scientific psychologist would to infer a stereotyper's intent.

LEGAL DEFINITIONS OF INTENT

Intent gives meaning to action in the law as well as in everyday life. For example, *Actus non facit reum, nisi mens sit rea* (An act does not render a person guilty, unless the mind is guilty), or *Intentio mea impornit nomen operi meo* (My intent gives a name to my act) (Burton, 1980). Because of its importance in legal settings, "intent" has various working definitions depending on the context, such as "premeditation," "malice aforethought," "fraudulent intent," and the like. In the law generally, "intent is treated as a purpose formed in the mind to do something maliciously or reckless of consequences, not accidentally," according to a central legal source on this topic (Marshall, 1968, p. 10). Because it is a mental state, intent usually must be inferred indirectly (Black, 1979). The law is concerned with perceived intent, so perhaps it is not surprising that many of the principles that laypeople use to infer intent are also used in legal settings (cf. Fincham & Jaspars, 1980; Hamilton, 1978). And, to some extent, these principles overlap with what scientific psychologists have written about intent.

Having Options, from a Legal Perspective

The defining criterion, having options, appears to be at the center of legal treatments of intent: "In law, intention is assumed to involve the making of choices. . . . Freedom of will is dependent on (1) the capacity of a particular individual to choose his action and (2) the choices which he perceives to be available to him" (Marshall, 1968, pp. 26–27). Although a person's perceived choices are not easy to determine, the law apparently deals with what a "reasonable person" would know and understand. Deciding what a reasonable person would perceive as choices is likely to rest on what the trier of fact (judge or jury) perceives as probable choices. In this way, "Law tends to direct its attention to the probable intent of *men* even when the probable intent of a given *man* is at issue" (Marshall, 1968, p. 11, italics in original). That is, a reasonable person would have considered alternatives to be available, so a particular person will be treated *as if* alternatives were available, whether that person actually considered them or not. One implication of this view is that an actual person can make decisions without consciously considering the alternatives, but if the trier of fact thinks that choices were potentially cognitively available, the person will be treated *as if* the actual choice were intentional. Hence, legal views of intent essentially focus on whether an act's consequences were foreseeable and quite possibly desirable to the actor (Holmes, 1881).

Making the Hard Choice, from a Legal Perspective

Legal discussions do not focus on the conditions under which laypeople are especially likely to perceive intent—that is, the obvious forms of intent, when the actor makes the hard choice, following the nondominant alternative. Perhaps analyzing lay perceptions is understandably a task best left to psychologists. In the opinion of one psychologically informed legal scholar, however, people's choices are best seen as the balance between, on the one hand, their inner needs, values, and perceptions, and, on the other, their need for external support from significant reference groups (Marshall, 1968). The inner and outer alternatives may conflict, as when a person who knows better is pressured by local racist norms. In such instances, people who cave in to the group norms may not view themselves as having made a choice, but "In the law it may be a situation in which conscious intent is presumed because a reasonable man would foresee the consequences" (Marshall, 1968, p. 108).

Paying Attention, from a Legal Perspective

Concerning the mechanism by which intent operates, legal sources concur with scientific and lay psychologies. Intent is revealed by what the actor has in mind, the focus of attention. It is the state of mind with which the act is committed or omitted (Black, 1979). *Quod factum est, cum in obscuro sit, ex affectione cujusque capit interpretationem* (When there is doubt about an act, it receives interpretation from the feelings or disposition of the actor) (Burton, 1980). The relationship of intent to attention is illustrated in one legal source by the Hebrew word for intent, *kavannah,* which means "the direction of the mind toward the accomplishment of a particular act, the state of being aware of what we are doing, of the task we are engaged in" (Heschel, 1955; cited in Marshall, 1968, p. 8). The implication is that intent presupposes attention. Whether intent also presupposes consciousness is less clear, given the contradiction between "the state of being aware," on the one hand, and the reasonable-person standard, which does not presuppose awareness on the part of that particular individual. In general, legal contexts centrally consider the direction of attention to an alternative (malice aforethought) or away from a potentially available alternative or consequence (negligence, recklessness), so attention plays a role in other guises.

Summary

Legal writing focuses on the definition of intent as having options—namely, the reasonable person's capacity to choose among cognitively available alternatives and the reasonably foreseeable consequences of those alternatives. Legal writing does not apparently differentiate the most obvious instances of intent (when a person makes the hard choice) from the less obvious forms of intent (when a person follows the dominant alternative). Finally, the direction of attention determines the central intent in legal writing, as elsewhere.

Legal Psychology's Implications for Stereotyping

In the legal setting most relevant to stereotyping and prejudice, intent is central to the psychological model underlying both constitutional and statutory discrimination law. The central question in discrimination law is whether an act or an omission causing harm to another person occurred because of that person's legally protected group membership (e.g., sex, race, or national origin). Translated into a psycholegal model, discriminatory *intent* ("because of another's group membership") can cause discriminatory *treatment* (the harmful act), which can cause discriminatory *impact* (the harmful outcome). If this intent–treatment–impact chain occurs, a legal wrong has occurred (e.g., Schlei & Grossman, 1983).

Intent has a central evidentiary role because it is the initial cause in this psycholegal model. If an individual admits that the harmful act occurred because of the (legally protected) group membership of the person harmed, this is sufficient proof that the harm arose from unlawful discrimination. The more difficult and common situation involves proving discrimination without direct proof of explicit intent—without an admission of discriminatory intent from the alleged discriminator. As noted, intent is a mental state that must be inferred. Moreover, because discrimination is now publicly unacceptable, people rarely admit openly that they acted because of prejudice or stereotypes about legally protected group members. Without direct admission of intent, discriminatory intent must be inferred from discriminatory treatment or discriminatory impact (the second and third links in the psycholegal model) and from the surrounding circumstances.

Some commentators advocate requiring direct proof of intent, and some advocate relying on circumstantial evidence drawn from observations of discriminatory treatment. Hence, direct proof of intent matters to a greater or lesser degree, depending on one's interpretation of discrimination law. A conservative interpretation of discrimination law tends to fall back on direct proof of intent, requiring the plaintiff to prove the decision makers' explicit discriminatory intent (Blumstein, 1984, p. 30). Because such an intent is of course publicly unacceptable, uncovering this type of evidence is a difficult enterprise at best. A liberal interpretation tends to read disparate treatment as indicating discriminatory intent (*International Brotherhood of Teamsters v. United States*, 1977), on the theory that a reasonable person should foresee that disparate treatment will lead to disparate outcomes.[7]

The difference between the conservative and liberal interpretations of the intent standard in discrimination law is crucial. The conservative direct-proof-of-intent stance allows the defendant to make a "good-faith" defense ("I did not intend to discriminate"); the stance thus means that any claim to unintentional discrimination would absolve alleged discriminators from responsibility for their actions. Clearly, it would be difficult to contradict such protestations, for few defendants would have previously articulated a discriminatory intent, given the prevailing legal and social norms. Hence, the "good-faith" claim is easy to make and hard to refute.

Moreover, decision makers' efforts to avoid discrimination are likely to depend on their understanding of which intent standard could apply. Decision makers who understand that they will be held responsible for disparate treatment, because their intent will be inferred from indirect proof, may try more readily to prevent disparate treatment and disparate impact. Decision makers who understand that the victim of potential discrimination must show that the decision maker deliberately meant to achieve discriminatory outcomes, on the other hand, may be less watchful, because the burden falls upon the party with the least access to the decision maker's state of mind. Thus, one's interpretation of intent makes a practical and legal difference.

CONCLUSIONS

Reviewing evidence from scientific, lay, and legal psychology has allowed us to synthesize some basic features of intent. One can judge whether a person intends something by whether the person has options (i.e., cognitively available alternatives). One can judge when intent will be most obvious by those circumstances under which people make the hard choice— namely, following a previously nondominant alternative. Note, however, that making the easy choice (following the dominant alternative) is still by definition intentional, although it may be a less obvious form of intent. Finally, intent operates when people attend to the chosen alternative.

Why might it be important to know that people intend the stereotypic or individuating processes by which they respond to other people? From an applied standpoint, I believe that it is dangerous to leave open the possible misinterpretation of cognitive approaches to stereotyping—namely, that social perceivers can't help it. If they can't help it, then no amount of incentive, pressure, or sanction will promote change. If stereotyping, prejudice, and discrimination result from unintentional and inevitable cognitive processes, then they are uncontrollable by the persons using them. The idea that such processes are unintentional may be used to justify releasing people from responsibility for their actions. Shaver (1985), for example, notes that intent is one of the key contributors to attributions of responsibility. Clearly, the role of intent in stereotyping and prejudice has potentially important legal, practical, and political implications.

Hence, it is important to address the potential misinterpretation of cognitive approaches to stereotyping—namely, that perceivers naturally categorize, and therefore that their stereotypes and prejudice are simply by-products of an unintentional and inevitable process. Given its potential importance, it seems premature to accept the unexamined assumption without closer study. This chapter is an attempt to begin that closer study.

From a psychological viewpoint, the examination of intent, with an emphasis on stereotyping, is also important. The idea that people have some control over stereotyping and prejudice is not new, but it has been ignored of late. Allport (1954) suggested that both knowledge and motivation are necessary to undercut bigotry. He suggested that one road to tolerance may be self-insight: People who are aware of their prejudices and ashamed of them are likely to be relatively tolerant (Allport & Kramer, 1946). Another road to tolerance that Allport suggested is the combination of knowledge and self-interest. That is, encountering a stereotype-discrepant individual usually does not change the stereotype of the group as a whole. However, when it is in the individual's self-interest to be accurate, then knowledge is more likely to lead to change. Both roads to tolerance suggest that conflict between cognitively available options—the still, small voice of tolerance versus the spontaneous drift toward prejudice—causes change and flexibility. Both self-insight and self-interest highlight the importance of motivational as well as cognitive pressure on stereotyping (cf. Erber & Fiske, 1984; Kruglanski & Freund, 1983; Neuberg & Fiske, 1987; Omoto & Borgida, 1988).

The psychology of intent and stereotyping suggests intriguing research possibilities. It would be well to examine the conditions of cognitive options: the ability to imagine alternatives, the ease of imagining such alternatives (as in the simulation heuristic; Kahneman & Tversky, 1982), the recency of considering alternatives, and similar issues, particularly as applied directly to stereotyping. It would be helpful, too, to investigate conditions under which stereotyping appears to be the easy or hard choice; elsewhere, my colleagues and I have made a start on the informational and motivational conditions that encourage stereotyping or individuating processes (see Fiske & Neuberg, in press, for a review). And the current concept of intent also emphasizes the role of attention as the primary mechanism for the operation of intent; research in our laboratory demonstrates the role of attention in stereotyping and individuating processes (see Fiske & Neuberg, in press).

If nothing else, we now have an answer for the cross-examining defense attorney in the nightmare about the discrimination case. The cognitive social psychologist could now reply that people probably can help it when they stereotype and prejudge. The idea that categorization is a natural and adaptive, even dominant, way of understanding other people does not mean that it is the only option available. Perceivers make the hard choice to individuate under a variety of circumstances (Fiske & Neuberg, in press). Because perceivers have options available, they may be said to intend the one they choose. If people stereotype and prejudge, reckless or careless of the consequences, they may be said to do so intentionally.

Because this examination of intent was partly catalyzed by legal concerns, a critic might ask whether the legal application has "pushed" the psychological investigation. In reply, I would say that it has done so no more than psychological researchers' values usually guide their work, and perhaps less, because the concern is more obvious here and has been a conscious issue from the outset. The breadth of material covered is one safeguard against bias; the concepts of having options, making the hard choice, and paying attention are all "out there" in the literature for anyone to examine, and I believe I have represented them accurately and logically. Of course, others may disagree, and it is their prerogative to delineate an alternative viewpoint. That is one way science proceeds. However, it is not as if legal psychology and scientific psychology operate at cross purposes. Legal psychology codifies society's long-term norms and common sense, a purpose related to social psychology's effort to examine systematically the operation of those norms and perceptions. Perhaps the primary difference between legal and scientific psychology is the former's problem-solving orientation. This is not necessarily a bad thing, for it encourages precision, concreteness, and accountability. In sum, if the legal concerns have pushed the psychological analysis, it is in the direction of clarity.

As a result of the concerns addressed and the literature examined, the definition of intent offered here is admittedly broad. Accordingly, one might ask whether any interesting social behavior is unintentional by this definition. The answer follows, as it must, from the central defining feature of intent: having cognitively available options. When an individual's culture or personal experience does not allow the person to conceive of alternatives, then that person's choices are explicitly not intentional. This suggests a broader contextual analysis of the person's situation as part of assessing possible intents, which seems a useful research agenda.

To reiterate the opening theme, it is clear that psychology's current emphasis on cognitive explanations has informed research on interpersonal behavior, personality, psychopathology, education, the environment, health, marketing, organizations, and the law, to name just a few areas. Notably, however, there is a particular spirit with which cognitive explanations have sometimes been adopted—namely, one that implies a lack of intent on the part of the actor. "Cognitive," applied outside basic research on human thinking, has often been equated with imperfect understanding caused by the inherent limitations of the human mind. Granted, this description of the applications oversimplifies them, but translations of cognitive principles to other settings frequently include an unstated assumption that actors lack knowledge of and control over their cognitive errors and biases. This is a mistaken assumption at worst, and certainly an inadequately examined one at best.

Social perceivers are flexible. By examining intent, one begins to see how motivational and cognitive factors may influence the different ways in which people control their social understanding and responding. Social perceivers have a healthy ability to function adaptively and effectively; they are not simply at the mercy of their cognitive limitations.

ACKNOWLEDGMENTS

I would like to thank the following individuals for their helpful comments: James Averill, John Bargh, Sarah Burns, David Hamilton, Sara Kiesler, George Levinger, Carolyn Mervis, Steven Neuberg, Shelley Taylor, Abraham Tesser, James Uleman, Daniel Wegner, and the fourth annual Nags Head Conference on Social Cognition. Preparation of this chapter was supported by National Science Foundation Grant Nos. BNS 8406913 and BNS 8569028; by National Institute of Mental Health Grant No. MH41801; and by my Carnegie-Mellon University sponsored leave, as a visiting scholar at the University of Michigan Research Center for Group Dynamics.

NOTES

1. Given that James's examples are behavioral and stereotyping is cognitive, one might wonder whether this analysis of intent applies equally to both types of process. However, according to James, they are closely linked. James discussed action as preceded by an idea of the action. The ideomotor idea creates the cognate action, unless a conflicting idea occurs simultaneously. Apart from reflexive, instinctual, or random actions, behavior is viewed as resulting from the idea of the behavior. Accordingly, if a person performs a discriminatory behavior, James would argue that the idea of the behavior precedes the action. Moreover, if a person has more than one idea about how to behave, including the idea to inhibit the behavior, then the person has both cognitive and behavioral options. One particularly

relevant type of deliberate action occurs, according to James, when, after indecision, we discover that "we can refer the case to a *class* upon which we are accustomed to act unhesitatingly in a certain stereotyped way" (p. 1138, italics in original). Hence, in other words, the person has the possibility of using or not using familiar stereotypes to guide behavior.

2. Lewin thus suggested a fundamental contrast between cognitive structure and motivation. Many of his contemporaries similarly contrasted dominant associations (cognitive structures) with overriding sets (intents), using a wide range of terms for "set," including "predisposition," "determining tendency," "attitude," "drive," and "purpose" (Boring, 1950). An apparently related message also emerged from the New Look in perception (Bruner, 1957; Erdelyi, 1974). That is, the New Look emphasized the ways in which motivational sets can override otherwise dominant perceptions. For example, perceptual vigilance and perceptual defense were posited to shape categorization far more than previously realized. The New Look supposed that these determining motivational processes were outside one's awareness and therefore outside one's control. However, in both the set and the New Look research traditions, the nature of intentional behavior was not the focal issue.

3. In an interesting repetition of history, instruction *(Aufgabe)* as determining intent *(Einstellung)* was the precise operationalization used by turn-of-the-century set psychology.

4. Lewin (1951) used the terms "controlled" and "uncontrolled" in a compatible but somewhat different sense, giving the following example:

> [W]hen a child decides to go past a dog of which he is afraid, the walking past is occasionally a controlled action; then the child passes the dog with a controlled and calm, though cautious, bearing. The intentional action is, however, often not a controlled action, or may show only little control. For instance, in the example given, the intention is often carried out in the form of entirely uncontrolled running past the dog. (Lewin, 1951, p. 147, original italics omitted)

5. Just as attention may be drawn to the dominant or nondominant alternative itself, attention may be distracted away from one or several consequences of an action alternative as well as the action itself. Clearly, one can intend an act but not all of its consequences. Attention may also be directed toward or distracted away from different purposes of an act (according to act identification theory; Vallacher & Wegner, 1987). For example, forming an impression of two people can simultaneously be considered "making a personnel decision," "choosing between a black candidate and a white candidate," or "picking the faster typist." Our focus here, however, is on the purposes and consequences cognitively available or potentially available to the person, as defined earlier.

6. Although usually interpreted as an analysis of how people attribute personality traits or other enduring dispositions, Jones's original paper "might better have been subtitled 'From Acts to Intentions' than 'From Acts to Dispositions' " (Jones & McGillis, 1976, p. 393).

7. The U.S. Supreme Court stated in the *Teamsters* decision that proof of intent is not absolutely required. However, under a conservative interpretation, proving a discrimination case could require intent. According to the required evidence in a

statutory discrimination case (*McDonnell Douglas Corp. v. Green*, 1973), the defendant must provide a legitimate nondiscriminatory reason (LNDR) for the alleged discriminatory treatment (e.g., someone else was promoted because of higher qualifications than the plaintiff). The plaintiff then must prove that the LNDR was merely a pretext and therefore that discriminatory intent was the real reason for the discriminatory treatment. Under a liberal interpretation, the pretext requirement might mean that the plaintiff merely had to show that the LNDR was not legitimate (e.g., that the plaintiff was better qualified). However, a conservative interpretation of the pretext requirement might mean that the plaintiff instead had to prove explicit discriminatory intent. Clearly, it would be harder to prove intent than it would be merely to prove that the alleged LNDR was in fact illegitimate.

REFERENCES

Allport, G. W. (1954). *The nature of prejudice*. Reading, MA: Addison-Wesley.

Allport, G. W., & Kramer, B. M. (1946). Some roots of prejudice. *Journal of Psychology, 22*, 9–39.

Anderson, C. A. (1982). Inoculation and counter-explanation: Debiasing techniques in the perseverance of social theories. *Social Cognition, 1*, 126–139.

Ashmore, R. D., & Del Boca, F. K. (1981). Conceptual approaches to stereotypes and stereotyping. In D. L. Hamilton (Ed.), *Cognitive processes in stereotyping and intergroup behavior* (pp. 1–36). Hillsdale, NJ: Erlbaum.

Bargh, J. A. (1984). Automatic and conscious processing of social information. In R. S. Wyer, Jr., & T. K. Srull (Eds.), *Handbook of social cognition* (Vol. 3, pp. 1–43). Hillsdale, NJ: Erlbaum.

Black, H. C. (1979). *Black's law dictionary* (5th ed.). St. Paul, MN: West.

Blumstein, J. F. (1984). Defining discrimination: Intent vs. impact. *New Perspectives, 16*, 29–33.

Boring, E. G. (1950). *A history of experimental psychology* (2nd ed). Englewood Cliffs, NJ: Prentice-Hall.

Brown, V., & Geis, F. L. (1984). Turning lead into gold: Evaluations of men and women leaders and the alchemy of social consensus. *Journal of Personality and Social Psychology, 46*, 811–824.

Brown v. Board of Education of Topeka, Kansas, 347 U.S. 483 (1954).

Bruner, J. S. (1957). Going beyond the information given. In H. E. Gruber, K. R. Hammond, & R. Jessor (Eds.), *Contemporary approaches to cognition: A symposium held at the University of Colorado* (pp. 41–69). Cambridge, MA: Harvard University Press.

Burton, W. C. (1980). *Legal thesaurus*. New York: Macmillan.

Deutsch, M. (1954). Field theory in social psychology. In G. Lindzey (Ed.), *Handbook of social psychology* (Vol. 1, pp. 181–222). Reading, MA: Addison-Wesley.

Erber, R., & Fiske, S. T. (1984). Outcome dependency and attention to inconsistent information. *Journal of Personality and Social Psychology, 47*, 709–726.

Erdelyi, M. H. (1974). A new look at the New Look: Perceptual defense and vigilance. *Psychological Review, 81*, 1–25.

Fincham, F. D., & Jaspars, J. M. (1980). Attribution of responsibility: From man the scientist to man as lawyer. In L. Berkowitz (Ed.), *Advances in experimen-*

tal social psychology (Vol. 13, pp. 81–138). New York: Academic Press.

Fiske, S. T., & Neuberg, S. L. (in press). A continuum model of impression formation, from category-based to individuating processes: Influences of information and motivation on attention and interpretation. In M. P. Zanna (Ed.), *Advances in experimental social psychology* (Vol. 23). New York: Academic Press.

Fiske, S. T., Neuberg, S. L., Beattie, A. E., & Milberg, S. J. (1987). Category-based and attribute-based reactions to others: Some informational conditions of stereotyping and individuating processes. *Journal of Experimental Social Psychology, 23,* 399–427.

Fiske, S. T., & Pavelchak, M. A. (1986). Category-based versus piecemeal-based affective responses: Developments in schema-triggered affect. In R. M. Sorrentino & E. T. Higgins (Eds.), *Handbook of motivation and cognition: Foundations of social behavior* (pp. 167–203). New York: Guilford Press.

Fiske, S. T., & Taylor, S. E. (1984). *Social cognition.* New York: Random House.

Hamilton, D. L. (1979). A cognitive–attributional analysis of stereotyping. In L. Berkowitz (Ed.), *Advances in experimental social psychology* (Vol. 12, pp. 53–84). New York: Academic Press.

Hamilton, D. L., & Trolier, T. K. (1986). Stereotypes and stereotyping: An overview of the cognitive approach. In J. Dovidio & S. L. Gaertner (Eds.), *Prejudice, discrimination, and racism* (pp. 127–163). New York: Academic Press.

Hamilton, V. L. (1978). Who is responsible? Toward a social psychology of responsibility attribution. *Social Psychology, 41,* 316–328.

Heider, F. (1958). *The psychology of interpersonal relations.* New York: Wiley.

Holmes, O. W., Jr. (1881). *The common law.* Boston: Little, Brown.

Hopkins v. Price-Waterhouse, 618 F. Supp. 1109, 111 (D.D.C. 1985).

International Brotherhood of Teamsters v. United States, 431 U.S. 324 (1977).

James, W. (1981). *The principles of psychology* (2 vols.). Cambridge, MA: Harvard University Press. (Original work published in 1890)

Jones, E. E., & Davis, K. E. (1965). From acts to dispositions: The attribution process in person perception. In L. Berkowitz (Ed.), *Advances in experimental social psychology* (Vol. 2, pp. 219–266). New York: Academic Press.

Jones, E. E., Farina, A., Hastorf, A. H., Markus, H., Miller, D. T., & Scott, R. A. (1984). *Social stigma: The psychology of marked relationships.* San Francisco: W. H. Freeman.

Jones, E. E., & McGillis, D. (1976). Correspondent inferences and the attribution cube: A comparative reappraisal. In J. H. Harvey, W. J. Ickes, & R. F. Kidd (Eds.), *New directions in attribution research* (Vol. 1, pp. 389–420). Hillsdale, NJ: Erlbaum.

Kahneman, D., & Tversky, A. (1982). The simulation heuristic. In D. Kahneman, P. Slovic, & A. Tversky (Eds.), *Judgment under uncertainty: Heuristics and biases* (pp. 201–208). Cambridge, England: Cambridge University Press.

Kimble, G. A., & Perlmuter, L. C. (1970). The problem of volition. *Psychological Review, 77,* 361–384.

Kruglanski, A. W., & Freund, T. (1983). The freezing and unfreezing of lay-inferences: Effects on impressional primacy, ethnic stereotyping, and numerical anchoring. *Journal of Experimental Social Psychology, 19,* 448–468.

Lewin, K. (1935). *A dynamic theory of personality* (D. K. Adams & K. E. Zener, Trans.). New York: McGraw-Hill.

Lewin, K. (1951). Intention, will, and need. In D. Rapaport (Ed. and Trans.), *Organization and pathology of thought* (pp. 95–153). New York: Columbia University Press.

Logan, G. D. (1980). Attention and automaticity in Stroop and priming tasks: Theory and data. *Cognitive Psychology, 12,* 523–553.

Logan, G. D., & Cowan, W. B. (1984). On the ability to inhibit thought and action: A theory of an act of control. *Psychological Review, 91,* 295–327.

Mandler, G. (1984). *Mind and body: Psychology of emotion and stress.* New York: Norton.

Marcel, A. J. (1983). Conscious and unconscious perception: An approach to the relations between phenomenal experience and perceptual processes. *Cognitive Psychology, 15,* 238–300.

Markus, H., & Zajonc, R. B. (1985). The cognitive perspective in social psychology. In G. Lindzey & E. Aronson (Eds.), *Handbook of social psychology* (2nd ed., Vol. 1, pp. 137–230). New York: Random House.

Marshall, J. (1968). *Intention in law and society.* New York: Funk & Wagnalls.

McDonnell Douglas Corporation v. Green, 411 U.S. 792, 5 FEP Cases 965 (1973).

Miller, G. A., Galanter, E., & Pribram, K. H. (1960). *Plans and the structure of behavior.* New York: Holt, Rinehart & Winston.

Mischel, W. (1974). Processes in delay of gratification. In L. Berkowitz (Ed.), *Advances in experimental social psychology* (Vol. 7, pp. 249–292). New York: Academic Press.

Neely, J. H. (1977). Semantic priming and retrieval from lexical memory: Roles of inhibitionless spreading activation and limited capacity attention. *Journal of Experimental Psychology: General, 106,* 226–254.

Neuberg, S. L., & Fiske, S. T. (1987). Motivational influences on impression formation: Outcome dependency, attention, and individuating processes. *Journal of Personality and Social Psychology, 53,* 431–444.

Nisbett, R. E., & Ross, L. (1980). *Human inference: Strategies and shortcomings of social judgment.* Englewood Cliffs, NJ: Prentice-Hall.

Nisbett, R. E., & Wilson, T. D. (1977). Telling more than we can know: Verbal reports on mental processes. *Psychological Review, 84,* 231–259.

Norman, D. A., & Shallice, T. (1986). Attention to action: Willed and automatic control of behavior. In R. J. Davidson, G. E. Schwartz, & D. Shapiro (Eds.), *Consciousness and self regulation: Advances in research and theory* (Vol. 4, pp. 1–18). New York: Plenum Press.

Omoto, A. M., & Borgida, E. (1988). Guess who might be coming to dinner: Personal involvement and racial stereotypes. *Journal of Experimental Social Psychology, 24,* 571–593.

Posner, M. I., & Snyder, C. R. R. (1975). Attention and cognitive control. In R. L. Solso (Ed.), *Information processing and cognition: The Loyola Symposium* (pp. 55–88). Hillsdale, NJ: Erlbaum.

Price-Waterhouse v. Hopkins, awaiting decision, U.S. Supreme Court No. 87-1167.

Schlei, B. L., & Grossman, P. (1983). *Employment discrimination law.* Chicago: American Bar Association.

Schneider, W., & Shiffrin, R. M. (1977). Controlled and automatic human information processing: I. Detection, search, and attention. *Psychological Review, 84,* 1–66.

Shallice, T. (1972). Dual functions of consciousness. *Psychological Review, 79,* 383–393.

Shaver, K. G. (1985). *The attribution of blame: Causality, responsibility, and blameworthiness.* New York: Springer-Verlag.

Shiffrin, R. M., & Schneider, W. (1977). Controlled and automatic human information processing: II. Perceptual learning, automatic attending, and general theory. *Psychological Review, 84,* 127–190.

Taylor, S. E., Fiske, S. T., Etcoff, N. L., & Ruderman, A. J. (1978). Categorical bases of person memory and stereotyping. *Journal of Personality and Social Psychology, 36,* 778–793.

Tolman, E. C. (1925). Purpose and cognition: The determiners of animal learning. *Psychological Review, 32,* 285–297.

Tolman, E. C. (1927). A behaviorist's definition of consciousness. *Psychological Review, 34,* 433–439.

Tolman, E. C. (1938). The determiners of behavior at a choice point. *Psychological Review, 45,* 1–41.

Vallacher, R. R., & Wegner, D. M. (1987). What do people think they're doing? Action identification and human behavior. *Psychological Review, 94,* 3–15.

PART III

REGAINING CONTROL OF UNINTENDED THOUGHT

9

Mental Control:
The War of the Ghosts
in the Machine

DANIEL M. WEGNER
Trinity University

DAVID J. SCHNEIDER
Rice University

Sometimes it feels as though we can control our minds. We catch ourselves looking out the window when we should be paying attention to someone talking, for example, and we purposefully return our attention to the conversation. Or we wrest our minds away from the bothersome thought of an upcoming dental appointment to focus on anything we can find that makes us less nervous. Control attempts such as these can meet with success, leaving us feeling the masters of our consciousness. Yet at other times we drift back to gaze out the window or to think again of the dentist's chair, and we are left to wonder whether mental control is real—and, if it is, how we might exercise it effectively.

THE NATURE OF MENTAL CONTROL

One way to approach this problem is to assume that mental control is a real phenomenon, ask people to exercise it, and see what happens. Some noteworthy regularities in the effects of mental control become evident on following this line of inquiry. This chapter is about experiments we have conducted in which people are asked to control their minds while they are describing the course of their thoughts. We begin by describing the course of our own thoughts.

A "Tumbling-Ground for Whimsies"

Mental control is connected to two of the most important controversial concepts in psychology—consciousness and the will. Even William James, a champion of the study of things mental, warned that consciousness has the potential to make psychology no more than a "tumbling-ground for whimsies" (1890, Vol. 1, p. 163). Psychology since James has echoed his concern. Although the idea of altogether abolishing consciousness from psychology only held sway at the peak of behaviorism, even after a cognitive revolution there remains a preference for the study of mind through its processes rather than its conscious content. The will, in turn, is relegated to the status of illusion by many—among them Gilbert Ryle, who called it the "ghost in the machine" (1949, p. 15). The question, then, of whether the will can operate upon consciousness is doubly troubling.

James held that we exert our wills by "effort of attention" (1890, Vol. 2, p. 562). He voiced the useful intuition that we do one thing as opposed to another by steering our consciousness. *How* we do this, however, is unclear. We appear to attend to one thing as opposed to another by—well, by just doing so. James's account only indicates that the willful movement of consciousness from one object to another feels like work, and that this movement can be contrasted with those cases in which our attention is drawn, seemingly without our effort, by forces beyond our will. Mental control is, in this light, one of the irreducible elements of conscious experience. This irreducibility is one of the puzzling aspects of mental control that has left those inclined to deal with this issue talking of ghosts and whimsies.

It is possible to study the operation of mental control in a useful way, however, without any further insight into this puzzle. One need only assume that there is a cognitive process responsible for activating and deactivating attentional mechanisms according to priorities that are reflected in conscious thoughts. A scientific understanding of this process does not require that we be able to see into it as we do it, any more than a science of movement requires that we have insight into the enervation of our muscles as we walk like a chicken. It is time to set aside the dissection of the conscious experience of willing, and study instead the observable circumstances and consequences of this experience.

There is one other feature of mental control that has given it a reputation as a phantom of the ganglia. Mental efforts sometimes fail, and we do not know enough about mental control to understand why this happens. Sometimes the right idea will not come, despite furrowed brows, squinted eyes, and all the deliberate concentration one can muster. This may not at first seem strange, because efforts of all sorts frequently fail.

But we find it surprising because whereas the effort to make a thought appear on command sometimes does not work, seemingly similar physical efforts rarely fail in the physically healthy. It is not odd to say that "I couldn't get it out of my mind" or "I couldn't concentrate on the idea," but it seems most peculiar to say that "I couldn't make my finger move."

Even mental control that is initially successful can subsequently falter. Unlike physical effort, which, once initiated, typically suffers few indigenous interferences (i.e., other than from physical restraint), our thoughts seem remarkably capricious. On good days our thoughts are as precise as a hawk gathering small rodents, but more often our thoughts seem like fluttery butterflies that not only fail to stay put for long but are subject to the winds of competing thought. Try as we may, we cannot concentrate on reading a novel or solving an equation when there are interesting distractions nearby. Or we may struggle to make particular thoughts go away in the midst of a sleepless night, only to have them return all too soon. And it is something of a universal tragedy that when we attempt to reject thoughts of hot fudge sundaes from our minds while dieting, we must usually watch as they then march through our imaginations again and again.

The Aims of Mental Control

There are two general goals to which we aspire in controlling our minds: having something in mind, and not having it in mind. Psychology gives us many terms for each. Having something in mind is "thinking," "attending," "retrieving," "perceiving," "encoding," and so on; not having something in mind is "forgetting," "denying," "repressing," "avoiding," "filtering," and so forth. The activities in which we engage when we consciously attempt to achieve one of these states are most generally called "concentration" and "suppression," respectively. Although there are other potential goals for mental control—one, perhaps, for each mental operation people can perform—it is clear that these are most fundamental. If we could not concentrate or suppress, it seems there would be little else we could do to our minds.

Normally, when we are thinking of one thing, we are not thinking of something else. Cognitive psychologists have often held that this dual function of the process of attending suggests the operation of two subprocesses, one that brings items to attention and one that filters out everything else (e.g., Broadbent, 1958). The central idea here is that *both* processes must be operating at all times in order to keep one thing in our conscious attention. If we assume that mental control processes are simply willful versions of such automatic processes, then we can suggest that concentration and suppression are typically associated. In concentrating on X, we suppress not-X; by the same token, in suppressing X, we concentrate on not-X.

By this logic, the two processes are always simultaneous. The reason we have different names for them and experience them as distinct is that we try to do one at a time (and the other follows). So, for instance, we may try to concentrate on writing a book chapter (and suppress thoughts of other things, such as going swimming). Alternatively, we may try to suppress a thought, say, of smoking a cigarette (and concentrate on other things, such as eating). In either case, we are primarily aware of intending only one of the processes, but we nevertheless must use the other process as well in order to fulfill our intention. This is true because both processes are versions of the "effort of attention" described by James, and we cannot move attention toward something without at the same time moving it away from something else.

The simultaneity of concentration and suppression suggests that there are two distinguishable forms of each process. First, there are primary and auxiliary forms of concentration; primary concentration is attending to something because we want to do so, whereas auxiliary concentration is attending to something because we wish to suppress attention to something else. In a similar vein, there are primary and auxiliary forms of suppression. Primary suppression is keeping attention away from something because we want to do so, whereas auxiliary suppression is keeping attention away as a means of concentrating on something else. Primary concentration is thus accompanied by an auxiliary suppression (as when one avoids thinking about the noise down the hall in order to study). And primary suppression brings with it an auxiliary concentration (as when one tries not to think of a broken romance by focusing on a television program).

Our studies of mental control have centered on the case of primary suppression with auxiliary concentration. This is the form of mental control that people appear most anxious to have, in large part because lapses of suppression announce themselves intrusively. We know quite clearly when an unwanted thought returns to consciousness. In a sense, our plan to suppress marks the thought as something of which we must be wary, and its return is thus heralded by an immediate reorientation to the suppression problem. By contrast, when we merely try to concentrate, it is quite possible to lose sight of the plan and mentally drift away, for minutes or perhaps even days. The only sign that we have failed to concentrate occurs if we happen in our mental meandering to stumble across the concentration target. And even then, the concentration target and our earlier failure do not seem to burst into our minds with nearly the force of a returning unwanted thought.

The reason for examining suppression rather than concentration, in short, is not too far removed from the sheer love of sport. When people concentrate, the purpose of mental control is to maintain a line of thought. In a sense, one part of the mind is cheering on another. But when people suppress, the purpose of mental control is to challenge a line of thought.

One part of the mind is set to defeat another. Skirmishes can break out on many mental fields of battle, and the most placid, unsuspecting states of mind can be ambushed from the blue by unwanted thoughts. Thought suppression is thus an occasion for mental conflict, a true war of the ghosts in the machine.

THE CASE OF THOUGHT SUPPRESSION

The fact that we sometimes suppress thoughts because they are painful is no surprise either to introspective laypeople or to readers of Freud. Sometimes mental pain seems as unbearable as its physical counterpart, and one does not have to be a committed hedonist to recognize that painful stimuli are typically avoided. Freud, of course, built much of his theory around such episodes. Although our work has not been much oriented toward Freudian ideas, he offered many masterful insights not only about the unconscious but the conscious part of mental life. We begin by considering his approach, and then turn to the basic problems of why people suppress, how they do it, what effect their efforts have, and how they might do it most competently.

Freud and Forgetting

Unfortunately, Freud was often most vague at the point where he should have been most precise, and it is hard to extract a consistent theory about the mental life from his work. This is especially true in the case of his accounts of suppression and repression. For example, it is commonly assumed that Freud made a sharp distinction between conscious "suppression" and unconscious "repression." In fact, he continuously and throughout his career used the terms interchangeably; furthermore, he never stated explicitly that repression referred only to pushing conscious material into the unconscious (cf. Erdelyi & Goldberg, 1979).

Freud preferred a broad definition of repression: "[T]he essence of repression lies simply in the function of rejecting and keeping something out of consciousness" (1915/1957, p. 105). It is certainly true that many (indeed, most) of the examples he used invoke a stronger and more popular sense of the term, involving the unconscious, but it is also true that he was generally perfectly explicit that removing cathexis (roughly, attention, in this context) from an idea was a sufficient condition for repression, defined as above. As far as we know, the closest he ever came to distinguishing between suppression and repression came in a long footnote in Chapter 7 of *The Interpretation of Dreams:* "For instance, I have omitted to state whether I attribute different meanings to the words 'suppressed' and 'repressed.' It should have been clear, however, that the latter lays more stress than the former upon the fact of attachment to the unconscious" (Freud, 1900/1953, Vol. 5, p. 606).

Psychoanalysts have now focused for many years on the notion of unconscious repression to the exclusion of simple suppression. Although Freud himself can surely be faulted for promoting this particular line of orthodoxy in psychoanalytic theorizing, his primary concern was in how we keep former ideas from recurring. This activity could involve suppression alone, and certainly need not depend on either unconscious motivation or memory erasure, the central features of classical repression. Each of these features of the concept of repression has served in its own way as a theoretical albatross.

The dogma of unconscious motivation, for example, requires that research on repression must typically arrive at the scene after the fact. We cannot know beforehand exactly what unconscious motive might be energized, nor when that motive might act, nor which particular conscious thought it might choose as a repression target; these things are all deeply unconscious. So, according to psychoanalysis, we must typically wait until after a repression has happened and then bring in the research crew to sift the ashes. For this reason, repression has seldom been approached as a cognitive process, and the research in this area has typically settled instead on the far weaker tactic of isolating individuals who tend to repress, and examining their other personality characteristics. This circuitous avenue of inquiry has met with some success (see, e.g., Davis, 1987), but of course cannot clarify the repression process itself.

Classical repression theory does make the strong prediction that memory can be erased, however, so much research has focused on this claim. It is in this domain that the Freudian notion of repression has received its most stunning disconfirmations. Holmes (1974) reviewed a long list of studies of repression and found no clear evidence for the occurrence of forgetting motivated by ego threat. Erdelyi (1985) sympathetically reviewed a series of his own and others' studies of hypermnesia (the retrieval of more information from memory than was retrievable at an earlier point), and concluded that no fully convincing demonstration had yet been made. Although there are many clinical cases of amnesia (e.g., Breznitz, 1983; Rapaport, 1959), and a variety of indications that physical illness or injury can render memory inaccessible (e.g., Yarnell & Lynch, 1973), there is little indication that the widespread and frequent memory losses Freud envisioned are at all so common in daily life. Studies of hypnotic amnesia (see Kihlstrom, 1983) and directed forgetting (e.g., Geiselman, Bjork, & Fishman, 1983) show instead that certain memory processes under voluntary control (e.g., the avoidance of rehearsal at encoding) may on occasion contribute to the occurrence of motivated forgetting.

What all this means is that the topic of thought suppression per se is relatively neglected and misunderstood. Consciously keeping a thought from consciousness is the task of suppression, and we know comparatively little about how such an activity proceeds. Do people control their minds, not by forgetting, but by failing to access thoughts that are nonetheless accessible in memory? Such "selective inattention" could perform many of the tasks that psychoanalysts have counted on unconscious repression to accomplish. Indeed, several theorists have argued that inattention is all we need to avoid painful affect (e.g., Klinger, 1982). One need not forget a thought forever, and also forget the forgetting, merely to remove the thought from one's focus of attention. All that is required is thinking of something else, and continuing to do so.

Why Do We Suppress?

There are many possible answers to the question of why a thought might be unwanted. Freud suggested several answers, but offered no unified picture of why people suppress. His most general theme was that those instinctually driven ideas that fail the censor's and/or superego's tests of acceptability will be suppressed. In Freud's earlier writing, he stressed the unacceptability of ideas as a direct motive for repression, whereas in his later work he was more inclined to stress the anxiety aroused by the ideas as the motive force behind repression. In any event, he never suggested (as did many of his followers) that suppression exists only for "dirty" thoughts. Indeed, in his work on dreams and his subsequent theoretical work, he often referred to pain in the broadest possible sense as a motive for repression.

A broad desire to avoid unpleasantness does not account fully, however, for a number of instances in which people tend to engage in suppression. It is possible to refine this global motive into at least three distinct categories (Wegner, 1988, 1989). One general class of such instances involves efforts at *self-control*. When people diet, try to quit smoking, attempt to get more exercise, try to stop using drugs, want to avoid alcohol, resolve to watch less television, or even attempt to break off a destructive or unhappy relationship, they usually find that they desire to suppress thoughts of the unwanted activity as well. Any straightforward definition of "pleasantness" would not class thoughts of food, alcohol, drugs, and the like as unpleasant, especially to the person who is feeling deprived; for this reason, it seems useful to suggest that instances of self-control can make thoughts *unwanted*, even though they may not be strictly unpleasant.

A dedicated psychoanalyst might note that the agonies of self-control are consistent in some respects with the struggles Freud envisioned between id and superego. We would concur with this, but expand this characterization to speak of self-control as a clash between habitual, automatic processes spawned by a history of appetitive contact with an entity, and enlightened, controlled processes attempting to redirect behavior. Mental control, in this analysis, is the first step toward any sort of self-control.

One must avoid thinking of the addictive object in order to stop the instigation of the addictive behavior. The only way to bypass the exercise of mental control in these circumstances is to act precipitously to prevent oneself from ever performing the unwanted behavior—padlocking the refrigerator in the case of food, perhaps, or avoiding alcohol by moving to Saudi Arabia.

A second source of suppression occurs in the need for *secrecy*. There is nothing that can instigate suppression faster than the threat that something normally private might be made public. The prototypical situation occurs when one encounters a person from whom a secret must be kept. With the person present, it is deeply tempting to blurt out the secret whenever it comes to mind—or at least one worries that this will happen. Thus, one makes a special point of suppressing the secret thought whenever the relevant person is around. The range of relevant people differs for different secrets, of course, and at the extreme one may find oneself suppressing a thought whenever anyone at all is present or even imagined.

This cause of suppression is strongly social in origin, forged in large part by the schism that inevitably develops between our private thoughts and our public lives. Self-deception is, in this sense, the child of social deception. We admire someone from a distance, for example, and because we fear our sentiments will not be reciprocated, we keep quiet about our feelings. We must hold this back each time we are in the person's presence, and we become a dithering caricature of ourselves as we work so hard to be-normal. Alternatively, there may be some occurrence in our childhood that we have never troubled to tell anyone about. It may not even be particularly traumatic (in the Freudian sense), but the secrecy alone is enough to make us try not to think of it when we encounter potential audiences (Pennebaker, 1988). Other instances occur when we harbor discriminatory opinions of someone and work extra hard at suppressing our usual disparaging thoughts to keep from appearing prejudiced when the person is around to notice (see Fiske, Chapter 8, this volume). The source of our secrets, in sum, can be concern about any social, moral, or personal blunder, but the most socially unacceptable secrets tend to spawn the greatest suppression.

The third wellspring of suppression can best be called a motive to find *mental peace*. Quite simply, we sometimes observe that we are thinking something too often for our liking. A dream is repeated several nights in a row; we notice we keep toying with a lock of our hair; the unnamed pain in our chest reappears each time we feel stressed; or the same worry about our family's safety comes up over and over. The mere repetition of a thought may be sufficient to suggest to us the need for mental control, and we try not to think of it. Such thoughts are not necessarily abhorrent because of any special unpleasantness, although they can be; rather, we hope to suppress them because we have decided we are thinking them too often. The decision that a thought occurs "too often" will often be based, of course, in some unwanted emotional reaction that the thought engenders. This motive thus can encompass a wide range of what Freud imagined as the beginnings of suppression or repression—all those thoughts that are too disturbing to think because they produce negative affect. For many such thoughts, even one occurrence is too many, and in search of mental peace we put them aside as soon as we can.

These sources of suppression—self-control, secrecy, and mental peace—are not mutually exclusive. Many cases of keeping secrets, for example, can be cast as instances of self-control as well, and the pursuit of mental peace may be the conscious desire that arises during mental control attempts originally set in motion by self-control or secrecy. Partitioning the sources of mental control in this way is not meant to provide an exhaustive system of independent motivational categories. Indeed, these three sources of the urge to suppress could well be seen as subservient to some more general motive, such as esteem maintenance, control, or the like. This partition is useful as a way of highlighting the principal everyday circumstances in which mental control is engaged: when we are dissatisfied with ourselves, when we hide things from others, and when we are not at peace in our minds.

How Do We Suppress?

The strategies people use to suppress unwanted thoughts can be described as either direct or indirect. A direct strategy, as noted earlier, is primary suppression through auxiliary concentration—actively trying to think of something else. The indirect strategies are many; they include such devices as using alcohol, engaging in strenuous physical activity, or performing some palliative action that makes the unwanted thought less intrusive (e.g., coming back home to check whether the stove was really left on). When suppression is auxiliary to the attempt at primary concentration, we may also call the suppression attempt indirect. Many forms of psychotherapy can also be classed as indirect forms of suppression, in that attempts at problem-solving, emotional expression, cognitive restructuring, and the like are commonly addressed toward the elimination of unwanted thoughts. Only "thought stopping" (Wolpe & Lazarus, 1966) verges on a direct therapeutic approach. With this technique, the client is taught to call out "stop" whenever an unwanted thought occurs in a therapeutic session, and is encouraged to continue this procedure covertly outside the session.

When people are asked to describe their own strategies for coping with everyday obsessions and worries, the most frequently mentioned tactic is the perfectly direct one—simple self-distraction (Rachman & de Silva, 1978). Respondents say they try to think about something else. People who report worrying too much appear to point to this tactic as well. They blame their worry on a personal inability to distract themselves, claiming that for them, worry subsides only in the presence of attention-demanding environmental events (Borkovec, Robinson, Pruzinsky, & DePree, 1983). The accuracy of self-reports of the relative usage of different tactics is debatable, however, because certain tactics may simply be more evident to the self-reporter than others, independent of their actual usage. Suffice it to say that in everyday life, the suppression of thoughts by direct mental control happens enough that people notice it.

In the laboratory, this tactic is easily observed as well. Subjects in our initial study of thought suppression were asked to spend a 5-minute period verbalizing the stream of their thoughts for tape recording (Wegner, Schneider, Carter, & White, 1987, Experiment 1). They were prompted to think aloud, verbalizing every thought, feeling, or image that came to mind, and were assured that the recordings would be completely confidential. The subjects were then asked to continue their reporting, but some were now to follow an additional instruction: "In the next 5 minutes, please verbalize your thoughts as you did before, with one exception. This time, try not to think of a white bear. Every time you say 'white bear' or have 'white bear' come to mind, though, please ring the bell on the table before you."

Subjects given this instruction typically began by describing their plan to suppress: "Okay, then, I'll think about the light switch instead," or "I guess I'll talk about my sister's operation." As a rule, this auxiliary concentration succeeded for some time, as the subject talked on about the chosen replacement for "white bear." But overall, the self-distraction tactic was not very successful: Subjects rang the bell a mean of 6.1 times in 5 minutes and mentioned a white bear a mean of 1.6 times in the period as well. The degree of thinking about a white bear did decrease over the experimental session, however, such that by the final minute of the period most subjects no longer reported more than one occurrence (mention or bell ring).

We made another observation in this study about how people suppress, and though it did not seem important at the time, it has turned out to be a crucial one. Most of the time, people carried out their suppression by concentrating in turn on each of a wide variety of different items; this seemed to be a kind of *unfocused self-distraction,* a wandering of thought to one item after another, seemingly in search of something that might be truly interesting. The flip side of this approach, then, was a tactic of *focused self-distraction,* always turning to one thing as a distracter whenever the unwanted thought intruded. This second sort of distraction is the only thing that psychologists encourage people to do in research on how distraction can dull pain, emotion, and the like (see McCaul & Malott, 1984), so no one has ever really considered the unfocused variety before—despite its apparently greater popularity. As it turned out, the subsequent effects of thought suppression are highly dependent on the difference between the focused and unfocused strategies.

With What Effect Do We Suppress?

The white-bear study was arranged to examine also what happens to thinking when the need for suppression is over. The subjects who were asked to suppress in the experiment were asked in a final time period to continue their stream-of-consciousness reports, this time with the instruction to think of a white bear. These subjects showed a level of thinking about a white bear (15.7 bells and 14.4 mentions) significantly greater than that shown by subjects in a comparison group who were asked from the start (immediately after the practice period) to think about a white bear (11.8 bells and 11.5 mentions). In short, the mere act of avoiding a thought for 5 minutes made subjects oddly inclined to signal a relative outpouring of the thought when thinking about it was allowed. We found not only that the absolute level of thinking of a white bear was greater in this group, but also that there was an accelerating tendency to think of a white bear over time. That is, whereas thinking about a white bear in all the other conditions of the experiment declined over the 5-minute session, in those subjects expressing after suppression, the level of thinking continued to increase.

This pattern suggests a "rebound" effect—an increase in preoccupation with a thought that was formerly suppressed. Much of our work on thought suppression has been prompted by the many parallels between this effect and a wide array of familiar phenomena in psychology. Certainly, Freud (1914/1958) was among the first to point out that an attempt to deny or repress a thought might lead to a subsequent obsession (conscious or unconscious) with that thought. But other observers have remarked on many kindred effects: The suppression of grief following a loss appears to hamper coping and amplify the later grieving that is exhibited (Lindemann, 1944); the suppression of thoughts about a surgery prior to its occurrence foreshadows great anxiety and distress afterwards (Janis, 1958); the suppression of thoughts about eating may be one of the features of dieting that leads to later relapse and binge eating (Polivy & Herman, 1985); the suppression of thoughts about early traumatic occurrences can portend later physical illness and psychological distress (Pennebaker, 1985; Silver, Boon, & Stones, 1983); the failure to express emotions can lead to subsequent emotional problems (Rachman, 1980). In short, the rebound effect in the white-bear study reminded us of many things, and we wondered whether it might provide a laboratory setting within which these phenomena might be explored.

The first step in such exploration must be the development of a theoretical understanding of the phenomenon. Why is it that suppression yields a later rebound of preoccupation? At this point, the distinction we observed between focused and unfocused self-distraction again becomes relevant. If someone spends the entire suppression period in unfocused self-distraction, it is likely that the person will think about many things, both in the laboratory setting and outside it. Each of these things will be concentrated on for a short time, usually as a replacement for a white-bear thought. All these topics will then become linked to a white bear in the person's mind by virtue of their single common quality—they are *not white bears*. Many different distractors, in short, become associated with the unwanted thought. It makes sense, then, that when these former distractors are encountered once more (say, in the later period when expression is invited), they serve as reminders of the earlier unwanted thought. The rebound may stem, then, from the special way in which people enlist their ongoing thoughts to help distract them from the thought they are trying to suppress.

We have tested this idea in several ways. In our first follow-up on the white-bear study (Wegner, Schneider, Carter, & White, 1987, Experiment 2), we tested this explanation by replicating the original experiment with one exception: Some of the subjects in the group who were asked to suppress white-bear thoughts were given a brief instruction to engage in *focused* self-distraction. They were told after the suppression instruction, "Also, if you do happen to think of a white bear, please try to think of a red Volkswagen instead." This group, when later given the chance to express thoughts of a white bear, did so at a significantly reduced level. Unlike the subjects in this study who were allowed to go their own way (and who typically used the unfocused, "think-about-anything" method), these individuals experienced a noteworthy drop in the rebound of the unwanted thought.

One lesson to be gleaned from this study is that wild-eyed ranging about for distractors is not a good method for thought suppression. True, this may be all that seems possible in the face of a particularly daunting unwanted thought. But it is more likely that one will defeat the rebound effect by choosing one special distractor and turning to it whenever the unwanted thought comes to mind. This tactic presumably prevents all the other things one might think about—whether they arise in memory or are instigated by observation of one's surroundings—from becoming cues to the unwanted thought. The focused distractor becomes the primary cue to that thought, and because it is not especially salient during the later expression period, there is no strong cuing of the unwanted thought to yield a rebound of preoccupation.

We find that in talking to people about this experiment, several have reported using their own versions of focused self-distraction. Often, the single distracter that is chosen in these cases is a religious one—thoughts of God, engaging in prayer, and so on. Others report doing arithmetic in their heads. In any case, we would predict that the single focused distractor might become a fairly strong reminder of the unwanted thought if suppression went on long enough, and thus could itself become unwanted (unless it were somehow absolved of its distressing tone by virtue of pairing with other, more positive experiences). We did not test these kinds of conjectures in the red-Volkswagen study, but they do suggest an interesting line of inquiry.

A different set of derivations from the observation of unfocused self-distraction was tested, however, in subsequent research (Wegner, Schneider, McMahon, & Knutson, 1989). This research examined the hypothesis that thought suppression in a particular context tends to "spoil" that context for the person; it makes that context an unusually strong reminder of the unwanted thought. This notion follows from the idea that when people engage in unfocused self-distraction, they pick many of the different distracters they will use from their current surroundings. These surroundings, later on, can become reminders of the unwanted thought and so may serve to cue the rebound of preoccupation when expression is allowed.

This research called for some subjects to complete the usual sequence of thought suppression followed by expression (or the comparison sequence of expression followed by suppression) in one context—a laboratory room in which a set of slides on a single theme was being shown. Subjects saw either a slide show of classroom scenes, or one of household appliances. Other subjects participated with different slide shows appearing during the initial and later periods of the experiment. We expected that subjects in this latter group who suppressed in the context of one slide show and then expressed in the context of another would show little of the rebound effect, and this is what happened. The degree to which the participants expressed the thought following suppression in a different context was reliably less than the amount of expression following suppression in a constant context. Therefore, the rebound effect was most pronounced when people distracted themselves by thinking about their surroundings, and then thought of the surroundings again when they were allowed to consider the formerly suppressed thought.

The implications of these findings are quite practical. The results suggest, for example, that residential treatment facilities for addictions, alcoholism, overeating, and the like may have a common benefit. Getting away from home during treatment may help, all by itself. Because people suppress thoughts of their forbidden behaviors in the strange surroundings of the facility, they may come to associate many of the features of the facility with their particular self-control problem. When they leave, however, these reminders are left behind, the rebound of preoccupation is disrupted, and there would seem to be a much greater likelihood of long-term success for the treatment. When we are bothered by unwanted thoughts at home or at work, though, it is tempting to suppress them right there. This strategy is likely to fail, for when we try to divest ourselves of a thought in a place, we seem in a sense to leave it there—only to find it again when we return.

Our work on suppression to date indicates, in sum, that people do not do it very well. The question that begins this section ("With what effect do we suppress?") must be met at this time with a disappointing reply: Apparently, we suppress with only temporary and incomplete success. Although our research subjects have been able to reduce their thinking about an innocuous item, a white bear, to relatively low levels in a short time, they nonetheless are not able simply to shut off the thought at will. And once the thought is suppressed, an invitation to return to it appears to have the ironic effect of prompting renewed preoccupation that proceeds at a level beyond what might have occurred had suppression never been started. This effect, too, can be overcome under certain circumstances, but it seems that people's natural proclivities (to use unfocused self-distraction and to stay in the same surroundings) work against them to make the task of long-term suppression most difficult. The effects of thought suppression, it seems, are not usually what we want them to be.

How Might We Suppress More Effectively?

Inevitably, the discussion of thought suppression comes around to home remedies: What should people do when they have unwanted thought? This is one of the great problems of our field, one of the main reasons why clinical psychology and psychotherapy were invented. It should be obvious that our research program is not yet mature enough even to have spawned clinical research, let alone to have yielded solid suggestions for psychotherapy or self-help. With this caveat out of the bag, we feel a bit better about offering our preliminary and untested nostrums.

Our simplest advice would be to avoid suppression, to stop stopping. The work we have conducted and the research by others we have reviewed seems to identify suppression as a strategy that can produce consequences every bit as discomfiting as the unwanted thoughts toward which it is directed. At the extreme, it may be that thought suppression can be the cause rather than the cure of unwanted thoughts, serving over time and in the right circumstances to produce "synthetic obsessions" that can be as painful as those derived from traumas (Wegner, 1988, 1989). Often people use thought suppression to deal with unwanted thoughts when a better strategy would be to work on the unwanted realities that those thoughts represent. We are not recommending that all suppression is nonsense, for there are some junctures at which it seems the only proper solution. When on the brink of a tall building one gets the urge to throw oneself off, it is surely best to suppress the thought. But we do believe that thought suppression is often a mental Band-Aid, a stopgap solution that can create its own problems.

If one must suppress, there are better and worse ways to do it. The research to this point suggests that suppression is likely to be more successful in the long run if we use a limited range of distracters—things we can focus on repeatedly, rather than sorting recklessly through every other thought that might be available. And in this enterprise, it may be best, too, if to do our suppression today, we get away from home or away from the environs we will have to inhabit later. There is the real possibility that the suppressed thoughts will be cued by the very context in which we suppressed them, climaxing our struggle to suppress with a very disappointing conclusion.

That's it. We hesitate to offer more advice at this point, because we believe there are enough unanswered questions that to offer advice now would be premature. We cannot be certain, after all, that white-bear-type studies capture the same processes that occur when people in everyday life attempt to suppress thoughts. The white-bear experiment adds the artificial requirement that people must report their thoughts aloud, for example, and it deals with thoughts that are not nearly as emotional as the ones people usually attempt to suppress.

Work on these things is currently underway. In one study (Chandler & Wegner, 1987), evidence of a rebound effect was found even when people were not asked to ring bells or report white-bear thoughts. It was arranged instead for them to talk freely "off the top of their heads" about any or all of five different topics written on a page before them. They did this during the usual white-bear experiment design: One group was asked first not to think of a white bear, then to think of it; another group did thinking first and then not thinking. The topics had been scaled ahead of time for their relevance to "white bear" ("iceberg" being very relevant, for example, and "gym shorts" being much less relevant). What we found was that subjects assigned to think of a white bear after suppression, as compared to those assigned to think about it from the outset, talked more about white-bear-relevant thoughts and less about thoughts irrelevant to white bears. So, even without the artificial thought-reporting requirement, an effect very much like the rebound effect was observed.

And in another recent set of experiments, the question of how people suppress more involving and emotional thoughts has been under scrutiny. Wenzlaff, Wegner, and Roper (1988) looked at how depressed and non-depressed people handle unwanted thoughts. Mildly depressed college students (as determined by the short form of the Beck Depression Inventory; Beck & Beck, 1972) and their nondepressed counterparts were asked to read a page-long story and imagine themselves in the starring role of either a very positive incident (e.g., finding a missing child) or a very negative one (e.g., being in a serious car accident). They were then asked to write their ongoing thoughts on three blank pages, and were paced through the pages to allow 3 minutes for each. In a column down the right side of each page, they were to make a check mark each time the thought of the story they had read came to mind.

Some subjects were put up to the task of suppression; they were asked not to think of the story, if they could. Others were not given any special instruction, and were merely told to describe whatever was on their minds. When we counted the marks subjects made, and also their written mentions of the target thought, we found that depressed subjects had a particularly difficult time suppressing negative thoughts. Nondepressed subjects were generally able to suppress both positive and negative thoughts, and depressed subjects did a fine job of suppressing positive thoughts. But when the depressed people tried to suppress a negative thought, they succeeded at first, only to experience a later resurgence of negative thinking. By the third page of writing, their reporting of the negative thought was back up to the same level as that of depressed subjects who had not even tried to suppress.

Further analyses of this study, and further experiments, have explored how this unusual resurgence takes place. What seems to happen is that depressed people distract themselves from negative thoughts by using *other negative thoughts*. These then serve as strong reminders of the thought that was first unwanted, and so return the depressed persons to the initial problem in short order. Nondepressed people, in turn, use positive distracters to get away from negative thoughts, and so leave the whole arena of negative thinking behind. This suggests again that the nature of the self-distraction strategy people use can be very important in determining how successful their thought suppression will be. So, if there is one last piece of advice we can sneak in, it is to look on the bright side. Positive self-distraction may be a generally useful technique whenever we have negative unwanted thoughts—even if we are not depressed at the time, but particularly if we are.

CONCLUSIONS

We should tie up at least one loose end before we draw the chapter to a close. We should explain the allusion to F. C. Bartlett that occurs in the odd mix of metaphors in the chapter subtitle. His story of the "War of the Ghosts" (1932) was used in his classic research on how people transform information in their minds. Although the story itself is not strictly relevant to our concerns, his general approach to psychology is right on target. One of the ideas that Bartlett championed was the role of motivation and affect in cognition, and that is a basic issue in this chapter.

Mental control must be counted as a central form of motivated cognition. Although motivation may affect our thoughts of many things, coloring our views of others and ourselves (see, e.g., Sorrentino & Higgins, 1986), its influence on thought is seldom held in such sharp relief as when we are motivated to control our thoughts directly. Mental control requires conscious motivation, and its success and failure can often appear in our conscious thoughts as well. So, although certain purists in both the cognitive and motivational camps of psychology would prefer not to use both explanatory networks at the same time in any domain of study, in the case of mental control this is simply impossible. Mental control is just too clear a case of motivated thought for either the motivation or the thinking to be ignored.

Our studies of thought suppression reveal that people engage in sensible activities when they are asked to suppress a thought in the laboratory. They try to think of other things, and over time they often can succeed. But thought suppression has ironic and troubling effects as well, in that the suppressed thought can return, sometimes to be more absorbing than it was at the start. It is therefore evident that motivated thinking may not have the clear-cut success we sometimes find with motivated physical activities. When we want to brush our teeth or hop on one foot, we can usually do so; when we want to control our minds, we may find that nothing works as it should. A war of the ghosts in the machine, it seems, may leave us with defeated spirits.

ACKNOWLEDGMENTS

We thank Toni Wegner, James Pennebaker, and the editors for helpful comments on an earlier draft.

REFERENCES

Bartlett, F. C. (1932). *Remembering.* Cambridge, England: Cambridge University Press.

Beck, A., & Beck, R. (1972). Screening depressed patients in family practice: A rapid technique. *Postgraduate Medicine, 52,* 81–85.

Borkovec, T. D., Robinson, E., Pruzinsky, T., & DePree, J. A. (1983). Preliminary exploration of worry: Some characteristics and processes. *Behaviour Research and Therapy, 21,* 9–16.

Breznitz, S. (Ed.). (1983). *The denial of stress.* New York: International Universities Press.

Broadbent, D. (1958). *Perception and communication.* Oxford: Pergamon Press.

Chandler, G., & Wegner, D. M. (1987). *The effect of thought suppression on preoccupation with associated thoughts.* Unpublished manuscript, Trinity University.

Davis, P. J. (1987). Repression and the inaccessibility of affective memories. *Journal of Personality and Social Psychology, 53,* 585–593.

Erdelyi, M. H. (1985). *Psychoanalysis: Freud's cognitive psychology.* San Francisco: W. H. Freeman.

Erdelyi, M. H., & Goldberg, B. (1979). Let's not sweep repression under the rug: Toward a cognitive psychology of repression. In J. F. Kihlstrom & F. J. Evans (Eds.), *Functional disorders of memory* (pp. 355–402). Hillsdale, NJ: Erlbaum.

Freud, S. (1953). The interpretation of dreams. In J. Strachey (Ed.), *The standard edition of the complete psychological works of Sigmund Freud* (Vol. 4, pp. 1–338; Vol. 5, pp. 339–627). London: Hogarth Press. (Original work published 1900)

Freud. S. (1957). Repression. In J. Strachey (Ed.), *The standard edition of the complete psychological works of Sigmund Freud* (Vol. 14, pp. 146–158). London: Hogarth Press. (Original work published 1915)

Freud, S. (1958). Remembering, repeating, and working-through. In J. Strachey (Ed.), *The standard edition of the complete psychological works of Sigmund Freud* (Vol. 12, pp. 145–150). London: Hogarth Press. (Original work published 1914)

Geiselman, R. E., Bjork, R. A., & Fishman, D. L. (1983). Disrupted retrieval in directed forgetting: A link with posthypnotic amnesia. *Journal of Experimental Psychology: General, 112,* 58–72.

Holmes, D. S. (1974). Investigation of repression: Differential recall of material experimentally or naturally associated with ego threat. *Psychological Bulletin, 81,* 632–653.

James, W. (1890). *The principles of psychology* (2 vols.). New York: Holt.

Janis, I. (1958). *Psychological stress.* New York: Wiley.

Kihlstrom, J. F. (1983). Instructed forgetting: Hypnotic and nonhypnotic. *Journal of Experimental Psychology: General, 112,* 73–79.

Klinger, E. (1982). On the self-management of mood, affect, and attention. In P. Karoly & F. H. Kanfer (Eds.), *Self-management and behavior change* (pp. 129–164). New York: Pergamon Press.

Lindemann, E. (1944). Symptomatology and management of acute grief. *American Journal of Psychiatry, 101,* 141–148.

McCaul, K. D., & Malott, J. M. (1984). Distraction and coping with pain. *Psychological Bulletin, 95,* 516–533.

Pennebaker, J. W. (1985). Inhibition and cognition: Toward an understanding of trauma and disease. *Canadian Psychology, 26,* 82–95.

Pennebaker, J. W. (1988). Confiding traumatic experiences and health. In S. Fisher & J. Reason (Eds.), *Handbook of life stress, cognition, and health* (pp. 669–682). Chichester, England: Wiley.

Polivy, J., & Herman, C. P. (1985). Dieting and binging: A causal analysis. *American Psychologist, 40,* 193–201.

Rachman, S. (1980). Emotional processing. *Behaviour Research and Therapy, 18,* 51–60.

Rachman, S., & de Silva, P. (1978). Abnormal and normal obsessions. *Behaviour Research and Therapy, 16,* 233–248.

Rapaport, D. (1959). *Emotions and memory.* New York: International Universities Press.

Ryle, G. (1949). *The concept of mind.* London: Hutchinson.

Silver, R. L., Boon, C., & Stones, M. H. (1983). Searching for meaning in misfortune: Making sense of incest. *Journal of Social Issues, 39,* 81–102.

Sorrentino, R. M., & Higgins, E. T. (Eds.). (1986). *Handbook of motivation and cognition: Foundations of social behavior.* New York: Guilford Press.

Wegner, D. M. (1988). Stress and mental control. In S. Fisher & J. Reason (Eds.), *Handbook of life stress, cognition, and health* (pp. 683–697). Chichester, England: Wiley.

Wegner, D. M. (1989). *White bears and other unwanted thoughts*. New York: Viking Press.

Wegner, D. M., Schneider, D. J., Carter, S., III, & White, L. (1987). Paradoxical consequences of thought suppression. *Journal of Personality and Social Psychology, 53*, 1–9.

Wegner, D. M., Schneider, D. J., McMahon, S., & Knutson, B. (1987). *Taking worry out of context: The enhancement of thought suppression effectiveness in new surroundings.* Manuscript submitted for publication.

Wenzlaff, R., Wegner, D. M., & Roper, D. (1988). Depression and mental control: The resurgence of unwanted negative thoughts. *Journal of Personality and Social Psychology, 55*, 882–892.

Wolpe, J., & Lazarus, A. A. (1966). *Behavior therapy techniques*. New York: Pergamon.

Yarnell, P. R., & Lynch, S. (1973). The "ding": Amnesic states in football trauma. *Neurology, 23*, 196–197.

10

Toward a Motivational and Structural Theory of Ruminative Thought

LEONARD L. MARTIN
ABRAHAM TESSER
University of Georgia

You know, when my father was alive, I didn't really think about him very much. But, as soon as he died, I couldn't stop thinking about him.

This remark, made to one of us, illustrates the phenomenon we address in this chapter. This phenomenon is called "rumination," and can be described very generally as conscious thinking directed toward a given object for an extended period of time. It is to be distinguished from other kinds of thinking, such as fleeting ideas that do not recur (e.g., noticing on a given day that the weather is nice) or brief thoughts directed toward transitory goals (e.g., deciding on a blouse to match the day's outfit). Rumination can be considered a broad class that includes such subclasses as problem solving, anticipation, and intrusive thinking.

Rumination is an important topic of investigation for several reasons. The occurrence of repetitive and unwanted thoughts is a major symptom of a number of mental disorders, and may even instigate and maintain some disorders, such as depression (Beck, 1983; Ellis, 1962; Nolen-Hoeksema, 1987; Pysczsynski & Greenberg, 1987). The study of rumination is also important because it may help us to gain a better understanding of the basic functioning of the cognitive system. In this regard, there are three features of rumination that make it a particularly useful topic of study: (1)

it occurs over relatively long periods of time, (2) it often appears to be counterproductive, and (3) it involves both automatic and controlled processes.

Ruminative behavior may occur over the course of years, and individuals may expend a great deal of cognitive energy in ruminating. For example, there are reports of widows having daily thoughts of their deceased husbands as much as decades after the husbands' deaths (Tait & Silver, Chapter 12, this volume). In short, ruminative thought can represent a particularly important and central component of a person's mental life.

Rumination often appears to be counterproductive in the sense that it seems most often to occur after the best chances for effective instrumental behaviors have passed. As in our opening example, a person may often think more about his or her father following the father's death than before it. In some perfectly logical, perfectly efficient world, such would not be the case. In this perfect world, the person would ignore the father's death (since it is a *fait accompli*) and invest his or her energies more productively in current events on which the person could have an impact. However, as already noted, people often think more about an event when it is too late to do anything about it, and they may continue thinking about it for years.

Finally, rumination appears to involve both controllable and uncontrollable components. For example, the person may make a controlled, conscious effort to analyze the implications of the father's death, in order to adapt himself or herself to the changed situation. Individuals may quite deliberately consider alternatives, construct contingency plans, and implement various behaviors designed to solve immediate problems. Alongside of these intended thoughts, however, may be some unwanted, intrusive thoughts that come without conscious design, and that may be difficult to suppress. For example, the person may suddenly and unintentionally find himself or herself thinking depressing thoughts about the father's death in the middle of a party.

In this chapter, we present a theory developed to answer three basic questions concerning rumination: What starts it? What stops it? And what determines its content? We begin with a brief overview of the theory, and follow that with a more explicit discussion of the assumptions underlying the theory. Finally, we discuss the implications of this theory for people's ability to determine the causes and direction of their thoughts.

A MOTIVATIONAL AND STRUCTURAL THEORY OF RUMINATIVE THOUGHT

Overview

The theory begins with the basic assumption that people's thoughts and actions are directed by goals. Failure to attain an important goal initiates two processes related to rumination: passive activation of goal-related information in memory (i.e., spreading activation) and motivationally driven activation of goal-related information (e.g., Zeigarnik, 1927/1938). The connections of spreading activation comprise the structural component of rumination, and the Zeigarnik charge is the motivational component. Rumination is assumed to be motivationally driven until individuals either satisfy the frustrated goal or disengage themselves from that goal. However, because repetition can "channelize" thought; environmental cues, even in the absence of motivation, may trigger rumination-like processes. Neither the goals nor their effects on thought and behavior are assumed to be always open to introspective awareness. Thus, the conscious content of rumination may not always be related to the particular unattained goal(s) that are driving the rumination. Rather, rumination may be related to goals that seem relevant only on the basis of naive, *a priori* theories or scripts.

Assumption 1: People's Thoughts and Actions Are Directed by Goals

We begin with the assumption that the functioning human organism can be conceived of as a cybernetic system (see Carver & Scheler, 1981; Miller, Galanter, & Pribram, 1960; Powers, 1973; von Bertalanffy, 1968). By this, we mean that people compare their current states with their desired goal states in order to assess their progress toward their goals. If they perceive no difference between their current state and the desired state, then they either continue doing what they are doing (Carver & Scheier, 1981) or exit the feedback loop and set up a new goal (Miller et al., 1960). When individuals perceive a discrepancy between the two states, they alter their behavior in an attempt to bring their current state closer to the desired one.

We assume that the cybernetic system is made possible because goals activate procedural knowledge (cf. Carver & Scheier, 1981; Srull & Wyer, 1986). That is, goals often (though not always) activate knowledge structures that tell individuals how to attain the goal and that allow them to gauge their progress toward the goal. As an example, consider a premedical student with the long-range goal of attending medical school. There are a number of prerequisites for getting into medical school. Knowledge of these prerequisites constitutes the procedural or "how to" knowledge. For example, the student must get good grades in undergraduate school, get good letters of recommendation, and do well on the Medical College Admissions Test (MCAT). Without knowledge of these contingencies, the student would be at a loss as to how to attain the goal.

Armed with this knowledge, however, the student not only knows what to do, but can also gauge how well he or she is doing it. For example, if the student is making good grades, then he or she is progressing toward the goal and does not need to alter his or her study habits. If the student is making poor grades, then his or her progress toward medical school is being threatened, and some behavior must be altered if the student is to attain the goal. Ideally, this behavioral alteration would take the form of increased studying, although cheating or bribery might accomplish the same end.

It is important to note that the cybernetic discrepancy (i.e., the completion–incompletion of the goal) is not objectively defined. A goal that has been reached objectively may not have been reached subjectively, and vice versa. A clear example of the distinction between objective and subjective goal attainment was presented by Marrow (1938) in research on the Zeigarnik effect. Marrow had two groups of subjects engage in a series of tasks. One group was instructed to "complete the task." A second group was told that they were to perform as well as they could, and that if they performed well enough, the experimenter would ask them to stop. Thus, in the first condition, objective completion of the task meant that subjects met their goal (i.e., completing the task), whereas in the second condition objective completion of the task meant that subjects had not reached their goal (i.e., satisfying the experimenter). All subjects were allowed to complete some tasks but not others. Then all subjects were asked to recall the tasks they had done.

Subjects who were instructed only to complete the task recalled more of the interrupted than of the completed tasks, thus replicating the traditional Zeigarnik effect. In contrast, subjects who believed that the experimenter would interrupt them when they had performed sufficiently well recalled more of the objectively completed than of the interrupted tasks. In other words, subjects recalled more *subjectively* incompleted tasks, regardless of the tasks' objective completion status.

We should also note that not all interruptions are disruptive. Interruptions are less disruptive if the individual has a "meta-plan" that includes getting interrupted on the subparts (Miller et al., 1960). For example, our premed student would be much more upset by continual interruptions while trying to write a paper if he or she had expected to be left alone than if he or she had anticipated that a friend or roommate would be coming by every few minutes.

Assumption 2: Goals Are Structured Hierarchically

Our second assumption is that the goals that guide people's day-to-day behaviors are somewhere in the middle of a hierarchy in which lower-order goals are pursued because they are instrumental to the attainment of higher-order goals. This hierarchy can be demonstrated by repeatedly asking "why" and "how" questions (Vallacher & Wegner, 1985). For example, if we ask our premed student why he or she is studying, the student may reply, "To do well on the biology test." Then, if we ask the student why he or she wants to do well on the test, the reply may be, "To get my degree." This can be followed by "why" questions until the student answers in the most abstract terms possible (e.g., "To live a happy life"). In short, "why" questions typically prompt people to think about higher-level concepts (Bower, Black, & Turner, 1979; Strack, Schwarz, & Gschneidinger, 1985; Vallacher & Wegner, 1987).

On the other hand, repeated "how" questions prompt individuals into thinking about the lower-order components of the goal hierarchy (Bower et al., 1979; Strack et al., 1985; Vallacher & Wegner, 1987). So, if we ask our premed student "how" he or she is studying, he or she may say, "I am looking over my notes." We may then ask, "How are you looking over your notes?" and the response may be, "I am considering only the highlighted parts." We can continue our questioning until we force the student into molecular, detailed answers (e.g., "I am scanning the page by flexing my eye muscles").

When the entire hierarchy is considered as a unit, it makes some sense to say that the student is flexing his or her eye muscles in order to get into medical school. Although such a statement may be logically sound, it is not psychologically sound. There are two reasons for this. First, naive explanations of actions tend to be made in terms of neighboring levels (Lalljee & Abelson, 1983). That is, the student is more likely to explain studying for an exam in terms of passing the exam than in terms of graduation or career aspirations. Second, people are not always conscious of all levels of the hierarchy. Rather, they may operate at some basic or midrange level (cf. Cantor & Mischel, 1979; Rosch, 1978), and identify the higher and lower components only when difficulties arise. More specifically, people tend to become aware of levels of action that are problematic and therefore require conscious control (see Carver & Scheier, 1981; Mandler, 1975; Vallacher & Wegner, 1987; Wicklund, 1986).

Before we leave this topic, it may be worth noting that although most thoughts and behaviors may be ultimately traceable to some abstract higher-order goal, not all of them are phenomenologically associated with such goals. Some behaviors appear to be performed solely for intrinsic reasons (i.e., to satisfy goals not distinctly linked to other goals). Behavior in the service of other goals appears to be driven by different processes than behaviors that are goals in and of themselves (Millar & Tesser, 1986a). For example, when individuals concentrate on why they like something, their attitudes are a good predictor of their behavior if their behavior is instrumental (i.e., a means to a further goal). By comparison, when individuals concentrate on how something makes them feel, their attitudes are a good predictor of behaviors that are undertaken for their own sake (i.e., consummatory/intrinsic behaviors). Moreover, making consummatory behaviors instrumental to another goal appears to reduce the satisfaction associated with performing those behaviors (Deci, 1971; Lepper, Greene, & Nisbett, 1973).

Assumption 3: Individuals Engage in a Relatively Specific Sequence of Behaviors Following Frustration of an Important Goal

Rumination has been defined as conscious thought that results from the disruption of goals. We believe, along with many other theorists (e.g., Bruner, 1957; Mandler, 1975, 1987; Wicklund, 1986), that consciousness is often a troubleshooting process. Much of people's behavior, even complex behavioral sequences, may be under nondeliberative control and may unfold without a great deal of conscious choice being involved (e.g., Abelson, 1981; Langer, 1978). Consciousness becomes consequential when the environment does not permit behavioral scripts to unfold in their expected way (Minsky, 1987). Under these circumstances consciousness overwhelms nonconscious control, and it does so for a very good reason: Nonconscious control has already failed.

We assume that rumination involves attempts to find alternate means to reach important unattained goals or reconciling oneself to not reaching those goals.[1] Moreover, the ruminative process may unfold in a rough sequence. We describe the sequence as "rough" because we do not wish to imply that persons necessarily go through a strict ordering of stages, that every stage is necessarily experienced, or that persons are necessarily either "in" one stage or another.

Any of these stages may be skipped, and they may be taken in any order. Moreover, the ruminative process associated with any particular goal disruption may at any point in time be dormant. Persons may actively distract themselves from thinking about the disruption, or other goals, needs, or environmental presses may become prepotent, thereby moving consciousness away from the ruminative content (Klinger, 1975). Thus, even though attainment of a goal may have been disrupted, the individual need not, at any given point in time, be in any of the stages connected to that particular disruption.

On the other hand, we believe that as a first approximation, the order we have suggested is sensible. This order is as follows: repetition of the initial instrumental behavior, problem solving (i.e., attempting to find alternate routes to the goal), end-state thinking, negotiation for goal abandonment, and "learned helplessness."

Repetition

When a goal is blocked, the simplest response is to repeat the same instrumental behavior, perhaps with greater intensity (cf. Mandler, 1975). To the extent that frustration is high, the response will be repeated with greater energy; the likelihood of a new, productive response will be diminished; and the response will be accompanied by increasing negative affect. On the other hand, if repetition allows individuals to attain their goals, then they are free to exit that cybernetic loop and pursue another goal. When repetition of the original behavior does not allow individuals to attain their goals, they abandon this strategy and move on to the next stage.

Problem Solving

The second stage associated with the nonattainment of goals is the search for alternative instrumental means to attain the goal. Such a search involves movement primarily in a horizontal direction through the goal hierarchy. For our hypothetical premed student, this would involve searching for an alternate study method, using a different textbook, working with a different tutor, cheating, and so on as a result of failing a test.

There is evidence consistent with the notion that thought following goal blockage goes in the direction of finding instrumental responses. For example, Atkinson and McClelland (1948) deprived people of food for various lengths of time and then asked them to make up stories about various pictures (the Thematic Apperception Test, or TAT). They found that greater hunger resulted in a greater incidence of stories that included a reference to successfully overcoming a source of food deprivation. Similarly, McClelland, Clark, Roby, and Atkinson (1949) found an increase in references to successful instrumental acts in TAT stories when need achievement had been aroused by blocking subjects' goal of successful test performance. More recently, Klinger (1978) has found that much ruminative content concerns the implementation of new behaviors intended to deal with "current concerns" or important personal goals.

If individuals have a number of instrumental responses available, elimination of any one does not thwart progress toward the goal. It is when alternative instrumental responses are threatened that rumination occurs. Thus, there should be an inverse relationship between the number of instrumental behaviors available to a person and their degree of rumination. Evidence to this effect was obtained by Millar, Tesser, and Millar (1988). These investigators questioned a number of women who were newly arrived on the college campus. The measures of interest concerned ruminations about a close person each woman had left behind when she came to college. Each subject was asked to indicate the activities she engaged in with this close other, and also to indicate which of these activities she continued to engage in after arriving at college. It was assumed that the greater the number of activities with the close other, the greater the number of potentially disrupted goals when the subject came to college. Hence, the greater should be the rumination about the close other when these behaviors were not continued. On the other hand, continued activities would represent the continued availability of instrumental responses. The presence of such responses should reduce ruminations about the close other. Consistent with this hypothesis, ruminations about the close other were a positive function of number of discontinued activities with the close other and a negative function of number of activities continued.

Instrumental thinking can also lead to vertical movement through the goal structure. Suppose that the premedical student from our earlier example has just failed a test in a biology course. In trying to find a new and productive instrumental behavior, the student may redefine the goal at a lower level: Instead of "passing the course," the goal may be reidentified as "passing tests," "studying," or "reading" (Vallacher & Wegner, 1986). This lower-level identity may be helpful in that the individual becomes more focused. But the adoption of such lower-level identities may cause a loss of flexibility with respect to what might satisfy the original goal. Thus, if one focuses on the goal of passing the test instead of passing the course, other means of passing the course (e.g., an extra-credit paper) may never be explored.

Furthermore, losing sight of the original (and higher-order) goals may make it more difficult to satisfy them or give them up, either of which is necessary for the ruminative process to stop. By losing sight of the higher-order goal, the individual is "locked in." That is, the student does not have the opportunity to redefine or refine the higher-order goal in a way that makes goal attainment possible. For example, focusing on passing the test does not allow for the possibility of substituting an easier course or taking it at a time when the student is less overloaded.

By being locked in on a lower level, the individual may also fail to give up the goal when goal attainment is impossible. For example, it may be possible to pass a particular test, but it may still be impossible to pass the course. Conversely, concentration on the lower-order goal may lead to premature goal disengagement. When effort expenditure is viewed as being in the service of a lower-order goal, it may not seem justified. However, the same effort viewed in terms of the higher-order goal may be amply justified (Seta & Seta, 1982).

Another possibility is that the ruminative search for instrumental behaviors following goal blockage may lead to the examination of higher-order goals. Upon failing a biology test, our premed student may think, "Why do I care if I pass this course? So I can graduate. Why do I care if I graduate? So I can go to medical school. What makes me think I am smart enough to get into medical school?" According to Wicklund (1986), goal blockage often results in persons' questioning the kind of individuals they are, their traits and attributes—the very stuff of higher-order goals. Such an examination can be useful if the higher-level goals are accurately identified, because it is ultimately the higher-order goals that will turn the ruminative process off. If, however, the higher-order goals are misidentified and instrumental behaviors that are enacted do not address the goals associated with the Zeigarnik tension, then the ruminations will not stop.

End-State Thinking

A third ruminative stage, end-state thinking, is likely to occur when individuals have difficulty in finding instrumental behaviors that will return them to the goal. At this stage, individuals think not about different ways of attaining the goal, but about the goal objects themselves and the feelings associated with them. For example, Sanford (1936) found that subjects tended to give more food responses on a word association task before a regular meal than after it. Brozek, Guetzkow, Baldwin, and Granston (1951) noted that "During starvation the thoughts of food, in all their ramifications, came to dominate the men's minds" (p. 250). McClelland et al. (1949), using the TAT, found that the arousal of a need for achievement increased the number of stories containing references to positive affect as a result of achievement.

End-state thinking can also encompass themes concerned with frustration and goal blockage. For example, Atkinson and McClelland (1948), in their study of the TAT as a function of food deprivation, found that as the incidence of central themes concerned with shortage of food or blockage of eating by an external agent increased; references to facilitative environmental circumstances and actual eating (i.e., goal activity) decreased. Similarly, under conditions designed to arouse a need for achievement, McClelland et al. (1949) found an increase in TAT themes in which the protagonist was having long-term achievement difficulty.

More recently, Wicklund and Braun (1987) have shown that experience makes a difference in ruminative responses. Persons who are experienced in a particular domain should have a larger repertoire of instrumental responses than persons with less experience. Since end-state thinking results when individuals run out of instrumental responses, we might expect a stronger (negative) association between task success and rumination among inexperienced actors than among experienced actors. Wicklund and Braun (1987, Study 3) asked experienced and inexperienced tennis players how much they thought about the kind of traits it takes to be a good tennis player. When they correlated these responses with expert ratings of each respondent's recent play, they found a substantial negative correlation between quality of play and trait thinking among inexperienced players ($r = -.59$), but not among experienced players ($r = .21$). The difference between these correlations was significant.

End-state thinking is also noteworthy because of its impact on feelings. The object of end-state thought sometimes has a positive valence (goal satisfying) and often a negative valence (goal blocking). A number of studies (e.g., Tesser, 1978) have shown that when persons simply think about something with either a positive or a negative valence, their feelings become polarized, even if they have no new information. That is, if feelings about the object of thought are initially positive, then they become even more positive; if initially negative, they become even more negative.

Particularly interesting, from the perspective of the present theoretical orientation, is the finding that this effect tends to be moderated by an individual's goal structure and the complexity of his or her thought processes (Millar & Tesser, 1986b). When an individual is committed to a particular evaluation of an object (i.e., has a goal involving that object), then the more complex the individual's structure for thinking about that object, the more rumination results in polarization. On the other hand, when the object of thought does not figure into the individual's goal structure, the greater the complexity, the less polarization as a result of rumination (Linville, 1982).

In some ways, end-state thinking tends to be the prototype of rumination: It is not instrumental, it tends to have a strong emotional overlay, and it appears to be nonadaptive. Eventually, individuals may realize that the goal is unattainable; consequently, they may try to disengage themselves from the goal. It is this latter stage of rumination to which we now turn.

Negotiation

As long as the goal remains "charged" (i.e., the goal remains unsatisfied), the individual will seek an adequate instrumental response or engage in end-state thinking, which, generally speaking, is not pleasant.[2] If, however, the individual gives up the goal or invests himself or herself in a substitute goal, then the Zeigarnik charge will disappear, and the fruitless search for adequate new behaviors and unpleasant end-state thinking can in principle be abandoned. Eric Klinger and his colleagues have shown in several studies (Klinger, 1975, 1978; Klinger, Barta, & Maxeiner, 1980) that indeed there is less frequent rumination, both in waking and in dreams, about abandoned goals than about current goals (see also Collins & Clark, 1987).

Giving up the goal may be difficult. First, because of the hierarchical structure of the goal system, giving up any particular goal without an adequate substitute may result in the continued disruption of the higher-level, more important goal that the abandoned goal serviced. For example, if our premed student drops out of college, then he or she can never be a doctor. This may mean that the student will be unable to please his or her parents, whose hopes are that he or she become a doctor. In short, if the student gives up the goal of completing college, he or she necessarily frustrates the higher-order goal of pleasing the parents.

There is a second difficulty in giving up a particular goal. Individuals may not always be aware of their own goal hierarchies (see "Awareness and Control," below). In identifying the goal structure, they may rely on implicit theories or schemata that may be wrong (Nisbett & Wilson, 1977). For example, a college degree may be a key to making a good living or a symbol that earns the respect of one's parents. On failing a course, the premed student may abandon the goal of seeking a college degree in favor of a high-paying job. If the student fails to recognize that earning the respect of his or her parents is an important goal, then he or she will continue to ruminate about college. The implications of this line of argument for clinical practice seem clear.

The timing of goal abandonment may have implications for subsequent rumination. Over time, a ruminative process may become "channelized." That is, the longer the ruminative process about some particular goal object, the more likely that the object will remain in conscious awareness even when the goal has been satisfied. There are at least two reasons for this. First, the longer the rumination, the greater the number of other cognitions to which the ruminative object is likely to become associated. With more associations, there is a broader net of entities that will call the ruminative object to mind. Second, the longer the rumination, the more frequently the ruminative object will be associated with its most common associates. Frequency of association is related to strength of association (Anderson, 1983). Thus, the longer the rumination, the easier it will be for common associations to elicit the ruminative object.

Thus, even if the appropriate goal is abandoned, there will be an extensive network of associations tied to it if it is abandoned after substantial rumination. This will result in goal-related thoughts' being easily and frequently cued from the environment. In other words, if the ruminative process concerning a particular object is engaged in frequently or for long periods of time, it will persist even if the driving goal is satisfied or given up. Giving up a goal dissipates the Zeigarnik charge but does not affect the associative structure among cognitions. This is what we mean by the ruminative process's becoming channelized.

Learned Helplessness

We suspect that eventually, if an individual cannot find a satisfactory way of meeting the goal or does not abandon the frustrated goal, he or she will experience depression (see Klinger, 1975; Pyszczynski & Greenberg, 1987). The cognitive overlay on the emotional response will be beliefs in one's own powerlessness and loss of control. Such a set of responses looks very much like what Seligman (1975) and his colleagues have termed "learned helplessness." More research is needed, however, to let us know whether the mapping of these responses onto the learned helplessness syndrome will ultimately prove useful.

In sum, we have suggested several stages of rumination. We believe that individuals will continue through the rumination sequence only to the extent that a prior step does not succeed in returning them to an attainable important goal. Individuals may cycle through the first four steps several times before they reach the learned helplessness stage. Each pass through the sequence, however, may be a little shorter and may result in a decreasing investment in the original goal.

AWARENESS AND CONTROL

We assume that people's thoughts and behaviors are directed by goals, but we do not assume that people are always aware of the impact of these goals on a given behavior. Indeed, we suspect that much of people's behavior occurs for reasons other than those they give in explanation of their behavior. This is a seeming paradox: How can conscious behaviors be directed by unconscious goals? The paradox can be resolved if certain distinctions are made clear.

First, we assume that a goal that has been interrupted does not directly produce ruminations about itself. In other words, the connection is not hard-wired.[3] Rather, interruption may cause a diffuse arousal response and a scanning of the environment (Mandler, 1975; Sokolov, 1963). One implication of this assumption is that the link between any given interruption and the onset of rumination must be inferred. To the extent that this is true, then such inferences may be susceptible to the same difficulties as other causal inferences and detections of covariation (see Nisbett & Wilson, 1977; Nisbett & Ross, 1980). Thus, our assertion that conscious ruminations have unconscious causes refers mainly to second-order consciousness (Bowers, 1987). That is, individuals may be aware of both their ruminations and their interrupted goal, but may not be aware of a causal connection between the two. There are several ways in which this faulty inference may come about.

One reason is people's reliance upon the representativeness heuristic (Kahneman & Tversky, 1972) and naive *a priori* causal theories (Nisbett & Wilson, 1977) in determining covariation. From this perspective, individuals may not see a causal connection between the occurrence of an event and the onset of their ruminations, because the connection is an implausible one according to their theory. Evidence to this effect was obtained by Nisbett and Wilson (1977). They asked subjects to tell which of four pairs of stockings they preferred and why. Subjects showed a preference for the pair that was presented last in the sequence, claiming that it had a better texture, appearance, and so on. In actuality, all four pairs of stockings were the same. They differed only in the order in which the subjects encountered them.

It would appear that subjects were conscious of the order of presentation, because they consciously considered each pair of stockings in sequence. Thus, their failure to mention order in their causal explanations could not have been due to the fact that order was out of first-order consciousness. Rather, it appears that subjects rejected order of appearance as an explanation because it did not represent a good naive explanation. A more plausible explanation (i.e., one more representative of a good naive rule for preferring one stocking over another) was that the stockings differed in quality.

By the same reasoning, a person may be aware of ruminating and aware of a disrupted goal, yet may deem a relation between the two to be implausible. For example, suppose that our premed student has two reasons for staying in school: to get a respectable job, and to please his or her parents. Suppose that this student finishes school and gets a respectable job, yet fails to please the parents. Although the student (now a practicing doctor) may generally rate his or her life as a happy one, and may have many indicators of success, he or she may also feel a continued source of discontent. However, the doctor may not immediately arrive at a correct identification of the source of this discontent. Failing to please one's parents may seem an implausible reason for a 35-year-old, otherwise successful professional to be discontent. A more plausible explanation may be that the condominiums in which the doctor invested are not selling as rapidly as he or she would like. So, despite the fact that the actual source of discontent is the failure to please his or her parents, the doctor may ruminate not about the parents but about the financial situation.

Another reason why it may be difficult for people to detect the relationship between a specific goal disruption and rumination is that goal disruption is subjective (e.g., Marrow, 1938). This means that there may be no consistent relationship between a given event and the onset of rumination. According to our theory, the hierarchical nature of the goal structure allows the frustration of a number of smaller goals to accumulate at higher-order goals. (For related work involving somewhat different assumptions, see Linville, 1982.) When that accumulation exceeds a certain threshold, ruminations about the higher-order goal will come into consciousness, even when the final precipitating event is not in itself very disruptive.

As an example, imagine that our premed student starts off the day by waking up late and then burning the breakfast toast. Then, imagine that as he or she leaves for school, the car won't start. Suppose, finally, that the student arrives at school, and then realizes that he or she was supposed to bring a book, but left it at home. None of these events in and of themselves may threaten the student's goal of being in control of his or her life. Yet, each of these may provide some activation toward that end. Consequently, by the end of the day, an unflattering but relatively innocuous remark by a friend may set off ruminations about the student's ability to control his or her own life, and these ruminations would appear to be beyond all bounds of the innocuous remark.

Moreover, because there is a great deal of disparity between the intensity of the innocuous remark and the degree of rumination, our student may be reluctant to conclude that the remark was the cause of the ruminations. And, in a sense, the student would be right. He or she is not responding to the remark in isolation, but to the accumulated frustrations that have activated the concept, "I am not in control of my life." However, to correctly ascertain this, the student would have to detect each of the subtle events, their relation to one another, and the relation of all of these to rumination. The difficulty in doing this may limit the number of times people will correctly identify the real cause of their ruminations (Wilson & Stone, 1985).

A third form of faulty inference may occur when individuals have theories that are only partially correct. Examples of this form of inference can be found in the literature on conditioning in adult humans (for a review, see Brewer, 1974). Dulany (1961), for example, asked subjects to emit single words and then rewarded them with "Um-hmm" for plural nouns. He found that this increased the frequency with which subjects said plural nouns. In assessing subjects' awareness after the experiment, however, he found that only those who were aware of a contingency between their verbal responses and the experiment's "Um-hmm's" showed any conditioning. Interestingly, though, most of these subjects had developed a hypothesis that was not the same as that which was being rewarded. Rather than giving more plural nouns, they increased the frequency with which they uttered more items of a given semantic category (e.g., "rubies," "pearls"), which happened to be plural.

We assume that rumination will continue until the individual correctly identifies (either deliberately or fortuitously) the goal that has been frustrated, because only identification of this goal allows the individual to find behaviors that lead reliably to goal attainment. Without correct identification of goals, individuals may reach goal attainment only fortuitously or sporadically.

EMPIRICAL CONSIDERATIONS

Throughout this chapter, we have cited studies that appeared relevant to rumination. However, no direct test of the theory has been reported. It is only now that a research program directly addressing these ideas is underway. In empirical work of this sort, there are two important problems: how to measure ruminations, and how to identify the goals that instigate ruminations when those goals may not be available to awareness.

The dependent-measure problem can be solved in a number of ways. For example, one can ask respondents to give a retrospective assessment of the extent to which they have ruminated about a particular aspect of their life (e.g., Millar et al., 1988; Tait & Silver, Chapter 12, this volume). Another possibility is to sample thoughts over the course of a respondent's day (Csikszentmihalyi & Kubey, 1981). A third possibility is to have respondents talk aloud about their conscious experiences or even to ring a bell when they think about a particular thing (Wegner, Schneider, Carter, & White, 1987).

There are also several indirect methods. Presumably, ruminating about a topic makes that and related information more accessible. Consequently, recognition times for degraded stimuli related to the topic of rumination should be faster when people are ruminating than when they are not. We obtained evidence to this effect (Martin & Tesser, 1988a, 1988b). We asked subjects to play the role of a corporation president. Subjects were presented with a series of business problems and asked to choose a course of action that would result in the most profit for the company. Subjects were also told that the ability to make good decisions was related to intelligence. All subjects were led to believe that they had made money for their company. However, some were told that their success was due to luck, whereas others were told that their success was due to their skills at decision making. Thus, subjects told that their success was due to luck did not reach their goal of demonstrating their intelligence.

Following the decision-making task, subjects engaged in a 5-minute distractor task (drawing a map of their campus), and then were presented with a series of asterisk strings on a computer screen. One by one in random order, the asterisks disappeared to reveal the letters of a word. The subjects' task was to recognize the word being revealed as quickly and as confidently as possible. It was assumed that failure to attain an important goal would engender rumination about the goal. As a result, words related to that goal should become more accessible. This meant that subjects whose success was due to luck (and who therefore did not reach their goal of demonstrating intelligence) should recognize intelligence-related words more quickly than subjects who were told that their success was due to skill. This was what happened.

Finally, because ruminations are conscious, they take up cognitive capacity. Thus, reaction times to unrelated materials should actually be slower when individuals are ruminating than when they are not (e.g., Britton & Tesser, 1982). These methods differ along a number of dimensions, including ease of use, precision, obtrusiveness, ecological validity, and social desirability. Choice of technique should depend on the nature of the specific question being addressed.

The second problem, the identification of nonconscious goals, can be dealt with in at least two ways. First, one can experimentally establish a nonconscious goal and measure the resulting ruminations when the goal has or has not been threatened. However, we know of no work that does this. A second possibility is to assume the presence of a goal, provide subjects with experiences that move them toward the presumed goal, and observe the resulting changes in rumination. Although we know of no work that has done this explicitly, the work of Claude Steele (e.g., Steele & Liu, 1983) provides a nice parallel example. Steele has suggested that behavior that appears to be directed by a consistency goal may actually be related to an even higher-order goal—namely, self-affirmation. To test this hypothesis, he had subjects engage in behavior that would disrupt this higher-order goal (i.e., they wrote a counterattitudinal essay with insufficient justification). Steele then provided subjects with a way to reattain the goal that was unrelated to the event of the initial disruption. Specifically, he gave subjects positive feedback on a personality test.

This feedback eliminated the attitude change that typically follows performance of counter attitudinal behavior under conditions of insufficient justification. The explanation was that subjects attained self-affirmation through the personality feedback, and therefore did not have to attain it through a justification of their counterattitudinal behavior. Regardless of whether one agrees or disagrees with Steele's interpretation of dissonance effects, our point remains the same: The strategy of assuming the existence of a goal and then providing experiences that interrupt or complete that goal allows one to make strong inferences about the influence of goals, even those of which subjects may be completely unaware.

CONCLUDING REMARKS

The investigation of ruminative processes raises some interesting questions concerning controlled and automatic processes. A number of theorists (e.g. Bargh, 1984; Posner & Snyder, 1975; Shiffrin & Schneider, 1977) have defined automatic processes as those processes that use no cognitive capacity, have no conscious component, are set into motion by the mere presence of the appropriate stimulus, are fixed and inflexible, and are not controllable. Controlled processes, on the other hand, are assumed to show the converse of each of these features. As Uleman (Chapter 14, this volume) aptly points out, not all processes (rumination included) can be clearly mapped onto one or the other of these categories. We agree with this (although we do not agree with his assertion that rumination is purposeless).

On the one hand, rumination is conscious and takes up capacity. On the other hand, it is often uncontrollable, and the instigating states may not be available to conscious awareness (i.e., the disrupted goals may be misidentified). In addition, people may be able to guide the content of ruminations to some degree, and they may be able to distract themselves from ruminating for a while. However, they may not be able to terminate the ruminations completely until they either satisfy or abandon the motivating goal. Thus, rumination lies somewhere between the extremes with regard to flexibility.

Finally, the theory proposed in this chapter seems to have some heuristic value for areas related to rumination that have not been fully articulated yet. For example, several theorists (Horowitz, 1986; Tait & Silver, Chapter 12, this volume) suggest that rumination continues until the individual finds "meaning" in the experience that triggered the ruminative process. As yet, however, there has been no clear theoretical statement of what constitutes "meaning." The present theory suggests that correctly identifying the goal and either abandoning it or finding an appropriate substitute for it constitutes the subjective experience of "finding meaning." We hope that this and other implications of the model will be useful in research, theorizing, and application.

ACKNOWLEDGMENTS

Work on this chapter was facilitated by a grant from the National Institute of Mental Health (No. R01MH414B7-0) to Abraham Tesser. We wish to thank John Bargh, Lawrence Calhoun, Leslie Clark, James Collins, Judith Cutshall, Fritz Strack, and James Uleman for helpful comments on previous drafts of this chapter. Aspects of this theory were first presented at the conference on Rumination, Self-Relevant Cognitions, and Stress, sponsored by the Memphis State University Center for Excellence, March 1987.

NOTES

1. Not all repetitive thoughts are initiated through the disruption of important, higher-order goals. Some stimulus events appear to be intrinsically compelling, and prompt repeated thinking through that quality. For example, if one were to witness a particularly gruesome automobile accident, one would probably have thoughts about the accident repeatedly over the course of the day. We would argue, however, that these thoughts would not be sustained over longer periods unless the event threatened attainment of an important, higher-order goal. Thus, sustained thinking should occur only if witnessing the accident threatens one's view of the world as a safe or just place, causes one to reconsider one's own mortality, and so on.

2. We recognize that there are occasions on which ruminations can be pleasant. For example, a particular scent may cause us to remember a past love affair. Reminiscence about the loved one may be quite pleasing. However, such reveries do not seem to have their genesis in goal frustration. Rather, they result from spreading activation of information cued by the environment. Their maintenance may be due to the pleasant affect they induce (Clark & Isen, 1982; Strack et al., 1985).

3. There is evidence from several strands of work to suggest that certain combinations of stimuli and responses have a biological advantage over arbitrary pairings. For example, Garcia and Koelling (1966) showed that rats more easily learned the pairing between food consumption and nausea than between food consumption and shock. Similarly, Ohman and Dimberg (1978) have shown that the pairing of shock with an angry face is more easily learned than is the pairing of shock with a smiling face. However, even where biological pairings are prepotent, the possibility of second-order unawareness (e.g., Bowers, 1987) remains. For example, people may become averse to foods with a particular smell after eating something that caused gastric distress, in spite of the fact that the smell played no causal role.

REFERENCES

Abelson, R. P. (1981). Psychological status of the script concept. *American Psychologist, 36,* 715–729.

Anderson, J. R. (1983). A spreading activation theory of memory. *Journal of Verbal Learning and Verbal Behavior, 22,* 261–295.

Atkinson, J. W., & McClelland, D. C. (1948). The effect of different intensities of the hunger drive on thematic apperception. *Journal of Experimental Psychology, 38,* 643–658.

Bargh, J. A. (1984). Automatic and conscious processing of social information. In R. S. Wyer, Jr., & T. T. Srull (Eds.), *Handbook of social cognition* (Vol. 3, pp. 1–43). Hillsdale, NJ: Erlbaum.

Beck, A. T. (1983). Cognitive therapy of depression: New perspectives. In P. J. Clayton & J. E. Barrett (Eds.), *Treatment of depression: Old controversies and new approaches* (pp. 315–350). New York: Raven Press.

Bower, G. H., Black, J. B., & Turner, T. J. (1979). Scripts in memory for texts. *Cognitive Psychology, 11,* 177–220.

Bowers, K. S. (1987). Revisioning the unconscious. *Canadian Psychology, 28,* 93–104.

Brewer, W. F. (1974). There is no convincing evidence for operant or classical conditioning in adult humans. In W. B. Weimer & D. S. Palermo (Eds.), *Cognition and the symbolc processes* (pp. 1–42). Hillsdale, NJ: Erlbaum.

Britton, B. K., & Tesser, A. (1982). Effects of prior knowledge on use of cognitive capacity in three complex cognitive tasks. *Journal of Verbal Learning and Verbal Behavior, 21,* 421–436.

Brozek, J., Guetzkow, H., Baldwin, M. V., & Granston, R. A. (1951). A quantitative study of perception and association in experimental semi-starvation. *Journal of Personality, 19,* 245–264.

Bruner, J. S. (1957). On perceptual readiness, *Psychological Review, 64,* 123–152.

Cantor, N., & Mischel, W. (1979). Prototypes in person perception. In L. Berkowitz (Ed.), *Advances in experimental social psychology* (Vol. 12, pp. 3–52). New York: Academic Press.

Carver, C. S., & Scheier, M. F. (1981). *Attention and self-regulation: A control-theory approach to human behavior.* New York: Springer-Verlag.

Clark, M. S., & Isen, A. M. (1982). Toward understanding the relationships between feeling states and behavior. In A. H. Hastorf & A. M. Isen (Eds.), *Cognitive social psychology* (pp. 73–108). New York: Elsevier.

Collins, J. E., & Clark, L. F. (1987). *Falling in and out of love: When do thoughts intrude?* Paper presented at the 95th annual conference of the American Psychological Association, New York.

Csikszentmihalyi, M., & Kubey, R. (1981). Television and the rest of life. *Public Opinion Quarterly, 45,* 317–328.

Deci, E. L. (1971). Effects of externally mediated rewards on intrinsic motivation. *Journal of Personality and Social Psychology, 18,* 105–115.

Dulany, D. E. (1961). Hypotheses and habits in verbal "operant conditioning." *Journal of Abnormal and Social Psychology, 63,* 251–263.

Ellis, A. (1962). *Reason and emotion in psychotherapy.* Secaucus, NJ: Lyle Stuart.

Garcia, J., & Koelling, R. A. (1966). Relation of cue to consequences in avoidance learning. *Psychonomic Science, 4,* 123–124.

Horowitz, M. J. (1986). *Stress response syndromes.* (2nd ed.). New York: Jason Aronson.

Kahneman, D., & Tversky, A. (1972). Subjective probability: A judgment of representativeness. *Cognitive Psychology, 3,* 430–454.

Klinger, E. (1975). Consequences to commitment to and disengagement from incentives. *Psychological Review, 82,* 223–231.

Klinger, E. (1978). Modes of normal conscious flow. In K. S. Pope & J. L. Singer (Eds.), *The stream of consciousness: Scientific investigations into the flow of human experience* (pp. 225–258). New York: Plenum.

Klinger, E., Barta, S., & Maxeiner, M. (1980). Motivational correlates of thought content. *Journal of Personality and Social Psychology, 39,* 1222–1237.

Lalljee, M., & Abelson, R. P. (1983). The organization of explanations. In M. Hewstond (Ed.), *Attribution theory: Social and functional extensions* (pp. 65–80). Oxford: Blackwell.

Langer, E. J. (1978). Rethinking the role of thought in social interaction. In J. Harvey, W. Ickes, & R. Kidd (Eds.) *New directions in attribution research* (Vol. 2, pp. 36–58). Hillsdale, NJ: Erlbaum.

Lepper, M. R., Greene, D., & Nisbett, R. E. (1973). Undermining children's intrinsic interest with extrinsic reward: A test of the "overjustification" hypothesis. *Journal of Personality and Social Psychology, 28,* 129–137.

Linville, P. W. (1982). Affective consequences of complexity regarding the self and others. In M. S. Clark & S. T. Fiske (Eds.), *Affect and cognition: The seventeenth annual Carnegie symposium on cognition* (pp. 79–109). Hillsdale, NJ: Erlbaum.

Mandler, G. (1975). *Mind and emotion.* New York: Wiley.

Mandler, G. (1987). Aspects of consciousness. *Personality and Social Psychology Bulletin, 13,* 299–313.

Marrow, A. J. (1938). Goal tension and recall. *Journal of General Psychology, 19,* 3–64.

Martin, L. L., & Tesser, A. (1988a). *Action-identification and self-identification: Stages of ruminative thought.* Poster session presented at the annual convention of the American Psychological Association, Atlanta, GA.

Martin, L. L., & Tesser, A. (1988b). *Goal hierarchies and the stages of ruminative thought.* Paper presented at the Nags Head Conference on the Direction of Thought and Emotion, Kill Devil's Hill, NC.

McClelland, D. C., Clark, R. A., Roby, T. B., & Atkinson, J. W. (1949). The effect of need for achievement on thematic apperception. *Journal of Experimental Psychology, 37,* 242–255.

Millar, K. U., Tesser, A., & Millar, M. (1988). The effects of a threatening life event on behavior sequences and intrusive thought: A self-disruption explanation. *Cognitive Therapy and Research, 12,* 441–457.

Millar, M., & Tesser, A. (1986a). Effects of affective and cognitive focus on the attitude–behavior relationship. *Journal of Personality and Social Psychology, 51,* 270–276.

Millar, M., & Tesser, A. (1986b). Thought induced attitude change: The effects of schema structure and commitment. *Journal of Personality and Social Psychology, 51,* 259–269.

Miller, G. A., Galanter, E., & Pribram, K. H. (1960). *Plans and the structure of behavior.* New York: Holt, Rinehart & Winston.

Minsky, M. (1987). *Societal structures of the mind.* London: Heinemann.

Nisbett, R. E., & Ross, L. (1980). *Human inference: Strategies and shortcomings of social judgment.* Englewood Cliffs, NJ: Prentice-Hall.

Nisbett, R. E., & Wilson, T. (1977). Telling more than we can know: Verbal reports on mental processes. *Psychological Review, 84,* 213–259.

Nolen-Hoeksema, S. (1987). Sex differences in unipolar depression: Evidence and theory. *Psychological Bulletin, 101,* 259–282.

Ohman, A., & Dimberg, V. (1978). Facial expressions as conditioned stimuli for electrodermal responses. A case of preparedness. *Journal of Personality and Social Psychology, 36,* 1251–1258.

Posner, M. I., & Snyder, C. R. R. (1975). Attention and cognitive control. In R. L. Solso (Ed.), *Information processing and cognition: The Loyola Symposium* (pp. 55–85). Hillsdale, NJ: Erlbaum.

Powers, W. T. (1973). *Behavior: The control of perception.* Chicago: Aldine.

Pyszczynski, T., & Greenberg, J. (1987). Self-regulatory perseveration and the depressive self-focusing style: A self-awareness theory of reactive depression. *Psychological Bulletin, 102,* 122–138.

Rosch, E. (1978). Principles of categorization. In E. Rosch & B. B. Lloyds (Eds.), *Cognition and categorization* (pp. 27–48). Hillsdale, NJ: Erlbaum.

Sanford, R. N. (1936). The effect of abstinence from food upon imaginal processes. *Journal of Psychology, 2,* 129–136.

Seligman, M. E. P. (1975). *Helplessness.* San Francisco: W. H. Freeman.

Seta, J. J., & Seta, C. E. (1982). Personal equity: An intrapersonal comparator system analysis of reward value. *Journal of Personality and Social Psychology, 43,* 222–235.

Shiffrin, R. M., & Schneider, W. (1977). Controlled and automatic human information processing: II. Perceptual learning, automatic attention, and a general theory. *Psychological Reviews, 84,* 127–190.

Sokolov, Y. N. (1963). *Perception and the conditioned reflex.* Oxford: Pergamon Press.

Steele, C. M., & Liu, T. J. (1983). Dissonance processes as self-affirmation. *Journal of Personality and Social Psychology, 45,* 5–19.

Strack, F., Schwarz, N., & Gschneidinger, E. (1985). Happiness and reminiscing: The role of time perspective, affect, and mode of thinking. *Journal of Personality and Social Psychology, 49,* 1460–1469.

Srull, T. K., & Wyer, R. S. (1986). The role of chronic and temporary goals in social information processing. In R. M. Sorrentino & E. T. Higgins (Eds.), *Handbook of motivation and cognition: Foundations of social behavior* (pp. 503–549). New York: Guilford Press.

Tesser, A. (1978). Self-generated attitude change. In L. Berkowitz (Ed.), *Advances in experimental social psychology* (Vol. 11, 289–338.). New York: Academic Press.

Tesser, A. (1980). When individual dispositions and social pressure conflict: A catastrophe. *Human Relations, 33,* 393–407.

Vallacher, R. R., & Wegner, D. M. (1987). What do people think they're doing? Action identification and human behavior. *Psychological Review, 94,* 3–15.

von Bertalanffy, L. (1968). *General systems theory.* New York: Braziller.

Wegner, D. M., Schneider, D. J., Carter, S. R., & White, T. L. (1987). Paradoxical effects of thought suppression. *Journal of Personality and Social Psychology, 47*, 237–252.

Wicklund, R. A. (1986) Orientation to the environment versus preoccupation with human potential. In R. M. Sorrentino & E. T. Higgins (Eds.), *Handbook of motivation and cognition: Foundations of social behavior* (pp. 64–95). New York: Guilford Press.

Wicklund, R. A., & Braun, O. L. (1987). Incompetence and the concern with human categories. *Journal of Personality and Social Psychology, 53*, 373–382.

Wilson, T. D., & Stone, J. I. (1985). Limitations of self-knowledge: More on telling more than we can know. In P. Shaver (Ed.), *Review of personality and social psychology* (Vol. 6, pp. 167–183). Beverly Hills, CA: Sage.

Zeigarnik, B. (1938). On finished and unfinished tasks. In W. D. Ellis (Ed. and Trans.), *A source book of gestalt psychology*. New York: Harcourt, Brace & World. (Original work published 1927)

11

Stream of Consciousness and Stress: Levels of Thinking

JAMES W. PENNEBAKER
Southern Methodist University

When jogging at a furious pace, I have a great deal of trouble thinking about complex issues.

When the spouse of one of my colleagues left him, he became obsessed with details. His reviews of manuscripts, which had formerly been broad and scholarly, now focused on sentence structure and grammar.

On learning that he had been unexpectedly fired from his job, a close friend immersed himself in playing pinball. Rather than think or talk about his experience, he devoted 10–12 hours per day to pinball for over 2 weeks.

The ways in which people think change dramatically when they are faced with massive stressors. Numerous laboratory and clinical studies clearly document that periods of psychological turmoil cause individuals to become distractible (e.g., Cohen, 1978; Cohen, Evans, Krantz, & Stokols, 1980), to make mistakes in the tasks that they are performing (e.g., Glass & Singer, 1972), and to become obsessed with detail (e.g., Teichman, 1966). By the same token, it is well documented that psychological upheavals alter autonomic activity such as heart rate and blood pressure (e.g., Obrist, 1981), hormonal levels (e.g., Frankenhauser, 1971; Selye, 1976), immune function (e.g., Kiecolt-Glaser & Glaser, 1988), cortical activity in the brain (e.g., Luria, 1980; Davidson, 1980), and health in general (e.g., Graham, 1972).

But there is more to the story. Although we know that stressors affect physiological activity and the ways we think, very few researchers have examined the links among stress, conscious thinking patterns, and physiological activity. As this chapter indicates, changes in our normal thinking patterns can affect biological changes, just as biological changes can affect our thinking processes.

The purpose of this chapter is to explore the dimensions of conscious thought that fluctuate during stressful periods. By "conscious thought processes," I mean those naturally occurring, ongoing thoughts that pop into our minds from second to second. These thought patterns have variously been described as the stream of thought (James, 1890), daydreaming (Singer, 1984), current concerns (Klinger, 1978), or the internal landscape (Csikszentmihalyi & Larson, 1984). Conscious thought, unlike perceptual or primary appraisal processes, is immediately accessible and usually language-based.

In this chapter, I first describe the changes that occur in thinking patterns during periods of stress. I then address various cognitive and motivational explanations for these changes. Finally, I point to the costs and benefits of changing thinking patterns during times of stress.

THINKING PATTERNS DURING STRESS

During times of physical or psychological stress, we think differently. Having worked with people whose spouses have unexpectedly died (e.g., Pennebaker & O'Heeron, 1984), I have been struck by the ways in which they guide ordinary conversation in one of two very different directions. The first, which is a confrontational strategy, involves their talking about various aspects of the loss. They may discuss their feelings of fear and anxiety, the circumstances surrounding the death, or the effects of the death on their own lives. Alternatively (and more likely), they often adopt an avoidant strategy, whereby they discuss the weather, the shirt I am wearing, or the groceries they must buy. Indeed, any mention of the death on my part may prompt them to discuss the weather with even greater intensity.

These differences are particularly dramatic when people who have recently suffered traumas are asked to talk or write in a stream-of-consciousness manner for 10 or 20 minutes as part of a general psychology study. The stream-of-consciousness transcripts of 12 individuals who had recently experienced major upheavals (e.g., death of spouse, parent, or child; breakup of a relationship; loss of job) indicated that 7 adopted avoidant strategies, 3 used confrontational strategies, and the remaining 2 alternated between avoidant and confrontational.

The use of avoidant, denial, and distracting strategies during or following stress has been discussed in detail by a number of thinkers (Freud, 1915/1963; Horowitz, 1976; Lazarus & Folkman, 1984; Rossi, 1986). A number of recent studies in our laboratory indicate that avoidant strategies can affect the entire domain of conscious thought. In this section, I first discuss the characteristics of conscious thought and then present a measurement strategy for capturing its occurrence. I conclude with laboratory evidence indicating how level of thinking changes during controllable versus uncontrollable stress.

Dimensions of Conscious Thought

Although people who have experienced a trauma may actively avoid discussing or thinking about all aspects of the trauma, their thinking is affected in a more profound way. Not only do they avoid the traumatic topic, but they also avoid talking and thinking about *any* significant or emotional topics in any depth. In this section, I first review three common changes in thinking that occur during stress. I then propose a general measure to assess these changes using a stream-of-consciousness methodology.

Changes in Thinking during Stress

Based on our own experience as well as the findings of others, my colleagues and I have isolated three important interrelated dimensions of thinking that change during stress:

1. *Breadth of perspective.* The more stress individuals endure, the narrower their perspective, both in time and in use of divergent information. That is, during periods of stress, people typically think about immediate issues and are less likely to consider historical precedents or long-term implications.

In discussing the role of attention, Easterbrook (1959) argued that when individuals are aroused (e.g., when they are under stress), their focus of attention narrows, with the result being that they are unable to process peripheral cues in their environment. In considering cognitive processes, Wyer and Srull (1986) have pointed out that individuals can process only a finite amount of information. During times of stress, or high information load, only the most recent and immediate types of cognitive materials are processed. Finally, research examining daydreaming indicates that the more individuals are engaged in complex tasks, the less their thoughts roam to task-irrelevant areas (Antrobus, Singer, Goldstein, & Fortgang, 1970; Klinger, 1978).

2. *Self-reflection.* When under stress, individuals are less likely to reflect on the causes and effects of their actions, thoughts, and feelings.

Wicklund (1975; Duval & Wicklund, 1972) has provided evidence that individuals alternate their attention between the environment and themselves. When people are self-focused, they examine their own motives, are attuned to their own inadequacies, and emit behaviors in line with their basic beliefs. In numerous studies, Wicklund and others have found that when individuals participate in complex tasks, they are much less aware of themselves, use fewer personal pronouns ("I," "me"), and report less extreme emotions. Similarly, the work of Schwartz (1983) and Carver and Scheier (1981) indicates that, when under stress, individuals are less self-conscious, which can undermine self-regulatory processes. Finally, in evaluating the results from patients with brain damage, Pribram's (1976) approach suggests that the more the brain is processing stress-relevant information, the less elaborate the verbal awareness of self is.

3. *Awareness of emotion.* When individuals must process a great deal of information, such as during times of stress, they are less aware of emotions or transient changes in mood.

The awareness of emotions and mood states is closely related to the processes of self-reflection. That is, to become aware of emotions, one must turn inwardly, at least briefly. Numerous studies indicate that when individuals are actively involved in a task, they are less aware of feelings of fatigue (Walster & Aronson, 1967) and negative moods (Pennebaker, 1982, Ch. 2; Pennebaker & Brittingham, 1982). In addition, numerous clinical investigators report that one of the hallmarks of coping with ongoing stress is an overall blunting of emotion (Rachman, 1980; Scurfield, 1985). Indeed, in studying communities that had been affected by the eruption of Mount St. Helens, Darren Newtson and I found that those people who were living closest to the volcano and who were thus in the most immediate danger of future eruptions reported significantly less negative and positive feelings about the volcano than those who lived further away and who had actually suffered significantly more damage from the ash of the original eruption (Pennebaker & Newtson, 1983).

Levels of Thinking: A General Assessment Tool

Over the past few years, my students and I have begun investigating naturally occurring thought processes using a stream-of-consciousness methodology. In reading hundreds of stream-of-consciousness transcripts, we have found that the dimensions of breadth, self-reflection, and emotion awareness are highly interrelated and represent a common dimension of thought. Our initial work indicates that the content of stream of consciousness can be viewed along a single continuum, called "level of thinking." According to this conception, high-level thinking is associated with a broad perspective, self-reflective thoughts, and reference to one's emotions and moods. Low-level thinking, on the other hand, is characterized by a narrow perspective, a total lack of self-reflection, and no awareness of moods.

Level of thinking is easily assessed by raters with a minimum of 5–10 minutes of training. In our studies, level of thinking is rated along a 5-

point scale, where 1 represents a low level of thinking and 5 a high level. Across four studies, where three raters independently judged stream-of-consciousness transcripts (usually 100–300 words), the mean intercorrelation among raters was .65, which translates to a Spearman–Brown reliability coefficient of .85. To indicate the ease of assessing levels of thinking, I include two examples:

> *High-level example:* I've been thinking about my parents. We recently had a fight about the car. It's not just the car, though. They won't accept that I'm 18, that I can think on my own. When I talk to them on the phone, I feel these powerful emotions of anger and love overpowering me. Have they forgotten their college years? I AM WORTHY. I AM MY-SELF. "Another identity crisis," I can hear the experimenter say when she reads this.

> *Low-level example:* Let's see. The wall is brown. The floor is a dirty gray. Hmmm, matches my shoes. Have to get them cleaned. As soon as this study is over, go to my room, sort the laundry, go to the laundromat. Don't forget the shoes. Where will I get the change for the machines? Maybe Jeannie (roomie). Got to get back by 4:30. Go to dinner at 5:00. Wonder what they'll serve for dinner tonight?

As would be expected, global ratings of level of thinking are correlated with the indirect measures of the components of thinking: breadth of perspective, self-reflection, and awareness of emotions. In one study involving 80 undergraduates who both wrote in a stream-of-consciousness mode for 15 minutes and talked into a tape recorder for 5 minutes on four separate occasions across a 2-month interval, independent raters coded the topics that subjects addressed, the raw number of self-references ("I," "me," "my"), and the number of emotion words used (from Pennebaker, Brumbelow, et al., 1987). Level of thinking was correlated with the breadth of the topic (e.g., .25 with sexuality, .24 with death, .27 with subjects' immediate families, and $-.23$ with the weather). In addition, the more personal pronouns used, the higher the level of thinking ($r = .39$). Finally, the more emotion words used, the higher the level ($r = .32$). (Unless noted otherwise, all correlations reported in this chapter are statistically significant at $p < .05$, two-tailed tests.)

In addition to being reliably rated and correlated with its components, level of thinking was reliable across modality (writing vs. talking) when separated a week apart ($r = .70$) and over a 2-month interval within the same modality ($r = .56$). In short, the level-of-thinking scoring technique demonstrated good psychometric properties.

Links to Related Constructs

In recent years, psychologists have suggested dimensions of thought that are relevant to our own. In this section, I briefly discuss models dealing with action identification, mindlessness, and cognitive complexity, and note their similarities to and differences from our own approach.

Vallacher and Wegner (1985) have found that individuals define their own behavior along a continuum ranging from low to high levels of action identification. For example, a person writing a manuscript could variously identify this action as "typing on a keyboard" (low level), "writing the introduction section" (moderate level), or "advancing knowledge" (high level). According to Vallacher and Wegner's theory of action identification, once an action is well learned, its identity tends to move from lower to higher levels. Furthermore, whenever an action is disrupted or becomes too complex, the identification of the action tends to move (at least temporarily) to a lower level. Although levels of action identification correlate with breadth of thoughts, they do not incorporate degree of self-reflection or awareness of affect.

Langer's (1987) work on mindlessness is also related to level of thinking. According to Langer, "mindless thinking" refers to the rigid use of information during which the individual is unaware of its potentially novel aspects. "Mindfulness," on the other hand, is associated with the active establishment of new cognitive categories that spur creative approaches to problem solving. Interestingly, mindlessness is more likely to occur during stress and is associated with adverse physical consequences. Although there are several similarities between the mindlessness–mindfulness and level-of-thinking dimensions, the measurement of thinking levels focuses on the content and direction of thoughts, rather than on the pre-existing or new schemata that dictate thoughts. Consequently, a person could be thinking creatively about ways to vacuum the carpet in a mindful way, while at the same time avoiding thoughts related to a personal trauma. Although this is an example of mindfulness, our group would judge the thoughts as reflecting a low level of thinking.

Finally, several researchers have pointed to the relevance of cognitive complexity in understanding thought processes. Research in the 1960s and 1970s found that individuals who were classified as high in psychological differentiation, or field independence, could easily break set, think creatively, and recall threatening information when under stress, compared to field-dependent subjects (Witkin, Goodenough, & Oltman, 1979). More recent work by Linville (1987) suggests that people who maintain greater distinctions among different aspects of themselves are better able to cope with stressors. Self-complexity, like psychological differentiation, assumes that the ability to organize and understand threats, negative emotions, and conflicting information is dependent on the existing schemata or sets available to the person. Indeed, the level-of-thinking characteristics of breadth of perspective and self-reflection are hallmarks of psychological differentiation and self-complexity.

Within the present context, our approach to levels of thinking has at least two distinct advantages to understanding thought processes. First, level of thinking is defined by the contents of ongoing thoughts, which are objectively rated. Unlike self-reports or manipulations of action identification, mindfulness, or cognitive complexity, level of thinking serves as a face-valid measure of thought. Second, it reflects a dynamic process that changes from situation to situation. In short, it can be viewed as an ongoing mediating process between external situational constraints or personality dimensions and physiological or cognitive effects.

Changes in Level of Thinking during Stress

Before evaluating the links between stream of consciousness and biological activities, we must first demonstrate that level of thinking does indeed change when individuals are under stress. The results of a recent experiment which examined changes in level of thinking resulting from uncontrollable versus controllable noise, are presented.

Based on our earlier speculations, my colleagues and I assumed that when individuals are faced with a stressor such as uncontrollable noise, they should move to a lower level of thinking. In the first study (from Pennebaker, Brumbelow, et al., 1987), 48 introductory psychology students tracked their thoughts in writing using a stream-of-consciousness technique on three 5-minute occasions. During the first writing period, all subjects sat quietly in a room and continuously wrote whatever came into their minds. Immediately afterwards, subjects again wrote for 5 minutes while listening to aversive, high-pitched (2,700 hertz), moderately loud (88 decibels), unpredictable noise bursts that were perceived to be either controllable or uncontrollable. After the noise period, subjects were escorted to an adjacent room where they again wrote in a stream-of-consciousness fashion for 5 minutes.

Subjects were randomly assigned to either the perceived-control or no-perceived-control conditions. Those in the perceived-control condition were told:

> If, at any time, you find the noise sufficiently unpleasant, simply press this button and it will stop. You are completely free to stop the noise at any time. Many people have, in fact, done so. I want to emphasize that you have complete control over the noise at all times.

Those in the no-perceived-control condition were informed:

> Once the noise begins, you must continue to listen to it. Do not try to stop the noise by tampering with the tape recorder. I want to emphasize that you do not have any control over the noise.

This technique, which was devised by Glass and Singer (1972), has been shown to be effective in manipulating perceptions of control, even though all subjects listen to the same aversive stimulus. As in previous studies, no subjects attempted to stop the noise during the study.

Three independent judges rated all of the writing samples for levels of thinking (Spearman–Brown reliabilities averaged .84) and counted the number of personal pronouns, emotion words, and physical symptom words (e.g., ringing ears, pounding heart). Because we were interested in studying changes in level of thinking, we excluded the data for subjects whose initial levels of thinking were in the top 16% and bottom 16% of the distribution. This was done because initial high levels and low levels were restricted by ceiling and floor effects, and therefore could change in only one direction. In short, only the middle 67% of the distribution was studied.

As can be seen in Figure 11.1, subjects wrote at lower levels in the no-perceived-control condition than in the perceived-control condition. A significant perceived control × time period interaction obtained ($p < .05$). Subjects who believed that they could control the noise maintained relatively constant thinking levels over the course of the study. Those who did not have perceived control, however, evidenced a marked drop in level of thinking both during and after the noise period.

Although no significant effects emerged for the total number of words written or for the number of physical symptom words, analyses of the negative-emotion words yielded an intriguing pattern of results. As depicted in Figure 11.2, a significant perceived control × time period interaction ($p < .01$) emerged, indicating that subjects in the no-perceived-control condition did not express negative emotions either during or following the noise. Those with perceived control, however, freely expressed emo-

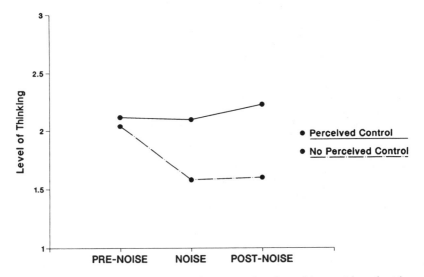

FIGURE 11.1. Level-of-thinking results across time for subjects with and without perceived control in the noise experiment.

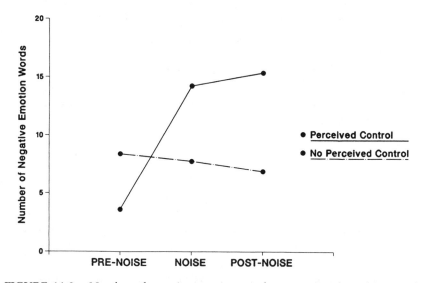

FIGURE 11.2. Number of negative-emotion words across time for subjects with and without perceived control in the noise experiment.

tions once the noise began and after it had stopped. A similar pattern emerged for number of self-references ($p < .01$). That is, perceived-control subjects increased their use of personal pronouns once the noise began, whereas the no-perceived-control subjects sharply decreased their use of personal pronouns during and following the noise.

The noise experiment is valuable in documenting the changes that occur in thinking levels during stressful periods. In many respects, the no-perceived-control subjects' lower levels of thinking following the noise are reminiscent of findings from the earlier studies of Glass and Singer (1972). In their studies, uncontrollable noise had its greatest impact—in terms of lack of task perseverance—following unpredictable or uncontrollable noise. If there is an overall trend toward lower-level thinking following uncontrollable experience, it could hamper one's abilities to think of task-relevant issues on a broader level. Indeed, Glass and Singer argued that decrements in performance following stress reflect the "psychic cost" of coping. The present results suggest that changes in level of thinking may be a pivotal factor in extracting the psychic cost.

Finally, the results concerning the use of emotion words indicate that individuals in perceived control of aversive experiences express emotions more freely than those not in perceived control. Although the lack of control is clearly aversive, individuals appear to withhold their expression of negative affect. Such a strategy may help people deny the immediate emotional consequences of their predicament.

COGNITIVE AND MOTIVATIONAL APPROACHES TO THINKING LEVELS

Why do people move to a lower level of thinking during periods of stress? Although a number of theoretical perspectives address this question, either directly or indirectly, this section discusses current trends in the areas of social cognition and motivation.

The Cognitive Approach

With the development and popularization of the computer, information-processing models based on both hardware and software design have become a dominant force. Although very few information-processing models have considered stream of consciousness per se, some have proposed the underlying processes behind the free flow of thought (Wyer & Srull, 1986) or remindings (Ross, 1984; Schank, 1982). One of the most comprehensive models using the computer as a metaphor, proposed by Wyer and Srull (1986), posits various cognitive functions complete with specifiable processing units, including a comprehender (for initial pattern recognition), an executor (for directing the flow of information), and various storage units that emphasize prior knowledge and current goals.

Whereas Wyer and Srull argue that most thought is oriented toward the completion of a hierarchy of goals, the free flow of thought can be seen when no specific goals exist (see also Martin & Tesser, Chapter 10, this volume). The central nervous system, which apparently is programmed in Fortran, enters a recursive feedback loop when no goal is present. During this time, a particular thought is semantically scanned. If no goal is specified, a random feature from the thought is sampled and a quick search for feature-relevant information is made, which then may result in retrieving a related thought. This process is repeated until a thought is found that has a specific goal, at which time a goal attainment subroutine is activated.

The Wyer and Srull model makes a number of predictions that are congruent with the level-of-thinking findings. Because these authors argue for a finite processing capacity, when too much information is available, the individual processes the most immediate information available. Apparently, the more stress a person is under (i.e., the more information to be processed), the more likely it is that he or she will fall into this "first in, first out" rule of processing. In a controllable situation, on the other hand, the mind should have more processing capacity to search for and examine more complex thoughts.

Particularly important is the model's ongoing search for sensory information and goal specification, which take precedence in being processed. Although discussed by William James (1890), this has also been a central feature of Jerome L. Singer's stream-of-consciousness models (Klos & Singer, 1981; Singer, 1975, 1984). According to Pope and Singer (1978), for example, individuals naturally process environmental and internal sensory information when it is available. However, if there is a paucity of this type of information (e.g., during sleep or in a boring situation), memories, associations, and images flow into the stream of consciousness. Using this assumption as a base, my colleagues and I would predict that controllable situations (relative to uncontrollable ones) that are boring or predictable would be conducive to elaborate daydreams and associated high-level thoughts.

Motivational Approaches

According to a motivational argument, individuals move to low levels of thinking to actively avoid aversive environmental stimulation and, perhaps, unpleasant internal thoughts or images. Although traditionally the domain of psychodynamic theorists, recent approaches that stress the importance of behavioral inhibition also indicate that low-level thinking can be motivated.

Freud (e.g., 1926/1959) was one of the first to seriously consider changes in thought processes as a function of stress and conflict. By studying the content of free association, everyday language, and dreams, Freud argued that individuals often adopt a variety of defenses that help them to avoid significant thoughts, memories, and emotions. Particularly important are Freud's discussions of obsessions and physical symptoms surrounding hysteria. According to Freud (1901/1960), individuals are able to distract themselves from unpleasant thoughts by focusing on trivial tasks or on subtle bodily sensations. When they do this, the aversive memories are temporarily suppressed. Interestingly, by using stream-of-consciousness techniques and in analyzing dreams and daily language, Freud found that these suppressed and repressed conflicts would surface, either symbolically or in slips of the tongue. Indeed, a number of studies indicate, for example, that individuals conflicted by sexuality are more likely to exhibit slips of the tongue that contain sexual overtones in controlled laboratory settings than nonconflicted individuals are (e.g., Baars, 1985; Motley, Camden, & Baars, 1979).

More recently, Daniel Wegner (1988; Wegner, Schneider, Carter, & White, 1987) has argued that individuals often use the natural strategy of unfocused self-distraction in order to try not to think of significant experiences. Wegner and his colleagues have found that when subjects are asked not to think of a particular object, they naturally try to focus on relatively simple and salient objects or events in their environment. Not only is this technique effortful, but it is usually unsuccessful, in that the self-distractors themselves become asociated with the object that they are not supposed to think about. In his discussion of "synthetic obsessions," Wegner (1988) argues that stress can exacerbate all forms of suppression, as well as unsuccessful attempts to control them. Extrapolating from his findings, then, we would predict that low-level thinking would be the strategy of choice that individuals would adopt to try to ignore unwanted thoughts or environmental stimuli.

Finally, work in our own laboratory indicates that, under certain circumstances, individuals actively attempt to inhibit ongoing thoughts, emotions, or behaviors. In many cases, individuals have experienced a significant trauma or event (e.g., rape, marital infidelity, arrest) that they attempt to hide from others and, on occasion, from themselves. When they do this, we have found that they are prone to numerous stress-related illnesses (Pennebaker & Susman, 1988), insomnia (Pennebaker, 1985), and reports of physical symptoms (Pennebaker, 1989). Indeed, as Freud suggested, many of these individuals have become obsessed about their bodies, including overconcern with physical attractiveness, weight, and health in general (Pennebaker, 1982, Ch. 7). Uncontrollable or stressful life circumstances cause individuals to think on a relatively lower level.

THE BIOLOGICAL AND COGNITIVE CONSEQUENCES OF LEVELS OF THINKING

As suggested by both cognitive and motivational approaches, dynamic changes in levels of thinking during and following stressful periods can be highly adaptive. Whereas low-level thinking can distract individuals from aversive stimulation (cf. McCaul & Malott, 1984), high-level thinking allows for considering new and creative ways of avoiding the stress. Unfortunately, both low and high levels of thought can extract physical and cognitive costs. In this section, we examine the potential consequences of adopting chronic low- or high-level thinking strategies over extended periods of time.

The Costs and Benefits of Low-Level Thinking

If we adopt a low-level thinking strategy in order to avoid significant experiences, most motivational and biological researchers would agree that we continue to process those things that we are trying not to think about. This active inhibition process, then, should be apparent in studies that directly or indirectly study brain activity as well as global somatic and cognitive activity.

Brain Processes Reflecting Low-Level Thinking

A personality construct that is associated with low-level thinking is that of the "repressive coping style" (Weinberger, Schwartz, & Davidson, 1979).

The repressive coping style is defined by high scores on the Marlowe–Crowne Social Desirability Scale (Crowne & Marlowe, 1964) and low scores on anxiety scales such as the Taylor Manifest Anxiety Scale (MAS). Our own research on 80 college students (Pennebaker, Brumbelow, et al., 1987) indicates that chronic level of thinking is negatively correlated with the Marlowe–Crowne ($r = -.22$) and positively correlated with anxiety measures, such as the Minnesota Multiphasic Personality Inventory (MMPI) Psychasthenia scale ($r = .31$). In short, low-level thinking can be viewed as a feature of the repressive coping style.

A number of recent studies suggest that repressors process threatening information in a fundamentally different way than do nonrepressors. Davis and Schwartz (1987) argue that the repressive coping style is characterized by the independent processing of verbal and emotional information in the two hemispheres of the brain. For example, repressors recall and respond to emotional information more slowly than nonrepressors (Epstein & Fenz, 1967; Weinberger et al., 1979). Recent electroencephalographic (EEG) studies provide similar evidence to suggest poorer correspondence in processing verbal and negative emotions among individuals with repressive coping styles (cf. Davidson, 1984, 1986).

Generalizing from the literature on repressive coping style, we think that low-level thinking during threat or stress allows for the effective blocking of emotional information. That is, by adopting a low-level thinking strategy, the person effectively (and usually temporarily) excludes affective information from linguistic processing. If there is independent processing of verbal and affective information, we would expect overall greater processing levels in the brain. Furthermore, this artificial form of processing should place greater demands on the body. Indeed, in a recent review, Lane and Schwartz (1987) hypothesize that independent cortical processing, which may be associated with repressive coping styles, could lead to lateralized, or uneven, neural stimulation of the heart. This uneven cardiac stimulation, then, could increase the chance of cardiac arrhythmias and fatal heart attacks. Specifically, failing to integrate the emotional and verbal systems throws the body into a state of disregulation. Lane and Schwartz (1987) point to the fact that people with highly lateralized EEGs (particularly in the frontal regions of the brain) are more likely to have cardiac problems because of an overall breakdown in the normal feedback systems of the body.

Somatic Effects of Low-Level Thinking

Whereas our understanding of brain activity associated with low-level thinking is largely speculative, recent studies in our laboratory point to more verifiable effects of level of thinking during stressful times on the body. In this section, I first examine the effects of low-level thinking on autonomic activity and then consider its long-term effect on health and immune function.

An interesting paradox of low-level thinking is that it allows individuals to distract themselves from physical and psychological discomfort. A number of studies indicate that repressors and low-level thinkers report fewer negative emotions and physical symptoms, while at the same time exhibiting higher autonomic levels (e.g., Notarius & Levenson, 1979; Weinberger et al., 1979). In short, correlational studies such as these indicate that low-level thinking is associated with the separation of verbal and physiological indicators of discomfort.

In a series of recent studies, we have attempted to manipulate low- and high-level thinking while at the same time measuring skin conductance, which has been shown to be a sensitive measure of inhibition or conflict (Fowles, 1980). In two similar studies, for example, students were instructed to talk about the most traumatic and upsetting experiences of their lives, as well as their plans for the remainder of the day (Pennebaker, Hughes, & O'Heeron, 1987). In other words, we attempted to manipulate high- and low-level thinking.

A number of interesting effects obtained. First, we found that people differed tremendously in the degree to which they disclosed personal and emotional information. When asked to divulge traumatic experiences, some subjects merely recounted specific facts with no insight, emotion, or breadth (essentially low-level thinkers or low disclosers). The other half of the subjects (high-level thinkers or high disclosers) readily revealed their deepest emotions, were self-reflective, and adopted a broader perspective. These two groups were defined by independent judges who listened to the tapes of all of the subjects.

Overall, when high-level thinkers talked about traumatic experiences, their skin conductance levels were quite low. However, when they were forced to think in low-level ways (i.e., plans for the afternoon), their skin conductance levels greatly increased. For naturally high-level thinkers, then, moving to a low level of thinking was physiologically stressful. A very different picture emerged for the naturally low-level thinkers: When they were addressing traumatic experiences, their skin conductance levels were higher than when they were discussing their plans for the day. To summarize, extremely high-level thinking appears to be psychologically painful, but at the same time is associated with lower skin conductance levels. If the high-level thinker is distracted from these painful thoughts by moving to a lower level of thinking, he or she exhibits greater physiological stress as measured by skin conductance.

Similar long-term effects of manipulated level of thinking have been found for measures of immune function and illness. We (Pennebaker, Kiecolt-Glaser, & Glaser, 1988) required 50 undergraduates to write about traumatic experiences or trivial events for 20 minutes a day for 4 consecutive days. In addition to measures of cellular immune function, we also monitored autonomic activity and health center visits for illness from before to 6 weeks after the writing phase of the study. Overall, forcing individuals to confront traumatic experiences (i.e., high-level thinking) was associated with improvements in T-lymphocyte activity and reduced health center visits, relative to low-level thinking instructions. (For a discussion of several comparable studies, see Pennebaker [1989], and Pennebaker and Beall [1986]).

More impressive were the results of internal analyses of the 25 subjects who wrote about traumas. In this group, subjects were asked to report the degree to which they wrote about experiences that they had actively held back in telling others. Based on our previous work, we reasoned that actively holding back in telling others about traumatic experiences represented a form of inhibition. Futhermore, the act of holding back should force an overall lower level of thinking. In dividing the trauma subjects at the median, we learned that those who wrote about things about which they had been previously inhibited were benefited by the writing far more than any other group. Not only were their T-lymphocyte responses increased the most, but measures of blood pressure and heart rate dropped significantly by the 6-week follow-up.

Cognitive Effects of Low-Level Thinking

As suggested earlier, when individuals must process a great deal of information from a variety of sources, they tend to move toward a lower level of thinking. By definition, they are less able to carefully weigh and elaborate upon the various sources of information impinging on them. A significant cost of low-level thinking, then, would be that individuals would have greater difficulty in making sophisticated judgments about the world around them.

Recently, Gilbert, Krull, and Pelham (1988) have suggested that the work of inhibition associated with suppressing behaviors and thoughts impedes people's abilities to draw accurate inferences about the causes of the behaviors of others. In two experiments, the authors found that individuals who actively inhibited their own eye movements or feelings made simplistic dispositional attributions about a target person's behaviors, compared to individuals who did not inhibit movements or feelings. Those who had the additional cognitive work of inhibiting their own behaviors ignored the situational cues that were clearly influencing the target person. Note that Gilbert et al. (1988) did not directly manipulate or measure level of thinking. Rather, their manipulations probably induced differential thinking levels by forcing subjects either to monitor or not to monitor specific inhibition-relevant cues. (See also Bargh & Thein, 1985, for a discussion of a conceptually similar study with comparable results.)

In addition to social judgments, we can also examine cognitive deficits among individuals with major clinical disorders that suggest low-level thinking. One disorder that has recently gained notoriety, called "alexithymia" (Sifneos, 1983), is characterized by the inability to perceive or express emotions. Individuals with alexithymia often have distorted body images, are unable to produce vivid images in their minds, have difficulty juggling complex thoughts, and are low in creativity. Interestingly, several investigators view this disorder as stemming from active attempts to exclude upsetting thoughts about traumatic experiences from consciousness (e.g., Bonanno & Singer, 1987; Henry & Stephens, 1977). Alexithymia is particularly relevant to our understanding of low-level thinking, in that its sufferers are remarkably obsessive, lack the ability to be self-reflective, and, of course, are unaware of their own emotions.

Summary

In this section, I have inferred thinking levels rather freely. I have variously defined the occurrence of low-level thinking by dispositional measures of repressive coping styles, manipulated topics of conversation, active inhibition of behaviors and feelings, or clinical symptoms of alexithymia. According to this loose definition, chronic or long-term low-level thinking in the face of stress or trauma is particularly deleterious. Low-level thinking per se when an individual is not stressed may not have any serious consequences, however.

An important point that I wish to emphasize is that there is a recursive causal relation between level of thinking and biological activity. Just as low-level thinking can trigger biological changes in the brain and body, so too can biological changes affect level of thinking. Indeed, psychological stressors should normally influence thinking level and somatic activity. Adaptively, the individual must physically prepare to fight or flee massive stressors, which will affect the body's physiological preparation; at the same time, the individual attempts to diminish the psychological or physical harm that the stressor brings about to the organism by changing the level of thinking. In the following section, I briefly consider some of the implications of high-level thinking during times of stress.

The Costs and Benefits of High-Level Thinking

To this point, I have given the false impression that low-level thinking is generally unhealthy, while at the same time suggesting that high-level thinking is good. As might be expected, however, there can be drawbacks to maintaining a high level of thinking during stress for extended periods of time. In this section, I first point to some of the potential psychological dangers of extended high-level thinking and then evaluate health implications.

Psychological Costs of High-Level Thinking

Because high-level thinking is associated with a confrontational approach to upsetting experiences, it will by definition arouse psychological conflict and negative emotions. Individuals who actively think about recent losses or their uncontrollable predicaments should be more motivated to resolve them, or, if that fails, should be more susceptible to depression (see Epstein, 1983). Indeed, the state of depression could be viewed in some circumstances as an extended period of high-level thinking.

Two of the features of high-level thinking, self-reflection and awareness of emotion, have recently been examined by David Watson and his colleagues as part of a general personality constellation called "negative affectivity," or NA (Watson & Clark, 1984; Watson & Pennebaker, in press; Watson & Tellegen, 1985). NA is a broad dimension of subjective distress that subsumes aversive mood states, including anger, anxiety, guilt, fearfulness, and depression. According to Watson and Clark (1984), high-NA individuals are introspective, dwell on the negative sides of themselves and others, and experience significant levels of distress and dissatisfaction at all times and in any given situation. Trait NA is a central feature of many common psychological scales that tap anxiety, repression–sensitization, depression, physical symptom reporting, and neuroticism (see also Costa & McRae, 1987).

In our own work, my colleagues and I have found level-of-thinking scores to be consistently related to various NA markers. In the Pennebaker, Brumbelow, et al. (1987) study of 80 undergraduates, level of thinking was significantly correlated with high scores on the Beck Depression Inventory (Beck, Ward, Mendelson, Mock, & Erbaugh, 1961) ($r=.30$), the MMPI Psychasthenia scale ($r=.39$), and the Pennebaker Inventory of Limbic Languidness (PILL; Pennebaker, 1982), a general symptom-reporting inventory ($r=.31$). Similarly, in the laboratory confession study described earlier (Pennebaker, Hughes, & O'Heeron, 1987), judges' ratings of degree of disclosure (which is virtually identical to level of thinking) correlated positively with measures of cognitive anxiety ($r=.44$) and somatic anxiety ($r=.33$), as well as the MMPI Psychasthenia scale ($r=.34$).

Given the parallel between level of thinking and NA, it is clear that high-level thinking is not a psychologically pleasant state. If it occurs in response to a transient stressor, it could serve as a powerful motive to learn more about the cause of the stress and the development of effective ways to resolve it. If high levels of thinking become chronic, however, individuals could manifest signs of depression or despair, such as substance abuse or even suicide.

Health Implications of High-Level Thinking

Chronic high-level thinking, like high NA, is associated with subjective distress, complaining, and physical symptom reporting. However, the links between objective health measures and thinking levels are less clear-cut.

In a recent review of dozens of studies that we and others have conducted using NA measures, David Watson and I concluded that NA is associated with health complaints but not with objective health markers

(Watson & Pennebaker, in press). Even though high-NA individuals report physical symptoms to a higher degree than do low-NA persons, there is no evidence that they visit health facilities more, or that they have any chronic physiological disturbances associated with blood pressure, immune function, cholesterol levels, uric acid levels, metabolism, or other cardio-vascular, pulmonary, kidney, or central nervous system difficulties. Indeed, among adult samples, there are weak but significant trends indicating that high-NA persons have lower resting blood pressures and uric acid levels than low-NA individuals.

The only evidence that we currently have on level of thinking and self-reported objective health measures (e.g., health center visits for illness, as-pirin and alcohol use) comes from the stream-of-consciousness study of 80 undergraduates (Pennebaker, Brumbelow, et al., 1987). In one analysis, the level-of-thinking scores across modality and time were averaged to yield a measure of chronic thinking level. Subjects were divided into three levels of thinking. Those scoring in the top 15% and bottom 15% of the chronic thinking levels were deemed extremely high-level and extremely low-level thinkers, respectively. The remaining 70% were considered moderate-level thinkers. Using an orthogonal contrast method for analyses of variance, we partitioned the two degrees of freedom to compare the moderate-level thinkers with the two extreme groups (referred to as the "moderate-level effect" in Table 11.1), and to compare the high versus low thinkers (re-ferred to as the "extremes effect").

As can be seen in Table 11.1, extremely high-level and extremely low-level thinkers were similar in their reports of health center visits, aspirins taken per month, and alcoholic drinks consumed each week. Each of these variables was significantly greater than for the moderate-level thinkers. This pattern of effects was in marked contrast to that for the NA measures, which were linearly related to thinking level. Note that Table 11.1 also includes the simple correlations between thinking level and these variables, as well as some supplemental findings of interest. For our purposes, how-ever, the most important conclusion is that chronic high-level thinking, like chronic low-level thinking, appears to be objectively unhealthy.

Summary

High-level thinking during times of stress is associated with reports of dis-comfort and unhappiness. Dispositionally, there appears to be a close par-allel between thinking level and high NA, which is associated with chronic levels of subjective distress. At this point, the links between high thinking levels and health problems are unclear. The NA research suggests no major physiological consequences of high-level thinking. Our one study of ex-tremely high-level thinkers, on the other hand, indicated that they reported visiting the health center for illness with the same frequency as extremely low-level thinkers.

TABLE 11.1. Means and Correlations between Levels of Thinking and Selected Variables

| | Chronic thinking level | | | | |
Variable	Low	Moderate	High	Effect[a]	Correlation[b]
Objective health markers					
Health center illness visits	1.22	0.77	1.67	M	.09
Aspirins/month	6.7	4.1	7.7	M	.14
Alcoholic drinks/week	10.5	5.5	10.7	M	.12
Negative affect markers					
Beck Depression Inventory	25.7	25.4	30.6	E	.30**
PILL symptom report	17.3	16.5	27.0	M, E	.39**
MMPI Psychasthenia	8.6	9.0	11.4		.31**
Other variables of interest					
Maudsley Obsession–					
Compulsion	10.2	6.5	9.2	M	.04
Marlowe-Crowne	15.1	14.4	11.2		−.22*
Religious upbringing (%):					
Protestant	53.9	54.4	30.0		−.12
Catholic	36.1	15.0	50.4	M	.10
All other	10.0	30.6	19.6		.05
Age	18.3	18.1	17.7	E	−.36**
Sex (% females)	45.1	52.0	54.9		.08
n	11	48	10		

[a] M denotes a significant moderate-level effect—that is, a significant difference between moderate-level thinkers and the two extreme groups. E represents a significant extremes effect, where high- and low-level thinkers' means are significantly different from each other.
[b] Simple Pearson correlations between the level-of-thinking continuous variable and each variable.
* $p = .08$ (two-tailed test).
** $p \leq .01$ (two-tailed test).

SUMMARY AND IMPLICATIONS

In this chapter, I have explored how conscious thinking patterns change during periods of stress. Three dimensions of conscious thought—breadth of perspective, self-reflection, and awareness of emotion—collectively make up the concept of "level of thinking." Normally, when faced with transient uncontrollable stressors, individuals move to a lower level of thinking. This phenomenon reflects information-processing demands and motives to psychologically escape the stressor.

In the last section of the chapter, I have focused on the psychological and physiological costs of low and high thinking levels. Despite some minor inconsistencies, my colleagues and I believe that there are fundamentally different problems associated with high- and low-level thinking in general. During stress, low-level thinking serves as a method by which individuals distract themselves from the cause and emotional consequences of the stressor. The significant disadvantages of low-level thinking, however, are that individuals are less likely to understand and cognitively resolve the stressors. Furthermore, low levels of thought place an undue burden on information-processing capacity, which may require additional biological resources to cope with the stressors. Low-level thinking, then, serves as a psychological Band-Aid with potentially damaging physiological costs. High-level thinking, on the other hand, is helpful in directly dealing with and understanding stressors. Psychologically, however, high-level thinking is associated with greater subjective distress, unhappiness, and possibly depression. The physiological costs appear to be less extreme than those of low-level thinking.

ACKNOWLEDGMENTS

The preparation of this chapter was supported by grants from the National Science Foundation (No. BNS 8606764) and the National Heart, Lung and Blood Institute of the National Institute of Health (No. HL32547). I am indebted to John Bargh, Jonathon Brown, Bob Emmons, Dan Gilbert, Ellen Langer, Jerome L. Singer, Jim Uleman, David Watson, and Dan Wegner for their helpful comments about the manuscript.

REFERENCES

Antrobus, J. S., Singer, J. L., Goldstein, S., & Fortgang, M. (1970). Mindwandering and cognitive structure. *Transactions of the New York Academy of Sciences, 32,* 242–252.

Baars, B. J. (1985). Can involuntary slips of the tongue reveal one's state of mind? In T. M. Shlechter & M. P. Toglia (Eds.), *New directions in cognitive science* (pp. 242–260). Norwood, NJ: Ablex.

Bargh, J. A., & Thein, R. D. (1985). Individual construct accessibility, person memory, and the recall–judgement link: The case of information overload. *Journal of Personality and Social Psychology, 49,* 1129–1146.

Beck, A. T., Ward, C. H., Mendelson, M., Mock, J., & Erbaugh, J. (1961). An inventory for measuring depression. *Archives of General Psychiatry, 4,* 561–571.

Bonanno, G. A., & Singer, J. L. (1987). *Repressive personality style: Theoretical and methodological implications for health and pathology.* Unpublished manuscript, Yale University.

Carver, C., & Scheier, M. F. (1981). *Attention and self-regulation.* New York: Springer-Verlag.

Cohen, S. (1978). Environmental load and the allocation of attention. In A. Baum,

J. E. Singer, & S. Valins (Eds.), *Advances in environmental psychology* (Vol. 1, pp. 253–268). Hillsdale, NJ: Erlbaum.

Cohen, S., Evans, G. W., Krantz, D. S., & Stokols, D. (1980). Physiological, motivational, and cognitive effects of aircraft noise on children: Moving from the laboratory to the field. *American Psychologist, 35,* 231–243.

Costa, P. T., & McRae, R. R. (1987). Neuroticism, somatic complaints, and disease: Is the bark worse than the bite? *Journal of Personality, 55,* 299–316.

Crowne, D. P., & Marlowe, D. (1964). *The approval motive: Studies in evaluative dependence.* New York: Wiley.

Csikszentmihalyi, M., & Larson, R. (1984). *Being adolescent: Conflict and growth in the teenage years.* New York: Basic Books.

Davidson, R. J. (1980). Consciousness and information processing: A biocognitive perspective. In J. M. Davidson & R. J. Davidson (Eds.), *The psychobiology of consciousness* (pp. 11–46). New York: Plenum.

Davidson, R. J. (1984). Affect, cognition, and hemispheric specialization. In C. E. Izard, J. Kagan, & R. Zajonc (Eds.), *Emotion, cognition, and behavior.* New York: Cambridge University Press.

Davidson, R. J. (1986). *Hemispheric specialization and emotion.* Paper delivered at the meeting of the Society for Psychophysiological Research, Montreal.

Davis, P. J., & Schwartz, G. E. (1987). Repression and the inaccessibility of affective memories. *Journal of Personality and Social Psychology, 52,* 155–162.

Duval, S., & Wicklund, R. A. (1972). *A theory of objective self-awareness.* New York: Academic Press.

Easterbrook, J. A. (1959). The effect of emotion on cue utilization and organization of behavior. *Psychological Review, 66,* 183–201.

Epstein, S. (1983). Natural healing processes of the mind. In D. Meichenbaum & E. M. Jeremco (Eds.), *Stress reduction and prevention* (pp. 39–66). New York: Plenum.

Epstein, S., & Fenz, W. (1967). The detection of areas of emotional stress through variations in perceptual threshold and physiological arousal. *Journal of Experimental Research in Personality, 2,* 191–199.

Fowles, D. C. (1980). The three arousal model: Implications of Gray's two-factor theory for heart rate, electrodermal activity, and psychopathy. *Psychophysiology, 17,* 87–104.

Frankenhaeuser, M. (1971). Behavior and circulating catecholamines. *Brain Research, 31,* 241–262.

Freud, S. (1960). The psychopathology of everyday life. In J. Strachey (Ed. and Trans.), *The standard edition of the complete psychological works of Sigmund Freud* (Vol. 6, pp. 1–310). London: Hogarth Press. (Original work published 1901)

Freud, S. (1963). Repression. In P. Rieff (Ed.), *General psychological theory* (pp. 104–115). New York: Collier. (Original work published 1915)

Freud, S. (1959). Inhibitions, symptoms and anxiety. In J. Strachey (Ed. and Trans.), *The standard edition of the complete psychological works of Sigmund Freud* (Vol. 20, pp. 77–174). London: Hogarth Press. (Original work published 1926)

Gilbert, D. T., Krull, D. S., & Pelham, B. W. (1987). *Of thoughts unspoken: Behavioral inhibition and social inference.* Unpublished manuscript, University of Texas at Austin.

Glass, D. C., & Singer, J. E. (1972). *Urban stress.* New York: Academic Press.

Graham, D. T. (1972). Psychosomatic medicine. In N. Greenfield & R. Sternbach (Eds.), *Handbook of psychophysiology* (pp. 839–926). New York: Holt, Rinehart & Winston.

Henry, J. P., & Stephens, P. M. (1977). *Stress, health, and the social environment.* New York: Springer-Verlag.

Horowitz, M. J. (1976). *Stress response syndromes.* New York: Jason Aronson.

James, W. (1890). *The principles of psychology* (Vol. 1). New York: Henry Holt.

Kiecolt-Glaser, J., & Glaser, R. (1988). Behavioral influences on immune function: Evidence for the interplay between stress and health. In T. Field, P. McCabe, & N. Schneiderman (Eds.), *Stress and coping* (Vol. 2). Hillsdale, NJ: Erlbaum.

Klinger, E. (1978). Modes of normal conscious flow. In K. S. Pope & J. L. Singer (Eds.), *The stream of consciousness.* New York: Plenum.

Klos, D. S., & Singer, J. L. (1981). Determinants of the adolescent's ongoing thought following simulated parental confrontation. *Journal of Personality and Social Psychology, 41,* 975–987.

Langer, E. J. (1987). *Mindlessness/mindfulness.* Reading, MA: Addison-Wesley.

Lane, R. D., & Schwartz, G. E. (1987). Induction of lateralized sympathetic input to the heart by the CNS during emotional arousal: A possible neurophysiological trigger of sudden cardiac death. *Psychosomatic Medicine, 49,* 274–284.

Lazarus, R., & Folkman, S. (1984). *Stress, appraisal, and coping.* New York: Springer.

Linville, P. W. (1987). Self-complexity as a cognitive buffer against stress-related illness and depression. *Journal of Personality and Social Psychology, 52,* 663–676.

Luria, A. R. (1980). *Higher cortical functions in man.* New York: Basic Books.

McCaul, K. D., & Malott, J. M. (1984). Distraction and coping with pain. *Psychological Bulletin, 95,* 516–533.

Motley, M. T., Camden, C. T., & Baars, B. J. (1979). Personality and situational influences upon verbal slips. *Human Communication Research, 5,* 195–202.

Notarius, C. I., & Levenson, R. W. (1979). Expressive tendencies and physiological response to stress. *Journal of Personality and Social Psychology, 37,* 1204–1210.

Obrist, P. A. (1981). *Cardiovascular psychophysiology: A perspective.* New York: Plenum.

Pennebaker, J. W. (1982). *The psychology of physical symptoms.* New York: Springer-Verlag.

Pennebaker, J. W. (1985). Traumatic experience and psychosomatic disease: Exploring the roles of behavioral inhibition, obsession, and confiding. *Canadian Psychology, 26,* 82–95.

Pennebaker, J. W. (1989). Confession, inhibition, and disease. In L. Berkowitz (Ed.), *Advances in experimental social psychology* (Vol. 22, pp. 211–243). New York: Academic Press.

Pennebaker, J. W., & Beall, S. K. (1986). Confronting a traumatic event: Toward an understanding of inhibition and disease. *Journal of Abnormal Psychology, 95,* 274–281.

Pennebaker, J. W., & Brittingham, G. (1982). Environmental and sensory cues affecting the perception of physical symptoms. In A. Baum & J. E. Singer (Eds.), *Advances in environmental psychology* (Vol. 4, pp. 115–136). Hillsdale, NJ: Erlbaum.

Pennebaker, J. W., Brumbelow, S., Cropanzano, R., Czajka, J., Ferrara, K., Thompson, R., & Thyssen, T. (1987). *Levels of thinking*. Unpublished manuscript, Southern Methodist University.

Pennebaker, J. W., Hughes, C., & O'Heeron, R. C. (1987). The psychophysiology of confession: Linking inhibitory and psychosomatic processes. *Journal of Personality and Social Psychology, 52*, 781–793.

Pennebaker, J. W., Kiecolt-Glaser, J. K., & Glaser, R. (1988). Disclosure of traumas and immune function: Health implications for psychotherapy. *Journal of Consulting and Clinical Psychology, 56*, 239–245.

Pennebaker, J. W., & Newtson, D. (1983). Observation of a unique event: The psychological impact of Mt. St. Helens volcano. In H. T. Reiss (Ed.), *Naturalistic approaches to studying social interaction* (pp. 93–110). San Francisco: Jossey-Bass.

Pennebaker, J. W., & O'Heeron, R. C. (1984). Confiding in others and illness rate among spouses of suicide and accidental death victims. *Journal of Abnormal Psychology, 93*, 473–476.

Pennebaker, J. W., & Susman, J. R. (1988). Disclosure of traumas and psychosomatic processes. *Social Science and Medicine, 26*, 327–332.

Pope, K. S., & Singer, J. L. (Eds.). (1978). *The stream of consciousness*. New York: Plenum.

Pribram, K. H. (1976). Self-consciousness and intentionality. In G. E. Schwartz & D. Shapiro (Eds.), *Consciousness and self-regulation* (Vol. 1). New York: Plenum.

Rachman, S. (1980). Emotional processing. *Behaviour Research and Therapy, 18*, 51–60.

Ross, B. H. (1984). Remindings and their effects in learning a cognitive skill. *Cognitive Psychology, 16*, 371–416.

Rossi, E. L. (1986). *The psychobiology of mind-body healing*. New York: Norton.

Schank, R. C. (1982). *Dynamic memory: A theory of reminding in computers and people*. Cambridge, England: Cambridge University Press.

Schwartz, G. E. (1983). Disregulation theory and disease: Applications to the repression/cerebral disconnection/cardiovascular disorder hypothesis. *International Review of Applied Psychology, 32*, 95–118.

Scurfield, R. M. (1985). Post-trauma stress assessment and treatment. In C. R. Figley (Ed.), *Trauma and its wake* (pp. 219–256). New York: Brunner/Mazel.

Selye, H. (1976). *The stress of life*. New York: McGraw-Hill.

Sifneos, P. E. (1983). Psychotherapies for psychosomatic and alexithymic patients. *Psychotherapy and Psychosomatics, 40*, 66–73.

Singer, J. L. (1975). *The inner world of daydreaming*. New York: Harper & Row.

Singer, J. L. (1984). The private personality. *Personality and Social Psychology Bulletin, 10*, 7–30.

Teichman, Y. (1966). The stress of coping with the unknown regarding a significant family member. In I. G. Sarason & C. D. Spielberger (Eds.), *Stress and anxiety* (Vol. 2, pp. 243–255). New York: Wiley.

Vallacher, R. R., & Wegner, D. M. (1985). *A theory of action identification*. Hillsdale, NJ: Erlbaum.

Walster, B., & Aronson, E. (1967). Effect of expectancy of task duration on the experience of fatigue. *Journal of Experimental Social Psychology, 3*, 41–46.

Watson, D., & Clark, L. A. (1984). Negative affectivity: The disposition to experience aversive emotional states. *Psychological Bulletin, 96*, 465–490.

Watson, D., & Pennebaker, J. W. (in press). Health complaints, stress, and distress: Exploring the central role of negative affectivity. *Psychological Review.*

Watson, D., & Tellegen, A. (1985). Toward a consensual structure of mood. *Psychological Bulletin, 98,* 219–235.

Wegner, D. M. (1988). Stress and mental control. In S. Fisher & J. Reason (Eds.), *Handbook of life stress, cognition, and health* (pp. 683–698). Chichester, England: Wiley.

Wegner, D. M., Schneider, D. J., Carter, S. R., & White, T. L. (1987). Paradoxical effects of thought suppression. *Journal of Personality and Social Psychology, 53,* 5–13.

Weinberger, D. A., Schwartz, G. E., & Davidson, R. J. (1979). Low-anxious, high-anxious, and repressive coping styles: Psychometric patterns and behavioral and physiological responses to stress. *Journal of Abnormal Psychology, 88,* 369–380.

Wicklund, R. A. (1975). Objective self-awareness. In L. Berkowitz (Ed.), *Advances in experimental social psychology* (Vol. 8, pp. 233–275). New York: Academic Press.

Witkin, H. A., Goodenough, D. R., & Oltman, P. K. (1979). Psychological differentiation: Current status. *Journal of Personality and Social Psychology, 37,* 1127–1145.

Wyer, R. S., & Srull, T. K. (1986). Human cognition in its social context. *Psychological Review, 93,* 322–359.

12

Coming to Terms with Major Negative Life Events

ROSEMARY TAIT
ROXANE COHEN SILVER
University of Waterloo

Remember Terry Howard? He's the University of Louisville guard who had made 28 of 28 free throws before going to the line in the final seconds of the NCAA Final Four game against UCLA in 1974–75. He missed the front end of a one-on-one, letting UCLA off the hook, and Louisville lost in overtime.

Asked not long ago if he ever thought of that fateful night, Howard said, "Every day of the week."

Now listen to Abel Kiviat, silver medalist in the Olympic 1,500 meters in 1912 at Stockholm. Kiviat had the race won until Britain's Arnold Jackson came from nowhere to beat him by one-tenth of a second.

Kiviat: "I wake up sometimes and say, 'What the heck happened to me?' It's like a nightmare."

Kiviat is 91 years old.

Los Angeles Times, January 15, 1984[1]

People experience a variety of negative life events over the course of their lives. No one is immune to their occurrence, and the longer the lifespan, the greater the number of undesirable events one is likely to encounter. It is also popularly assumed in our society that "Time heals all wounds," and that psychological recovery will occur within a relatively brief period of time (Silver & Wortman, 1980). However, an increasing body of research evidence is calling these assumptions into question (see Silver & Wortman, 1980; Tait & Silver, 1989; Wortman & Silver, 1987, for re-

351

views of this literature). In fact, evidence has begun to accumulate indicating that the psychological impact of negative life events may persist for many years for a significant proportion of the population.

Although theoretical and empirical attention devoted to the long-term effects of negative life events has increased steadily over the past few decades, no comprehensive view has yet emerged of the nature, prevalence, or chronicity of their psychological impact. In fact, the extent to which persistent effects can be seen as abnormal or normative consequences of these events remains unclear. However, one of the major impediments to the development of a model to predict or explain the long-term psychological impact of negative life events has been the wide range of interindividual variability in responses to a similar type of event (cf. Silver & Wortman, 1980; Wortman & Silver, 1987, 1989). The fact that people respond so differently to the same type of event suggests that the type of event per se may be less relevant to psychological impact and its persistence than are factors that influence how the event is experienced. In this chapter, we first describe the ways in which we feel major negative life events may continue to have an impact on those who encounter them. We then describe in some detail a study we recently conducted to examine the long-term impact of undesirable life experiences (Tait & Silver, 1989). Finally, we consider a number of situational, psychological, and social factors that may contribute to individuals' continuing cognitive and emotional involvement in the major events of their lives.

A GENERAL MEASURE OF IMPACT: EVENT-RELATED RUMINATIONS

Much of the past research on the psychological effects of negative life events has been concerned with clinical or dysfunctional levels of emotional impact. In contrast, our work has focused on a more subtle form of impact, which is believed to constitute a relatively common pattern of response to these events, at least over the short term. Previous work has pointed to a tendency among those who have undergone major negative events to experience involuntary, intrusive, and distressing ruminations (i.e., thoughts, memories, and/or mental images related to the event; see Silver, Wortman, & Klos, 1982). Horowitz (1975) has described such ruminations as a general stress response tendency. Their occurrence has been documented across different nonclinical populations with varying predispositions; following low, moderate, and high levels of stress; and for both natural and contrived stressors (see Horowitz, 1976, 1982, and Wegner, 1988, for reviews of this work). The experience of these ruminations tends to be correlated positively with the degree of reported stress and with levels of negative affect, and inversely related to indices of positive emotion (Horowitz,

1975). Though less extreme, the general stress response tendency is similar in many respects to the intrusive element of Posttraumatic Stress Disorder (PTSD), as observed clinically and described in the *Diagnostic and Statistical Manual of Mental Disorders,* third edition (DSM-III; American Psychiatric Association, 1980). PTSD may persist for extended time periods (see, e.g., Brende & Parson, 1985; Horowitz, Wilner, Kaltreider, & Alvarez, 1980); however, with few exceptions (e.g., Lehman, Wortman, & Williams, 1987; Silver, Boon, & Stones, 1983), the general stress response has tended to be examined only over the short term. We believe that continuing ruminations about major stressful events constitute a rich but largely untapped source of information about the psychological aftereffects of negative life experiences.

Event-Related Ruminations and the Process of Recovery

Event-related ruminations have been linked to the Freudian theory of the compulsive repetition of reminiscences subsequent to traumatic events (see, e.g., Horowitz, 1979). In clinical investigations, Breuer and Freud (1895/1955) considered them to be hysterical symptoms precipitated by a traumatic event or series of events, and noted in particular the inordinate length of time they may persist. Breuer and Freud interpreted this persistence as symptomatic of an event that has not been sufficiently "abreacted" or discharged, due either to the nature of the event itself or to the psychological state of the individual confronted with it.

Although event-related ruminations of the type described by Horowitz and his colleagues occur involuntarily, they are believed to play an integral role in the "working through" or processing of a negative life event whereby an individual gradually comes to terms with it (Horowitz, 1976, 1985; Janis, 1971; Parkes, 1972; Silver et al., 1983). It is hypothesized that the occurrence of these ruminations, in alternation with periods of denial, allows the individual to come gradually to tolerate increasing doses of distressing aspects of the event. Event-related ruminations are believed to diminish over time as the event is worked through or resolved. Distressing ruminations are seen as falling within normal limits when they occur and subside within a relatively brief period of time following a disturbing event (Horowitz, 1985; Parkinson & Rachman, 1981a, 1981b, 1981c; Rachman, 1979, 1981); the persistence or recurrence of these ruminations is regarded as "the central, indispensable index of unsatisfactory . . . processing" (Rachman, 1979, p. 51).

However, the nature of this "working-through" process is unclear. Horowitz (1975) describes a cognitive process, involving "matching and integrating . . . new or massive information about the self or world," including "the assessment of the meaning, interpretations and implications of [the] incoming information" (p. 1462). Rachman (1979) favors an emotional-processing view, whereby "emotional disturbances are absorbed, and decline to the extent that other experiences and behavior can proceed without disruption" (p. 51). It seems most probable that cognitions and emotions are equally essential, and that the working-through process involves a dynamic interplay between them. Thus, thoughts, memories, or mental images related to a negative life event may elicit certain types of affect (Folkman, Schaefer, & Lazarus, 1979; Lazarus, Kanner, & Folkman, 1980; Singer, 1978), and certain moods or feelings may evoke event-related ruminations (e.g., Bower, 1981; Clark & Isen, 1982; Snyder & White, 1982; Wenzlaff, Wegner, & Roper, 1988; Zajonc, 1980). The general measure of psychological impact adopted in our work—the experience of involuntary, intense, intrusive, and distressing ruminations related to a negative life event—addresses the extent of ongoing cognitive and emotional involvement with an event's occurrence.

TRIGGERS OF ONGOING COGNITIVE AND EMOTIONAL INVOLVEMENT IN EVENTS

The literature has suggested three factors that may be particularly relevant to understanding reasons for the persistence of psychological impact over time. They include the ongoing implications of the event (i.e., changes in life circumstances brought about by its occurrence); the need to interpret or appraise the meaning or personal significance of the event; and social responses to the occurrence of the event and/or to the expression of event-related difficulties or distress. Each of these is considered in turn below.

The Ongoing Implications

The occurrence of a major negative event may engender changes in an individual's life circumstances (e.g., alterations in social roles and/or relationships) or in related considerations (e.g., finances, environment). Studies by Pearlin and his colleagues (see, e.g., Pearlin, 1983; Pearlin & Lieberman, 1979; Pearlin, Lieberman, Menaghan, & Mullan, 1981) have demonstrated the importance of these changes as possible enduring sources of strain. This work suggests that the psychological impact of major negative events is largely channeled through the persistent situational difficulties that may follow them (see also Antonovsky, 1982; Parkes, 1971; Thoits, 1983; Vachon et al., 1982). From this perspective, the negative implications of an event can be seen as referring to the loss of important aspects of the past—that is, of life prior to the event's occurrence.

However, the negative implications of an event may also include the loss of important aspects of the future. For example, an event's occurrence may preclude the realization of plans, possibilities, or aspirations in which an individual may be heavily invested (cf. Carr, 1975; Neugarten, 1979; Parkes, 1971; see, e.g., Kaltreider, Wallace, & Horowitz, 1979; Szybist,

1978). Although they cannot be considered aspects of one's actual life circumstances at the time of an event's occurrence, the preclusion of these
possibilities may nonetheless represent a significant loss.

The ongoing negative implications of an event may differ widely in
both nature and salience even among individuals confronting the same type
of event, and may be experienced as part and parcel of an event's occurrence. We believe that they constitute an integral aspect of the experience
of an event, and that without consideration of their implications, the psychological impact of an event can only partially be understood. In addition
to coming to terms with the event itself, one must also come to terms with
these implications. As long as they are salient and problematic, cognitive
and emotional involvement in the event may persist. The continuing salience of an event's negative implications may be represented by ongoing
unfavorable comparisons between aspects of one's life given the event's
occurrence, and life as it might have been had the negative event not occurred (cf. Glick, Weiss, & Parkes, 1974; Kahneman & Tversky, 1982).

The Need to Find Meaning

Meaning has been described as the crucial organizing principle of human
behavior (Marris, 1986). The need to find meaning in events—that is, to
construe their personal significance in cognitive and affective terms—has
been proposed as a fundamental and universal motive (see, e.g., Frankl,
1963; Marris, 1986). The search for a meaningful perspective of, or rationale for, the occurrence of a negative life event is believed to play an integral role in the process of adjustment (Benner, Roskies, & Lazarus, 1980;
Bulman & Wortman, 1977; Moos & Tsu, 1977; Silver et al., 1983; Taylor, 1983). Since individuals respond not to events in and of themselves,
but to their interpretations of events (cf. Beck, 1975; Epstein, 1983, in
press; Frankl, 1963; Kelly, 1955; Lazarus & Folkman, 1984; Parkes &
Weiss, 1983), we believe that the ability to find meaning in an event plays
a key role in influencing psychological impact and the process of recovery.
Moreover, meaning must also be found in an event's negative implications—that is, in life given its occurrence (see also Epstein, in press; Frankl,
1963). Thus, thoughts about an event's ongoing implications may be related to a continuing search for meaning in the event. When a meaningful
and acceptable interpretation is not forthcoming, the search may persist
for extended time periods, contributing to ongoing cognitive and emotional involvement in the event. A persistent search for meaning has been
found to be inversely related to psychological recovery and positively related to the occurrence of involuntary, intrusive, and distressing event-related ruminations (Silver et al., 1983).

Social Responses to the Need for Discussion

Individuals confronting major negative events frequently report feeling a
need to discuss the event or their responses to it with others (Coates &

Wortman, 1980; Coates, Wortman, & Abbey, 1979; Dunkel-Schetter & Wortman, 1981, 1982; Silver & Wortman, 1980; Wortman & Dunkel-Schetter, 1979). The persistence of such a need has been described as a direct sign of incomplete processing of the event (Rachman, 1979). There is some evidence that ruminating about an event and discussing its occurrence or related concerns with others may represent personal and social aspects of the same process of "working through" the event (Pennebaker & O'Heeron, 1984; see also Breuer & Freud, 1895/1955). Thus, a persistent need for discussion may be related to the continuing salience of an event's negative implications, and/or to an ongoing search for meaning in the event's occurrence.

When an ongoing need for discussion is met by a supportive environment, adjustment or acceptance may be facilitated in a number of ways (cf. Silver & Wortman, 1980). For example, free discussion may allow a cathartic discharge of emotion. Even in the absence of such a discharge, the act of putting the experience into words may provide useful insight or increase one's sense of control (cf. Pennebaker, 1989; Pennebaker & Hoover, 1985). Most importantly, perhaps, confiding in others about the event or related concerns or difficulties can serve to clarify and convey relevant coping needs. This may increase the probability that the support provided will be appropriate to these needs, and therefore effective (cf. Thoits, 1985; Wortman & Lehman, 1985).

However, the literature suggests that the need for discussion may frequently go unmet (see, e.g., Dunkel-Schetter & Wortman, 1982, for a review of this literature). In these cases, cognitive and emotional involvement in the event may continue. Moreover, it appears that social responses to the expression of event-related difficulties or distress are often negative (e.g., derogation and rejection; see Coates et al., 1979; Lazarus, 1985; Strack & Coyne, 1983). We would expect this to be particularly the case when these expressions persist over or after extended time periods (see, e.g., Coyne, 1976a, 1976b). We believe that the dynamics of the social situation that arise when continuing distress is communicated may not only fail to facilitate the process of recovery, but may also enhance the difficulty of that process. That is, the individual who consults a friend, relative, or colleague about one event-related problem may find himself or herself returning from the interaction with two problems.

In short, persistent thoughts about an event's negative implications, involvement in a continuing search for meaning, and feeling a need to discuss the event or related concerns or difficulties with others can all be seen as aspects of ongoing cognitive and emotional involvement with an event's occurrence. We believe that each of these responses reflects a particular dimension of the experience of a major negative event—situational, psychological, and social—that may account for continuing difficulties in coming to terms with it. We also see these responses as likely to be dynamic, transactional, and reciprocal in nature.

Recently, we have made an initial attempt to explore some of these issues in the context of a study of the long-term impact of stressful life events. In this research (Tait & Silver, 1989), we chose to examine the prevalence of the aforementioned responses and of persistent ruminations across a number of different types of major negative life events—"major" not according to any predetermined or objective criteria, but in terms of our respondents' subjective, relative assessments. Given our interest in time as a factor potentially related to impact and recovery, we also chose to examine effects across a wide range of time periods since an event's occurrence. Finally, we chose to assess long-term psychological effects among a group of people who continue to function more or less successfully in their day-to-day social roles. With these purposes in mind, we approached senior citizens residing in the community for our study (Tait & Silver, 1989). We assumed that respondents aged 60 and over would have experienced a variety of negative life events, one of which would be perceived by each individual as his or her "most negative event," providing us with a wide range of types of major negative events and of time periods elapsed since their occurrence.

THE STUDY

In our study, we sought to explore the association between our measures of continuing impact and subjects' self-assessed recovery from their most negative event, their overall level of life satisfaction, and the number of years that had passed since the event's occurrence. Potential respondents were contacted initially by means of a letter describing our research as an investigation of the long-term impact of major life events (see Tait & Silver, 1989, for a more detailed discussion). Structured interviews were conducted in respondents' homes, lasting an average of 2 hours. The interview consisted of a series of open- and closed-ended questions, many of which were developed for the particular purposes of our research.

Following completion of a measure of psychological well-being (Neugarten, Havighurst, & Tobin, 1961), respondents were asked to describe the negative events they had experienced over the course of their lives, and to state when each event had occurred. From this list, subjects were asked to select the particular event they considered to have been "the worst thing that had ever happened" to them. The questions that followed focused on the ongoing psychological effects of this particular event.

Closed-ended questions assessed the general frequency of ruminations about the most negative event and the frequency of deliberate event-related ruminations, as well as the frequency, intensity, and intrusiveness of involuntary ruminations and the kinds of affect associated with their occurrence. Closed-ended questions were also used to assess the persistence of thoughts about the event's negative implications, involvement in a continuing search for meaning in the event's occurrence, and an ongoing need to discuss the event or one's responses to it with others. Open-ended questions explored the content of ongoing event-related ruminations.

The 45 respondents who met our eligibility requirements ranged in age from 60 to 93; the mean age of the final sample was 76. The gender composition of the sample was 76% female and 24% male. The various types of major events reported by our respondents included the death of a spouse, other family member or friend; desertion by a spouse; health problems; and the like (see Tait & Silver, 1989, for a more detailed discussion). The average time period that had elapsed since the occurrence of these events was 22.8 years; the range was from 2 to 50 years.

Thematic Content of Typical Event-Related Ruminations

For the purposes of our research, event-related ruminations were described to respondents as "thoughts, mental images, or memories related to the [reported most negative] event or to the person or people associated with it." Respondents' descriptions of "typical" event-related ruminations were assessed for thematic content. Rumination themes fell into three major categories. Forty-nine percent of these ruminations centered on the event itself. This type of rumination is exemplified by the following, in which a widow of 10 years described a rumination related to her husband's death:

> When he was in the hospital, I used to visit him every night. The week before he died, he said, "We have to talk." I said, "Why?" He said, "Because I'm going to die." I said, "Don't talk silly." I didn't let him speak. I always wonder what he would have said if I had let him talk.

Twenty-one percent of the ruminations described referred to aspects of life prior to the event that had changed as a result of its occurrence. An illustration of this type of rumination is provided in the following statement, in which a widow of 7 years described ongoing ruminations about her deceased spouse:

> I think about him every day. I never go to bed at night without thinking of him before I settle down. We'd go out together a lot, go for walks. We'd usually talk together for an hour before going to sleep.

Nine percent of the typical ruminations reported focused on aspects of life at present that might have been different had the event not occurred. Exemplifying this type of rumination is the following statement by a respondent who had lost his only child in an automobile accident 20 years earlier:

If she was living, it'd give me something to get out of life—I'd have her, and grandchildren, which would mean a lot to me.

The remaining 21% of the ruminations described by our respondents involved a combination of two of these three themes.

Characteristics of Event-Related Ruminations

A number of aspects of event-related ruminations were examined in our study, including the general frequency of ruminations related to the given event and the frequency of deliberate ruminations about it. Of particular interest, however, were the frequency, intensity, and intrusiveness of involuntary ruminations related to the respondent's most negative event. Each of the latter three characteristics was tapped by two separate items, which are described below. Table 12.1 presents a breakdown of subjects' responses to each of these questions.

TABLE 12.1. Characteristics of Event-Related Ruminations: Percentage of Sample Reporting in Each Response Category

Frequency	Never	Rarely	Sometimes	Frequently	All the time
General	4	24	47	20	4
Deliberate	83	5	10	2	—
Involuntary					
Thinking without meaning to	19	24	41	12	5
Thoughts "pop into mind"	9	33	33	23	2

Intensity	Not at all	Just a little	Somewhat	Quite a bit	A great deal
How "real," vivid, clear	2	14	19	35	30
How absorbing, involving	21	33	26	14	7

Intrusiveness	Never	Rarely	Sometimes	Frequently	All the time
Difficulty dispelling	63	16	12	9	—
Trouble doing other things	84	2	7	7	—

Note. Adapted from *The Long-Term Psychological Impact of Major Negative Life Events* by R. Tait and R. C. Silver, 1989, manuscript submitted for publication. Adapted by permission of the authors.

General Frequency of Ruminations

An average of 22.8 years following their most stressful experience, 71% of our sample reported that they continued to experience thoughts, memories, and/or mental images related to their most negative event at least sometimes. This percentage included 47% who sometimes had ruminations about the experience, 20% who ruminated frequently, and 4% for whom these ruminations occurred all the time. Only 4% of the sample reported never experiencing ruminations about their most negative life event. The frequency of event-related ruminations in general was inversely related to both self-assessed recovery from the event, r (40) $= -.51$, $p \leq .001$, and current life satisfaction, r (41) $= -.48$, $p \leq .001$, but was not significantly related to the number of years that had passed since the event occurred.

Frequency of Deliberate Thoughts, Memories, or Mental Images

Deliberate thoughts, memories, or mental images related to the most negative event were relatively infrequent: 12% of the sample reported intentionally ruminating about the event at least sometimes; 83% reported never doing so. The frequency of deliberate thoughts, memories, or mental images was not related significantly to the frequency of involuntary event-related ruminations. In addition, no significant relations emerged between deliberate ruminations and self-assessed recovery, current life satisfaction, or the number of years elapsed since the occurrence of the event.

Frequency of Involuntary Ruminations

Two questions examined the frequency of involuntary event-related ruminations. Fifty-seven percent of the sample reported at least sometimes finding themselves ruminating about the event without really meaning to, including 12% for whom this happened frequently and 5% for whom these ruminations occurred all the time. Fifty-eight percent of respondents reported that thoughts, memories, and/or mental images related to the event "popped into" their minds at least sometimes, including 23% for whom this occurred frequently, and 2% for whom this happened all the time.

These two items were significantly related, r (40) $= .33$, $p < .05$, and were combined into an index representing the frequency of involuntary event-related ruminations. This index was negatively correlated with both self-assessed recovery from the event, r (39) $= -.51$, $p \leq .001$, and current life satisfaction, r (40) $= -.56$, $p < .001$. No significant association emerged between the frequency of involuntary ruminations and the amount of time that had passed since the event's occurrence.

The Intensity of Ongoing Ruminations: Vividness and Absorption

The intensity of event-related ruminations was conceptualized as involving two components: their perceived vividness or clarity, and the extent to which the individual reported becoming absorbed or "caught up" in them.

Eighty-four percent of the sample described their ruminations as at least somewhat clear or vivid, including 35% who described them as quite vivid and 30% who reported them as extremely vivid. Forty-seven percent of the sample reported becoming at least somewhat caught up or absorbed in them, including 14% who became quite absorbed and 7% who became extremely absorbed.

The perceived clarity of and absorption in these ruminations were significantly related, $r(41) = .53$, $p < .001$, and were combined into an index of intensity. This index was inversely related to both self-assessed recovery from the event, $r(41) = -.45$, $p < .01$, and current life satisfaction, $r(41) = -.33$, $p < .05$. However, the intensity of event-related ruminations was not significantly related to the number of years that had elapsed since the event's occurrence.

Intrusiveness: Difficulty Dispelling Ruminations and Interference with Other Activities

Intrusiveness was assessed through the use of two items examining respondents' perceived difficulty in dispelling ongoing event-related ruminations and the degree of interference with other activities that was experienced when they occurred. Twenty-one percent of the sample reported at least sometimes having difficulty dispelling event-related ruminations, including 9% for whom this difficulty occurred frequently. Fourteen percent reported at least sometimes having trouble engaging in other activities when these ruminations occurred, including 7% for whom this was frequently the case. Difficulty in dispelling ruminations and in engaging in other activities when they occurred were significantly related, $r(41) = .58$, $p < .001$, and were combined into an index of intrusiveness. This index was only marginally related to self-assessed recovery, $r(40) = -.27$, $p = .08$, but was negatively related to current life satisfaction, $r(41) = -.50$, $p \le .001$. The intrusiveness of ongoing ruminations was, however, unrelated to the amount of time that had passed since the event.

Types of Affect Associated with Event-Related Ruminations

Six closed-ended questions assessed the frequency of a variety of emotions experienced in conjunction with ruminations related to the most negative event. The specific types of affect examined included feelings of sadness, upset, anger, and anxiety, as well as feelings of happiness and of being "at peace." For 67% of the sample, feelings of sadness were at least sometimes associated with event-related ruminations, including 10% for whom sadness occurred frequently and 19% who always felt sad when these ruminations occurred. Thirty percent of respondents reported finding these ruminations upsetting at least sometimes, including 7% who were frequently upset and 9% who were always upset. Smaller proportions of our sample reported that feelings of anger and anxiety at least sometimes accompanied these ruminations (17% and 21%, respectively).

These four emotions (sadness, upset, anger, anxiety) were significantly interrelated (Cronbach's alpha for interitem reliability = .73), and were combined into an index representing general distress. This index was inversely related to both self-assessed recovery, r (40) = −.52, $p<.001$, and current life satisfaction, r (41) = −.57, $p<.001$, but was unrelated to the amount of time that had passed since the event.

Sixty-two percent of the sample reported that feelings of happiness were at least sometimes associated with event-related ruminations, including 7% who reported feeling happy frequently and 19% who always felt happy when these ruminations occurred. Seventy-two percent reported at least sometimes feeling "at peace" (26% frequently, 31% always). Feelings of happiness and feeling "at peace" were positively related, r (40) = .26, $p = .05$, and these two items were combined into an index representing the degree to which ruminations were associated with positive emotions. This index was positively related to both self-assessed recovery, r (40) = .39, $p \le .01$, and current life satisfaction, r (41) = .30, $p \le .05$. It was also inversely related to the number of years that had elapsed since the event, r (41) = −.38, $p \le .01$.

Additional Dimensions of Ongoing Cognitive and Emotional Involvement

Thirty-nine percent of our sample at least sometimes found themselves thinking about ways in which life might have been different had the event not occurred. Thirty-seven percent of the sample reported still searching at least sometimes for a meaningful perspective from which to view their most negative life event. Twenty-one percent frequently or always felt a need to discuss the event or their responses to it with others. These three variables were positively interrelated and were combined into an index representing aspects of ongoing cognitive and emotional involvement with the given event.

This index of ongoing involvement was negatively related to both self-assessed recovery from the event, r (39) = −.41, $p<.01$, and current life satisfaction, r (40) = −.48, $p<.01$, but was unrelated to the number of years that had passed since the event's occurrence. This index was positively related to the frequency of involuntary event-related ruminations, r (39) = .45, $p<.01$; to their intensity, r (40) = .32, $p<.05$, and their intrusiveness, r (40) = .47, $p<.01$; and to the experience of distress in association with them, r (39) = .72, $p<.001$.

In summary, for a considerable proportion of the cases examined in our study, the psychological impact of major negative events persisted after an extended period of time had passed. In fact, the ongoing experience of involuntary, intense, intrusive, and distressing ruminations related to our subjects' most negative life events was inversely related to both perceived recovery from the event and life satisfaction, after an average of more than 22 years since the events' occurrence. Moreover, the negative relations observed between these ruminations and subjective assessments of recovery provide some support for the validity of the former as a measure of persistent impact. With the single exception of the experience of positive emotions in association with event-related ruminations, which was inversely related to the number of years that had elapsed since the event, none of these measures of impact were significantly related to the amount of time that had passed since the event.

Since change over time was not examined in our study, it remains unclear to what extent the ruminations described by our respondents reflected a fairly steady perseverance as opposed to widely fluctuating levels of impact during the years between the occurrence of the event and our interview. Our data indicate only that, for many of our subjects, cognitive and emotional involvement in the event was ongoing. For these individuals, in Lewin's (1951) terminology, the event still "had existence"; that is, it was not a closed issue, but remained a part of psychological reality, exerting demonstrable influence that was measurable in both quantitative and qualitative terms.

Despite evidence of ongoing cognitive and emotional impact, our respondents appeared to be functioning at least adequately in their day-to-day social roles. Exactly half the sample reported that they felt they had completely recovered from the event in question, and the mean life satisfaction score compared favorably with established norms (see Tait & Silver, 1989). Nonetheless, the pattern of significant relations that emerged between self-assessed recovery and life satisfaction and our measures of ongoing impact underscores the importance of considering the various factors that may contribute to or maintain psychological impact or impede the process of recovery.

Our research addressed such factors through the examination of three additional indicators of ongoing cognitive and emotional involvement in a negative life event. Persistent thoughts about the negative implications of the event, a continuing search for meaning in the event's occurrence, and feeling a need to discuss the event or related concerns or distress with others were conceptualized as referring to aspects of ongoing difficulty in coming to terms with the given event. As was the case for our more general measure of impact, the index formed by combining these responses was inversely related to both self-assessed recovery and life satisfaction, and unrelated to the amount of time that had passed since the event.

RUMINATIONS, LIFE SATISFACTION, AND THE CONTINUING IMPLICATIONS OF AN EVENT

Since the correlational nature of the relations examined in our work precludes the formulation of causal statements, it remains unclear whether event-related ruminations contribute to or arise from lower levels of life satisfaction, or whether the inverse relation between them is attributable to the influence of other factors. However, studies by Schwarz and Strack and their colleagues (see, e.g., Schwarz & Clore, 1983; Strack, Schwarz, & Gschneidinger, 1985) provide some evidence that ruminations about a past event can influence current evaluations of life satisfaction. Their analysis suggests that a key factor determining the nature of this influence is the kind of affect elicited by these ruminations in the present. Thus, negatively valenced ruminations about a past event may bias judgments of life satisfaction downward, whereas positively valenced ruminations may exert the opposite effect. Because of its focus on voluntary rather than involuntary ruminations, it is unclear to what extent valid extrapolations can be made from this work to our research. Nonetheless, it may be the case that distressing event-related ruminations, regardless of their voluntary or involuntary nature, can exert a considerable negative influence on judgments of satisfaction with life.

Perhaps a clearer argument can be made that factors contributing to lower levels of life satisfaction may directly or indirectly enhance the likelihood of distressing event-related ruminations, particularly when these factors are attributed to the occurrence of the given event, as in the case of its ongoing negative implications. Some evidence for the relevance of an event's implications to long-term psychological impact and life satisfaction can be found in the results of the thematic analysis of the content of the "typical" event-related ruminations described by subjects in our study. In addition to thoughts, memories, or mental images centering on the event itself, respondents described ruminations about negative implications of the event in terms of either aspects of life prior to the event that had changed as a result of its occurrence, or aspects of life in the present that might have been different had the event not occurred. Responses to our question specifically addressing the experience of thoughts about the ongoing implications of the most negative event also suggest the importance of this consideration to both psychological recovery and satisfaction with life.

When the continuing salience of an event's negative implications results in unfavorable comparisons between aspects of the past (i.e., of life prior to the event's occurrence) and one's present circumstances (cf. Brickman, Coates, & Janoff-Bulman, 1978; Strack et al., 1985), even pleasant thoughts, memories, or mental images may be a source of current distress. In the words of one of our respondents,

> Sometimes I remember the good times we used to have, and how good he was to me and the children. He certainly was a very good husband. He had his temper, like any man; we had our ups and downs, and our quarrels. But most of them are very good memories. They hurt now, too. They hurt since he died. Although they are good memories, they still hurt me.

Aspects of one's present life circumstances may also be unfavorably compared against plans, hopes, or goals that were precluded by the occurrence of the negative event. In discussing thoughts about the implications of the death of her husband after his decision to postpone retirement for 2 years, another of our respondents described them in the following terms:

> We would have gone to Europe. We would have tried to enjoy life without working: the friends, the relatives, a better social life. I'd still be living with him in the same house; I wouldn't have to live in Ontario [Public] Housing. . . . These things keep coming back.

The continuing negative implications of an event, when they result in unfavorable comparisons between life as it is and life as it might have been had the event not occurred, may make a substantial contribution to lower life satisfaction, and may also act as persistent triggers of distressing event-related ruminations.

An event's implications may contribute to ongoing cognitive and emotional involvement in three ways. First, the implications of an event may remain salient and problematic over time. It is also possible that an event's implications may only become salient and problematic with the passing of time. Such a case has been illustrated earlier by the respondent in our study who described ongoing ruminations related to the death of his adolescent daughter 20 years earlier; his ruminations centered on the loss not only of his only child, but also of the grandchildren he could have expected had her death not occurred (see also Carr, 1975; Parkes, 1971). A final possibility is suggested by the significant inverse relation observed in our study between the experience of positive emotions (happiness, feeling "at peace") in association with event-related ruminations and the number of years that had passed since the event. In explaining these positive emotions, many of our subjects referred to the fact that the event was over, and with it had terminated the suffering of a loved one. It is possible that this type of positive implication, while potentially of great salience in the immediate aftermath of an event, may decrease in salience over time relative to negative implications that remain or become salient or problematic.

Salient negative implications of an event that remain operative in the individual's current life situation represent potential sources of ongoing psychological impact above and beyond the occurrence of the event. Through these implications, an event may continue, long after its termination, to exert considerable influence on one's life. However, as is the case for the occurrence of the event itself, the actual implications of an event may be of less importance to understanding psychological impact and recovery than the interpretation of their meaning or personal significance.

PSYCHOLOGICAL RECOVERY: INTERPRETATION AND INTEGRATION

The process of "working through" a negative life event (cf. Freud, 1914/ 1958), optimally leading to resolution or recovery, has been described as involving two interrelated tasks: the interpretation of the event in meaningful terms, and the integration of this information into a coherent, stable, and adaptive conceptual framework (see, e.g., Marris, 1986; Piaget, 1926, 1952). The conceptual framework represents the individual's assumptive world (Janoff-Bulman, 1985, in press; Janoff-Bulman & Timko, 1987; Parkes, 1975), models or theories of reality (Bowlby, 1980; Epstein, 1973, 1979, 1981; Parkes, 1971, 1972, 1975; Parkes & Weiss, 1983), or structures of meaning (Marris, 1986; see also Horowitz, Wilner, Marmar, & Krupnick, 1980). It consists of descriptive and prescriptive postulates, interwoven into a system of beliefs, assumptions, or expectations related to oneself, others, and the world, and of various emotions associated with them. It functions as a frame of reference, guiding both interpretations of the data of experience and the selection of appropriate responses, and providing a sense of coherence, predictability, and control over reality. The need to interpret and integrate experience into constructions of reality has been described as a fundamental and universal motive related to adaptation and survival (e.g., Marris, 1986; see also Frankl, 1963).

Events are interpreted in light of the existing conceptual structure. Aspects of the extant framework may preclude the appraisal of an event as stressful, even when it is considered to be objectively so (see, e.g., Baluk & O'Neill, 1980; May, 1977; Wortman & Silver, 1987, 1989). Conversely, an event that may be considered objectively innocuous may yet be appraised as quite stressful by the individual confronted with its occurrence.[2]

Integration of the information inherent in an event's interpretation may occur in two ways, as a function of its consistency or incompatibility with the existing system. When an event is interpreted in terms that are consistent with operative conceptual models or theories of self, others, and the world, this information may be assimilated relatively easily into the extant framework. When the event's interpretation is inconsistent or incompatible with aspects of the conceptual framework, either these aspects of the existing system must be altered to accommodate the information, or the event must be reinterpreted in terms that are more assimilable (see also Horowitz, 1975; Lazarus, 1966; Lazarus & Folkman, 1984; Lerner, 1980; May, 1977). Persistent event-related ruminations are believed to represent attempts to integrate such inconsistent information (cf. Epstein, 1987).

Complications in the Process

Several types of complications may arise in the process of formulating a meaningful and acceptable interpretation of a negative life event. First, an event may prove to be difficult to interpret in meaningful terms. Since the conceptual framework is built up as a function of direct and vicarious experience, it may be that problems in interpretation can arise in particular for events that are beyond the range of common experience. Examples of such events include incest (Silver et al., 1983); the accidental, suicidal, or homicidal death of a loved one (Lehman et al., 1987; Rynearson, 1986); and catastrophic events, such as natural or human-caused disasters (e.g., Eitinger, 1980; Lifton, 1968; Titchener & Kapp, 1976). Individual characteristics or motives may also influence the search for a meaningful interpretation; for example, a need for validity (Kruglanski, Baldwin, & Towson, 1983) may prolong the search for extended periods of time.

A second type of complication may arise when an event is interpreted in terms that are meaningful, but inconsistent with aspects of the existing system—challenging or violating, for example, fundamental beliefs, assumptions, or expectations (e.g., Janoff-Bulman, 1985, in press; Lerner, 1980). In these cases, the information may be integrated by altering the existing belief system to accommodate it. However, the process of accommodation may prove to be both time-consuming and distressing. Marris (1986) has proposed the influence of a general "conservative impulse," an initial and potentially persistent resistance against change in aspects of the prevailing conceptual structure, which have probably established some validity over time. Dissonance between an event's interpretation and operative beliefs, theories, or models has been associated with a sense of discontinuity or disorganization, a sense of incoherence or unpredictability, and feelings of the loss or absence of control (cf. Antonovsky, 1982; Epstein, 1982; Festinger, 1957; Kruglanski et al., 1983). Again, individual characteristics or motives may play an important role in determining the extent of resistance to inconsistent information. Resistance may be stronger, for example, with higher levels of the need for structure or of the need for specific conclusions (Kruglanski et al., 1983).

Factors that may influence the process of accommodation include the nature and centrality of the threatened or violated construct, and its interrelatedness with other aspects of the existing system. We would expect that the more central or deeply embedded the relevant belief or model, the more difficult and prolonged the process is likely to be. For example, applying Bem's (1970) hierarchical model of cognitive structures, one might anticipate that zero-order beliefs would be more resistant to alteration than first- or second-order beliefs. On the other hand, the greater the individual's cognitive complexity—that is, the greater the extent to which beliefs or models are compartmentalized or discrete—the easier the process may be (see, e.g., Linville, 1985). The influence of individual characteristics or motives may also come into play in the accommodation process. For example, a high need for structure (Kruglanski et al., 1983) may intensify the distress associated with dissonance between an event's interpretation and aspects of the existing conceptual framework.

When the interpretation of an event is inconsistent or incompatible with the extant conceptual framework, integration may also be achieved by reinterpreting the event in terms that are assimilable within the given structure (see, e.g., Frankl, 1963; Lerner, 1980). In some cases, reinterpreting an event in terms that are acceptable may prove to be as difficult as, or more difficult than, the initial formulation of meaning. As long as a meaningful and acceptable interpretation remains elusive, the search for meaning may continue for extended time periods. Moreover, we believe that the implications of an event constitute an integral aspect of its overall meaning or personal significance, and that long-term psychological resolution requires the development of a meaningful and acceptable interpretation not only of the event, but also of its ongoing implications (i.e., of life given the occurrence of the event). The positive relation that emerged in our research (Tait & Silver, 1989) between ruminations about an event's implications and a continuing search for meaning suggests that this may be the case. Whether a continuing search for meaning elicits thoughts about an event's implications, or whether problematic implications cause one to consider the meaning of an event, is unclear. It may be, however, that the clearest interpretation of a major negative event can be made only from a long-term perspective, in light of its full range of negative and positive implications.

PSYCHOLOGICAL IMPACT AND THE SOCIAL MILIEU

Lazarus (see, e.g., Lazarus & Folkman, 1984) has suggested that an individual confronting a major negative life event may face two sources of threat or stress—that arising from the event itself, and that arising from his or her responses to the event. The literature indicates that people are frequently surprised by the nature and intensity (and, perhaps, persistence) of their own responses to these events (cf. Horowitz, 1985; Silver & Wortman, 1980). In fact, the need to discuss an event or one's responses to it with others has been linked to the need to receive validation—that is, feedback from others indicating that these responses are normal and appropriate to the circumstances (e.g., Dunkel-Schetter & Wortman, 1981, 1982).

Individuals who experience major negative life events or difficulty in coming to terms with them may frequently turn to significant others in the social milieu for assistance or support. Prior work has identified various forms of social support that may facilitate the process of recovery by reducing the demands associated with an event's occurrence or by enhancing the individual's ability to meet these demands (for reviews, see Cohen & Wills, 1985; Kessler & McLeod, 1985; Kessler, Price, & Wortman, 1985; Turner, 1983). In order for social support to be effective, however, it must be appropriate to the particular needs or difficulties experienced by the individual (cf. Lehman, Ellard, & Wortman, 1986; Thoits, 1985; Wortman & Lehman, 1985). Ineffective or inappropriate responses can contribute to the maintenance of psychological impact, or may add to the complexity of the recovery process by increasing the sources of strain with which the individual must cope. The likelihood of effective support may be a direct function of the individual's ability to communicate openly with others about the event and/or event-related difficulties or distress. We believe that social responses to these communications may play an integral role in the mediation or moderation of psychological impact (cf. Strack & Coyne, 1983).

Whether social responses effectively enhance or impede the process of recovery, we believe that they may be more clearly understood by drawing a parallel between the sources of threat or stress that may be faced by the individual and those that may be faced by members of his or her social milieu (cf. Thoits, 1985). That is, the occurrence of a negative event or of continuing event-related difficulties or distress may pose a threat not only for the individual directly confronted with the event, but also for members of the social network. This parallel is based on empirical evidence that people respond not only to their own events and outcomes, but also to those of relevant others. When these events or outcomes involve another's suffering or distress, observers frequently respond with physiological and psychological arousal (see, e.g., Lazarus, Speisman, Mordkof, & Davison, 1962; Lerner, 1980). Merely viewing a film depicting the suffering and distress of an unknown other may result in marked mood changes (Tannenbaum & Gaer, 1965) or in the experience of involuntary and distressing ruminations related to the material observed (Horowitz, 1975, 1976; Horowitz & Wilner, 1976; Wilner & Horowitz, 1975), or both. The personal experience of witnessing the ongoing event-related difficulties or distress of a significant other may have considerably greater impact.

Given some basic degree of perspective-taking ability, observing another's suffering and distress can also elicit two qualitatively different and apparently independent kinds of empathic arousal (Coke, Batson, & McDavis, 1978; see also Davis, 1983). Observers may experience personal distress (feelings of fear, apprehension, or discomfort) or empathic concern (feelings of warmth and compassionate concern for the other's welfare). Lerner (1980) has described a similar dichotomy in responses to another's suffering, distinguishing "empathy," defined as the automatic arousal experienced in response to evidence of another's suffering, from "sympathy," described as the compassionate concern that may be elicited when one identifies with the distressed individual.

We believe that these two forms of empathic arousal (cf. Batson & Coke, 1981) may be particularly useful in explaining social responses to the need to discuss the event or event-related difficulties or distress. The experience of personal distress in response to these communications may be more likely to result in responses of flight (i.e., avoidance of the individual or of attempts to discuss the event or related problems), fight (i.e., hostility toward or rejection of the individual or his or her attempts at discussion), or freezing (no response or "cliche" response). All of these reactions may serve to inhibit expressions of the need for discussion. In comparison, the experience of empathic concern may result in greater openness to manifestations of this need—that is, in more willingness to confront evidence of continuing difficulty or distress, and in a higher probability that attention will be directed to relevant contributing factors.

To some extent, these two basic empathic responses may reflect underlying differences in general orientations to stress or threat (i.e., avoidance vs. approach or confrontation; Roth & Cohen, 1986). However, other factors may also influence the nature and extent of arousal elicited by observing another's ongoing distress. Most relevant to the present analysis are the nature and extent of the threat that may be posed to the observer by the occurrence of the event and/or of continuing event-related difficulties or distress, or, more precisely, by the interpretation of the event and/or of its persistent impact.

Drawing a parallel between the sources of threat that may be faced by the individual and those that may be posed for members of the social milieu broadens our perspective on the psychological impact of a negative event. This broader perspective allows us to look beyond the individual confronted with its occurrence, and to consider the event's potential impact on members of the social milieu, the relation between this impact and social responses, and the potential effects of these responses on the individual's experience of the event. From this perspective, the model of psychological impact and recovery described above may be extended to members of the individual's social network. That is, the occurrence of a major negative event and/or of ongoing difficulties in coming to terms with it may threaten or violate important beliefs, assumptions, theories, or models of self, others, or the world, not only for the individual, but also for members of his or her social environment. To the extent that this is the case, both parties may experience direct threat or stress, and both may be faced with similar tasks of interpretation, assimilation, accommodation, or reinterpretation. The basic motive to find meaning in events or outcomes characterizes both parties of a social relationship, and extends beyond one's own outcomes to include those of significant others. Thus, for both parties, the actual event or outcome may be of less relevance to the process of recovery than their interpretation of its meaning or personal significance, and the consistency or inconsistency of this interpretation with important aspects of existing conceptual frameworks or structures of meaning. In cases of inconsistency, significant others may be directly, rather than just vicariously, threatened by the occurrence of the event and/or evidence of persistent difficulty in resolving it. The experience of direct threat or stress may increase the likelihood of responding to the event or to evidence of its continuing impact with personal distress rather than with empathic concern.

As in the case of the individual, the extent of threat directly experienced among members of the social milieu may be a function of the nature and centrality of the particular beliefs, assumptions, theories, or models that are challenged or violated by the interpretation of these events or outcomes, and the degree of inconsistency between them. One kind of belief, assumption, or expectation of particular relevance has been identified as the "assumption of invulnerability" (i.e., the belief that major negative events are unlikely to happen to us; Janoff-Bulman & Frieze, 1983; Perloff, 1983; Perloff & Fetzer, 1986), and as the "optimistic bias" (i.e., the tendency to underestimate the probability of personally experiencing major negative events; Weinstein, 1980, 1984; Weinstein & Lachendro, 1982). We believe that this kind of assumption or expectation may also extend to one's perceived probability of experiencing persistent event-related difficulties or distress (Olshansky, 1962; Wikler, Wasow, & Hatfield, 1981). That is, the motives or processes underlying the tendency to assume invulnerability to, or to underestimate the probability of, the occurrence of negative events in one's own life may contribute to a similar tendency to minimize the perceived likelihood of experiencing persistent event-related difficulties or distress. Indeed, since we are generally held less responsible for the events that happen to us than for our responses to these events (cf. Brickman et al., 1982), there may be an even greater tendency to underestimate the likelihood of experiencing persistent distress. Moreover, this same tendency toward underestimation may exert a similar biasing influence with regard to one's beliefs about the probability of major negative events occurring and of their persistent impact among those who are closest to us—that is, those with whom we share an identity relationship (cf. Lerner, 1981). This tendency may make a substantial contribution to a more general belief, assumption, or expectation that the psychological impact of these events is normally limited within relatively narrow temporal parameters, and that persistent psychological impact represents an "abnormal" outcome of these events.

THE INDIVIDUAL'S RESPONSES TO SOCIAL RESPONSES

When the need for discussion is inhibited by members of the social milieu, the individual may find himself or herself caught in a conflict between the need to discuss a major negative event or related concerns or distress with others, and the need to maintain stable and harmonious social relations (Epstein, 1985). The individual may respond by persisting in his or her attempts to involve others in discussion, or may acquiesce to strong social sanctions against the persistent expression of event-related distress. In the former case, others may respond with increasing hostility toward, or rejection or avoidance of, the individual or his or her communications (e.g.,

Coates et al., 1979; Strack & Coyne, 1983), or with a complex sequence of mixed responses, some positively reinforcing the need to talk, others inhibiting this need (Coyne, 1976a, 1976b). Some social responses may effectively eliminate attempts at discussion. However, mixed responses may contribute to the persistence of these attempts, and to an escalating cycle of mutual hostility, frustration, and perhaps alienation.

Alternatively, negative social responses to the expression of continuing difficulty or distress may result in a split between the private experience and the public expression of ongoing impact. Together with the paucity of clear norms, roles, or guidelines outlining effective behavior for either the distressed individual or members of the social milieu, and with the influence of frequent media depictions of "super copers" (Wood, Taylor, & Lichtman, 1985) who deal with major negative events quickly, effectively, and with little apparent need for continuing social support, the stigma that may be associated with persistent psychological impact can result in the adoption of self-presentational strategies that are more in line with social expectations (see, e.g., Goffman, 1959, 1963), and perhaps with one's own prior expectations. Insofar as these strategies are effective, the actual extent or persistence of psychological impact may be underrepresented in the perceptions of members of the social milieu.

Both of these responses to the inhibition of the need for discussion may ultimately contribute to the belief that persistent psychological impact represents an "abnormal" outcome. The findings of our research, as well as of related work, strongly suggest that this is not the case. The attribution of abnormality to what is essentially a normal response (see, e.g., Goin, Burgoyne, & Goin, 1979; Szybist, 1978) by health care professionals, laypersons, and distressed individuals alike may make a significant contribution to the maintenance or enhancement of ongoing psychological impact.

Because members of the social milieu may exert a significant influence in mediating or moderating the impact of negative events, and may also directly or vicariously share in the psychological impact of these events, it may be that psychological recovery is most appropriately conceptualized not as an individual but as a social process. However, recognizing persistent impact as a "normal" outcome of major negative events does not imply that the best response for either the individual or members of the social network would be one of passive acquiescence to an inevitable outcome. We cannot prevent the occurrence of these events; speaking in relative and subjective terms, everyone will experience a "most negative event" over the course of his or her life. Nonetheless, awareness of continuing impact as a relatively normal response to these events can reduce or eliminate a potential source of stress for both the individual and members of his or her social milieu, and may enhance the ability of both parties to deal effectively with the factors contributing to its persistence.

CONCLUSIONS

The purpose of this chapter has been to contribute to a normative view of the long-term psychological impact of major negative life events, and to apply to this description a theoretically based explanation. In attempting to do so, we have adopted a broader frame of reference than is usually the case in studies of the psychological impact of events. Rather than examining impact within a given type of event, we have attempted to establish some basis for comparison across different types of events, according to subjective and relative judgments of severity. Comparison across event types is not a novel approach. For example, Parkes (1972) compared the psychological impact of the loss of a limb, the death of a spouse, and forced relocation due to urban renewal. Marris (1986) points to the commonalities in patterns of response to bereavement, slum clearance, and the experience of colonization and industrialization in Third World countries. Similarly, Parkes and Weiss (1983) suggest that studies of the process of recovery from bereavement and the ways in which this process may be impeded can provide a viable model of recovery from any irremediable loss.

The experience of loss may represent a significant common denominator among the major negative events described by respondents in our research (Tait & Silver, 1989). This loss may be literal (e.g., the loss of a particular person, environment, role, or relationship) and/or symbolic (e.g., the loss of future possibilities, cherished hopes, goals, or plans). Our basic emphasis is on the meaning of events, situations, or responses, and represents a symbolic interactionist approach. From this perspective, any event that threatens or violates important models or theories of self, others, or the world may represent a loss (cf. Viorst, 1986). Moreover, dissonance between the meaning of experience and central models or theories of reality may pose a significant threat or loss, insofar as they undermine the predictability of one's situational and/or social experience (cf. Marris, 1986; Simos, 1979).

Rather than concentrating primarily on the occurrence of the event as the single determinant of impact, the focus of our work has been on the nature and influence of potential contributing factors that are dependent on the event's occurrence and widely variable across individuals and over time. These factors (i.e., the ongoing negative implications of an event, the need or motive to find meaning in it, and social responses to the occurrence of the event and/or to expressions of continuing difficulty or distress) may be thought of as referring to situational, psychological, and social dimensions of the experience of a major negative event. Persistent cognitive and emotional involvement along these dimensions has been considered as indicative of ongoing difficulty in resolving the experience. This view of impact and recovery is essentially transactional, assuming that the individual and his or her situational and social environment are involved in a continuing dynamic and reciprocal relation (cf. Lazarus & Folkman, 1984).

Our concern with normative long-term psychological responses to negative life events reflects a developmental as opposed to a disease perspective (cf. Sugarman, 1986). Rather than viewing these events as pathological causes of dysfunctional impact, we see them as normative transitions that carry the potential for growth and development, as well as for persistent difficulty or distress. Normative data provide a description of average or typical impact, and do not refer to optimal or ideal responses or effects. It is important to distinguish between normative and prescriptive approaches; in acknowledging lasting impact as a normal outcome, it is necessary to avoid contributing to the belief that a brief, uncomplicated recovery is in any way abnormal.

The individual confronted with a major negative event may encounter a number of obstacles on the road to recovery, and there is considerable potential for associated impact to persist for years or even decades. However, it is also possible for such an individual to meet the demands of the event's negative implications and to develop a meaningful and acceptable interpretation of the experience over the short or long term. It is also possible for members of the social milieu to respond to the event and its continuing impact with maximal empathic concern and a minimum of personal distress. The probability of these latter outcomes may be significantly enhanced by recognition of the prevalence of persistent psychological impact of negative life events. We believe that the absence of clear normative information about the possible long-term effects of these events has played a major role in the perpetuation of overly optimistic beliefs, assumptions, or expectations regarding the potential complexity and duration of the recovery process. Ironically, these optimistic assumptions or expectations may themselves make a substantial contribution to the persistence of distress.

NOTES

1. We wish to thank David Hamilton for bringing this item to our attention.

2. Is the type of negative event that occurs an adequate basis for arriving at objective ratings of its severity? In addition, is there a relation between these objective assessments and the individual's subjective experience of a given type of event? Because of potential differential access to relevant information (see, e.g., Jones & Nisbett, 1971), we would expect to find a considerable discrepancy in assessments of the severity of various types of events between the individuals confronted with them and those viewing the events from an outsider's perspective. Our study (Tait & Silver, 1989) provided some evidence that this is, in fact, the case. Two independent raters were presented with a list of all negative events each subject had

reported having experienced over the course of his or her life, and were asked to select for each subject the particular event they believed would have been the most negative. These raters agreed in their initial selections of most negative events in only 55% of the cases. In only 50% of the cases did the raters' final selection of the most negative events correspond with the events reported by the respondents as the most severe. This finding calls into question the viability of attempts to predict or explain the impact of negative life events as a function of objective group ratings of the severity or stressfulness of various types of events (e.g., Holmes & Rahe, 1967).

REFERENCES

American Psychiatric Association. (1980). *Diagnostic and statistical manual of mental disorders* (3rd ed.). Washington, DC: Author.

Antonovsky, A. (1982). *Health, stress, and coping.* San Francisco: Jossey-Bass.

Baluk, U., & O'Neill, P. (1980). Health professionals' perceptions of the psychological consequences of abortion. *American Journal of Community Psychology, 8,* 67–75.

Batson, C. D., & Coke, J. S. (1981). Empathy: A source of altruistic motivation for helping. In J. P. Rushton & R. M. Sorrentino (Eds.), *Altruism and helping behavior* (pp. 167–187). New York: Academic Press.

Beck, A. T. (1975). *Depression: Causes and treatment.* Philadelphia: University of Pennsylvania Press.

Bem, D. J. (1970). *Beliefs, attitudes, and human affairs.* Monterey, CA: Brooks/Cole.

Benner, P., Roskies, E., & Lazarus, R. S. (1980). Stress and coping under extreme conditions. In J. E. Dimsdale (Ed.), *Survivors, victims and perpetrators: Essays on the Nazi Holocaust* (pp. 219–258). Washington, DC: Hemisphere.

Bower, G. H. (1981). Mood and memory. *American Psychologist, 36,* 129–148.

Bowlby, J. (1980). *Attachment and loss: Vol. 3. Loss: Sadness and depression.* New York: Basic Books.

Brende, J. E., & Parson, E. R. (1985). *Vietnam veterans: The road to recovery.* New York: Plenum.

Breuer, J., & Freud, S. (1955). Studies on hysteria. In J. Strachey (Ed. and Trans.), *The standard edition of the complete psychological works of Sigmund Freud* (Vol. 2, pp. 1–305). London: Hogarth Press. (Original work published 1895)

Brickman, P., Coates, D., & Janoff-Bulman, R. (1978). Lottery winners and accident victims: Is happiness relative? *Journal of Personality and Social Psychology, 36,* 917–927.

Brickman, P., Rabinowitz, V. C., Karuza, J., Coates, D., Cohn, E., & Kidder, L. (1982). Models of helping and coping. *American Psychologist, 37,* 203–212.

Bulman, R. J., & Wortman, C. B. (1977). Attributions of blame and coping in the "real world": Severe accident victims react to their lot. *Journal of Personality and Social Psychology, 35,* 351–363.

Carr, A. C. (1975). Bereavement as a relative experience. In B. Schoenberg, A. Wiener, A. H. Kutscher, D. Peretz, & A. C. Carr (Eds.), *Bereavement: Its psychosocial aspects* (pp. 3–8). New York: Columbia University Press.

Clark, M., & Isen, A. (1982). Toward understanding the relationship between feeling states and social behavior. In A. H. Hastorf & A. M. Isen (Eds.), *Cognitive social psychology* (pp. 73–108). New York: Elsevier.

Coates, D., & Wortman, C. B. (1980). Depression maintenance and interpersonal control. In A. Baum & J. Singer (Eds.), *Advances in environmental psychology* (Vol. 2, pp. 149–182). Hillsdale, NJ: Erlbaum.

Coates, D., Wortman, C. B., & Abbey, A. (1979). Reactions to victims. In I. H. Frieze, D. Bar-Tal, & J. S. Carroll (Eds.), *New approaches to social problems* (pp. 21–52). San Francisco: Jossey-Bass.

Cohen, S., & Wills, T. A. (1985). Stress, social support, and the buffering hypothesis. *Psychological Bulletin, 98,* 310–357.

Coke, J., Batson, D., & McDavis, K. (1978). Empathic mediation of helping: A two-stage model. *Journal of Personality and Social Psychology, 36,* 752–766.

Coyne, J. C. (1976a). Depression and the response of others. *Journal of Abnormal Psychology, 85,* 186–193.

Coyne, J. C. (1976b). Toward an interactional description of depression. *Psychiatry, 39,* 28–40.

Davis, M. H. (1983). Measuring individual differences in empathy: Evidence for a multidimensional approach. *Journal of Personality and Social Psychology, 44,* 113–136.

Dunkel-Schetter, C., & Wortman, C. B. (1981). Dilemmas of social support: Parallels between victimization and aging. In S. B. Kiesler, J. N. Morgan, & V. K. Oppenheimer (Eds.), *Aging: Social change* (pp. 349–381). New York: Academic Press.

Dunkel-Schetter, C., & Wortman, C. B. (1982). The interpersonal dynamics of cancer: Problems in social relationships and their impact on the patient. In H. S. Friedman & M. R. DiMatteo (Eds.), *Interpersonal issues in health care* (pp. 69–100). New York: Academic Press.

Eitinger, L. (1980). The concentration camp syndrome and its late sequelae. In J. E. Dimsdale (Ed.), *Survivors, victims and perpetrators: Essays on the Nazi Holocaust* (pp. 127–162). Washington, DC: Hemisphere.

Epstein, S. (1973). The self-concept revisited, or a theory of a theory. *American Psychologist, 28,* 404–416.

Epstein, S. (1979). The ecological study of emotions in humans. In P. Pliner, K. R. Blankenstein, & I. M. Spigel (Eds.), *Advances in the study of communication and affect: Vol. 5. Perceptions of emotions in self and others* (pp. 47–83). New York: Plenum.

Epstein, S. (1982). Conflict and stress. In L. Goldberger & S. Breznitz (Eds.). *Handbook of stress* (pp. 49–68). New York: Free Press.

Epstein, S. (1983). Natural healing processes of the mind. In D. Meichenbaum & M. E. Jaremko (Eds.), *Stress reduction and prevention* (pp. 39–66). New York: Plenum.

Epstein, S. (1985). The implications of cognitive–experiential self-theory for research in social psychology and personality [Special issue]. *Journal for the Theory of Social Behavior, 15,* 283–310.

Epstein, S. (1987). Implications of cognitive self-theory for psychopathology and psychotherapy. In N. Cheshire & H. Thomae (Eds.), *Self, symptoms and psychotherapy* (pp. 43–58). New York: Wiley.

Epstein, S. (in press). The self-concept, the traumatic neurosis, and the structure of personality In D. Ozer, J. M. Healy, & A. J. Stewart (Eds.), *Perspectives on personality* (Vol. 3). Greenwich, CT: JAI Press.

Festinger, L. (1957). *A theory of cognitive dissonance*. Evanston, IL: Row-Peterson.

Folkman, S., Schaefer, C., & Lazarus, R. S. (1979). Cognitive processes as mediators of stress and coping. In V. Hamilton & D. M. Warburton (Eds.), *Human stress and cognition: An information-processing approach* (pp. 265–298). Chichester, England: Wiley.

Frankl, V. E. (1963). *Man's search for meaning: An introduction to logotherapy*. New York: Washington Square Press.

Freud, S. (1958). Remembering, repeating, and working-through. In J. Strachey (Ed. and Trans.), *The standard edition of the complete psychological works of Sigmund Freud* (Vol. 12, pp. 145–150). London: Hogarth Press. (Original work published 1914)

Glick, I. O., Weiss, R. S., & Parkes, C. M. (1974). *The first year of bereavement*. New York: Wiley.

Goin, M. K., Burgoyne, R. W., & Goin, J. M. (1979). Timeless attachment to a dead relative. *American Journal of Psychiatry, 136,* 988–989.

Goffman, E. (1959). *The presentation of self in everyday life*. New York: Doubleday.

Goffman E. (1963). *Stigma: Notes on the management of a spoiled identity*. Englewood Cliffs, NJ: Prentice-Hall.

Holmes, T. H., & Rahe, R. H. (1967). The Social Readjustment Rating Scale. *Journal of Psychosomatic Research, 11,* 213–218.

Horowitz, M. J. (1975). Intrusive and repetitive thoughts after experimental stress: A summary. *Archives of General Psychiatry, 32,* 1457–1463.

Horowitz, M. J. (1976). *Stress response syndromes*. New York: Jason Aronson.

Horowitz, M. J. (1979). Psychological response to serious life events. In V. Hamilton & D. M. Warburton (Eds.), *Human stress and cognition: An information-processing approach* (pp. 235–263). Chichester, England: Wiley.

Horowitz, M. J. (1982). Stress response syndromes and their treatment. In L. Goldberger & S. Breznitz (Eds.), *Handbook of stress* (pp. 711–732). New York: Free Press.

Horowitz, M. J. (1985). Disasters and psychological response to stress. *Psychiatric Annals, 15,* 161–167.

Horowitz, M. J., & Wilner, N. (1976). Stress films, emotion, and cognitive response. *Archives of General Psychiatry, 33,* 1339–1344.

Horowitz, M. J., Wilner, N., Kaltreider, N., & Alvarez, W. (1980). Signs and symptoms of posttraumatic stress disorder. *Archives of General Psychiatry, 37,* 85–92.

Horowitz, M. J., Wilner, N., Marmar, C., & Krupnick, J. (1980). Pathological grief and the activation of latent self-images. *American Journal of Psychiatry, 137,* 1157–1162.

Janis, I. L. (1971). *Stress and frustration*. New York: Harcourt Brace Jovanovich.

Janoff-Bulman, R. (1985). The aftermath of victimization: Rebuilding shattered assumptions. In C. R. Figley (Ed.), *Trauma and its wake* (pp. 15–35). New York: Brunner/Mazel.

Janoff-Bulman, R. (in press). Assumptive worlds and the stress of traumatic events: Applications of the schema construct. *Social Cognition*.

Janoff-Bulman, R., & Frieze, I. H. (1983). A theoretical perspective for understanding responses to victimization. *Journal of Social Issues, 39*(2), 1–17.

Janoff-Bulman, R., & Timko, C. (1987). Coping with traumatic life events: The role of denial in light of people's assumptive worlds. In C. R. Snyder & C. E. Ford (Eds.), *Coping with negative life events: Clinical and social psychological perspectives* (pp. 135–159). New York: Plenum.

Jones, E. E., & Nisbett, R. E. (1971). The actor and the observer: Divergent perceptions of the causes of behavior. In E. E. Jones, D. Kanouse, H. H. Kelley, R. E. Nisbett, S. Valins, & B. Weiner (Eds.), *Attribution: Perceiving the causes of behavior* (pp. 79–94). Morristown, NJ: General Learning Press.

Kahneman, D., & Tversky, A. (1982). The simulation heuristic. In D. Kahneman & A. Tversky (Eds.), *Judgment under uncertainty: Heuristics and biases* (pp. 201–208). Cambridge, England: Cambridge University Press.

Kaltreider, N. B., Wallace, A., & Horowitz, M. J. (1979). A field study of the stress response syndrome. *Journal of the American Medical Association, 242,* 1499–1503.

Kelly, G. A. (1955). *The psychology of personal constructs* (Vol. 1). New York: Norton.

Kessler, R. C., & McLeod, J. D. (1985). Social support and mental health in community samples. In S. Cohen & S. L. Syme (Eds.), *Social support and health* (pp. 219–240). New York: Academic Press.

Kessler, R. C., Price, R. H., & Wortman, C. B. (1985). Social factors in psychopathology: Stress, social support, and coping processes. *Annual Review of Psychology, 36,* 531–572.

Kruglanski, A. W., Baldwin, M. W., & Towson, S. M. J. (1983). The lay-epistemic process in attribution-making. In M. Hewstone (Ed.), *Attribution theory: Social and functional extensions* (pp. 81–95). Oxford: Blackwell.

Lazarus, R. S. (1966). *Psychological stress and the coping process.* New York: McGraw-Hill.

Lazarus, R. S. (1985). The trivialization of distress. In J. C. Rose & L. J. Solomon (Eds.), *Primary prevention of psychopathology: Vol. 8. Prevention in Health Psychology* (pp. 279–298). Hanover, NH: University Press of New England.

Lazarus, R. S., & Folkman, S. (1984). *Stress, appraisal, and coping.* New York: Springer.

Lazarus, R. S., Kanner, A. D., & Folkman, S. (1980). Emotions: A cognitive–phenomenological analysis. In R. Plutchik & H. Kellerman (Eds.), *Theories of emotion* (pp. 189–214). New York: Academic Press.

Lazarus, R. S., Speisman, J. C., Mordkof, A. M., & Davison, L. A. (1962). A laboratory study of psychological stress produced by a motion picture film. *Psychological Monographs, 76*(34, Whole No. 553).

Lehman, D. R., Ellard, J. H., & Wortman, C. B. (1986). Social support for the bereaved: Recipients' and providers' perspectives on what is helpful. *Journal of Consulting and Clinical Psychology, 54,* 438–446.

Lehman, D. R., Wortman, C. B., & Williams, A. F. (1987). Long-term effects of losing a spouse or child in a motor vehicle crash. *Journal of Personality and Social Psychology, 52,* 218–231.

Lerner, M. J. (1980). *The belief in a just world: A fundamental delusion.* New York: Plenum.

Lerner, M. J. (1981). The justice motive in human relations: Some thoughts on what we know and need to know about justice. In M. J. Lerner & S. C. Lerner (Eds.), *The justice motive in social behavior: Adapting to times of scarcity and change* (pp. 11–35). New York: Plenum.

Lewin, K. (1951). *Field theory in social science.* New York: Harper & Brothers.

Lifton, R. J. (1968). *Death in life: Survivors of Hiroshima.* New York: Random House.

Linville, P. W. (1985). Self-complexity and affective extremity: Don't put all of your eggs in one cognitive basket. *Social Cognition, 3,* 94–120.

Los Angeles Times. (1984, January 15). Morning Briefing, Part III, p. 3.

Marris, P. (1986). *Loss and change* (rev. ed.). London: Routledge & Kegan Paul.

May, R. (1977). *The meaning of anxiety.* New York: Washington Square Press.

Moos, R. H., & Tsu, V. D. (1977). The crisis of physical illness: An overview. In R. H. Moos (Ed.), *Coping with physical illness* (pp. 3–21). New York: Plenum.

Neugarten, B. L. (1979). Time, age, and the life cycle. *American Journal of Psychiatry, 136,* 887–894.

Neugarten, B. L., Havighurst, R. J., & Tobin, S. S. (1961). The measurement of life satisfaction. *Journal of Gerontology, 16,* 134–143.

Olshansky, S. (1962). Chronic sorrow: A response to having a mentally defective child. *Social Casework, 43,* 190–193.

Parkes, C. M. (1971). Psychosocial transitions: A field for study. *Social Science and Medicine, 5,* 101–115.

Parkes, C. M. (1972). Components of the reaction to loss of a limb, spouse or home. *Journal of Psychosomatic Research, 16,* 343–349.

Parkes, C. M. (1975). What becomes of redundant world models? A contribution to the study of adaptation to change. *British Journal of Medical Psychology, 48,* 131–137.

Parkes, C. M., & Weiss, R. S. (1983). *Recovery from bereavement.* New York: Basic Books.

Parkinson, L., & Rachman, S. (1981a). Intrusive thoughts: The effects of an uncontrived stressor. *Advances in Behaviour Research and Therapy, 3,* 111–118.

Parkinson, L., & Rachman, S. (1981b). The nature of intrusive thoughts. *Advances in Behaviour Research and Therapy, 3,* 101–110.

Parkinson, L., & Rachman, S. (1981c). Speed of recovery from an uncontrived stress. *Advances in Behaviour Research and Therapy, 3,* 119–123.

Pearlin, L. I. (1983). Role strains and personal stress. In H. B. Kaplan (Ed.), *Psychosocial stress: Trends in theory and research* (pp. 3–32). New York: Academic Press.

Pearlin, L. I., & Lieberman, M. A. (1979). Social sources of emotional distress. In R. Simmons (Ed.), *Research in community and mental health* (Vol. 1, pp. 217–248). Greenwich, CT: JAI Press.

Pearlin, L. I., Lieberman, M. A., Menaghan, E. G., & Mullan, J. T. (1981). The stress process. *Journal of Health and Social Behavior, 22,* 337–356.

Pennebaker, J. W. (1989). Confession, inhibition, and disease. In L. Berkowitz (Ed.), *Advances in experimental social psychology* (Vol. 22, pp. 211–244). Orlando, FL: Academic Press.

Pennebaker, J. W., & Hoover, C. W. (1985). Inhibition and cognition: Toward an understanding of trauma and disease. In R. J. Davidson, G. E. Schwarz, & D.

Shapiro (Eds.), *Consciousness and self-regulation* (Vol. 4, pp. 107–136). New York: Plenum.

Pennebaker, J. W., & O'Heeron, R. C. (1984). Confiding in others and illness rate among spouses of suicide and accidental-death victims. *Journal of Abnormal Psychology, 93,* 473–476.

Perloff, L. S. (1983). Perception of invulnerability to victimization. *Journal of Social Issues, 39*(2), 41–61.

Perloff, L. S., & Fetzer, B. K. (1986). Self–other judgements and perceived vulnerability to victimization. *Journal of Personality and Social Psychology, 50,* 502–510.

Piaget, J. (1926). *The language and thought of the child.* New York: Harcourt.

Piaget, J. (1952). *The origins of intelligence in children.* New York: International Universities Press.

Rachman, S. (1979). Emotional processing. *Behaviour Research and Therapy, 18,* 51–60.

Rachman, S. (1981). Unwanted intrusive cognitions. *Advances in Behaviour Research and Therapy, 3,* 89–99.

Roth, S., & Cohen, L. J. (1986). Approach, avoidance and coping with stress. *American Psychologist, 41,* 813–819.

Rynearson, E. K. (1986). Psychological effects of unnatural dying on bereavement. *Psychiatric Annals, 15,* 272–275.

Schwarz, N., & Clore, G. (1983). Mood, misattribution, and judgments of well-being: Informative and directive functions of affective status. *Journal of Personality and Social Psychology, 45,* 513–523.

Silver, R. L., Boon, C., & Stones, M. H. (1983). Searching for meaning in misfortune: Making sense of incest. *Journal of Social Issues, 39*(2), 81–102.

Silver, R. L., & Wortman, C. B. (1980). Coping with undesirable life events. In J. Garber & M. E. P. Seligman (Eds.), *Human helplessness* (pp. 279–340). New York: Academic Press.

Silver, R. L., Wortman, C. B., & Klos, D. S. (1982). Cognition, affect, and behavior following uncontrollable outcomes: A response to current human helplessness research. *Journal of Personality, 50,* 480–514.

Simos, B. G. (1979). *A time to grieve: Loss as a universal human experience.* New York: Family Service Association of America.

Singer, J. L. (1978). Experimental studies of daydreaming and stream of thought. In K. S. Pope & J. L. Singer (Eds.), *The stream of consciousness* (pp. 187–223). New York: Plenum.

Snyder, M., & White, P. (1982). Moods and memories: Elation, depression, and the remembering of the events of one's life. *Journal of Personality, 50,* 149–167.

Strack, S., & Coyne, J. C. (1983). Shared and private reactions to depression. *Journal of Personality and Social Psychology, 44,* 798–806.

Strack, F., Schwarz, N., & Gschneidinger, E. (1985). Happiness and reminiscing: The role of time perspective, affect, and mode of thinking. *Journal of Personality and Social Psychology, 49,* 1460–1469.

Sugarman, L. (1986). *Life-span development: Concepts, theories and interventions.* New York: Methuen.

Szybist, C. (1978). Thoughts of a mother. In O. J. Z. Sahler (Ed.), *The child and death* (pp. 283–288). St. Louis: C. V. Mosby.

Tait, R., & Silver, R. C. (1989). *The long-term psychological impact of major negative life events.* Manuscript submitted for publication.

Tannenbaum, P. H., & Gaer, E. P. (1965). Mood changes as a function of stress of protagonist and degree of identification in a film viewing situation. *Journal of Personality and Social Psychology, 2,* 612–616.

Taylor, S. E. (1983). Adjustment to threatening events: A theory of cognitive adaptation. *American Psychologist, 38,* 1161–1173.

Thoits, P. A. (1983). Dimensions of life events that influence psychological distress: An evaluation and synthesis of the literature. In H. B. Kaplan (Ed.), *Psychosocial stress: Trends in theory and research* (pp. 33–103). New York: Academic Press.

Thoits, P. A. (1985). Social support as coping assistance. *Journal of Consulting and Clinical Psychology, 54,* 416–423.

Titchener, J. L., & Kapp, F. T. (1976). Family and character change at Buffalo Creek. *American Journal of Psychiatry, 133,* 295–299.

Turner, R. J. (1983). Direct, indirect, and moderating effects of social support on psychological distress and associated conditions. In H. B. Kaplan (Ed.), *Psychosocial stress: Trends in theory and research* (pp. 105–155). New York: Academic Press.

Vachon, M. L. S., Sheldon, A. R., Lancee, W. J., Lyall, W. A. L., Rogers, J., & Freeman, S. J. J. (1982). Correlates of enduring distress patterns following bereavement: Social network, life situation and personality. *Psychological Medicine, 12,* 783–788.

Viorst, J. (1986). *Necessary losses.* New York: Simon & Schuster.

Wegner, D. M. (1988). Stress and mental control. In S. Fisher & J. Reason (Eds.), *Handbook of life stress, cognition, and health* (pp. 685–699). Chichester, England: Wiley.

Weinstein, N. D. (1980). Unrealistic optimism about future life events. *Journal of Personality and Social Psychology, 39,* 806–820.

Weinstein, N. D. (1984). Why it won't happen to me: Perceptions of risk factors and susceptibility. *Health Psychology, 3,* 431–457.

Weinstein, N. D., & Lachendro, E. (1982). Egocentrism as a source of unrealistic optimism. *Personality and Social Psychology Bulletin, 8,* 195–200.

Wenzlaff, R. M., Wegner, D. M., & Roper, D. W. (1988). Depression and mental control: The resurgence of unwanted negative thoughts. *Journal of Personality and Social Psychology, 55,* 882–892.

Wikler, L., Wasow, M., & Hatfield, E. (1981). Chronic sorrow revisited. *American Journal of Orthopsychiatry, 51,* 63–70.

Wilner, N., & Horowitz, M. J. (1975). Intrusive and repetitive thoughts after a depressing film: A pilot study. *Psychological Reports, 37,* 135–138.

Wood, J. V., Taylor, S. E., & Lichtman, R. R. (1985). Social comparison in adjustment to breast cancer. *Journal of Personality and Social Psychology, 49,* 1169–1183.

Wortman, C. B., & Dunkel-Schetter, C. (1979). Interpersonal relationships and cancer: A theoretical analysis. *Journal of Social Issues, 35*(1), 120–155.

Wortman, C. B., & Lehman, D. R. (1985). Reactions to victims of life crises: Support attempts that fail. In I. G. Sarason & B. R. Sarason (Eds.), *Social support: Theory, research and applications* (pp. 463–489). Dordrecht, The Netherlands: Martinus Nijhoff.

Wortman, C. B., & Silver, R. C. (1987). Coping with irrevocable loss. In G. R. VandenBos & B. K. Bryant (Eds.), *Cataclysms, crises, and catastrophes: Psychology in action* (Master Lecture Series, Vol. 6, pp. 189–235). Washington, DC: American Psychological Association.

Wortman, C. B., & Silver, R. C. (1989). The myths of coping with loss. *Journal of Consulting and Clinical Psychology, 55,* 349–357.

Zajonc, R. (1980). Feeling and thinking. *American Psychologist, 35,* 151–175.

13

Automatic and Dysfunctional Cognitive Processes in Depression

MARLENE M. MORETTI
University of Waterloo

BRIAN F. SHAW
University of Toronto
Toronto General Hospital

Intrusive negative thoughts are among the most distressing symptoms of depression. The content of these thoughts can vary widely from one depressed person to another: Some individuals may complain that they are preoccupied with thoughts of failure in their career, whereas others are plagued with intrusive thoughts concerning their inability to establish close relationships. Although the content of these thoughts varies among depressed patients, the theme of negative self-evaluation and self-reproach remains constant. Depressed individuals also complain that their negative thoughts "have a life of their own"—their onset occurs without intention, and their relation to environmental events is unclear. In addition, depressed individuals often regard their negative thoughts as "uncontrollable," since their attempts to inhibit or suppress them are futile. For example, a patient may report that while he or she is engaged in a conversation with a close friend, thoughts of personal inadequacy and rejection (e.g., "I'm boring," "I know they don't like me") intrude into awareness, even though the negative content of these thoughts seems incongruent with the situation. And the depressive thoughts persist "like a broken record," despite attempts to inhibit or distract attention away from them.

The intrusive nature of depressive thought has led researchers and clinicians to label these thought processes as "automatic" (Beck, 1967; Beck, Rush, Shaw, & Emery, 1979). Clinical observations suggest that automatic cognitive processes may be symptomatic of depression. But it is important to note that similar cognitive processes are found in a number of different psychological disorders. For example, intrusive and dysfunctional thoughts are found in patients suffering from anxiety disorder (Beck, 1986; Glass, Merluzzi, Biever, & Larsen, 1982; Ingram & Kendall, 1987; Sutton-Simon & Goldfried, 1979), and the inability to control thought processes is even more pronounced in obsessive–compulsive disorder (Salkovskis, 1985). Hence, it is clear that intrusive and automatic cognitive processes are not diagnostic of depression per se. In fact, automatic cognitive processes may not be indicative of psychopathology at all. Research in the areas of cognition and social cognition has indicated that many on-line cognitive processes operate automatically. The onset of these processes occurs without intention and awareness of triggering stimuli, and these processes may be difficult to inhibit when attentional resources are limited (Bargh, 1984; Bargh & Pratto, 1986; Logan, 1980, 1985; Posner & Snyder, 1975; Schneider & Shiffrin, 1977; Shiffrin & Schneider, 1977; Uleman, 1987). Such automatized cognitive processes are not necessarily dysfunctional. As cognitive psychologists have pointed out, automatic processes can be highly efficient and advantageous in many circumstances (Glass & Holyoak, 1986; Shiffrin & Schneider, 1977).

Even though automatic cognitive processes are not unique to the disorder of depression, and are not always a cause of dysfunctional information processing, the operation of such processes under certain conditions may exacerbate and prolong periods of depression. Under what conditions might automatic cognitive processes have dysfunctional consequences? This is the question we address in this chapter. Before turning directly to this issue, however, we briefly review the characteristics that distinguish automatic from controlled cognitive processes, and identify factors that may contribute to automatic and dysfunctional modes of information processing.

CONTROLLED VERSUS AUTOMATIC PROCESSING MODES

The distinction between cognitive processes that operate "automatically" and those that require our direct attention and monitoring—"controlled" processes—has been of long-standing interest to cognitive psychologists. Almost a century ago, researchers noted that repeated exposure to a stimulus led to a reduction in both attention and effort required for effective responding (Bryan & Harter, 1899; James, 1890). This effect is now well documented (Logan, 1980). Shiffrin and Schneider (1977) have proposed that frequent exposure to a task or event results in the development of a cognitive "set," or organized representation of information in memory pertaining to a sequence of stimulus features and responses. If frequently activated, this cognitive set directs processing with little demand on limited attentional capacity. Consequently, automatic processes can be initiated when attention is allocated to the performance of other tasks. In contrast, controlled processes require considerable attention and usually cannot be initiated when individuals are engaged in the performance of other tasks that require attention.

In recent years, the term "automaticity" has been used to describe a broad range of cognitive processes. As Bargh (Chapter 1, this volume) notes, this has led to some confusion regarding the definition and essential characteristics of automaticity. However, several characteristics have been consistently identified that distinguish automatic from controlled processes. First, as we have noted, automatic processes place a considerably lighter demand on attentional resources than do controlled processes. Second, whereas the onset of automatic processes can be triggered by stimuli without an individual's awareness, the onset of controlled processes can only be initiated with intention (Bargh, 1984; Shiffrin & Schneider, 1977). Third, research in both cognitive and social psychology has indicated that under certain conditions automatic processes may be difficult to inhibit. In contrast, controlled processes can be interrupted and altered with little difficulty. Finally, even though controlled processes place high demands on attentional resources, memory appears to be better for stimuli processed in controlled modes than in automatic modes (Fisk & Schneider, 1984; Shiffrin & Schneider, 1977; Smith & Lerner, 1986). Thus, the adoption of controlled processing modes is advantageous when performance requires learning new stimulus–response patterns.[1]

Functional versus Dysfunctional Automatic Processes

There are many circumstances in which the development of automatic processes is advantageous (Glass & Holyoak, 1986; Shiffrin & Schneider, 1977). For example, the development of automatized strategies can maximize processing efficiency when response demands remain stable for the performance of a task. Under these conditions, automatized strategies allow attention to be directed to other aspects of functioning, such as the performance of concurrent tasks (LaBerge & Samuels, 1974). However, automatized processing strategies may be dysfunctional when individuals are required to alter well-established patterns of attending and responding to stimuli, because previously established automatized processes may be difficult to inhibit. The repeated demonstrations of the Stroop effect are evidence of the adverse consequences of automatic processing when subjects are required to inhibit well-established response patterns (e.g., reading color names) and attend to other aspects of a stimulus (e.g., naming the color of the ink in which color names are printed) (Logan, 1980; Posner, 1978; Stroop, 1935).

How seriously is performance impaired by interference from automatized processes? Although it is often assumed that interference from automatic processes results in substantial negative effects on performance, research indicates that performance in such situations is only minimally affected (Hasher & Zacks, 1979; Jonides, 1981; Logan, 1978, 1979; Posner & Snyder, 1975; Shiffrin & Schneider, 1977). Logan (1985) notes that the error rate on the Stroop task is typically very low, and subjects usually experience only small increases in reaction time (less than 10%) as a result of interference from automatic processes. Furthermore, when errors do occur during the performance of tasks that have been loosely categorized as automatic (e.g., typing, speaking), they are usually detected quickly, and a shift to controlled processing is made to correct these errors (Hasher & Zacks, 1979; Levelt, 1983; Logan, 1979, 1982; Posner & Snyder, 1975). Thus, it appears that interference from automatic processes has only a limited negative effect on the performance of simple cognitive tasks. Such findings have prompted Logan (1985) to conclude that there is no clear association among automaticity, higher error rates in performance, and loss of control over information processing.

An important finding of this research is that on simple cognitive tasks, individuals easily identify errors in their performance and readily *shift* from automatic to controlled processing modes to correct these errors. This pattern of results suggests that maximum efficiency is most likely to be achieved when subjects are able to (1) identify inaccuracy or error that has occurred while performing a task automatically, and (2) flexibly alternate between automatic and controlled processes to correct these errors. Although the recognition that existing processing strategies are producing inaccuracy or error may be relatively straightforward in some domains of performance (e.g., speech, typing), this may be difficult to establish in other areas of information processing, or under some processing conditions. In addition, the interruption of automatic processes and shift to controlled processing modes may sometimes be difficult to achieve. Finally, there may be individual-difference factors that increase vulnerability to processing information in a dysfunctional and automatic manner. More specifically, we propose that the probability of dysfunctional automatized processing will increase under the following conditions:

1. Criteria for detecting dysfunction in processing are ambiguous and performance feedback is not readily available (i.e., individuals are unaware of the dysfunctional consequences of automatic information processing).
2. Automatized processes are utilized in the performance of complex

rather than simple stimulus–response sequences, and consequently individuals are unable to detect the source of dysfunction in processing.

3. Processing conditions, such as the presence of heightened affective arousal and limited attentional resources, prevent an interruption of automatic processes and a shift to controlled processing strategies.

4. Contextual and/or individual-difference factors heighten the accessibility of particular constructs for processing information.

Criteria for Detecting Accuracy or Error in Processing

When criteria for identifying dysfunctional consequences of automatic processing are unclear, subjects are unlikely to recognize that performance should be altered. As we have noted, this is not typically a problem in the performance of simple cognitive tasks. However, this problem may arise in contexts requiring the processing of social or self-relevant information, because (1) criteria for what is functional and dysfunctional in these situations are usually ambiguous, and (2) feedback regarding dysfunctional information processing is not typically available. Consider how readily subjects make spontaneous trait inferences about others on the basis of limited information (e.g., Smith & Lerner, 1986; Uleman, 1987; Winter & Uleman, 1984; Winter, Uleman, & Cunniff, 1985). Subjects who interpret the behavior of targets in a stereotyped or biased manner may not doubt the validity of their interpretations and hence may not alter their impressions. Even if criteria for accuracy could be established, direct feedback about accuracy in social perception is not usually available in real-life social interactions. The impressions that we form about others are not typically discussed explicitly during social interaction, and one's behavior toward a target may elicit confirmatory behavior (Darley & Fazio, 1980). Hence, not only is feedback about the bias in one's interpersonal perceptions difficult to obtain, but there may be reasons to doubt the validity of feedback that is elicited.

A similar problem exists for detecting bias[2] in the processing of self-relevant information. For example, is it negatively biased to interpret the neutral expression of your colleague following your colloquium as evidence of disappointment in your presentation? There may be many reasons for the display of a neutral expression by your colleague that have nothing to do with the nature of your colloquium. However, if you assume that this is a reflection of your colleague's disappointment, this bias may go undetected, because this interpretation often deters attempts to seek out clarification. Since bias in social and self-referent information processing is difficult to detect, individuals are unlikely to interrupt automatic or habitual modes of processing information and shift to controlled processing modes. Quite simply, it may be that individuals do not shift to controlled

processing modes because they have no reason to suspect that their interpretations of self-referent and social information are biased.

Complex versus Simple Automatized Sequences

A second factor that may be associated with dysfunctional automatic processing is the complexity of automatized sequences. Dysfunctional automatic processes may arise and persist when complex stimulus–response
sequences become automatized, because individuals are unable to detect
the *source* of dysfunction in their performance. When automatic processes
are developed for the performance of relatively simple stimulus–response
sequences, identifying the source of performance error in the sequence is
usually straightforward. For example, a a typist who strikes the wrong key
can often determine the source of error in performance. In contrast, consider the difficulties that an athlete or musician may encounter in altering
well-established but dyfunctional automatized stimulus–response sequences. Because the performance of these individuals is likely to reflect
complex automatized sequences, it may be extremely difficult to identify
the source or sources of dysfunction in performance. Hence, altering these
patterns may be very difficult.

It may also be the case that individuals who are informed that their
processing of interpersonal information is dysfunctional experience difficulty identifying the source of inaccuracy or bias in on-line processing because of the complexity of these processes. Consequently, they may be
unable to adjust for this bias in their current and future interpersonal evaluations. Similarly, individuals who are made aware of biases in their interpretations of self-relevant information may be unable to identify the cause
or causes of inaccuracy or bias in on-line processing. If this is the case,
these biases are likely to persist as a source of dysfunction in self-referent
information processing.

Affective Arousal and Limited Attentional Resources

There are several reasons to suspect that dysfunctional automatic processing may occur more frequently when individuals process information under conditions of heightened affective arousal. First, there is evidence that
affective states heighten the accessibility of similarly valenced constructs
for information processing (Higgins & King, 1981; Isen, 1984; Johnson
& Tversky, 1983). For example, Isen and her colleagues have demonstrated that the induction of positive mood via exposure to positive experiences increases the positivity of subsequent evaluations of events and the
likelihood of prosocial behavior (Isen, 1970; Isen & Levin, 1972). Johnson
and Tversky (1983) suggest that the influence of affect on processing is
independent of semantic association. Their results demonstrated that judgments of events were influenced by subjects' mood even when these events

were unrelated to the cause of mood (but see Erdley & D'Agostino, 1988, in which priming did not depend on the valence of information).

There may be other reasons for the relationship of affect to dysfunctional automatic processing. One possibility is that affective arousal impinges on limited attentional resources, reducing an individual's capacity to monitor information processing. A reduction in attentional resources may result in the failure to detect dysfunction associated with automatized processing, and consequently the failure to initiate or maintain corrective controlled processing strategies. This proposal is consistent with the recent findings of Kim and Baron (1988). In this study, subjects experiencing high levels of physiological arousal were more likely to use stereotypic adjectives to describe individuals in occupations than were subjects experiencing low levels of arousal. Kim and Baron (1988) suggest that heightened arousal reduces cognitive capacity and increases the likelihood that information will be processed automatically in accord with stereotypes and schemata. The effect of emotional arousal on cognitive capacity may be similar to that of physiological arousal. It may also be the case that affect both increases the accessibility of similarly valenced constructs in memory for processing, and reduces attentional resources for monitoring automatic processing and initiating controlled modes of information processing.

Heightened or Chronic Accessibility of Constructs

Construct accessibility, or the "readiness with which a stored construct is utilized in information processing" (Higgins & King, 1981, p. 71), is influenced by both temporary and chronic factors (Bargh, Bond, Lombardi, & Tota, 1986). Increased frequency and/or recency of construct activation via the adoption of specific processing goals or exposure to particular types of experiences can temporarily increase the accessibility of constructs during processing (Higgins, 1987; Higgins & King, 1981; Higgins, Kuiper, & Olson, 1980; Wyer & Srull, 1981). For example, exposure to situations that involve high levels of interpersonal threat may temporarily increase or "prime" the accessibility of constructs associated with this situation (e.g., mistrust, defense).

Several studies have demonstrated that subjects' processing of interpersonal information is strongly influenced by priming manipulations that temporarily heighten the accessibility of constructs. Using the unrelated-studies paradigm, Higgins, Rholes, and Jones (1977) demonstrated that incidental presentation of trait-related adjectives influenced subjects' judgments about a target in a presumably unrelated subsequent experiment. Studies using similar research paradigms have replicated and extended this finding (Higgins, Bargh, & Lombardi, 1985; Smith & Lerner, 1986; Srull & Wyer, 1979, 1980). Bargh and his colleagues (Bargh et al., 1986; Bargh & Pietromonaco, 1982) have demonstrated that *subliminal* presentation of trait-related stimuli influenced subsequent judgments about a target person. These results clearly indicate that subjects need not be aware of the priming of constructs in order for it to influence the processing of subsequent information.

Long-term or chronic expectancies, needs, and values, or chronic exposure to particular types of experiences, can result in relatively stable individual differences in construct accessibility (Bruner, 1957; Higgins & King, 1981; Postman & Brown, 1952). Several studies have demonstrated that individual differences in the chronic accessibility of constructs exert a significant influence on the encoding, interpretation, and recall of interpersonal information. For example, Bargh and Pratto (1986) found that subjects automatically attended to information that corresponded to chronically accessible constructs on a Stroop color-naming task. Chronically accessible constructs have also been found to influence on-line impressions of others under conditions of information overload, but not when subjects are given control over the presentation of information about others (Bargh & Thein, 1985). In addition, Higgins, King, and Mavin (1982) have found that chronic construct accessibility (as measured by the frequency of construct use in descriptions of others) predicts how the behavior of others is interpreted and recalled. It is important to note that chronic and temporary sources of construct accessibility may operate jointly to determine automaticity in processing information (Bargh et al., 1986).

There are many reasons to believe that the heightened accessibility of constructs, as a function of either chronic situational or individual-difference factors, may lead to dysfunctional automatic processing. Higgins and Moretti (1988) suggest that chronic construct accessibility results in the following:

1. The utilization of chronically accessible constructs to evaluate an *increasing range* of events or performances.
2. The introduction of chronically accessible constructs at early stages of information processing.

Range of Utilization

When constructs are highly accessible, they are likely to be automatically utilized as standards or guides for interpreting a wide range of experiences. In some instances, the use of such constructs will be appropriate or normative for the interpretation of an event; that is, the construct that is utilized will be one that is commonly used by others to evaluate the event. However, because chronically accessible constructs are likely to be utilized across a wide range of events, they may be applied inappropriately or nonnormatively on some occasions. For example, if an individual's experiences have led to the chronic accessibility of the construct of independence–dependence, he or she is likely to apply this construct in interpreting his or her behavior across a wide range of situations. In some situations, the use of this construct will be normative for self-evaluation (e.g., one's ability to independently generate innovative solutions to problems at work, one's capacity to tolerate being alone), but in other situations the application of this construct would be less normative (e.g., the decision to ask for directions when lost in a new city becomes an issue that is related to independence–dependence). Processing is likely to be dysfunctional to the extent that chronically accessible constructs dominate the processing of information in contexts where the application of these constructs is non-normative.

Stage of Utilization

Information processing can be conceptualized as a multistage process beginning with the simple registration and representation of a stimulus (stimulus representation) and proceeding to the stages of identification, interpretation, and appraisal (for a more detailed description of this process, see Higgins & Moretti, 1988; Higgins, Strauman, & Klein, 1986). Normatively, factual standards (i.e., beliefs about the *actual* performance or attributes of one or more persons) determine how individuals interpret an event. For example, a grade of 65% on an exam is interpreted as a "success" when evaluated in relation to the mean on an exam of 40% (social category reference point). In contrast, personal standards or acquired guides (i.e., internalized standards associated with the self) determine how individuals appraise or feel about an event. For example, even though a grade of 50% may be interpreted as a pass, it may not be appraised positively because it falls short of an internal guide for self-evaluation.

Higgins and Moretti (1988) have proposed that when constructs are chronically accessible, they displace the application of factual standards at the stage of interpretation. For example, the chronic accessibility of the construct of intelligence may lead an individual to automatically apply this personal standard for self-evaluation rather than a factual standard at the stage of interpretation. Hence, a grade of 65% on an exam may be interpreted as "unsuccessful," despite the fact that the mean on the exam was 40%. That is, the automatic intrusion of this chronically accessible construct displaces the application of a factual standard of interpretation that would indicate the performance was a "success." With increasingly high levels of construct accessibility, it is conceivable that the application of factual standards at even earlier stages of processing (i.e., identification and encoding) could be displaced. The displacement of factual standards at early stages of processing may lead to very unusual and even bizarre percepts and interpretations.

This analysis suggests that the chronic accessibility of self-relevant constructs may be a vulnerability factor that predisposes one to dysfunctional automatic processing. Highly accessible self-relevant constructs may automatically intrude during the processing of a wide range of events and at early stages of information processing.

One question to consider is whether chronic construct accessibility and dysfunctional automatic processing are more likely to be found in relation to self-referent information processing than to other domains of information processing. Although the significance of the self per se in determining the efficiency of information processing has been questioned (Higgins & Bargh, 1987), there are several reasons to believe that dysfunctional automatic processing is more likely to be found when individuals are processing self-relevant information than when they are processing other types of information. First, as previously noted, there are few "checks and balances" to ensure that self-referent information processing is not biased. Consequently, individuals may persist in utilizing chronically accessible constructs in an inappropriate manner without an awareness of the bias that is introduced in self-referent information processing.

Second, self-referent constructs are likely to be among the most frequently utilized during information processing (Higgins et al., 1982). To the extent that the self is frequently activated during processing, it is likely that some constructs will become highly associated with the self (Bargh & Tota, 1988; Markus, 1977). These constructs are likely to be highly accessible during the processing of self-referent information. This analysis of the role of the self in processing need not imply that the self is a *unique* cognitive structure (Higgins & Bargh, 1987; Segal, 1988), but simply a representation of constructs that are, to a greater or lesser degree, associated with the self.

A third reason why self-referential information processing may be characterized by automaticity and dysfunction is that information related to the self is typically more affectively charged than are other types of information (Markus & Sentis, 1982; Zajonc, 1984). The activation of similarly valenced information is likely to maintain automatic and dysfunctional patterns of information processing. In addition, affective arousal may reduce available attentional resources for initiating controlled processing strategies.

IMPLICATIONS FOR UNDERSTANDING DEPRESSION

What are the implications of the distinction between automatic and controlled processes, and our analysis of risk factors associated with dysfunctional automatic processing, for understanding information processing in depression? There are many facets of depressive thought processes that appear to be automatic. The onset of dysfunctional patterns of attention, interpretation, and memory occurs effortlessly and without intention during depressed states. These negatively biased cognitive processes are often initiated without awareness of triggering stimuli. Although depressed patients may be unaware of the stimuli that precipitate the onset of automatic and dysfunctional cognitive processes, and of the chronically accessible constructs or beliefs that guide these processes (Beck, 1976; Beck et al., 1979), they are painfully aware of the *products* (Ingram & Hollon, 1986) of automatic processes (i.e., negative thoughts and feelings). It is at this level that automatic processes are experienced as intrusive. It is important to note that although the on-line operation of dysfunctional automatic processes in depression may not place demands on limited attentional resources, the feelings and thoughts that are produced by these processes dominate depressed patients' attention and may interfere with performance on other tasks (Beck, 1967, 1976). As previously noted, depressed individuals experience great difficulty inhibiting dysfunctional automatic processes or distracting attention away from the products of these processes.

Our discussion of risk factors that may be associated with dysfunctional automatic processing leads us to propose that depressed individuals are most likely to experience dysfunctional automatic processing when the following hold true:

1. The dysfunctional consequences of automatic information processes are not readily apparent, such as in the processing of social and self-relevant information.
2. Automized processes involve complex rather than simple stimulus–response sequences.
3. Information processing is associated with high rather than low affective arousal.

In addition, it is likely that the presence of chronically accessible negative self-constructs in depressed individuals is associated with the likelihood that they will experience dysfunctional patterns of automatic information processing. Finally, the risk factors for automatic and dysfunctional information processing we have presented may *interact* to increase the probability of dysfunctional automatic processing. The assumption that dysfunctional information processing is determined by multiple risk factors raises the possibility that the likelihood of depressive information processing may vary across individuals and across situations. Under some conditions, all individuals may process information in a dysfunctional manner (e.g., self-referent processing of highly emotional information; see Bradley, 1978; Greenwald, 1980). However, some individuals may be more vulnerable to engage in automatic and dysfunctional information processing under conditions that do not lead others to process information dysfunctionally.

A number of these risk factors for dysfunctional automatic processing have been discussed by depression researchers and clinicians, although the role of automaticity in these models of depression is not always clearly explicated. In the next section of this chapter, we review contemporary models of depression that have incorporated the notion of automatic and dysfunctional information processing, and the empirical support for these positions.

The Role of Automaticity in Contemporary Models of Depression

According to Beck, depression stems from the activation of pathological cognitive structures or "schemata" that develop early in life in response to particularly stressful experiences (e.g., perceived rejection, deprivation). Schemata are organized representations of both episodic and abstract information. Not only do they embody information about specific stressful experiences, but they also contain information about beliefs that have been abstracted from experiences (Higgins & Bargh, 1987). Once established, negative schemata about the self, the world, and the future become active in response to periods of stress, particularly from events that are thematically related to issues of deprivation or rejection (e.g., "No one cares," "I'm not good enough"). Beck postulates that the activation of negative schemata displaces other cognitive processes that are critical to reality testing and to attaining self-objectivity. As depression worsens, processing becomes increasingly dominated by "hyperactive" negative schemata (Kovacs & Beck, 1978). Consequently, negative schemata are evoked in response to more diverse and less logically related information and experiences; that is, "the orderly matching of an appropriate schema to a particular stimulus is upset by the intrusion of these overly active idiosyncratic schemas" (Beck et al., 1979, p. 13).

Beck has proposed that that activation of negative schemata increases the likelihood of several types of cognitive errors. These include "paralogical," "stylistic," and "semantic" errors. Paralogical errors occur when conclusions are drawn (1) in the absence of evidence or in the face of contradictory evidence; (2) on the basis of irrelevant details often interpreted out of context; or (3) from an inadequate or nonrepresentative data base. Stylistic errors involve the systematic magnification or minimization of events or information and lead to negative self-evaluations. Finally, semantic errors occur when events are erroneously or inappropriately labeled on the basis of affective reactions, rather than on the basis of the actual intensity or importance of the event. Beck views these errors in cognitive functioning as distinct from the occasional inaccuracy and inconsistency that characterize everyday cognitive processes, because these errors represent a *systematic negative bias* against the individual.

Beck claims that cognitive errors associated with the activation of depressive schemata occur automatically. This proposal is based on his observations indicating that negative thoughts in depression do "not arise as a result of deliberation, reasoning, or reflection about an event or topic," but rather "just happen" and are difficult to "turn off" (Beck, 1976, p. 36). Because he has observed that negative thoughts "appeared to emerge automatically and extremely rapidly" (Beck, 1976, p. 35), he has labeled them "automatic thoughts."

Higgins and King (1981) have also suggested that automaticity plays an important role in depressive information processing, although their conceptualization of this process is somewhat different from that offered by Beck. According to Higgins and King (1981), it is unlikely that depressed persons differ in the *availability* (Bruner, 1957; Tulving & Pearlsone, 1966) of positive and negative constructs for processing information—that is, whether or not positive or negative constructs are stored in memory. However, the activation of the self may result in different patterns of positive- and negative-construct *accessibility* for depressed and nondepressed individuals. Whereas self-reference in nondepressed individuals may be associated with a greater accessibility of positive than of negative constructs for information processing, self-reference in depressed individuals may be associated with an inhibition of positive relative to negative constructs for information processing. An important difference between the models of Beck (1967, 1976) and Higgins and King (1981) is that the former view is based on the concept of a "self-schema," which implies the presence of a structurally interconnected cognitive representation; the latter perspective is not. In this regard, the Higgins and King (1981) model of depression is more congruent with the present status of research on self-referent information processing, which generally does not support the notion that self-information is *structurally* interconnected (for reviews of this issue, see Higgins & Bargh, 1987; Segal, 1988).

The use of the notions of automaticity and construct accessibility by Teasdale (1983) differs from that of both Beck (1976) and Higgins and King (1981). He suggests that depressed mood and stressful events activate concepts, interpretations, and memories that have been encoded during previous periods of depression. This "spread of activation" heightens the probability that negative constructs will influence on-line processing. Hence, information that is made accessible by negative mood contributes to the exacerbation and maintenance of the disorder by exerting a negative bias on the processing of information from new experiences (see also Isen, 1984).

The concept of automatic and dysfunctional patterns of information processing also emerges in the work of Kuiper and his colleagues (Derry & Kuiper, 1981; Kuiper & Derry, 1982; Kuiper & MacDonald, 1982; MacDonald & Kuiper, 1985). Kuiper proposes that the content of the self-schema leads to greater efficiency in processing schema-congruent than schema-incongruent information. He also suggests that depth of processing will be greater for information that is congruent rather than incongruent with the content of the self-schema. These propositions have led him to predict that the depressed individual will process negative self-referent information more quickly than will the nondepressed individual. In addition, he predicts that the depressed person will display greater recall for negative self-referent information than will the nondepressed person. Kuiper's model suggests that the depressed individual's attention to and processing of schema-congruent information are unintentional and difficult to inhibit.

More recently, Bargh and Tota (1988) have proposed that depressed and nondepressed individuals do not differ in the content of the self-concept so much as in the accessibility of positive and negative constructs associated with the self. They suggest that depressive information processing occurs because of the strong links between the self-concept and depressive constructs that develop during periods of depression. Once an individual has made the decision to process information from a self-referent perspective, constructs associated with the self exert an automatic and pervasive influence over information processing. For the depressed individual, the decision to process information from a self-referent perspective leads to the heightened accessibility of depressed-content constructs. In contrast, the nondepressed individual's decision to process information from a self-referent perspective is associated with the heightened accessibility of nondepressed-content constructs. It is important to note that Bargh and Tota (1988) view automaticity in depressive information processing as "context-dependent"; that is, a controlled decision to engage in self-referential thought precedes the automatic activation of self-related constructs. Hence, they do not view depressive information processing as automatic in the strictest sense of the term. Nonetheless, once initiated, depressive cognitive processes appear to operate automatically.

Although these models of depressive information processing present somewhat different perspectives on the role of automaticity in depression, they share the views that dysfunctional cognitive processes in depression operate without intention, are uncontrollable, and lead to negative interpretations of self-relevant information. All models also propose that the activation of a cognitive representation or pattern of self-related constructs underlies dysfunctional information processing.

Only a subset of the risk factors for automatic and dysfunctional information processing that we have identified is represented in these models. Most of the models of depressive information processing identify the "self" or self-reference as a vulnerability factor in depression. However, few have explicitly discussed the interactions among self-reference, affect, task ambiguity, and complexity in determining the probability of automatic and dysfunctional information processing. Let us now turn to a review of the empirical evidence for the role of automatic and dysfunctional information processing in depression.

Empirical Support for the Role of Dysfunctional Automatic Processes in Depression

In reviewing this literature, it is important to keep in mind that very few studies have actually been conducted in such a way as to allow for a direct test of the automaticity hypothesis. What type of evidence is relevant to the hypothesis that depressive information processing occurs automatically? First, it is important that studies show that depressed subjects, in comparison to nondepressed subjects, process negative information more efficiently and without placing demands on limited attentional resources. Research demonstrating that depressed individuals process negative information more quickly than do nondepressed individuals is consistent with the automaticity hypothesis. However, such studies do not provide direct evidence of the automaticity of depressive information processing, since the attentional demands associated with information processing are not assessed. For this reason, it is important that studies show that the processing of negative information by depressed subjects is not impaired by the concurrent performance of another task that demands attention (i.e., the presence of a concurrent memory-load task; see Bargh & Tota, 1988).

The second type of evidence that is directly relevant to the automaticity hypothesis comes from research that has investigated the extent to which the onset of automatic and dysfunctional information processing in depression is unintentional (i.e., not due to controlled processes) and the degree to which such processes are controllable (i.e., can be inhibited). Relatively few studies have been designed to evaluate these aspects of depressive information processing. The bulk of existing research investigates whether depressive information processing is negatively biased rather than automatic. For this reason, many studies provide only circumstantial evidence about the role of automaticity in processing information during depression. With this caveat in mind, let us now examine the research that has been completed to date.

Is Negative Information Processed Efficiently during Periods of Depression?

There is strong evidence of a negative bias in self-referent information processing during depressed states. Depressed individuals are more likely to evaluate themselves negatively under almost all conditions and with regard to both interpersonal and achievement-related tasks than are nondepressed individuals (Beck, 1967; Gotlib, 1982; Gotlib & Olson, 1983; Hammen & Krantz, 1976; Loeb, Beck, & Diggory, 1971; Lobitz & Post, 1979; Sacco & Hokanson, 1978; Smolen, 1978; Wollert & Buchwald, 1979; Zarantonello, Johnson, & Petzel, 1979). In contrast to nondepressed individuals, depressed individuals are also more likely to anticipate failure (Garber & Hollon, 1980; Golin, Terrell, & Johnson, 1977; Golin, Terrell, Weitz, & Drost, 1979; Klein & Seligman, 1976; Miller & Seligman, 1973), and to underestimate the quality of their performance (Dobson & Shaw, 1981; Nelson & Craighead, 1977). Finally, whereas nondepressed individuals are more likely to assume personal responsibility for positive events (i.e., to make internal, stable, and global causal attributions) and to attribute responsibility for negative events to external factors (i.e., to make external, unstable, and specific causal attributions), depressed individuals show an "evenhandedness" in their causal attributions for positive and negative events (for a review, see Miller & Moretti, 1987). This pattern of causal attribution suggests that depressed individuals process information related to negative events quite differently than do nondepressed individuals.

Depressed individuals' view of the past appears to be as negative as their view of the present and future. Depressed individuals tend to recall previous periods of performance more negatively than do nondepressed individuals (Dobson & Shaw, 1981), and they are more likely to recall negative personal memories than are nondepressed persons. For example, Lishman and his colleagues (Lishman, 1972; Lloyd & Lishman, 1975) have demonstrated that depressed psychiatric patients, unlike nondepressed patients, show shorter latencies for the recall of unpleasant than of pleasant events. Similar results have been found in nonclinical populations (Bower, Giligan, & Monterio, 1981) and in individuals exposed to negative mood inductions (Teasdale & Fogarty, 1979; Teasdale, Taylor, & Fogarty, 1980).

It is important to note that, although depressed individuals view themselves more negatively than do nondepressed individuals, they do not necessarily view others as negatively as they view themselves. Indeed, research examining depressed individuals' evaluations of themselves versus their evaluations of others indicates that they view themselves as unique in their suffering and inadequacy (Hoen-Hyde, Schlottman, & Rush, 1982; Margin, Abramson, & Alloy, 1984; Tabachnik, Crocker, & Alloy, 1983).

Cumulatively, these studies support the notion that the products of self-relevant information processing in depressed states are highly negative. These cognitions can be viewed as dysfunctional, insofar as they promote negative affect and inhibit adaptive functioning. However, none of the studies reviewed thus far provide evidence that the cognitive processes that give rise to these cognitions can be classified as automatic.

Is Negative Information Processed Automatically during Periods of Depression?

One source of evidence for the automaticity of depressive information processing comes from studies conducted by Kuiper and his colleagues (Derry & Kuiper, 1981; Kuiper & Derry, 1982; Kuiper & MacDonald, 1982). It will be recalled that Kuiper has proposed that schema-congruent information is processed more efficiently than schema-incongruent information. On the basis of this model, Kuiper predicted that depressed subjects would have shorter response latencies for decisions about the self-descriptiveness of depressed-content than nondepressed-content words. He also predicted that depressed subjects would display greater recall of depressed-content than nondepressed-content information, because of the greater depth of processing (Craik & Tulving, 1975) of negative information that occurs in depression. The basic methodology employed in these studies involved instructing depressed and nondepressed subjects to make forced-choice decisions about the self-descriptiveness of depressed-content and nondepressed-content adjectives.

In the first of a series of studies, Derry and Kuiper (1981) found that clinically depressed patients and nondepressed subjects did not differ in their response latencies for identifying depressed- and nondepressed-content adjectives as self-descriptive. However, nondepressed subjects displayed superior recall of nondepressed-content adjectives, whereas depressed subjects displayed superior recall for depressed-content adjectives. These results were interpreted as evidence of the greater depth of processing of negative self-relevant information in clinically depressed patients than in nondepressed subjects.

Kuiper and Derry (1982) examined recall of self-referent information by mildly depressed and nondepressed subjects. Consistent with earlier findings, nondepressed subjects displayed better recall for self-referenced nondepressed-content adjectives than for depressed-content adjectives. Mildly depressed subjects did not differ in their recall of nondepressed-content versus depressed-content adjectives. Similar findings were reported by Kuiper and MacDonald (1982). In this study, nondepressed subjects demonstrated better recall of nondepressed-content than of depressed-content words, but mildly depressed subjects showed no difference in recall. Nondepressed subjects also displayed significantly shorter reaction times for self-referent decisions for nondepressed-content adjectives than for depressed-content adjectives. Response latencies for self-referent decisions for nondepressed-content and depressed-content adjectives were not significantly different for mildly depressed subjects.

According to Kuiper and his colleagues, these findings indicate that the self-schema of the clinically depressed patient facilitates more efficient or automatic processing of negative than of positive information, and that the self-schema of the mildly depressed individual facilitates equal efficiency in processing of positive and negative information. However, Bargh and Tota (1988) have challenged Kuiper's conclusions on conceptual and methodological grounds. Bargh and Tota's (1988) most pressing concern with Kuiper's research (specifically, Kuiper & MacDonald, 1982) is that raw response latencies were interpreted as pure measures of automaticity, even though this dependent variable is potentially confounded by numerous factors involved in controlled processing, such as self-presentational biases and judgment confidence. Bargh and Tota (1988) suggest that researchers need to utilize concurrent memory-load tasks or similar procedures in studies of automaticity, in order to rule out the possibility that biases due to controlled processing have contributed to response latencies.

In their most recent research, MacDonald and Kuiper (1985) did use a memory-load condition to investigate automatic processing of depressed-

content and nondepressed-content adjectives by clinically depressed patients and nondepressed subjects. As previously noted, if information is
processed automatically, the presence of a memory-load condition should
not influence response latencies. Hence, in the MacDonald and Kuiper study,
one would predict that the response latencies of depressed subjects for self-
referent decisions about depressed-content words (i.e., schema-congruent
information) should not differ under memory-load and non-memory-load
conditions. If one assumes, as Kuiper and his colleagues do, that nondepressed-content information is not processed automatically by clinically
depressed individuals (i.e., schema-incongruent information), the response
latencies of depressed subjects for self-referent decisions about nondepressed-content words should be significantly longer in the memory-load
than in the non-memory-load condition.

MacDonald and Kuiper (1985) found that clinically depressed subjects displayed significantly longer response latencies for "no" decisions to
depressed-content adjectives than did nondepressed subjects. However, they
did not find that the presence of a memory-load condition influenced the
response latencies of depressed subjects' decisions for depressed-content or
nondepressed-content adjectives. MacDonald and Kuiper (1985) note that
if the automaticity of depressive information processing is to be truly established, content specificity (i.e., depressed content vs. nondepressed content) of automatic processing must be established. Nonetheless, they interpret the lack of an interaction among memory load, adjective content, and
depression as evidence of automatic processing of schema-congruent information.

Bargh and Tota (1988) argue that MacDonald and Kuiper's (1985)
failure to find a memory-load effect indicates either that all self-referent
decisions for depressed-content and nondepressed-content adjectives were
automatic for depressed and nondepressed subjects, or that all self-referent
decisions were equally nonautomatic. They conclude that MacDonald and
Kuiper's (1985) study fails to provide a clear indication of whether schema-
congruent information is processed automatically. They also point out that
MacDonald and Kuiper (1985) failed to record response latencies precisely
(response latencies were measured only to the nearest second), and this
might have been related to their failure to find a memory-load effect.

In light of these criticisms, Bargh and Tota (1988) altered the procedures used in Kuiper's research and attempted to test the automaticity hypothesis of depression more directly. Depressed and nondepressed subjects
were asked to make forced-choice decisions as to whether depressed-content or nondepressed-content adjectives were structurally or semantically
similar to other adjectives, either self-descriptive or descriptive of an "average" person. Subjects completed this task in either a memory-load or a
non-memory-load condition. In the memory-load condition, the subjects
were required to remember a six-digit number while they made decisions
about the adjectives. In contrast, subjects in the non-memory-load condi-

tion were simply required to make decisions about the adjectives. Bargh and Tota (1988) reasoned that if processing negative information is automatized in depression, response latencies for self-referential judgments of depressed-content adjectives should be unaffected by the memory-load condition. Consistent with this prediction, they found that the response latencies for self-referential judgments of depressed-content adjectives were similar for depressed subjects in the memory-load and non-memory-load conditions, but self-referential judgment latencies of nondepressed-content adjectives were greater in the memory-load than in the non-memory-load condition. Nondepressed subjects displayed an opposite pattern of results in which memory load increased latencies for depressed adjectives. Furthermore, both depressed and nondepressed subjects displayed longer response latencies for judgments of other-referent negative adjectives under the memory-load than under the non-memory-load condition. This pattern of results suggests that although depressed individuals process negative self-relevant information automatically, they do not process negative information that is directed at others automatically. In other words, automaticity in processing negative information during depressed states occurs only within the context of self-reference.

Additional support for the notion that depressed individuals process self-referent negative information automatically comes from studies that have assessed the performance of depressed and nondepressed subjects on a modified version of the Stroop color–word test (Stroop, 1935). This task requires that subjects attend to and report on one of two conflicting aspects of a stimulus. In the traditional version of the Stroop test, subjects report on the color of the ink of incongruent-color words. In the modified version of the Stroop test used by Gotlib and McCann (1984), subjects reported on the color of the ink of neutral, depressed-content, and manic-content words. The use of this task to assess automaticity of information processing in depression was based on the reasoning that the heightened accessibility of negative constructs associated with the self in depression would lead to greater interference between the semantic meaning of depressed-content words and the color-naming task. Hence, depressed subjects, unable to inhibit the automatic processing of depressed-content information, would demonstrate longer response latencies when naming the color of depressed-content words than of manic-content or neutral words. Consistent with this prediction, Gotlib and McCann (1984) found that depressed college students showed longer response latencies for color naming of depressed-content words than of manic-content or neutral words. In contrast, nondepressed subjects did not demonstrate significantly different response latencies for color naming of the three categories of words. Recently, this effect has been replicated by Williams and Nulty (1986).

These studies are consistent with the hypothesis that negative information is automatically processed during states of depression. One question that is raised by the studies reviewed thus far is whether depressed individuals automatically and dysfunctionally process emotional information about social interactions in the same manner in which they dysfunctionally process adjectives that are descriptive of the self. In an attempt to investigate this question, Moretti and Miller (1988) had depressed and nondepressed subjects in self-referent, other-referent, and control conditions view pictures of targets displaying different types of emotional expressions. Two photographs of the same target person (one neutral expression; one positive or negative expression) were simultaneously presented to subjects for a very brief period (300 milliseconds). In the self-referent condition, subjects were asked to imagine that the target's expressions were responses to something the subjects had said or done. Subjects indicated which of the two pictures "told them the most about how the target felt about" them. In the other-referent condition, subjects were asked to imagine that the target's expressions were responses to someone else. Subjects indicated which of the two pictures "told them the most about how the target felt about someone else." In the control condition, subjects were simply asked to identify the picture with the more emotional expression.

Moretti and Miller (1988) predicted that the speed and accuracy[3] of responses would depend on the accessibility of positive relative to negative constructs associated with self-reference versus other-reference. Self-reference for nondepressed individuals has been associated with greater accessibility of positive than of negative constructs. Hence, it was predicted that nondepressed subjects in the self-reference condition would identify pictures of targets with positive expressions more quickly and more accurately than pictures of targets displaying negative expressions. Nondepressed individuals have also been shown to view themselves more positively than they view others. Therefore, a positivity bias in construct accessibility was not expected to arise for nondepressed subjects in the other-referent condition.

In contrast to nondepressed individuals, numerous studies have shown that depressed individuals are "evenhanded" in their processing of positive and negative self-referent information (see Miller & Moretti, 1988). The evenhandedness of depressed individuals may reflect the equal accessibility of positive and negative constructs related to the self. This reasoning led to the prediction that depressed individuals would identify pictures of targets displaying positive and negative expressions with equal speed and accuracy; that is, depressed subjects would be evenhanded in their efficiency of processing positive and negative information. As previously noted, depressed individuals tend to see themselves more negatively than do others (Hoehn-Hyde et al., 1982; Martin et al., 1984; Tabachnik et al., 1983). This tendency may reflect the greater accessibility of positive than of negative constructs associated with other-reference for depressed subjects. Hence, it was predicted that depressed subjects in the other-referent condition would identify targets displaying positive expressions more quickly and more accurately than targets displaying negative expressions.

As predicted, Moretti and Miller (1988) found a significant three-way interaction among subject depression (depressed, nondepressed), reference (self-reference, other-reference, control), and type of target expression (positive, negative) for both speed and accuracy of performance. Simple-effects analyses indicated that nondepressed subjects in the self-referent condition identified pictures of targets displaying positive expressions significantly more quickly and accurately than pictures of targets displaying negative expressions. In contrast, nondepressed subjects in the other-referent condition were not significantly different in the speed or accuracy with which they identified pictures of targets displaying positive versus negative expressions (see Figures 13.1 and 13.2).

In contrast, depressed subjects in the self-referent condition were evenhanded in their processing of positive and negative information. Specifically, depressed subjects identified pictures of targets displaying positive expressions no more quickly or accurately than pictures of targets displaying negative expressions. However, depressed subjects in the other-referent condition tended to identify pictures of targets displaying positive expressions more quickly and accurately than pictures of targets displaying negative expressions (see Figures 13.3 and 13.4).

Of course, it was important to establish whether the differences between those depressed and nondepressed subjects in processing positive and negative information in self-referent and other-referent conditions were due to differences in construct *accessibility* (i.e., the readiness with which constructs are utilized during processing) or differences in construct *availabil-*

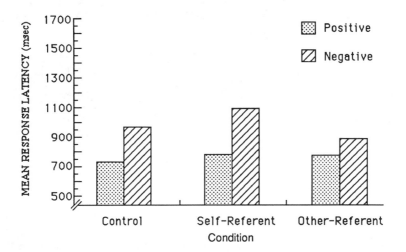

FIGURE 13.1.   Mean response latency (in milliseconds) of nondepressed subjects for identification of targets displaying positive and negative expressions in the control, self-referent, and other-referent conditions. From *Processing Positive and Negative Information in Depression* (p. 34) by M. M. Moretti and D. T. Miller, 1988, unpublished manuscript, University of Waterloo. Reprinted by permission of the authors.

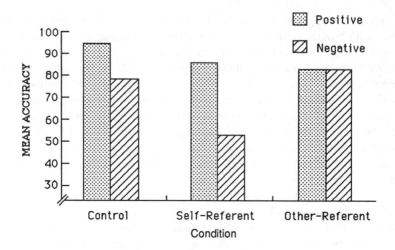

FIGURE 13.2. Mean accuracy of nondepressed subjects for the identification of targets displaying positive and negative expressions in the control, self-referent, and other-referent conditions. From *Processing Positive and Negative Information in Depression* (p. 35) by M. M. Moretti and D. T. Miller, 1988, unpublished manuscript, University of Waterloo. Reprinted by permission of the authors.

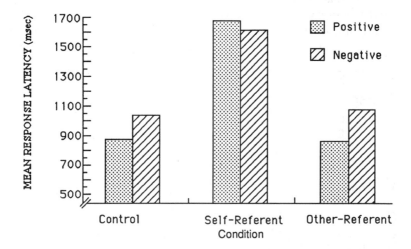

FIGURE 13.3. Mean response latency (in milliseconds) of depressed subjects for identification of targets displaying positive and negative expressions in the control, self-referent, and other-referent conditions. From *Processing Positive and Negative Information in Depression* (p. 36) by M. M. Moretti and D. T. Miller, 1988, unpublished manuscript, University of Waterloo. Reprinted by permission of the authors.

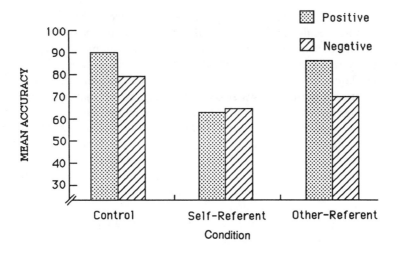

FIGURE 13.4. Mean accuracy of depressed subjects for the identification of targets displaying positive and negative expressions in the control, self-referent, and other-referent conditions. From *Processing Positive and Negative Information in Depression* (p. 37) by M. M. Moretti and D. T. Miller, 1988, unpublished manuscript, University of Waterloo. Reprinted by permission of the authors.

ity (i.e., whether or not constructs are present in memory). Moretti and Miller (1988) reasoned that if depressed and nondepressed subjects differed in the *availability* of positive and negative constructs, they would differ in the speed and accuracy with which they identified pictures of targets displaying positive and negative expressions when they were simply asked to identify the more emotional expression—that is, in the control condition. Results indicated that this was not the case. All subjects in the control condition, regardless of depression, identified pictures of targets displaying positive expressions more quickly and accurately than pictures of targets displaying negative expressions. These results suggest that depressed and nondepressed subjects did not differ in the *availability* of positive and negative constructs, and that the differences noted between the two groups in the self-referent and other-referent conditions were due to differential patterns of construct *accessibility*.

As Bargh and Tota (1988) noted, it is important to determine whether raw response latencies reflect only the automaticity of processing and not controlled response strategies or biases. Thus, in a separate study, Moretti and Miller (1988) asked depressed and nondepressed subjects to identify pictures of targets displaying more emotional expressions or to identify pictures of targets displaying more neutral expressions. If a response bias were to exist either toward or against the identification of targets with a particular type of emotional expression, the response latencies and accuracy of subjects identifying the more emotional expressions should differ from the response latencies and accuracy of subjects identifying neutral expressions. Results indicated that depressed and nondepressed subjects did not differ in these two conditions. Although this procedure does not completely rule out the possibility that response biases contributed to the response latencies and accuracy scores in the self-referent and other-referent conditions, these findings suggest that such biases may not have contributed significantly to the variance across the conditions.

This review highlights several important points in the existing literature. First, despite the theoretical importance of the notion of automatic processing in contemporary cognitive models of depression, relatively few studies have directly investigated this phenomenon. Indeed, many studies that are often cited as support for the notion of dysfunctional automatic processing only provide evidence that the self-referent information processing in depression is negatively biased. Although the results of these studies are consistent with the automaticity hypothesis, this research should be viewed as circumstantial evidence of automaticity, because it does not evaluate the nature of the cognitive processes that give rise to negative cognitions. Second, it is important to note that several of the studies designed to test the automaticity hypothesis are methodologically flawed. The most serious problem is that researchers frequently interpret raw response latencies as measures of automaticity without ruling out alternative sources of variance in these scores. Finally, research has yet to investigate several important aspects of automaticity in depressive information processing. For example, the ability of depressed subjects to inhibit or control automatized processes has yet to be examined. In addition, it would be interesting to investigate whether depressed individuals are more likely to experience difficulty with dysfunctional thought processes in some conditions than in others (e.g., high vs. low emotional arousal). Future research in these areas will help to delineate the context in which dysfunctional automatic processing is most likely to occur.

In summary, even though there remain many unanswered questions in this area of research, studies completed to date are generally consistent with the notion that self-referent information processing in depression is automatic and dysfunctional. The products of these cognitive processes are highly negative, intrusive, and distressing. In the final section of this chapter, we discuss the types of therapeutic interventions that might alter these dysfunctional cognitive patterns.

CLINICAL INTERVENTIONS AND THE PROCESS OF CHANGE

Our analysis of dysfunctional cognitive processes in depression has important treatment implications. Not only may it enhance our understanding of *why* current therapeutic interventions are helpful to patients (i.e., clarify the underlying mechanisms of therapeutic change), but it may also increase our appreciation of the difficulties that patients experience when they attempt to alter their cognitive processes.

As we have pointed out, it is common for depressed patients to complain about negative self-related thoughts that seem to occur spontaneously. Their attempts to inhibit these negative thoughts are unsuccessful. Not surprisingly, these experiences contribute to a sense of helplessness, hopelessness, and loss of control. There are several different clinical perspectives on the role of negative thoughts in depression and how they are most effectively treated in therapy. Psychodynamic models assume that the direct reports of patients, including negative intrusive thoughts, are of limited significance. They are important only insofar as they represent transformed and disguised expressions of unconscious conflicts and impulses, or defensive maneuvers. Hence, from a psychodynamic perspective, the negative thoughts that accompany depression are not an appropriate target of intervention, but rather are "stepping stones" to underlying dynamic conflicts (Beck, 1976).

Although behavioral models of depression do not view the negative cognitions that characterize the depressed state as important in the etiology and maintenance of depression (Lewinsohn, 1974), behavioral techniques have been developed to treat intrusive and distressing thoughts. "Thought stopping," a technique developed for the treatment of ruminations by Wolpe and Lazarus (1966), basically involves the therapist's directing the patient to verbalize distressing ruminative thoughts; when the patient indicates that he or she has done so, the therapist shouts, "Stop!" This procedure is repeated several times in the therapy session, and the patient is taught to say "Stop!" subvocally each time a rumination comes to mind. Although single-case reports suggest that this technique is effective for the treatment of a variety of obsessive ruminations, including persistent negative thoughts (Campbell, 1973; Hays & Waddell, 1976; Stern, 1970), the results of controlled studies have not been supportive (Emmelkamp & Kwee, 1977; Hackman & McLean, 1975; Stern, 1978; Stern, Lipsedge, & Marks, 1973).

There are reasons to believe that the use of thought-stopping techniques may actually increase rather than decrease the frequency of intrusive thoughts. The research of Wegner and his colleagues (Wegner, Schneider, Carter, & White, 1987; Wegner, Wenzlaff, Kerker, & Beattie, 1981; see Wegner & Schneider, Chapter 9, this volume) indicates that instructing individuals *not* to think about a particular thought has the paradoxical effect of increasing the frequency of the not-to-be-thought-about thought. It may be that drawing attention to a dysfunctional thought in order to suppress it increases the accessibility of the thought in memory, and consequently decreases the probability that it can be inhibited.

Both Wegner et al. (1987) and Fennell and Teasdale (1984) have demonstrated that thought suppression using a distractor as a replacement for the not-to-be-thought-about thought was effective in reducing the frequency with which this thought intruded into awareness. However, it is questionable whether the use of distractors is effective for inhibiting highly accessible and distressing thoughts. Although depressed patients sometimes find relief from their distressing thoughts in distraction, this approach to controlling negative thoughts would seem limited, simply because such individuals may have difficulty finding a constant stream of distractors to evade their distressing thoughts. Depressed patients also experience a reduction of interest in previously enjoyable activities; consequently, engaging in such activities may not effectively distract their attention from distressing thoughts. Most importantly, the introduction of distractors seems to depend on the ability of individuals to maintain controlled processing, and it is likely that intrusive thoughts will return when attention is turned to other tasks. For these reasons, therapeutic approaches that are aimed at identifying negative automatic thoughts and simply replacing these thoughts with more adaptive thoughts (Meichenbaum, 1977) are unlikely to produce more than momentary relief from feelings of depression, unless the suppression of negative thoughts lead to experiences that alter underlying dysfunctional beliefs (Safran, Vallis, Segal, & Shaw, 1986).

Cognitive therapy represents an alternative approach to treating dysfunctional thought processes (Beck, 1967, 1976; Beck et al., 1979). The fundamental goal of cognitive therapy is to help patients regain control over their thought processes. The first step in this process involves helping patients to become aware of their automatic thoughts about themselves, the underlying beliefs or salient constructs that guide their processing of self-related information, and the internal and external precipitants that trigger automatic and dysfunctional cognitive processes.

Although most patients come to therapy with an awareness of the products of dysfunctional processes (feelings of dysphoria, negative thoughts about the self), few are aware of the self-relevant beliefs or constructs that lead to these negative products. For example, one patient reported that he frequently felt lonely and miserable because he was "nothing but a great big sad bore, undynamic and uninteresting." He was so overwhelmed by these negative feelings and his thoughts of worthlessness that he felt hopeless about the future. The first task in cognitive therapy for this patient was to use his negative feelings as a cue to carefully monitor his thoughts about himself. In doing so, he came to realize that many of his automatic thoughts of personal inadequacy were related to his fundamental belief that in order for others to find him interesting, he needed to "conform to today's image of the successful male." More generally, this belief incorporated the notion that he had to live up to extremely high standards to be an adequate male. If he was unable to live up to these standards, he risked humiliation and rejection by others. He noted that this belief or self-relevant construct was extremely significant to him, seemed to pervade his evaluation of himself in every domain of his life, and contributed to intense feelings of dysphoria. In this sense, this self-guide appeared to be highly self-relevant and chronically accessible. As the patient attended to his thought processes, he began to notice that his feelings of inadequacy could be triggered by media images of attractive men as handsome, intelligent, fascinating, vigorous, and unbothered by feelings of unworthiness and low self-esteem. He also noticed that his dysfunctional thought processes could be triggered by stimuli that were only remotely related to the construct of competence. At this point, the patient felt he had more control over his thought processes simply because he could identify stimuli that precipitated his negative thoughts, and he could understand the relation among the precipitants, his beliefs, and his thoughts and feelings.

As this example illustrates, many interventions in cognitive therapy rest on the ability of therapists to help patients shift from automatic to controlled processing modes. In the preceding example, the patient was required to carefully monitor his thought processes by using his negative feelings as a cue to shift from automatic to controlled processing. When he felt lonely and worthless, he was instructed to stop what he was doing and carefully make note of his thoughts and of the activities he was currently engaged in. His ability to shift to a controlled processing mode made it possible for him to examine his thought processes and to become aware of the stimulus–response sequences that typically occurred automatically without his awareness.

Once patients have become aware of their self-relevant beliefs and thoughts, they are encouraged to evaluate the effects of these beliefs on the self-evaluative process rather than simply to inhibit or replace these thoughts, as in thought stopping or self-statement modification. In the example above, the patient began to consider how his standards for self-worth had led him to evaluate himself chronically and inappropriately in relation to an unrealistic image of a "perfect" male. He recognized that his negative self-evaluations were based on inferences in ambiguous social and self-relevant situations. For example, noting that he was one of a few single males at a party suggested to him that the reason he was alone was his complete failure to live up to the standard of an acceptable male. The failure of the receptionist at his workplace to greet him in the morning was evidence of her opinion that she considered him inadequate. When his car broke down, he interpreted others as laughing at him for his inadequacy. As these examples suggest, this patient chronically utilized the construct of competence to evaluate himself in a wide variety of highly emotional contexts, some of which were clearly non-normative. He experienced these self-evaluations as entirely legitimate and consistent with his depressed mood. Consequently, he had not bothered to consider alternative explanations for these events. However, when he reconsidered the receptionist's behavior, he realized that she greeted few employees and that he had never taken it upon himself to greet her first.

This patient's experiences were consistent with our suggestion that automatic processes are most likely to have negative consequences when feedback about performance and legitimacy of interpretations is not readily available. Not only had he never seriously considered that his interpretations might be biased, but the nature of his interpretations had led him to avoid engaging in activities that might have disconfirmed his beliefs. Once he became aware of his beliefs and the questionable evidence upon which they were based, he was able to consider alternative interpretations and to test out these new hypotheses by engaging in some behaviors that he had previously avoided (e.g., saying hello to the receptionist). In addition, he began to wonder about the validity of using a media image as a guide to evaluate himself. When he examined the evidence for the use of this guide for self-evaluation, he noted that he could not think of one male that he knew who lived up to this guide; nevertheless, many of these men seemed reasonably happy with themselves. This patient's reconsideration of his beliefs, and the events that he experienced as a function of his questioning his beliefs, led him to change a central guide that he had used to evaluate himself. The alteration of this dysfunctional and chronically accessible guide decreased his tendency to negatively bias his interpretations of his experiences and to reach negative conclusions about himself.

Of course, the alteration of dysfunctional thought processes is not always as straightforward as our example suggests. Many patients have great difficulty shifting from automatic to controlled processing modes, so that they are unable to become aware of chronically accessible beliefs that lead to negative thoughts about themselves. This problem may occur for many reasons. Patients who are overwhelmed by their emotional distress sometimes appear to be unable to initiate controlled processes. We have suggested that this may occur because patients in this state do not have sufficient attentional resources to direct toward monitoring automatic processes. On the other hand, some patients experience difficulty in cognitive therapy because they lack awareness and differentiation of their emotional states and are unable to track variations in their feelings that might cue them to attend to underlying thought processes. Even if patients can become aware of dysfunctional self-relevant beliefs, this does not necessarily imply that they will be successful in altering their beliefs. Despite the lack of evidence and obvious irrationality of beliefs, some patients simply will not abandon dysfunctional self-relevant beliefs. In such cases, patients are encouraged to consider the emotional and behavioral consequences of holding such beliefs. Sometimes this is a sufficient incentive for developing coping strategies to counteract the effects of adherence to dysfunctional beliefs.

A common problem for patients in cognitive therapy is that even when dysfunctional beliefs have been identified and reconsidered, they continue to automatically influence the processing of self-relevant information. In such situations, patients report that they know their interpretations are biased, yet they are unable to intervene in the process while it is happening. This problem is not surprising in light of the difficulties that may accompany attempts to inhibit automatic processes. In addition, depressed patients may have difficulty avoiding the types of self-focus and self-referent information processing that have been associated with automatic and dysfunctional information processing (Bargh & Tota, 1988; Pyszczynski & Greenberg, 1987). In such cases, it is important to realize that patients are confronted with inhibiting a chronic cognitive process that is triggered by many environmental cues. Altering this process requires time, experience, and practice. Even if patients are unable to document and alter their cognitive processes immediately when they occur, because of high levels of emotional arousal associated with dysfunctional beliefs, they can often review their thought processes shortly thereafter and consider alternative interpretations for distressing events. This often brings relief from negative feelings and thoughts, weakens dysfunctional self-relevant beliefs, and offers the patients an opportunity to process self-relevant information in a functional rather than a dysfunctional manner.

The high rate of effectiveness of cognitive therapy for treating depression (Beck et al., 1979; Hollon & Beck, 1978; McLean & Hakstian, 1979; Rush, Beck, Kovacs, & Hollon, 1977) may be related to the fact that, although therapeutic interventions were not developed on the basis of research in the areas of cognition and social cognition, they are consistent with what is known about the operation of automatic and controlled processing modes. Cognitive therapy techniques are directed at the central complaints of depressed patients. The depressed patients' intrusive and negative thoughts are viewed as the end product of dysfunctional automatic processes, and therapeutic techniques are designed to help patients to shift from automatic to controlled processing modes. Instead of simply encouraging patients to inhibit or replace highly accessible thoughts, cognitive therapists help patients to reconsider the self-relevant beliefs or constructs that lead to negative thoughts about the self. Patients' reconsideration of their beliefs, and of alternative interpretations for their experiences, helps them to alter or modify dysfunctional aspects of their thought processes.

CONCLUSIONS

In this chapter, we have examined the concept of dysfunctional automatic processing as a source of emotional distress and dysfunction. Although automatic processing may lead to adaptive and efficient functioning in some contexts, it may lead to dysfunction in other situations. Specifically, automatic processing may become dysfunctional when criteria for the identification of bias in information processing are ambiguous and/or performance feedback is not readily available. In these circumstances, individuals may not be able to detect the dysfunctional consequences of automatic processing and to shift to controlled processing modes to correct errors. Automatic processing may also be a source of dysfunction when processing involves complex rather than simple response sequences, because the source of error in processing becomes difficult to locate. In addition, individuals may be more likely to engage in automatic information processing under conditions of high than of low affective arousal, because of the reduction in attentional resources that may accompany emotional arousal. Finally, when individuals suffer from the chronic accessibility of negative self-relevant constructs, these constructs are likely to be applied automatically and non-normatively during self-referent information processing. Cognitive therapy is designed to help patients to become aware of and alter their beliefs or chronically accessible constructs associated with dysfunctional processing.

Even though contemporary models of information processing in depression acknowledge the central role of automaticity in dysfunctional processing, relatively few studies have directly evaluated this concept. Research to date supports the role of automaticity as a source of dysfunction in depressive cognition. However, further studies are needed to determine the contexts that are most likely to give rise to dysfunctional processing, the role of affect in dysfunctional automatic processing, and the extent to which dysfunctional processes can be interrupted and altered.

Several other questions regarding the role of dysfunctional automatic processing in depression have not yet been addressed. The most important issue is whether dysfunctional processing occurs as a result of depression, or whether the tendency to process information dysfunctionally represents a stable vulnerability factor that precedes and precipitates the onset of depression. One possibility is that dysfunctional automatic processing characteristics found in depression simply reflect the increased accessibility of negative constructs associated with negative mood. This model of dysfunctional processing is consistent with the recent study of Gotlib and Cane (1987). These researchers found that patients demonstrated longer latencies for color naming of depressed-content words than for color naming of other words *only* while they were depressed. Once the depression had remitted, previously depressed patients did not show differences in their response latencies for color naming of depressed-, nondepressed-, and neutral-content words. These results suggest that dysfunctional automatic processing in depression is transitory.

However, it is premature to rule out the possibility that there are stable individual differences in construct accessibility that increase vulnerability to depression. Higgins and his colleagues (Higgins, Chapter 3, this volume; Higgins, 1989; Moretti & Higgins, 1989) have suggested that exposure to particular parental socialization practices may lead to the development of self-system vulnerabilities in construct accessibility. This view is consistent with clinical theory and research that links parental socialization practices to the development of psychopathology across the lifespan (e.g., Aber &

Cicchetti, 1984; Cicchetti & Rizley, 1981; Maccoby & Martin, 1983; Main, Kaplan, & Cassidy, 1985; Main & Weston, 1981; Sroufe, 1979).

The study of vulnerability factors in psychopathology has been plagued with methodological difficulties (see Alloy, Abramson, Metalsky, & Hartlage, 1988, for an analysis of vulnerability models), and the results of research in this area have been extremely disappointing (see Coyne & Gotlib, 1983; Miller & Moretti, 1987, for reviews). It is paramount that researchers carefully examine the assumptions that are made in vulnerability models of depression, and the methodological problems inherent in testing these models. In this regard, it is very important to realize that depressed patients are probably not alone in experiencing periods of automatic and dysfunctional information processing; it is likely that we all process self-relevant information in an automatic and dysfunctional manner on occasion, and that we temporarily suffer from feelings of dysphoria and agitation. What may be unique about the vulnerable individual is that the activation of dysfunctional automatic processing precipitates a self-perpetuating cycle of negative construct accessibility that maintains feelings of depression.

ACKNOWLEDGMENTS

We wish to thank the editors of this book, Jim Uleman and John Bargh, for their insightful comments and very helpful editorial assistance. Thanks also to Tory Higgins, Ian McBain, and Pat Bowers for their thoughtful comments while this chapter was prepared. Preparation of this manuscript was supported by Social Sciences and Research Council of Canada Grant No. 410-88-0908 to Marlene M. Moretti.

NOTES

1. Our use of the term "stimulus–response sequence" refers to cognitive, affective, and behavioral responses to stimuli.

2. A discussion of accuracy in self-referent and social information processing is beyond the scope of the current chapter (see Higgins & Bargh, 1987; Nisbett & Kunda, 1985). However, our discussion of depressive bias in self-referent and social information processing is not intended to imply that nondepressed individuals are less biased, or more accurate, in their processing of self-referent or social information. It is also not intended to convey the impression that depressed individuals may lack biases that are typically found in nondepressed populations, and are therefore more accurate than nondepressed individuals. Our current position is that it is extremely difficult to establish theoretically or empirically the criteria for "accuracy" of self-referent or social information processing, and that both depressed and nondepressed individuals are likely to demonstrate biases in information processing. It is the functional or dysfunctional consequences of these biases rather than their relative accuracy that is of interest to us in the current chapter.

3. "Accuracy" was defined in terms of whether or not subjects correctly identified targets with more emotional expressions as more informative, regardless of the valence of their emotional expression. The degree and type of emotional expression displayed by targets were established in earlier studies.

REFERENCES

Aber, J. L., & Cicchetti, D. (1984). The socio-emotional development of maltreated children: An empirical and theoretical analysis. In H. Fitzgerald, B. Lester, & M. Yogman (Eds.), *Theory and research in behavioral pediatrics* (Vol. 2, pp. 147–205). New York: Plenum.

Alloy, L. B., Abramson, L. Y., Metalsky, G. I., & Hartlage, S. (1988). The hopelessness theory of depression: Attributional aspects. *British Journal of Clinical Psychology, 27,* 5–21.

Bargh, J. A. (1984). Automatic and conscious processing of social information. In R. S. Wyer, Jr., & T. K. Srull (Eds.), *Handbook of social cognition* (Vol. 3, pp. 1–43). Hillsdale, NJ: Erlbaum.

Bargh, J. A., Bond, R. N., Lombardi, W. J., & Tota, M. E. (1986). The additive nature of chronic and temporary sources of construct accessibility. *Journal of Personality and Social Psychology, 50,* 869–878.

Bargh, J. A., & Pietromonaco, P. (1982). Automatic information processing and social perception: The influence of trait information presented outside of conscious awareness on impression formation. *Journal of Personality and Social Psychology, 43,* 437–449.

Bargh, J. A., & Pratto, F. (1986). Individual construct accessibility and perceptual selection. *Journal of Experimental Social Psychology, 22,* 293–311.

Bargh, J. A., & Thein, R. (1985). Individual construct accessibility, person memory, and the recall–judgment link: The case of information overload. *Journal of Personality and Social Psychology, 49,* 1129–1146.

Bargh, J. A., & Tota, M. E. (1988). Context-dependent processing in depression: Accessibility of negative constructs with regard for self but not others. *Journal of Personality and Social Psychology, 54,* 924–939.

Beck, A. T. (1967). *Depression: Clinical, experimental and theoretical aspects.* New York: Harper & Row.

Beck, A. T. (1976) *Cognitive therapy and the emotional disorders.* New York: International Universities Press.

Beck, A. T. (1986). Cognitive approaches to anxiety disorder. In B. F. Shaw, Z. V. Segal, T. M. Vallis, & F. E. Cashman (Eds.), *Anxiety disorders: Psychological and biological perspectives.* New York: Plenum.

Beck, A. T., Rush, A. J., Shaw, B. F., & Emery, G. (1979). *Cognitive therapy of depression.* New York: Guilford Press.

Bower, G. H., Gilligan, S. G., & Monterio, K. P. (1981). Selectivity of learning caused by affective states. *Journal of Experimental Psychology: General, 110,* 451–473.

Bradley, G. W. (1978). Self-serving biases in the attribution process: A reexamination of the fiction question. *Journal of Personality and Social Psychology, 36,* 56–71.

Bruner, J. S. (1957). On perceptual readiness. *Psychological Review, 64,* 123–152.

Bryan, W. L., & Harter, N. (1899). Studies of the telegraphic language: The acquisition of a hierarchy of habits. *Psychological Review, 6,* 345–375.

Campbell, L. M. (1973). A variation of thought-stopping in a twelve-year-old boy: A case report. *Journal of Behavior Therapy and Experimental Psychiatry, 4,* 69–70.

Cicchetti, D., & Rizley, R. (1981). Developmental perspectives on the etiology, intergenerational transmission and sequelae of child maltreatment. In R. Rizley & D. Cicchetti (Eds.), *Developmental perspectives on child maltreatment* (pp. 31–55). San Francisco: Jossey-Bass.

Coyne, J. C., & Gotlib, I. H. (1983). The role of cognition in depression: A critical appraisal. *Psychological Bulletin, 94,* 472–505.

Craik, F. I. M., & Tulving, E. (1975). Depths of processing and the retention of words in episodic memory. *Journal of Experimental Psychology: General, 104,* 268–294.

Darley, J. M., & Fazio, R. H. (1980). Expectancy confirmation processes arising in the social interaction sequence. *American Psychologist, 35,* 867–881.

Derry, P. A., & Kuiper, N. A. (1981). Schematic processing and self-reference in clinical depression. *Journal of Abnormal Psychology, 90,* 286–297.

Dobson, K. S., & Shaw, B. F. (1981). The effects of self-correction on cognitive distortions in depression. *Cognitive Therapy and Research, 5,* 391–403.

Emmelkamp, P. M. G., & Kwee, K. G. (1977). Obsessional ruminations: A comparison between thought-stopping and prolonged exposure in imagination. *Behaviour Research and Therapy, 15,* 441–444.

Erdley, C. A., & D'Agostino, P. (1988). Cognitive and affective components of automatic priming effects. *Journal of Personality and Social Psychology, 54,* 741–747.

Fennell, M. J. V., & Teasdale, J. D. (1984). Effects of distraction on thinking and affect in depressed patients. *British Journal of Clinical Psychology, 23,* 65–66.

Fisk, A. D., & Schneider, W. (1984). Memory as a function of attention, level of processing, and automatization. *Journal of Experimental Psychology: Learning, Memory, and Cognition, 10,* 181–197.

Garber, J., & Hollon, S. D. (1980). Universal versus personal helplessness: Belief in uncontrollability or incompetence? *Journal of Abnormal Psychology, 89,* 56–66.

Glass, A. L., & Holyoak, K. J. (1986). *Cognition.* New York: Random House.

Glass, C. R., Merluzzi, T. V., Biever, J. L., & Larsen, K. H. (1982). Cognitive assessment of social anxiety: Development and validation of a self-statement questionnaire. *Cognitive Therapy and Research, 6,* 37–55.

Golin, S., Terrell, F., & Johnson, B. (1977). Depression and the illusion of control. *Journal of Abnormal Psychology, 86,* 440–442.

Golin, S., Terrell, F., Weitz, J., & Drost, P. (1979). The illusion of control among depressed patients. *Journal of Abnormal Psychology, 88,* 454–457.

Gotlib, I. H. (1982). Self-reinforcement and depression in interpersonal interaction: The role of performance level. *Journal of Abnormal Psychology, 90,* 521–530.

Gotlib, I. H., & Cane, D. B. (1987). Construct accessibility and clinical depression: A longitudinal investigation. *Journal of Abnormal Psychology, 96,* 199–204.

Gotlib, I. H., & McCann, C. D. (1984). Construct accessibility and depression: An examination of cognitive and affective factors. *Journal of Personality and Social Psychology, 93,* 19–30.

Gotlib, I. H., & Olson, J. M. (1983). Depression, psychopathology and self-serving attributions. *Journal of Personality and Clinical Psychology, 22,* 309–310.

Greenwald, A. G. (1980). The totalitarian ego: Fabrication and revision of personal history. *American Psychologist, 35,* 603–618.

Hackman, A., & McLean, C. (1975). A comparison of flooding and thought-stopping in the treatment of obsessional neurosis. *Behaviour Research and Therapy, 13,* 263–269.

Hammen, C. L., & Krantz, S. (1976). Effect of success and failure on depressive cognitions. *Journal of Abnormal Psychology, 85,* 577–586.

Hasher, L., & Zacks, R. T. (1979). Automatic and effortful processes in memory. *Journal of Experimental Psychology: General, 108,* 356–388.

Hays, V., & Waddell, K. J. (1976). A self-reinforcing procedure for thought-stopping. *Behavior Therapy, 7,* 559.

Higgins, E. T. (1987). Self-discrepancy: A theory relating self and affect. *Psychological Review, 94,* 319–340.

Higgins, E. T. (1989). Continuities and discontinuities in self-regulatory and self-evaluative processes: A developmental theory relating self and affect. *Journal of Personality.*

Higgins, E. T., & Bargh, J. A. (1987). Social cognition and social perception. *Annual Review of Psychology, 38,* 369–425.

Higgins, E. T., Bargh, J. A., & Lombardi, W. (1985). Nature of priming effects on categorization. *Journal of Experimental Psychology: Learning, Memory, and Cognition, 11,* 59–69.

Higgins, E. T., & King, G. (1981). Accessibility of social constructs: Information processing consequences of individual and contextual variability. In N. Cantor & J. Kihlstrom (Eds.), *Personality, cognition, and social interaction* (pp. 69–121). Hillsdale, NJ: Erlbaum.

Higgins, E. T., King, J. A., & Mavin, G. H. (1982). Individual construct accessibility and subjective impressions on recall. *Journal of Personality and Social Psychology, 43,* 35–47.

Higgins, E. T., Kuiper, N. A., & Olson, J. M. (1981). Social cognition: A need to get personal. In E. T. Higgins, C. P. Herman, & M. P. Zanna (Eds.), *Social cognition: The Ontario Symposium* (Vol. 1, pp. 395–420). Hillsdale, NJ: Erlbaum.

Higgins, E. T., & Moretti, M. (1988). Standard utilization and the social-evaluative process: Vulnerability to types of aberrant beliefs. In T. Oltman (Ed.), *Delusional beliefs: Theoretical and empirical perspectives* (pp. 110–137). New York: Wiley.

Higgins, E. T., Rholes, W. S., & Jones, C. R. (1977). Category accessibility and impression formation. *Journal of Personality and Social Psychology, 13,* 141–154.

Higgins, E. T., Strauman, T., & Klein, R. (1986). Standards and the process of self-evaluation. Multiple affects from multiple stages. In R. M. Sorrentino & E. T. Higgins (Eds.), *Handbook of motivation and cognition: Foundations of social behavior* (pp. 23–63). New York: Guilford Press.

Hoen-Heyde, D., Schlottman, R. S., & Rush, A. J. (1982). Perception of social interaction in depressed psychiatric patients. *Journal of Consulting and Clinical Psychology, 50,* 209–212.

Hollon, S. D., & Beck, A. T. (1978). Psychotherapy and drug therapy: Comparison and combinations. In S. L. Garfield & A. E. Bergin (Eds.), *Handbook of psy-*

chotherapy and behavior change: An empirical analysis (2nd ed., pp. 437–490) New York: Wiley.

Ingram, R. E., & Hollon, S. D. (1986). Cognitive therapy for depression from an information processing perspective. In R. E. Ingram (Ed.), *Information processing approaches to clinical psychology* (pp. 259–281). New York: Academic Press.

Ingram, R. E., & Kendall, P. C. (1987). The cognitive side of anxiety. *Cognitive Therapy and Research, 11,* 523–536.

Isen, A. M. (1970). Success, failure, attention and reaction to others: The warm glow of success. *Journal of Personality and Social Psychology, 15,* 294–301.

Isen, A. M. (1984). Toward understanding the role of affect in cognition. In R. S. Wyer, Jr., & T. K. Srull (Eds.), *Handbook of social cognition* (Vol. 3). Hillsdale, NJ: Erlbaum.

Isen, A. M., & Levin, P. F. (1972). On helping: Cookies and kindness. *Journal of Personality and Social Psychology, 21,* 384–388.

James, W. (1890). *The Principles of psychology* (2 vols.). New York: Holt.

Johnson, E. J., & Tversky, A. (1983). Affect, generalization, and the perception of risk. *Journal of Personality and Social Psychology, 45,* 20–31.

Jonides, J. (1981). Voluntary versus automatic control over the mind's eye movement. In J. Long & A. D. Baddeley (Eds.), *Attention and performance IX* (pp. 187–203). Hillsdale, NJ: Erlbaum.

Kim, H., & Baron, R. S. (1988). Exercise and the illusory correlation: Does arousal heighten stereotypic processing? *Journal of Experimental Social Psychology, 24,* 366–380.

Klein, D. C., & Seligman, M. E. P. (1976). Reversal of performance deficits and perceptual deficits in learned helplessness and depression. *Journal of Abnormal Psychology, 37,* 1798–1809.

Kovacs, M., & Beck, A. T. (1978). Maladaptive cognitive structures in depression. *American Journal of Psychiatry, 135,* 525–533.

Kuiper, N. A., & Derry, P. (1982). Depressed and nondepressed-content self-reference in mild depressives. *Journal of Personality, 50,* 67–80.

Kuiper, N. A., & MacDonald, M. R. (1982). Self and other perception in mild depression. *Social Cognition, 1,* 223–239.

LaBerge, D., & Samuels, S. J. (1974). Toward a theory of automatic information processing in reading. *Cognitive Psychology, 6,* 293–323.

Levelt, W. J. M. (1983). Monitoring and self-repair in speech. *Cognition, 14,* 41–104.

Lewinsohn, P. M. (1974). A behavioral approach to depression. In R. J. Friedman & M. M. Katz (Eds.), *The psychology of depression: Contemporary theory and research.* New York: Wiley.

Lishman, W. P. (1972). Selective factors in memory: Part 2. Affective disorders. *Psychological Medicine, 2,* 248–253.

Lloyd, G. G., & Lishman, W. P. (1975). Effect of depression on the speed of recall of pleasant and unpleasant experiences. *Psychological Medicine, 5,* 173–180.

Loeb, A., Beck, A. T., & Diggory, J. (1971). Differential effects of success and failure on depressed and nondepressed patients. *Journal of Nervous and Mental Disease, 152,* 106–114.

Lobitz, W. C., & Post, R. D. (1979). Parameters of self-reinforcement and depression. *Journal of Abnormal Psychology, 88,* 33–41.

Logan, G. D. (1978). Attention in character classification: Evidence for the automaticity of component stages. *Journal of Experimental Psychology: General,* *107,* 32–63.

Logan, G. D. (1979). On the use of concurrent memory load to measure attention and automaticity. *Journal of Experimental Psychology: Human Perception and Performance, 5,* 189–207.

Logan, G. D. (1980). Attention and automaticity in Stroop and priming tasks: Theory and data. *Cognitive Psychology, 12,* 523–553.

Logan, G. D. (1982). On the ability to inhibit complex movements: A stop-signal study of typewriting. *Journal of Experimental Psychology: Human Perception and Performance, 8,* 778–792.

Logan, G. D. (1985). Skill and automaticity: Relations, implications and future directions. *Canadian Journal of Psychology, 39,* 367–386.

Maccoby, E. E., & Martin, J. A. (1983). Socialization in the context of the family: Parent–child interaction. In E. M. Hetherington (Vol. Ed.), *Handbook of child psychology* (4th ed.): Vol. 4. *Socialization, personality, and social development.* (pp. 643–691). New York: Wiley.

MacDonald, M. R., & Kuiper, N. A. (1985). Efficiency and automaticity of self-schema processing in clinical depressives. *Motivation and Emotion, 9,* 171–184.

Main, M., Kaplan, N., & Cassidy, J. (1985). Security in infancy, childhood, and adulthood: A move to the level of representation. In I. Bretherton & E. Waters (Eds.), *Growing points in attachment theory and research. Monographs of the Society for Research in Child Development, 50* (1–2, Serial No. 209), 66–104.

Main, M., & Weston, D. (1981). The quality of toddler's relationship to mother and to father: Related to conflict behavior and the readiness to establish new relationships. *Child Development, 52,* 932–940.

Markus, H. (1977). Self-schemata and processing information about the self. *Journal of Personality and Social Psychology, 35,* 63–78.

Markus, H., & Sentis, K. (1982). The self in social information processing. In J. Suls (Ed.), *Psychological perspectives on the self* (Vol. 1, pp. 41–70). Hillsdale, NJ: Erlbaum.

Martin, D. J., Abramson, L. Y., & Alloy, L. B. (1984). Illusion of control for self and others in depressed and nondepressed college students. *Journal of Personality and Social Psychology, 46,* 125–136.

Meichenbaum, D. (1977). *Cognitive behavior modification.* New York: Plenum.

McLean, P. D., & Hakstian, A. R. (1979). Clinical depression: Comparative efficacy of outpatient treatments. *Journal of Consulting and Clinical Psychology, 47,* 818–836.

Miller, D. T., & Moretti, M. M. (1988). The causal attributions of depressives: Self-serving or self-disserving? In L. B. Alloy (Ed.), *Cognitive processes in depression* (pp. 266–286). New York: Guilford Press.

Miller, W. R., & Seligman, M. E. P. (1973). Depression and the perception of reinforcement. *Journal of Abnormal Psychology, 82,* 62–73.

Moretti, M. M., & Miller, D. T. (1988). *Processing positive and negative information in depression.* Unpublished manuscript, University of Waterloo.

Moretti, M. M., & Higgins, E. T. (1989). The development of self-system vulnerabilities: Social and cognitive factors in developmental psychopathology. In

R. J. Sternberg & J. Kolligian (Eds.), *Perceptions of competence and incompetence across the lifespan*. New Haven, CT: Yale University Press.

Nelson, R. E., & Craighead, W. E. (1977). Selective recall of positive and negative feedback, self-control behaviors and depression. *Journal of Abnormal Psychology, 36*, 379–388.

Nisbett, R. E., & Kunda, Z. (1985). The perception of social distributions. *Journal of Personality and Social Psychology, 48*, 297–311.

Posner, M. I. (1978). Chronometric explorations of mind. New York: Oxford University Press.

Posner, M. I., & Snyder, C. R. R. (1975). Attention and cognitive control. In R. L. Solso (Ed.), *Information processing and cognition: The Loyola Symposium* (pp. 55–58). Hillsdale, NJ: Erlbaum.

Postman, L., & Brown, D. R. (1952). The perceptual consequences of success and failure. *Journal of Abnormal and Social Psychology, 47*, 213–221.

Pyszczynski, T., & Greenberg, J. (1987). Self-regulatory perseveration and the depressive self-focusing style: A self-awareness theory of reactive depression. *Psychological Bulletin, 102*, 122–138.

Rush, A. J., Beck, A. T., Kovacs, M., & Hollon, S. (1977). Comparative efficacy of cognitive therapy and imipramine in the treatment of depressed outpatients. *Cognitive Therapy and Research, 1*, 17–37.

Sacco, W. P., & Hokanson, J. E. (1978). Performance satisfaction under high and low success conditions. *Journal of Clinical Psychology, 34*, 907–909.

Safran, J. D., Vallis, M. T., Segal, Z. V., & Shaw, B. F. (1986). Assessment of core cognitive processes in cognitive therapy. *Cognitive Therapy and Research, 10*, 509–526.

Salkovskis, P. M. (1985). Obsessional–compulsive problems: A cognitive–behavioural analysis. *Behaviour Research and Therapy, 23*, 571–583.

Segal, Z. V. (1988). Appraisal of the self-schema construct in cognitive models of depression. *Psychological Bulletin, 103*, 147–162.

Schneider, W., & Shiffrin, R. M. (1977). Controlled and automatic processing human information processing: I. Detection, search and attention. *Psychological Review, 84*, 1–66.

Shiffrin, R. M., & Schneider, W. (1977). Controlled and automatic human information processing: II. Perceptual learning, automatic attending, and a general theory. *Psychological Review, 84*, 127–190.

Smith, E. R., & Lerner, M. (1986). Development of automatism of social judgments. *Journal of Personality and Social Psychology, 50*, 246–259.

Smolen, R. C. (1978). Expectancies, mood, and performance of depressed and nondepressed psychiatric inpatients on chance and skill tasks. *Journal of Abnormal Psychology, 87*, 91–101.

Sroufe, L. A. (1979). The coherence of individual development: Early care, attachment and subsequent developmental issues. *American Psychologist, 34*, 834–841.

Srull, T. K., & Wyer, R. S., Jr. (1979). The role of category accessibility in the interpretation of information about persons: Some determinants and implications. *Journal of Personality and Social Psychology, 37*, 1660–1672.

Srull, T. K., & Wyer, R. S., Jr. (1980). Category accessibility and social perception: Some implications for the study of person memory and interpersonal judgments. *Journal of Personality and Social Psychology, 38*, 841–856.

Stern, R. (1970). Treatment of a case of obsessional neuroses using a thought-stopping technique. *British Journal of Psychiatry, 117*, 441–442.

Stern, R. (1978). Obsessive thought: The problem of therapy. *British Journal of Psychiatry, 132*, 200–205.

Stern, R., Lipsedge, M. S., & Marks, I. M. (1973). Obsessive ruminations: A controlled trial of thought-stopping techniques. *Behaviour Research and Therapy, 11*, 652–659.

Stroop, J. R. (1935). Studies of interference in serial verbal reactions. *Journal of Experimental Psychology, 19*, 643–662.

Sutton-Simon, K., & Goldfried, M. R. (1979). Faulty thinking patterns in two types of anxiety. *Cognitive Therapy and Research, 3*, 193–203.

Tabachnik, N., Crocker, J., & Alloy, L. B. (1983). Depression, social comparison and the false consensus effect. *Journal of Personality and Social Psychology, 45*, 688–699.

Teasdale, J. D. (1983). Negative thinking in depression: Cause, effect, or reciprocal relationship? *Advances in Behaviour Research and Therapy, 5*, 3–25.

Teasdale, J. D., & Fogarty, S. J. (1979). Differential effects of induced mood on retrieval of pleasant and unpleasant events from episodic memory. *Journal of Abnormal Psychology, 88*, 248–257.

Teasdale, J. D., Taylor, R., & Fogarty, S. J. (1980). Effects of induced elation–depression on the accessibility of memories of happy and unhappy experiences. *Behaviour Research and Therapy, 18*, 339–346.

Tulving, E., & Pearlstone, Z. (1966). Availability versus accessibility of information in memory for words. *Journal of Verbal Learning and Verbal Behavior, 5*, 381–391.

Uleman, J. S. (1987). Consciousness and control: The case of spontaneous trait inferences. *Personality and Social Psychology Bulletin, 13*, 337–354.

Wegner, D. M., Schneider, D. J., Carter, S. R., & White, T. L. (1987). Paradoxical effects of thought suppression. *Journal of Personality and Social Psychology, 53*, 5–13.

Wegner, D. M., Wenzlaff, R. Kerker, R. M., & Beattie, A. E. (1981). Incrimination through innuendo: Can media questions become public answers? *Journal of Personality and Social Psychology, 40*, 822–832.

Williams, J. M. G., & Nulty, D. D. (1986). Construct accessibility, depression and the emotional Stroop task: Transient mood or stable structure? *Personality and Individual Differences, 7*, 485–491.

Winter, L., & Uleman, J. S. (1984). When are social judgments made? Evidence for the spontaneousness of trait interferences. *Journal of Personality and Social Psychology, 47*, 237–252.

Winter, L., Uleman, J. S., & Cunniff, C. (1985). How automatic are social judgments? *Journal of Personality and Social Psychology, 49*, 904–917.

Wollert, R. W., & Buchwald, A. M. (1979). Subclinical depression and performance expectations, evaluations of performance, and actor performance. *Journal of Nervous and Mental Disease, 167*, 237–242.

Wolpe, J., & Lazarus, A. A. (1966). *Behavior therapy techniques: A guide to the treatment of neurosis.* New York: Pergamon.

Wyer, R. S., Jr., & Srull, T. K. (1981). Category accessibility: Some theoretical and empirical issues concerning the processing of social stimulus information. In

E. T. Higgins, C. P. Herman, & M. P. Zanna (Eds.), *Social cognition: The Ontario Symposium* (Vol. 1, pp. 395–420). Hillsdale, NJ: Erlbaum.

Zarantonello, M. W., Johnson, J. E., & Petzel, T. P. (1979). The effects of ego involvement and task difficulty on actual and perceived performance of depressed college students. *Journal of Clinical Psychology, 5,* 273–281.

Zajonc, R. B. (1984). On the primacy of affect. *American Psychologist, 39,* 117–123.

PART IV

SUMMARIES AND CONCLUSIONS

14

A Framework for
Thinking Intentionally
about Unintended Thoughts

JAMES S. ULEMAN [1]
New York University

In this chapter, I begin by developing the case for the importance of spontaneous inferences and their two defining characteristics: the absence of intentions and awareness. I then discuss how they differ from automatic and from "controlled" processes, and propose a framework for differentiating among several kinds of cognitive processes in terms of personal control. Finally, I attempt to illustrate the utility of this framework by briefly characterizing some of the cognitive processes involved in text comprehension.

SPONTANEOUS INFERENCES

Spontaneous inferences occur without intentions to make them, and usually without awareness that they have been made.[2] They were first demonstrated and singled out for special attention in a study of trait inferences (Winter & Uleman, 1984). Subjects read a series of behavior descriptions implying traits (e.g., "The librarian carries the old woman's groceries across the street" implies that the librarian is "helpful"). Subjects were told that they were in a memory experiment, and were asked to study the sentences carefully for a subsequent memory test. There was no instruction to infer traits or form impressions of the sentence actors. In a subsequent cued-recall test of memory for the sentences, the implied traits (e.g., "helpful")

425

were more effective retrieval cues than much stronger semantic associates to the major words or phrases in the sentences (e.g., "books" to "librarian" and "bag" to "carries groceries"). This was interpreted as indicating that the implicit traits had been inferred and encoded along with the sentences, even though there was no reason to infer traits at encoding. This paradigm and interpretation are based on Tulving's (Tulving & Thompson, 1973) research on encoding specificity, in which appropriate control conditions rule out alternative explanations that rely only on retrieval processes.

When subjects were asked about their encoding and retrieval processes, they showed no awareness of having made trait inferences. And those few subjects who did report thinking about the actors' traits or personalities showed no better trait-cued recall of the sentences than did other subjects. (For a fuller summary of research on spontaneous trait inferences, see Uleman, 1987. For a discussion of when spontaneous trait inferences may occur and their possible role in other social cognitive phenomena, see Newman & Uleman, Chapter 5, this volume.)

This initial research suggested that spontaneous inferences may be the result of automatic processes, which occur "without intention, without giving rise to any conscious awareness, and without producing interference with other ongoing mental activity" (Posner & Snyder, 1975, p. 56). Automatic processing has also been characterized as "a fast, parallel, fairly effortless process that is not limited by short-term memory (STM) capacity, is not under direct subject control, and is responsible for the performance of well-developed skilled behaviors" (Schneider, Dumais, & Shiffrin, 1984, p. 1). The first study to examine any of these other criteria for automatic processing suggested that spontaneous trait inferences may be automatic, in the sense of being unaffected by limitations in STM capacity (Winter, Uleman, & Cunniff, 1985). This study found that apparent variations in a concurrent memory load, and hence in STM capacity, had no effect on trait-cued recall. However, subsequent work has shown that actual reductions in STM capacity can interfere with spontaneous trait inferences (Uleman, Newman, & Winter, 1987), indicating that spontaneous trait inferences are not automatic by this criterion.

In both of these studies (Uleman et al., 1987; Winter et al., 1985), trait-implying sentences were presented as distractors in "a study of memory for digits." The subsequent cued-recall test of sentence memory was completely unexpected. Thus, subjects did not have even a memory goal to provide a reason for elaborative encoding, which might include making trait inferences. Nevertheless, trait inferences still occurred, in that trait-cued recall still exceeded semantic-cued recall. Subjects also showed no awareness of having made trait inferences, even though they were questioned about this immediately after they read the last "distractor" sentence.

In addition to not being limited by STM capacity, automatic processes are often characterized as difficult to inhibit or modify. "Automatic processes tend to run to completion. . . . If an automatic process does not result in attention demands or [overt motor] actions, then it is difficult to see why one would want to halt or change it prior to completion" (Shiffrin & Dumais, 1981, pp. 121–122). Of course, control processes may override or suppress the results of automatic processes after they have run to completion (Bargh, 1984; Posner & Synder, 1975), but this is different from halting them in midstream after they have begun. The Stroop effect (e.g., Dyer, 1973) probably provides the best-known example of difficult-to-inhibit, largely automatic processing. When subjects are asked to rapidly name the color of ink in which words are printed, they are invariably slowed down by words referring to different colors (e.g., the word "white"). People seem to be unable to prevent activation of the conflicting color concepts while naming the ink colors.

If spontaneous trait inferences are automatic, it should be difficult or impossible for subjects to examine a trait-implying sentence without inferring a trait. This should be particularly true because they are unaware of the trait inference process, so they should have no reason "to halt or change it prior to completion." However, we (Uleman & Moskowitz, 1987) found that several sentence-processing goals sharply reduced the frequency of spontaneous trait inferences, as indexed by the level of trait-cued recall. A graphemic goal required some subjects to pick out H's. A phonemic goal required others to decide whether the sentence contained words that rhymed with target words. And a semantic goal required others to identify the gender of each personal noun and pronoun. Even though his last goal involved semantic analyses of individual words and anaphoric inferences, trait inferences were much less common than under memory instructions.

So by at least two criteria that have been used to define automatic processes, spontaneous trait inferences do not seem to be automatic. However, they are not "controlled" or "intentional," or "conscious" either, in any sensible way. How can subjects be said to "control" a cognitive process they do not intend or even notice? If "control" is taken to mean anything other than simply "not automatic," we must entertain the possibility that some cognitive processes, such as spontaneous trait inferences, are *neither* automatic *nor* controlled (intentional, conscious, strategic, or whatever).

AUTOMATIC PROCESSES

In most current usage of these terms, if a cognitive process is not automatic, it is controlled (or intentional, conscious, strategic, or attentive). What are the defining features of automatic processes? In his recent review of theory and research on attention, Shiffrin (1988) concluded that "Attempts to define necessary and sufficient criteria to distinguish automatic and attentive processes in complete generality have not yet proven success-ful . . . different answers may be obtained when the size of the unit of analysis is changed. Furthermore, in practice, many processes that have the potential to become fully automatic will have been trained only to some degree of partial automatism" (p. 775). Each of these three points deserves further comment, beginning with the last.

A cognitive process can be characterized as automatic or nonauto-matic only at a particular point in the thinker's training history. Training can change a process's status in either direction, though interest is usually in processes' becoming more automatic. One might imagine that very com-plex processes would always be nonautomatic, but there is no agreement in the literature on whether there is an upper bound on the complexity of processes that may become automatic (e.g., Neisser, 1976; Shiffrin & Du-mais, 1981, p. 123). Some spontaneous inference processes may be those that "have been trained only to some degree of partial automatism," and would become completely automatic with further appropriate training (Shiffrin, 1988, p. 775).

Second, the unit of analysis is critical. In the least ambiguous case, one deals with single processes. Of course, what constitutes a single pro-cess depends on the task and one's analysis of it. But in the literature of concern to us here, "single processes" such as automatic concept activa-tion require 300 milliseconds *or less* (e.g., Neely, 1977). Longer durations almost certainly indicate that several processes are operating. As Shiffrin and Dumais (1981, p. 112) noted, "virtually all complex and interesting processes of significant duration involve a mixture of automatic and con-trol processes, often taking place in parallel, with each being able to initi-ate a process of the same type, or of the other type." Such a mixed process is usually characterized as controlled. But this characterization does not say very much, and leaves unspecified whether there is control over initi-ating, guiding, inhibiting, or terminating the process (Uleman, 1987) and whether or not the control is conscious.

At the level of analysis appropriate for most social, personality, and clinical phenomena, virtually all cognitive processes are mixes of auto-matic and nonautomatic processes. Thus "controlled" (or strategic or at-tentive) is too broad a category to be descriptively useful. A potentially more useful framework that distinguishes among four kinds of nonauto-matic processes is sketched below.

Shiffrin's third point is that there is no agreement on the defining criteria for automatic processes, even at the level of the most elemental process. Bargh (1984, pp. 6–14) has lucidly outlined the major theorists' positions, two central disagreements, and his own preferences. For clarity's sake, I will do the same. The first disagreement concerns the classification of Shiffrin and Schneider's (1977) automatic attentional processes as "au-tomatic." These are processes that cause consistently mapped (trained) tar-gets to uncontrollably "pop out" of a display in a visual search task. Such targets pop out even when they are no longer intended targets, in spite of subjects' best effort to ignore them, and this interferes with other search tasks (Schneider & Shiffrin, 1977). So this is a different kind of "automatic" process—not an automatic "process that does not use general nonspecific processing resources and does not decrease the general nonspecific capacity available for other processes," but one that "always utilizes general resources and decreases general processing capacity whenever a given set of external initiating stimuli are present, regardless of a subject's attempt to ignore or bypass the distraction" (Shiffrin & Dumais, 1981, pp. 116–117).

Although classifying such processes as automatic may appear to contradict Posner and Snyder's (1975) and Logan's (1980) views that control processes can override automatic ones, this depends on one's level of analysis and time frame. Because automatic processes are faster than controlled processes, one may find both uncontrollable automatic attentional processes at brief latencies (<300 milliseconds), and controlled processes that override their effects at longer latencies, as in the Stroop effect. So automatic processes are uncontrollable in the short run, but eventually controllable. Logan and Cowan (1984) go so far as to reject control as a criterion relevant to automatism, and propose instead a subordinate–executive dichotomy to describe control: "All goal-directed activity is controlled, whether it is carried out by the executive or by the subordinates. It may be appropriate to call work done by subordinates automatic, but it need not be uncontrolled" (p. 323). Their choice of terms makes clear the importance of one's level of analysis in discussing questions of control and automatism. But whether or not all goal-directed activity is controlled depends upon what is meant by "controlled" (see below).

The second disagreement Bargh discusses concerns the utility of limiting automatic processes to those initiated by external stimuli. Although most theorists (Logan & Cowan, 1984; Posner & Snyder, 1975; Shiffrin, 1988; Shiffrin & Schneider, 1977) have not favored such a limitation, Bargh and others have. Bargh (1984) cogently notes

> [There are] problems inherent in defining as automatic mental processes that are started by intention but then proceed without awareness. It is not that the automaticity of such processes is questioned so much as that the utility of the *automatic/conscious* distinction is essentially lost in this definition, given one's *general* lack of awareness of one's cognitive processes. For these reasons the "stimulus-driven" definition [of automatic] is strongly advocated here. (p. 14, first emphasis added)

But this is merely a reason to reject the automatic–conscious dichotomy. Bargh's more general point is a good one: Processes that are driven directly by external stimuli and proceed completely outside of awareness must be automatic, by any definition. It is also true that less restrictive definitions can result in theoretical confusion and operational anarchy. Whatever their defining criteria, automatic processes must be carefully and restrictively defined if the concept is to retain any precision and utility. Even so, I prefer the position that processes that summon awareness or that are not stimulus-driven may still be automatic, as with Schneider and Shiffrin's (1977) automatic attentional processes, and automatic subordinate processes initiated intentionally by controlling executive processes. Bargh's preference was reasonable for his research program on preattention cognitive processes. It is too restrictive for my research program on spontaneous, "preintentional" cognitive processes.

Finally, this brief overview of automaticity would not be complete without noting that some recent treatments discuss the use of a central-capacity criterion in relative terms (Kahneman & Treisman, 1984).

To summarize, nearly all researchers in this field conceive of an automatic process as a "fast [<300 milliseconds], parallel, fairly effortless process that is not limited by short-term memory (STM) capacity, is not under direct subject control" (Schneider et al., 1984, p. 1), is not itself intended, and is difficult to inhibit because it tends "to run to completion" (Shiffrin & Dumais, 1981, p. 121). However, I see no reason to exclude Schneider and Shiffrin's automatic attentional processes—which may give rise to conscious awareness and produce interference with other ongoing cognitive processes that require attentional resources—or intentionally initiated, postattentive processes. Processes that are not automatic are not necessarily controlled (or intentional or conscious). The degree to which, and the sense in which, a process is controlled depends heavily on the level of analysis. At levels of analysis appropriate for most phenomena of interest to social and personality psychologists, cognitive processes are almost always mixtures of the automatic and nonautomatic. Finally, if we are to understand the control of cognitive processes, we need concepts more differentiated, and more appropriate to hierarchical organized processes, than automatic versus whatever.

CONTROL AND AWARENESS

What does it mean to control one's own thoughts, and how is this related to awareness? To "control" something means to regulate it, direct it, or guide it. So control requires a standard or goal in terms of which something is regulated or guided. This goal is discrepant from the current state, and a controlling process operates to reduce the discrepancy. Miller, Galanter, and Pribram's (1960) "Test–Operate–Test–Exit" (TOTE) unit comes to mind, as does Newell's (1973) more recent concept of a production system with its tests and actions. Consider the TOTE unit. In its simplest version, input information enters the test procedure of the TOTE unit and is tested against some standard or goal. If the input does not match the standard, an operation is triggered to reduce the discrepancy between the input and the standard. The result provides new input for the test, which is carried out again. The operation is performed again, if necessary, and so on until the criterion or goal is reached. Then an output signal exits from the unit, passing control to the next processing unit.

One example that Miller et al. (1960) discuss extensively is hammering a nail into a board. Beginning with the nail sticking out of the board, one first tests whether its head is flush with the board. If it is not, one operates by striking the nail with the hammer. Then one tests again, operates if necessary, and so on until the nail's head is flush and one can exit from the nail-driving TOTE. As this illustration suggests, TOTE is the shortest form; more generally, it is a TO[TO[TO . . .]]TE unit, where bracketed cycles are optional and depend on the outcome of the test. Furthermore, the tests and operations may themselves consist of TOTE units. For instance, before one can perform the operation of hammering, one must test to see whether the hammer is raised. If it is, one can operate by bringing it down onto the nail. If it is not, one must first raise it. So TOTEs are often hierarchically nested within each other.

Thus, at a minimum, control requires a Test (goal) and an Operation (procedure for attaining the goal, or for reducing the discrepancy between the input or current state and the goal). Figure 14.1 depicts hierarchically organized TOTE units. The superordinate TOTE's Operation$_1$ is itself described as a TOTE unit. This two-level system could be extended indefinitely, with Tests and Operations each being broken down into TOTEs that are composed of TOTEs that are composed of TOTEs . . . , to whatever level of specificity is required by one's symbolic language or hardware. The resulting regress is not infinite, though it may be extensive. And

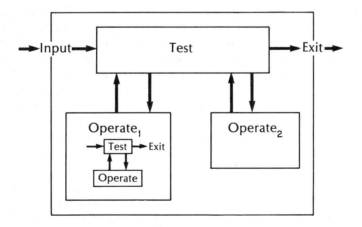

FIGURE 14.1. A Test–Operate–Test–Exit (TOTE) model of intentional control, with a conditional test, and one operation depicted as another TOTE.

the somewhat startling result of such a detailed decomposition of a control process is that it solves the "homunculus" problem.

The homunculus problem is this: If control is being exercised, *who* is ultimately in control? Doesn't there have to be a homunculus, or little person, inside the system somewhere to monitor what is going on, select which TOTE units operate at a particular time, set priorities, and so forth? The answer is "No, the homunculus is an emergent property of the entire organized system." In describing the characteristics of data structures developed in artificial intelligence, Dennett (1978) has put the argument quite clearly:

> A flow chart is typically the organizational chart of a committee of homunculi (investigators, librarians, accountants, executives); each box specifies a homunculus by prescribing a function *without saying how it is to be accomplished* (one says, in effect: put a little man in there to do the job). If we then look closer at the individual boxes we see that the function of each is accomplished by subdividing it via another flow chart into still smaller, more stupid homunculi. Eventually this nesting of boxes within boxes land you with homunculi so stupid (all they have to do is remember whether to say yes or no when asked) that they can be, as one says, "replaced by a machine." One *discharges* fancy homunculi from one's scheme by organizing armies of such idiots to do the work. (pp. 123–124)

Of course, none of this requires consciousness, as illustrated by thermostats and other servomechanisms, homeostatic biological systems, and computer programs. However, homunculi also come up in discussions of control because we usually mean "conscious" control, and our intuition is that "someone" in the system has to be conscious. (See Dennett, 1984, for a brilliant and entertaining discussion of the implicit meanings—often insupportable and mutually incompatible—that we attach to such terms as "control" and "free will.") Without attempting to specify what consciousness is or to designate a part of the system to be conscious of events, consider the variety of ways in which control may be conscious in Figure 14.1. Imagine that "the person" (a superordinate control level not shown in Figure 14.1, or an emergent property of the system of which Figure 14.1 is a part) is consciously controlling his or her thoughts and is aware of "everything," at some level of analysis. This would mean that the person is aware of, or can easily become aware of, (1) the current state, or Input; (2) the goal, or Test; (3) the way to attain the goal, or Operation; and (4) the fact that a TOTE unit is operating (a metacognition that an Exit is pending).

In addition, conscious control implies choice among goals or among ways of reaching a goal (see Fiske, Chapter 8, this volume). Both kinds of choices could be represented in Figure 14.1; only the latter is shown, to keep the figure simple. The Test is conditional and has two Operates associated with it: If Test $= O_1$, then Operate$_1$; if Test $= O_2$, then Operate$_2$.

So conscious control also connotes awareness of (5) available alternatives that were not chosen. As is always the case for awareness, this is a matter of degree. Being aware of "the road not taken" (Frost, 1949) does not require traveling down it, or even knowing where it goes.

Thus there are at least five different aspects of which one may be aware in controlling one's thoughts, all depicted in Figure 14.1. First is awareness of the current content of one's thoughts, the input (1) above. Second and third are awareness of one's current cognitive goals and means to attain them, (2) and (3) above, respectively. It is important to note that awareness of content, goals, and means may exist at many levels of the TOTE model, from a microscopic analysis for some purposes to the most molar level for others (see Wegner & Vallacher, 1986). Each additional level of a TOTE hierarchy that is included adds its own content, goals, and means to the potential contents of awareness. Fourth is a metacognition, (4) above: awareness of the existence of thought processes whatever their content or goals, as in "I'm thinking." Fifth is awareness of foregone alternative means and/or goals, at whatever level of the TOTE model, (5) above.

And there are at least two other noteworthy aspects of consciously controlling one's thoughts that are not shown in Figure 14.1. One of these (6) is awareness of oneself as a thinker, as in "I think, therefore I am." This is consciousness of a capability, not necessarily a current state of affairs. Another aspect (7), of particular interest to social and clinical psychologists, is awareness of other people's view of oneself as a thinker, one's reputation as thinker. Both (6) and (7) refer to capabilities and past performances, and thus represent more general theories about the self than do (1) through (5). But as Nisbett and Wilson (1977) have noted, such general theories can and do influence beliefs (awareness) about one's current cognitive processing.

So there are at least seven senses in which one may intentionally control one's thoughts, or seven elements of control of which one may be aware. A minimal set of five elements (1 through 5 above) is depicted in Figure 14.1. Input is from internal sources because it follows preattentive processing of external stimuli or internally generated stimuli. Intentional control of thoughts includes awareness of the Input, and conscious selection from among at least two processing goals or methods (awareness of Test and both Operation$_1$ and Operation$_2$). It includes awareness of the nature of the selected method and its goal (T), the operation (O) used to attain that goal, and awareness that attaining that goal will terminate or Exit the process at some appropriate nested level of the process. In Figure 14.1, one would usually think of Operation$_1$ as the intentional process itself. The presence and awareness of Test and Operation$_2$ are what make it intentional, because they allow conscious choice. So if the person is (or can easily become) aware of all of these elements in Figure 14.1, the process should be described as completely intentional.

The last two metacognitive elements (6 and 7) may condition the intentionality of cognitions. If the thinker does not experience self as thinker—if the thoughts seem to "think themselves," or if the thinker feels that he or she is "not myself" or is "beside myself" for whatever reasons—one might not call the thought intentional. The thinking should be done by the person in his or her normal state. Finally, the thoughts may have such moral, legal, or other reputational implications that they produce a sincere denial of intentionality: "I had those thoughts, but I didn't mean to."

Thus far, we have implicitly considered only the selection or initiation of cognitive processes. However, this framework can also be used to represent two other important and distinct aspects of the intentional control of thought suggested by the literature on automatic and controlled processing: termination and inhibition (see Uleman, 1987). Termination may occur naturally when the Exit conditions are met. But what if they are never met? What will prevent the process from continuing indefinitely? To do this job, some kind of override termination capability is necessary. This capability may be a general one that can be applied to many different cognitive operations (see Logan, Chapter 2, this volume), or it may be operation-specific. Without it, the process would be intentionally initiated but subsequently uncontrollable.

"Control" of thought may also refer to the capacity to inhibit it before it begins—that is, prevention. One of the characteristics of automatic processes is that they cannot be inhibited or prevented. If the triggering stimuli are presented and registered at all, they always initiate the process. Automatic attentional processes (Schneider & Shiffrin, 1977) illustrate this. The activation of color concepts by color words in the Stroop phenomenon (see above) is another example of this. If color concept activation were controlled rather than automatic in this prevention or inhibition sense, people could preset their cognitive systems to prevent the activation of such interfering concepts. But the activation of competing color concepts is uncontrollable in the sense that it cannot be inhibited.[3]

In short, a completely intentional cognitive process is one that can be intentionally initiated, terminated, and inhibited. And it is one for which the thinker's most complete description of what they are doing (the global TOTE) and how they are doing it (T and O in Operation$_1$) can be mapped onto each of the elements in Figure 14.1. And, finally, it is a cognitive process for which the thinker ordinarily accepts responsibility.[4]

RELATIONS AMONG SPONTANEOUS, AUTOMATIC, AND INTENTIONAL THOUGHT

So far, I have described three kinds of thought that can be roughly distinguished in terms of awareness and control: spontaneous, automatic, and intentional. These characterizations can be sharpened by indicating how they might be related to one another, and to other kinds of thought that differ from them in controllability.

Five kinds of thought are shown in the overlapped boxes in Figure 14.2. They are arrayed from the simplest to the most complex kind of personal control. In the simplest (extreme left), an external stimulus (S) triggers an automatic process such as concept activation in the Stroop task. In general, awareness increases from the left to the right of Figure 14.2. So people are unaware of most automatically activated concepts. However, people may be aware of the stimulus (S), and may even exercise intentional control over selecting among stimuli or seeking them out or generating them (internally or externally), as indicated by the arrows to Automatic and to S from the more complex processes at the right. Thus, people may control automatic processes by controlling the stimuli that initiate them. But once that initiation has occurred, the automatic process runs to completion uncontrollably . The automatic process itself could presumably be described in more detail—as a series of nested TOTE units, for example. This is true of the other process types as well, not just intentional processes. What distinguishes intentional processes is *awareness* of the TOTE elements noted in Figure 14.1.

Also note that although the flow of time and processing is generally from left to right in such figures, this need not be the case in Figure 14.2.

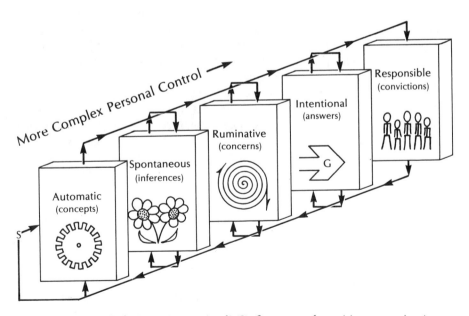

FIGURE 14.2. Relations among stimuli (S), five types of cognitive processing (automatic, spontaneous, ruminative, intentional, and responsible), and their typical outputs (concepts, inferences, concerns, answers, and convictions).

Arrows go in both directions, with each process type potentially providing input to all the others and receiving output from them. The whole thing is a loop, so "the beginning" can be anywhere and depends on the theorist's analytic purposes.

Typical or illustrative output is noted for each process (e.g., concepts for automatic concept activation), both to enhance heuristic clarity and to indicate that not all output from a process must serve simply as input for other processes. Presumably, some output does not "go" anywhere, but simply fades or is stored in memory. That is, I am explicitly *not* making the teleological assumption that every output has some "purpose" in being relevant to other processes, or that output only occurs if it is "needed" by some subsequent processing stage. Incidental outputs may be just as interesting as those leading to conscious or intended thoughts, as we develop ways to detect them.

The results of automatic processes typically trigger spontaneous processes. Like automatic processes, spontaneous processes occur largely without intentions or awareness. But unlike automatic processes, they require some cognitive capacity; they produce more complex output, such as inferences; they combine the output of several automatically activated concepts; and they can be inhibited and terminated rather than merely initiated by output from more controllable processes to the right.

Ruminative processes lie between spontaneous and intentional processes. They produce conscious concerns (or daydreams or obsessions) that serve no conscious purpose or goal. They may be instigated by the output from intentional processes, but are not themselves intentional in the full sense I have described above. So both spontaneous and ruminative processes are typically uncontrolled, though they may be controllable if the person is aware of them (see Uleman, 1987).

Clearly, not all ruminations are the same. Daydreams seem to be much more controllable than obsessions. Thoughts that we would not even have had, had we not been trying to suppress them, seem to be different from these (see Wegner & Schneider, Chapter 9, this volume). Thus simply classifying thought processes into one or another of these types does *not* mean that they are identical to all others in the category. These categories are fuzzy, and every example also has unique characteristics. But ruminative concerns share the features of being conscious but not consciously goal directed (see Martin & Tesser, Chapter 10, this volume). They are phenomenologically important and can have important noncognitive consequences (see Pennebaker, Chapter 11, and Tait & Silver, Chapter 12, this volume).

Intentional processes produce conscious output directed toward clear goals (hence the G in Figure 14.2), such as providing answers or solutions or explanations. Intentional processes are fully controlled, even though they may be made up of automatic and spontaneous subprocesses. (Remember that the characterization of any process depends on the level and unit of analysis the theorist adopts.) And, like other processes, their output may also serve as stimuli that trigger further automatic processes.

The last kind of processing depicted at the far right of Figure 14.2 is what I call "responsible" processing. It consists of intentional processes and outputs for which the thinker claims responsibility, such as convictions. Responsible processing is engaged when the person is consciously concerned about his or her *reputation* as a thinker and actor (see above). So these outputs are typically public, and the processing includes additional layers of intentional control (for checking, filtering, censoring, elaboration, and/or integration) to ensure that the output meets public (in addition to private) accountability standards. If it does, someone will judge the output and the thinker to be "responsible"; if it does not, they will be judged "irresponsible." We seem to be able to distinguish responsible thought from intentional thought, in that someone can be intentionally irresponsible. Unintentionally responsible thought is also possible, as when the accountability standards have become so internalized and chronic that they operate without intent. In such cases, their operation is usually inferred from contrasts with other people's behavior.

Responsible processing may include some kinds of systematic processing (Chaiken, 1980; Chaiken, Liberman, & Eagly, Chapter 7, this volume) and central processing (Petty & Cacioppo, 1986) of persuasive messages. It clearly includes the judgment and decision processes invoked by Tetlock's (1983; Tetlock & Kim, 1987) manipulation of social accountability. And we may also want to include the effects of pragmatics in language production, such as cognitive tuning (Zajonc, 1960) and other aspects of the "communication game" (Higgins, 1981). "Responsible processes" give an explicit place in our framework to socially responsive and responsible, rather than merely self-controlled, thought processes. (See Fiske, Chapter 8, this volume, for an illustration of being held responsible for thoughts.)

The output of responsible processes includes public positions, beliefs, and attitudes (i.e., convictions held with varying amounts of conviction). Abelson (1988) examined several measures of the conviction with which people hold attitudes, and unexpectedly found that conviction is multidimensional. However, the three most important factors suggest how central personal, public responsibility is to the meaning of conviction(s). The first factor is emotional conviction, in which a person's attitudes reflect "the real *me*" enough that the person would "spend a day a month working for a group supporting *my* views." The second factor is ego preoccupation, in which the person thinks "about the issue often" and the "belief is important to *me*." And the third factor is cognitive elaboration, indicated by agreeing that "several other issues could come up *in a conversation*" about the issue, and that "it's easy to explain *my* views" (p. 273, italics added). Responsible thought is personally and publicly owned.

Although I do not mean to imply that all the lines of research that illustrate responsible processing concern the same phenomena, they do seem collectively important enough and similar enough to justify singling out responsible processes as a distinct fifth category, particularly because of its highly social nature. It represents cognitive processes that are subject to the most extensive set of controls (i.e., those representing social as well as personal standards).

Notice that these five processing types, instead of being diagrammed in a series with feedback as in Figure 14.2, could be stacked up with processes on the right placed above and "controlling" those on the left. This would be consistent with the descriptions above, and with the general practice of characterizing an organized set of processes in terms of the most complex ones in the set. Thus, if the set includes automatic and spontaneous processes, it is called "spontaneous." If it includes everything to the left of responsible processes, it is called "intentional."

But the most important thing about the distinctions in Figure 14.2 is not how the processes are connected, because essentially everything is connected to everything else. Rather, the important things are the distinctions among processes themselves; the insistence that stimulus control (maximal at the left) differs from intentional or personal control (maximal at the right; see, e.g., Dennett, 1978; Harré & Secord, 1973); and the assertion that it is fruitful to differentiate among nonautomatic processes. The types are suggested for their intuitive heuristic value, not as established logical or empirical realities. Additional types are no doubt possible. But these five seem to be the minimal set for discussing automatic, spontaneous, and intentional processes; what they are and are not; and their possible relations with one another.

SPONTANEOUS INFERENCES IN TEXT COMPREHENSION

Having outlined some preliminary ideas on what automatic, spontaneous, and intentional inferences are and are not, I want to suggest the ubiquity and importance of spontaneous inferences by briefly describing some research from a rather intensively studied domain of cognitive activity: text comprehension. Referring to the comprehension of social events generally, Lichtenstein and Srull (1987, p. 98) have noted that there "are several reasons to believe that ordinary comprehension is the most important and yet least well-understood processing objective that characterizes social information processing. It is important because it is probably the most dominant 'set' that people use outside the laboratory." Comprehending text is also ubiquitous and important (especially for such readers as the present audience). But it is particularly relevant because my colleagues and I have used textual stimuli in our research on spontaneous trait attributions. And we have assumed (along with Mandler, 1984; Schank & Abelson, 1977; and others) that many of the same knowledge structures, schemata, and procedures involved in text comprehension are also involved in comprehending *in vivo* social events (even though this clearly involves other processes as well; e.g., Brewer, 1988; Kassin & Baron, 1985).

Many lines of evidence on text comprehension demonstrate inference processes that are neither automatic nor intentional, in the sense described in Figure 14.1. Such inferences may be best characterized as spontaneous.

Single Words' Meanings

Single words often seem to activate their meanings automatically. The Stroop effect described above is usually understood as a case of color words automatically activating color concepts. The work of Bargh and his colleagues with subliminal concept activation (Bargh, Bond, Lombardi, & Tota, 1986; Bargh & Pietromonaco, 1982), in which the subjects do not even realize that they are being shown trait-related adjectives that then affect their subsequent impression formation, provides other examples (see Bargh, Chapter 1, this volume).

Single words may also automatically activate meanings—thematic associates such as "king–queen" (see reviews by Fischler, 1981, and Foss, 1982), associates of associates (Balota & Lorch, 1986), and superordinate categories (Barsalou & Ross, 1986; Fisk & Schneider, 1983, 1984). It has even been suggested that the appropriate meanings of ambiguous words can also be selected by textual context automatically (Glucksberg, Kreuz, & Rho, 1986; but see also Burgess, Tanenhaus, & Seidenberg, 1987), though this is a large and complex literature. Simpson's (1984) extensive review of it concludes that "the major remaining issue of controversy is whether these effects of meaning frequency and context [on meaning selection] are characteristics of [automatic] lexical access itself or [nonautomatic, strategic] postaccess decision processes" (p. 327).

There are other cases in which the activation of meanings does not seem to be automatic, yet is not really intentional either. For example, Barsalou (1982) has distinguished between context-independent (CI) and context-dependent (CD) properties of nouns. CI properties are invariably and automatically activated by the noun, because the noun and property have been frequently and consistently paired in the past (e.g., "basketball" and "round"). CD properties are not automatically activated by the word, but depend on context for activation (e.g., the property that a basketball will "float" is activated by "The basketball bounced into the swimming pool"). Subjects were given 6 seconds to fully comprehend each context sentence and read it aloud; then they verified a property of the target word in the sentence. CI properties' reaction times (RTs) were unaffected by context in the property verification task, indicating that they were invariably and rapidly activated; however, CD properties' RTs were affected by context.

Note that both CI and CD property activation took place during an intentional activity. The former was deemed automatic on the basis of its speed and insensitivity to context. But establishing that CD property activation was not an automatic result of reading the target word does not make it intentional. No one would say that subjects read the sentences with an intention to infer targets' properties. Such properties are innumerable, and inferring properties could be interminable. It is more accurate and useful to say that subjects intended to comprehend the sentences, but they did not know and could not say what processes that involved, how they went about them, or even when or how they decided they had finished (exited) "comprehending." There are many ways to comprehend sentences, some of which people can roughly describe (e.g., visually, empathetically, stylistically), just as there are many ways people can intentionally "memorize" words (e.g., rote repetition, visualization, semantic elaboration). Indeed, there is a fairly large literature on the differences in how good and poor readers comprehend text. So "intending to comprehend" something does not make the *particular processes* involved in comprehension any more intentional (chosen with awareness) than "intending to memorize" something makes those processes intentional.

In general, one may carry out a superordinate intention without knowing how one does it. In fact, it may be impossible to "choose" subprocesses in advance, because they may depend upon unforeseeable features of the task. At the conscious level, most of us have had the experience of intending to write something in a particular way, following an outline, only to have the material "take over" when we actually began writing, so that we have to depart significantly from our prior intention, the outline. If the intention to comprehend always or necessarily invoked the same processes, we might call those processes intentional as well. But comprehension is an amorphous, fuzzy goal operating in an ill-defined problem space, and invoking a variety of optional procedures that psychologists are only beginning to map. If the procedure is not a logically necessary or actuarially common consequence of the more molar, conscious intention, then it should not be called intentional. It seems quite unlikely that CD property activation is intentional in the sense of being consciously chosen. Nor is it intentional through being a logically necessary consequence of intentional comprehension. Its logical necessity arises from an interaction between the global intention to comprehend and a particular text's structure. It is probably nonconscious, but it is also not automatic. Thus, in terms of the framework sketched out in Figure 14.2, CD property activation is neither automatic nor intentional; it is best characterized as spontaneous.

It is interesting to note Barsalou's (1982) observation:

> CD properties may become available in two ways. First, they may actually be stored in a concept and be activated by contexts containing similar or associated information. . . . Just how contexts activate these

properties is a topic worthy of future interest. [Second, they] may be computed with various inference procedures. . . . The range and nature of these inference processes . . . appear to present a problem for theories of semantics, which usually try to characterize word meanings with finite sets of properties. (pp. 87–88)

That is, some CD properties may be activated by spontaneous inference processes, computed on the spot.

Backward and Forward Inferences

Backward inferences in text comprehension connect current text with text presented earlier, and are important in establishing the text's coherence. Forward inferences predict or anticipate text that has not been encountered yet.

One extensively studied backward inference is "anaphoric reference," in which a word (a pronoun or general concept name) refers back to some preceding specific referent (e.g., "A *burglar* surveyed the garage set back from the street. . . . The *criminal* slipped away from the street lamp"). In order to understand the anaphor "criminal," the referent "burglar" must be activated and connected to it. McKoon and Ratcliff (1980) have used probe recognition RTs to show that referent activation is automatic (RTs < 250 milliseconds). Dell, McKoon, and Ratcliff (1983) have shown that an anaphor automatically activates the entire proposition containing the referent, and that the parts of the proposition relevant to establishing text coherence remain active while irrelevant parts fade. So, within the intentional task of text comprehension, anaphoric references seem to be automatic.

"Instrument inferences" occur when the text describes an action that is apparently performed with a previously mentioned instrument. These are also backward inferences, but evidence suggests that they do not always occur automatically. When people read, "Bobby got a saw, hammer [or mallet], screwdriver, and square from his toolbox. . . . Then Bobby pounded the boards together with nails" (McKoon & Ratcliff, 1981, pp. 674 & 676), do they infer that he used the hammer, or the mallet if they read that version? Surprisingly, using a probe recognition RT procedure, McKoon and Ratcliff found that "only instruments highly related [semantically] to an action [e.g., hammer] were activated [within 250 milliseconds] by reading a sentence containing the action and that only instruments highly related to the action were connected to the action in the memory representation of the text" (1981, p. 671). They suggest that unlike anaphoric inferences, instrument inferences may not be made automatically because they are not required for comprehension.

Forward inferences, such as events' consequences, are usually not required for text coherence. Singer and Ferreira (1983) found that subjects took about 200 milliseconds longer to answer questions about paraphrases and forward inferences than they took for questions about backward inferences, suggesting that backward inferences are made more quickly and reliably during comprehension.

McKoon and Ratcliff (1986) investigated the automaticity of forward inferences about highly predictable events (e.g., inferring that someone is "dead" after "falling off a 14th-story roof"). In Experiment 1, subjects responded as quickly as possible to recognition probe words, indicating whether or not they had appeared in the text. The text implied events (e.g., "dead") without stating them explicitly. It took subjects about 30 milliseconds longer to correctly respond "no" to such words as "dead" than to event words that were not implied by the paragraphs, suggesting that the predictable events had been inferred. However, these RTs were too long (>800 milliseconds) to rule out the alternative explanation that strategic context checking had produced the longer delay. Therefore, in Experiment 4, subjects were forced to respond in less than 350 milliseconds, thus precluding strategic processes. This increased the error rate for the probes, suggesting that the highly predictable events were inferred automatically.

Thus backward inferences that are required to establish the coherence of text seem to occur automatically. Other backward inferences, such as instrument inferences, are either less likely, or less likely, to be automatic. There is also evidence that some kinds of forward inferences occur automatically, so that for highly predictable events, people automatically "go beyond the information given" and draw at least the most obvious conclusions. These automatic inferences are probably not conscious and not intended either explicitly or as a logically necessary part of text comprehension. In terms of the framework in Figure 14.2, they are distinguished from spontaneous inferences by being faster.

The occurrence of automatic backward and forward inferences that are not logically necessary for text comprehension indirectly supports the plausibility of spontaneous inferences. Spontaneous inferences are also unconscious and unintended, but they require more time and some central processing capacity. They are lumped together with other "strategic" processes by the current nomenclature. They may be more common than automatic inferences, because they should require less practice to become relatively effortless but not-yet-automatic procedures (e.g., Smith & Lerner, 1986). But they may also be less common in task environments that put a premium on the efficient use of limited central processing resources, and thereby eliminate ultimately irrelevant processes. Of course, what is "ultimately irrelevant" depends on the task. When there is no task, or the task is ill defined (e.g., a "task" of playing), spontaneous inferences would not be eliminated by such competition for resources. This suggests that spontaneous inferences should be most common in the least constrained and task-like, and the most "playful," environments.

Structural Inferences

Text comprehension involves other kinds of inferences as well: inferences about such things as causality, actors' plans and goals (Mandler, 1984; Schank & Abelson, 1977), and the overall structure of the text (vanDijk, 1980; vanDijk & Kintsch, 1983). Black, Galambos, and Read's (1985) review gives some sense of how complex these inferences are, and how elaborate the activated knowledge structures may be that are required for text comprehension.

Most research in this area seeks evidence that these structures are inferred, or exist and are activated, during text comprehension. Reading times, probe recognition RTs, or lexical decision RTs are measured, but these times are much too long to distinguish between automatic and strategic processes. Very little research has focused on possible effects of readers' intentions, because the intention to read "for comprehension" is usually given or assumed.

One interesting exception to this neglect of intentions is the studies by Seifert, McKoon, Abelson, and Ratcliff (1986). They investigated the conditions under which readers inferred stories' global thematic abstraction units (TAUs), such as "closing the barn door after the horse is gone." Subjects were quicker to verify a test sentence from one story if they had just read a test sentence from a thematically similar story, but only if they read the stories with an intention to rate their similarity. Similar effects were obtained with more vague instructions to study each story extensively. But no such effects were obtained with simple comprehension instructions. Seifert et al. concluded that thematic story information may activate "similar episodes and formation of connections in memory," but not automatically. Rather, TAU activation "depends on subjects' strategies and task difficulty" (1986, p. 220).

It is possible that some global structural inferences are automatic. But it seems likely that many are not, though they can be obtained with appropriate instructions. Should these be called intentional? Subjects usually do not intend to make them in the course of comprehension, and are probably not aware that they have made them when they do, so they are not intentional in any straightforward way or in the comprehensive way described in Figure 14.1. Perhaps they are intentional in the sense that they are logically necessary components of an intentional process, such as "comprehending" or "studying extensively." Though this may be true for some texts and structures, it cannot be generally true, because "comprehension" and "studying" (like "thinking" and "playing" and "working") can be done in too many ways to *require* particular procedures. These terms describe relatively amorphous activities, rather than well-defined goal-directed procedures that we could map into TOTEs. Thus, most global structural inferences are probably neither automatic not intentional in any meaningful sense. Readers are probably no more aware of making them than they are of following the rules of syntax when they speak. Thus, most of these inferences are probably best described as spontaneous.

CONCLUSIONS

This chapter presents a general classification of cognitive processes, and focuses on intentional, spontaneous, and automatic processes. Other process types that are briefly described are either beyond the scope of this chapter (e.g., ruminative processes; but see the chapters in this volume by Martin & Tesser, Pennebaker, Tait & Silver, and Wegner & Schneider) or beyond the scope of a book on unintended thought, and have been presented chiefly to sharpen the meaning of the major types by contrast with them. Readers will have to judge the utility of this framework for whatever goals they have in mind. I have found it useful, and would be happy to see it added to and amended to make it more useful. It is offered primarily for its heuristic value, rather than as a powerful analytic tool or definitive description of research in this area.

Nevertheless, it seems to me that the research cited here points to several conclusions about how we should think about thought. Most of them are not novel. But they all seem important, if we are to successfully communicate and identify the central issues for research on unintended thought.

1. Spontaneous trait inferences are neither automatic nor controlled.

2. Automatic processes are fast (<300 milliseconds), effortless, relatively unaffected by limiting cognitive capacity, not controlled by the person, and unintended. Thus, most complex cognitive processes are mixes of automatic and nonautomatic processes.

3. There is disagreement in the literature regarding other criteria for automaticity. But "nonautomatic" is not the same as "controlled."

4. Intentional control of cognitions requires awareness of alternative processing goals and choice among them, as well as awareness of operations that can be performed to attempt to attain those goals (Figure 14.1). Not all thought is consciously goal-directed, so not all thought is under intentional control.

5. How a process is described depends upon the level of analysis. Within an intentional, controlled process, there may be automatic, spontaneous, and even ruminative processes.

6. It is useful to distinguish among at least five types of cognitive processes, in terms of degrees of intentional or personal control: automatic, spontaneous, ruminative, intentional, and responsible (Figure 14.2). In general, processes at the left of the figure are embedded within those at the right.

ACKNOWLEDGMENT

Preparation of this chapter was facilitated by National Institute of Mental Health Grant No. BSR 1 R01 MH43959.

NOTES

1. Portions of this chapter appeared as "Unconscious Processes in Inferring Traits from Behavior" by J. S. Uleman, 1987, in J. A. Bargh (Chair), *Nonconscious processes in social cognition.* Symposium conducted at the annual convention of the Society for Experimental Social Psychology, Charlottesville, VA.

2. It may be informative that these two characteristics co-occur. Awareness or knowledge that we have done something may often be inferred from the combination of an intention to do it and incomplete information about outcomes that does not disconfirm goal attainment. That is, we may sometimes decide we have done something, especially if it is covert and does not offer many clear outcomes, by saying to ourselves, "I must have done it because I meant to, and I have no reason to believe otherwise." Langer's (1978, pp. 39–40) example of "Did you flush the toilet the *last time* you went to the bathroom?" comes to mind. Of course, we may require more detailed contextual episodic memory to answer such awareness questions, especially about overt behaviors in real-world settings. But internal operations (cognitions) may be relatively deficient in generating such contextual cues, on which to base judgments that an event actually occurred. So we may be especially likely to rely on memory of our own intentions.

3. In fact, the situation is more complex than this, because there is evidence that "automatic" Stroop effects depend on the intent to respond with color names, which preactivates color concepts. Shiffrin (1988, p.766) cites "a study in which the subject must emit digit names as well as color names; in such a case printed names of digits produce as much interference with the ink color naming as do printed color words (Neumann, 1984)." But the simpler view of the Stroop is a better illustration of my point.

4. Now that I have laid out this long list of the defining features of intentional thought, this is probably the most appropriate place to confess my suspicion that our categories of cognitive processes are actually fuzzy (Rosch, 1978) and metaphorical (Lakoff & Johnson, 1980), with the metaphor here based on overt intentional actions. Thus some instances of thought processes will be more "typical" than others of any proposed category, and not all aspects of these metaphors will prove to be useful or appropriate.

REFERENCES

Abelson, R. P. (1988). Conviction. *American Psychologist, 43,* 267–275.
Balota, D. A., & Lorch, R. F., Jr. (1986). Depth of automatic spreading activation: Mediated priming effects in pronunciation but not in lexical decision. *Journal*

of Experimental Psychology: Learning, Memory, and Cognition, 12, 336–345.

Bargh, J. A. (1984). Automatic and conscious processing of social information. In R. S. Wyer, Jr., & T. K. Srull (Eds.), *Handbook of social cognition* (Vol. 3, pp. 1–43). Hillsdale, NJ: Erlbaum.

Bargh, J. A., Bond, R. N., Lombardi, W. J., & Tota, M. E. (1986). The additive nature of chronic and temporary sources of construct accessibility. *Journal of Personality and Social Psychology, 50,* 869–878.

Bargh, J. A., & Pietromonaco, P. (1982). Automatic information processing and social perception: The influence of trait information presented outside of conscious awareness on impression formation. *Journal of Personality and Social Psychology, 43,* 437–449.

Barsalou, L. W. (1982). Context-independent and context-dependent information in concepts. *Memory and Cognition, 10,* 82–93.

Barsalou, L. W., & Ross, B. H. (1986). The roles of automatic and strategic processing in sensitivity to superordinate and property frequency. *Journal of Experimental Psychology: Learning, Memory, and Cognition, 12,* 116–134.

Black, J. B., Galambos, J. A., & Read, S. J. (1984). Comprehending stories and social situations. In R. S. Wyer, Jr., & T. K. Srull (Eds.), *Handbook of social cognition* (Vol. 3, pp. 45–86). Hillsdale, NJ: Erlbaum.

Brewer, M. B. (1988). A dual process model of impression formation. In T. K. Srull & R. S. Wyer, Jr. (Eds.), *Advances in social cognition* (Vol. 1, pp 1–36). Hillsdale, NJ: Erlbaum.

Burgess, C., Tanenhaus, M. K., & Seidenberg, M. S. (1987). *Context and lexical access: Implications of nonword interference for lexical ambiguity resolution.* Unpublished manuscript, University of Rochester.

Chaiken, S. (1980). Heuristic versus systematic information processing and the use of source versus message cues in persuasion. *Journal of Personality and Social Psychology, 39,* 752–766.

Dell, G. S., McKoon, G., & Ratcliff, R. (1983). The activation of antecedent information during the processing of anaphoric reference in reading. *Journal of Verbal Learning and Verbal Behavior, 22,* 121–132.

Dennett, D. C. (1978). *Brainstorms: Philosophical essays on mind and psychology.* Cambridge, MA: Bradford Books.

Dennett, D. C. (1984). *Elbow room: The varieties of free will worth wanting.* Cambridge, MA: Bradford Books.

Dyer, F. N. (1973). The Stroop phenomenon and its use in the study of perceptual, cognitive and response processes. *Memory and Cognition, 1,* 106–120.

Fischler, I. (1981). Research on context effects in word recognition: 10 years back and forth. *Cognition, 10,* 89–95.

Fisk, A. D., & Schneider, W. (1983). Category and word search: Generalizing search principles to complex processing. *Journal of Experimental Psychology: Learning, Memory, and Cognition, 9,* 177–195.

Fisk, A. D., & Schneider, W. (1984). Memory as a function of attention, level of processing and automatization. *Journal of Experimental Psychology: Learning, Memory, and Cognition, 10,* 181–197.

Foss, D. J. (1982). A discourse on semantic priming. *Cognitive Psychology, 14,* 590–607.

Frost, R. (1949). The road not taken. In *Complete poems of Robert Frost* (p. 131). New York: Holt, Rinehart & Winston.

Glucksberg, S., Kreuz, R. J., & Rho, S. H. (1986). Context can constrain lexical access: Implications for models of language comprehension. *Journal of Experimental Psychology: Learning, Memory, and Cognition, 12*, 323–335.

Harré, R., & Secord, P. F. (1973). *The explanation of social behavior.* Totowa, NJ: Littlefield, Adams.

Higgins, E. T. (1981). The "communication game": Implications for social cognition and persuasion. In E. T. Higgins, C. P. Herman, & M. P. Zanna (Eds.), *Social cognition: The Ontario Symposium* (Vol. 1, pp. 343–392). Hillsdale, NJ: Erlbaum.

Kahneman, D., & Treisman, A. (1984). Changing views of attention and automaticity. In R. Parasuraman & D. R. Davies (Eds.), *Varieties of attention* (pp. 29–61). New York: Academic Press.

Kassin, S. M., & Baron, R. M. (1985). Basic determinants of attribution and social perception. In J. H. Harvey & G. Weary (Eds.), *Attibution: Basic issues and application* (pp. 37–64). New York: Academic Press.

Lakoff, G., & Johnson, M. (1980). *Metaphors we live by.* Chicago: University of Chicago Press.

Langer, E. J. (1978). Rethinking the role of thought in social interaction. In J. H. Harvey, W. Ickes, & R. F. Kidd (Eds.), *New directions in attribution research* (Vol. 2, pp. 35–58). Hillsdale, NJ: Erlbaum.

Lichtenstein, M., & Srull, T. K. (1987). Processing objectives as a determinant of the relationship between recall and judgment. *Journal of Experimental Social Psychology, 23*, 93–118.

Logan, G. D. (1980). Attention and automaticity in Stroop and priming tasks: Theory and data. *Cognitive Psychology, 12*, 523–553.

Logan, G. D., & Cowan, W. B. (1984). On the ability to inhibit thought and action: A theory of an act of control. *Psychological Review, 91*, 295–327.

Mandler, J. M. (1984). *Stories, scripts, and scenes: Aspects of schema theory.* Hillsdale, NJ: Erlbaum.

McKoon, G., & Ratcliff, R. (1980). The comprehension processes and memory structures involved in anaphoric reference. *Journal of Verbal Learning and Verbal Behavior, 19*, 668–682.

McKoon, G., & Ratcliff, R. (1981). The comprehension processes and memory structures involved in instrumental inferences. *Journal of Verbal Learning and Verbal Behavior, 20*, 671–682.

McKoon, G., & Ratcliff, R. (1986). Inferences about predictable events. *Journal of Experimental Psychology: Learning, Memory, and Cognition, 12*, 82–91.

Miller, G. A., Galanter, E., & Pribram, K. H. (1960). *Plans and the structure of behavior.* New York: Holt, Rinehart & Winston.

Neely, J. H. (1977). Semantic priming and retrieval from lexical memory: Roles of inhibitionless spreading activation and limited-capacity attention. *Journal of Experimental Psychology: General, 106*, 226–254.

Neisser, U. (1976). *Cognition and reality.* San Francisco: W. H. Freeman.

Neumann, O. (1984). Automatic processing: A review of recent findings and a plea for an old theory. In W. Prinz & A. F. Sanders (Eds.), *Cognition and motor processes* (pp. 255–294). Berlin: Springer-Verlag.

Newell, A. (1973). Production systems: Models of control structures. In W. C. Chase (Ed.), *Visual information processing* (pp. 465–526). New York: Academic Press.

Nisbett, R. E., & Wilson, T. D. (1977). Telling more than we can know: Verbal reports on mental processes. *Psychological Review, 84,* 231–259.

Petty, R. E., & Cacioppo, J. T. (1986). The elaboration likelihood model of persuasion. In L. Berkowitz (Ed.), *Advances in experimental social psychology* (Vol. 19, pp. 123–206). New York: Academic Press.

Posner, M. I., & Snyder, C. R. R. (1975). Attention and cognitive control. In R. L. Solso (Ed.), *Information processing and cognition: The Loyola Symposium* (pp. 55–85). Hillsdale, NJ: Erlbaum.

Rosch, E. (1978). Principles of categorization. In E. Rosch & B. B. Lloyd (Eds.), *Cognition and categorization* (pp. 27–48). Hillsdale, NJ: Erlbaum.

Schank, R. C., & Abelson, R. (1977). *Scripts, plans, goals and understanding.* Hillsdale, NJ: Erlbaum.

Schneider, W., Dumais, S. T., & Shiffrin, R. M. (1984). Automatic and control processing and attention. In R. Parasuraman & D. R. Davies (Eds.), *Varieties of attention* (pp. 1–27). New York: Academic Press.

Schneider, W., & Shiffrin, R. M. (1977). Controlled and automatic human information processing: I. Detection, search, and attention. *Psychological Review, 84,* 1–66.

Seifert, C. M., McKoon, G., Abelson, R. P., & Ratcliff, R. (1986). Memory connections between thematically similar episodes. *Journal of Experimental Psychology: Learning, Memory, and Cognition, 12,* 220–231.

Shiffrin, R. M. (1988). Attention. In R. C. Atkinson, R. J. Herrnstein, G. Lindzey, & R. D. Luce (Eds.), *Stevens' handbook of experimental psychology* (2nd ed., pp. 739–811). New York: Wiley.

Shiffrin, R. M., & Dumais, S. T. (1981). The development of automatism. In J. R. Anderson (Ed.), *Cognitive skills and their acquisition* (pp. 111–140). Hillsdale, NJ: Erlbaum.

Shiffrin, R. M., & Schneider, W. (1977). Controlled and automatic human information processing: II. Perceptual learning, automatic attending and a general theory. *Psychological Review, 84,* 127–190.

Simpson, G. B. (1984). Lexical ambiguity and its role in models of word recognition. *Psychological Bulletin, 96,* 316–340.

Singer, M., & Ferreira, F. (1983). Inferring consequences in story comprehension. *Journal of Verbal Learning and Verbal Behavior, 22,* 437–448.

Smith, E. R., & Lerner, M. (1986). Development of automatism of social judgments. *Journal of Personality and Social Psychology, 50,* 246–259.

Tetlock, P. E. (1983). Accountability and complexity of thought. *Journal of Personality and Social Psychology, 45,* 74–83.

Tetlock, P. E., & Kim, J. I. (1987). Accountability and judgment processes in a personality prediction task. *Journal of Personality and Social Psychology, 52,* 700–709.

Tulving, E., & Thomson, D. M. (1973). Encoding specificity and retrieval processes in episodic memory. *Psychological Bulletin, 30,* 352–373.

Uleman, J. S. (1987). Consciousness and control: The case of spontaneous trait inferences. *Personality and Social Psychology Bulletin, 13,* 337–354.

Uleman, J. S., & Moskowitz, G. B. (1987). *Spontaneous and strategic social inferences.* Unpublished manuscript, New York University.

Uleman, J. S., Newman, L., & Winter, L. (1987). *Making spontaneous trait inferences uses some cognitive capacity at encoding.* Unpublished manuscript, New York University.

vanDijk, T. A. (1980). *Macrostructures: An interdisciplinary study of global structures in discourse, interaction, and cognition.* Hillsdale, NJ: Erlbaum.

vanDijk, T. A., & Kintsch, W. (1983). *Strategies of discourse comprehension.* New York: Academic Press.

Wegner, D. M., & Vallacher, R. R. (1986). Action identification. In R. M. Sorrentino & E. T. Higgins (Eds.), *Handbook of motivation and cognition: Foundations of social behavior* (pp. 550–582). New York: Guilford Press.

Winter, L., & Uleman, J. S. (1984). When are social judgments made? Evidence for the spontaneousness of trait inferences. *Journal of Personality and Social Psychology, 47,* 237–252.

Winter, L., Uleman, J. S., & Cunniff, C. (1985). How automatic are social judgments? *Journal of Personality and Social Psychology, 49,* 904–917.

Zajonc, R. B. (1960). The process of cognitive tuning and communication. *Journal of Abnormal and Social Psychology, 61,* 159–167.

15

Intentional Chapters
on Unintended Thoughts

MICHAEL I. POSNER
MARY K. ROTHBART
University of Oregon

Freud's original goal was the development of a theory linking brain systems to the thought processes of daily life, although later he favored the independence of his psychoanalytic theory from brain systems (Sulloway, 1979). There is no doubt of the Freudian influence on the present volume. Social psychologists have found that our reactions to others are often constructed unconsciously. They also know from their work and from the last two decades of cognitive studies that the unconscious nature of these mental constructions does not prevent psychologists from studying them and their relation to consciousness.

The continuing success of social psychologists in this enterprise will likely rest upon their understanding of cognitive methods that can be used to study the unconscious. In addition, their work may also be aided by new ideas of how these methods relate to underlying neural mechanisms. It is the main theme of this chapter that current studies in social psychology, cognition, and neuroscience provide the basis for an increasingly unified view of the mind. In this chapter, we try to relate some of the issues raised in this volume to recent progress in related areas of cognition, neuroscience, and development.

Freud's concern with the unconscious was so strong that he only rarely explored the shallower depths of the conscious mind. The study of the conscious mind was one of the great contributions of the cognitive psychology stemming from Herbert Simon's (1979) work. His model of bounded rationality gave impetus to the study of those mental events we intentionally control. A number of cognitive psychologists following in Simon's tradition have been chiefly concerned with conscious processes reportable in protocol analyses and the search strategies that control them. In the cognitive writings most strongly influenced by computer metaphors, there has been relatively little concern with the unconscious (but see Kihlstrom, 1987, for a review of the continuing interest in unconscious processes by other cognitive psychologists).

Discussions of unconscious processes in the cognitive literature have often been hidden under the study of parallel preattentive processes and automaticity, and both of these approaches serve as operational methods for exploring processes for which we have poor awareness. Only rather slowly are cognitive psychologists coming to understand that much of our mental life is structured outside of consciousness and that our intentional control of mental events represents only one, perhaps small, part of the mind.

In neuroscience, the importance of unconscious events in ordering mental life has been brought home forcefully in studies of split-brain patients. What Gazzaniga (1985) calls the "interpreter system" can thus be disconnected from other systems that carry on very complex processing but cannot report it, at least by conventional means. The split brain is just one of many conditions producing dissociations between unconscious and conscious information processing. The study of amnesia suggests that unconscious memories can be preserved while the ability to form conscious ones is lost, due to hippocampal damage (Squire, 1986). Occipital damage may spare orienting toward an object, while its appearance in consciousness is completely blocked, in the "blindsight" phenomenon (Weizkrantz, 1977). The preverbal infant also appears to have mature processing systems well in advance of the development of the attention system that supports much of our conscious problem solving (Weizkrantz, 1988). These studies indicate that unconscious processes need be neither simple nor fleeting, as is sometimes assumed from the use of cognitive methods. Instead, as Freud claimed, these processes can carry on a sophisticated cognition of their own.

These results suggest that a combined cognitive–neuroscience viewpoint may provide an enlarged perspective for understanding unconscious influences upon thought. Of particular importance for this understanding are efforts to understand deficits in attention in such disorders as schizophrenia or depression. We have found that a joint consideration of cognitive and anatomical constraints provides a much better approach to some of these deficit states than the cognitive approach alone (Posner, 1988; Posner, Petersen, Fox, & Raichle, 1988).

Several chapters of this book are concerned with the idea that thoughts about ourselves and others may arise without deliberate intention, and we review these chapters in the section that follows. We then review automaticity in light of cognitive and neuroscience findings on selective attention, followed by a discussion of chapters that deal with the relationship of cognition and affect. Here the application of cognitive theory has already proven inadequate to the satisfactory discussion of the issues (Rothbart, 1983; Tucker, 1985). We examine the possible advantages of linking cognition and affect through studies of underlying neural systems and their development. Finally, we examine the effort to control automatic processes. Here, instead of dealing directly with the adult social-psychological literature, we turn to infant development as a model of how central control over automatic processes begins. We believe that careful studies of the development of attentional mechanisms will provide needed insight into the problems and mechanisms of control.

UNBIDDEN THOUGHTS

The importance of awareness within cognition is brought out in several chapters dealing with the issue of how thoughts come to mind either without our bidding (i.e., without a deliberate search or intention) or structured in a way we may not have intended. The chapters by Tait and Silver (Chapter 12) and by Martin and Tesser (Chapter 10) deal with the general importance of what they label "ruminative thoughts." It is unsurprising that such thoughts often deal with the traits of others or even of ourselves (see Newman & Uleman, Chapter 5; Gilbert, Chapter 6; and Chaiken, Liberman, & Eagly, Chapter 7, this volume). The importance of trait attribution to social psychology makes critical the extent to which evaluations of self and others are imposed automatically upon us. Fiske (Chapter 8) raises this problem in wondering whether the concept of automatic categorization (stereotyping) might not be used as a legal excuse for bigotry against minorities, and we return to this issue later in this commentary. There may thus be serious social issues involved in the extent to which our thought processes are structured outside our current intentions.

Higgins (Chapter 3) argues for the importance of priming in manipulating cognitive structures outside of the subject's awareness. This kind of semantic priming follows rules of recency and repetition well known in cognitive psychology (Morton, 1969). Chronic accessibility (e.g., word frequency) and temporary availability (e.g., primary, recency) appear to combine to influence the likelihood that a concept will be activated. Of great importance to the work described in this book is the person's lack of awareness that external (sensory) activation and internal activation (from previous thought) are separate processes. Thus the experimenter knows that the thoughts of his or her subject are controlled by a prime, but the subject does not. This same idea has been incorporated into many parallel activation models (see Rumelhart & McClelland, 1986), an example of which is the "synapse" model described by Higgins in Chapter 3.

The effort to understand the rules by which these unconscious inferences are made is a major aspect of the study of trait inference revealed in this book. While Higgins stresses accessibility and spreading activation, Gilbert (Chapter 6) opts for a set of criteria developed by Helmholtz to describe unconscious inference in the study of perception. Automatic processes in unconscious inference are environmentally triggered, outside awareness, and not cognitively penetrable (see also Bargh, Chapter 1, this volume). Automatic processes seem most effective in governing behavior when the subject is otherwise preoccupied and thus less able to employ a qualifying context.

What these assertions argue is that traits of self and others are influenced by a cognitive network of concepts constructed from one's culture and individual past learning. The network appears to obey the same rules as those found in nonsocial experiments. The complexity of mental processing of which such networks are capable is a subject of intense study in many disciplines (Rumelhart & McClelland, 1986). Helmholtz may have been correct about the simple basic rules of unconscious inference, but not about their lack of creativity. Networks may in fact be capable of the kind of rules of systematic distortion implied by the ego defenses. Perhaps the methods used to study simple inferences outside of awareness will eventually reveal whether such complex distortion is within the capability of the unconscious. In any case, some of the simpler unconscious mechanisms have been elucidated within both cognitive and neuropsychology, and we now turn to these analyses.

BASIC PROCESSES

A major theme of this book is that there are varieties of automaticity. The chapters by Bargh (Chapter 1), Logan (Chapter 2), and Uleman (Chapter 14) are mainly involved with this issue, while those of Moretti and Shaw (Chapter 13), Chaiken et al. (Chapter 7), Newman and Uleman (Chapter 5), Gilbert (Chapter 6), Martin and Tesser (Chapter 10), and Higgins (Chapter 3) deal with it in passing. We learn that automatic processes can be conditional upon context, controlled, and intended, all without being available to awareness. Several years ago, Posner and Snyder (1975) proposed an operational distinction between automatic and conscious processes. In this 1975 paper, frequently cited in this book, they began by raising exactly the issue considered in the current volume: "To what extent are our conscious intentions and strategies in control of the way information is processed in our minds?" (p. 64).

It is a pleasure to see how energetically this issue is currently being addressed within social psychology. The Posner–Snyder approach provided three criteria for distinguishing automatic from conscious processes, suggesting that automatic operations are not limited in capacity, occur without intention, and occur without awareness. The importance of this idea is that there are measurable consequences of attending to an item that are not present when the same item is processed automatically, without attention. It was assumed that attention has limited capacity and that automatic activation of the semantic network has no similar limitation. In Posner and Snyder's experiments, activation of a node within the semantic network by a word was found to facilitate reactivation by a related word, but had no negative (inhibitory) influence on the efficiency of handling any other word. However, if a node was activated by attending to it, the capacity limit of attention meant that unrelated items not sharing that pathway would be inhibited from attention, and thus nonhabitual responses made to it, such as making classifications by pressing keys, would be less efficient.

Inhibitory control was the sign of attention. Thus, if semantic priming was obtained without attention, benefits from activation of the semantic pathway were demonstrated, but no general inhibition was seen. If a subject attended to the prime, facilitation due to pathway activation was accompanied by inhibition, due to the use of a limited-capacity system. In 1977, Neely performed a well-known series of experiments that confirmed this dissociation between automatic and attended activations. This work was summarized in 1978 (Posner, 1978) and defended in 1982 (Posner, 1982).

Automatic Networks

Much of this literature can be summarized by the concept of "pathway activation." This concept was thought to underlie the phenomenon of "spreading activation" formulated by Collins and Loftus (1975). The activation of a pathway can occur without intention or awareness, since this is the property of a separate system. However, there is ample opportunity for control by context. First, activations sum, so that when the activation of the word "palm" follows the word "tree," items such as "elm" or "oak" have stronger and longer-lasting activation than if "tree" had not been presented. Second, the attention system can use context, including goals, to guide its interaction with the automatic network (Neely, 1977).

At the time of our original findings, the concept of pathway activation was entirely based on studies of performance. More recently, however, by use of neural imaging techniques, it has been possible to show that the physical, phonological, and semantic codes of words activate quite separate neural areas (Posner, Petersen, et al., 1988). This set of areas and their linking fiber tracts now serve as the physical realization of one system of pathways.

Both Bargh (Chapter 1) and Logan (Chapter 2) raise important qualifications and objections to the network idea. They argue that a process may be automatic in some senses of the term but not in others. Logan offers the argument that what is automatic is retrieval from memory, whereas operations on this retrieved information, such as making responses or using retrieval cues for gathering further information, are controlled by attention. This is a view that Keele (1973) developed in considerable detail; it has merits for many situations, including many social situations where memory retrieval is basic. However, it begins with the object as the basic unit of analysis, and many studies of sensory processing (Treisman, 1987) have shown that the construction of the object from the visual array has both automatic and attended components, many of which do not depend upon stored information. This restriction and the close identification of memory with a particular theory (instance selection) in Logan's chapter make the general idea problematic, but allowing control to influence otherwise automatic processes is certainly compatible with much that has been found in cognitive studies.

Automaticity is a construct that can be likened to the concept of the reflex. Sherrington (1906) argued at the turn of the century that a reflex is a tool of analysis that is never really observed in pure form. Although we like to think of reflexes as automatic, they can, as Logan argues, be easily modified by context and through attention. Thus many automatic processes are conditional and can be controlled. For example, there is a strong tendency to move one's eyes to a visual stimulus, but if one is given an instruction to maintain fixation, a peripheral stimulus that might elicit an eye movement under usual conditions will not do so. One can control eye movements by attention just as one can control respiration, but it is nevertheless possible to breathe and move the eyes automatically, depending upon the situation and one's goal. Thus Bargh's argument that one needs to look at the goal state in determining whether a process will be automatic is correct. It is also true, as Bargh argues (see Chapter 1, this volume), that activation of a pathway may follow active attention to a word. For example, when one thinks about items related to a stimulus, activation of the related nodes will remain even when attention is diverted elsewhere (McLean & Shulman, 1978).

Despite its limitations as identified by Sherrington, the idealized reflex has been of great importance both to physiology and to psychology. Similarly, the idea of a purely automatic process that meets all three criteria is a convenient fiction that allows us to explore the internal systems responsible for our awareness of stimuli and our feeling of control. There has been substantial progress in this enterprise (Posner, 1988; Posner, Petersen, Fox, & Raichle, 1988), and it may be possible in the future to parcel the criteria of limited capacity, intention, and awareness into the properties of various underlying brain systems that constitute portions of the human selective attention system. We know that these criteria can be remarkably dissociated in nervous and mental disorders. Patients with schizophrenia, for example, are perfectly aware of ideas they feel they cannot control. Patients with posterior brain lesions may lose awareness of stimuli in conflict situations, but when the stimuli are present alone, they are able to shift attention and be aware of the same stimuli (Posner, 1988). Patients unable to use semantic information deliberately may show powerful effects of semantic priming (Milberg & Blumstein, 1981).

As an example of a combined cognitive–anatomical approach to automaticity, consider two forms of priming. One form ("repetition priming") comes from repeating the same item twice, reactivating the same pathway. The second form ("semantic priming") comes from presenting a semantically related target following a prime. Work in cognitive psychology has suggested that priming occurs in both cases and that either may be automatic. Studies of visual word recognition using positron emission tomography (PET; Petersen, Fox, Posner, Mintun, & Raichle, 1988) to image the areas of cerebral blood flow indicate that visual word forms are developed in the ventral occipital lobe, whereas semantic tasks uniquely activate a left-lateralized set of areas that appear to be involved in semantic memory. The word form areas can be activated even when the subject is entirely passive (i.e., when the subject is instructed to simply look at a word but not to do anything with it), and by this criterion seem to be automatic. On the other hand, the semantic area is never seen to have increased blood flow unless subjects process the words actively (i.e., name a word aloud or make a silent classification).

Of course, the PET method does not have a clearly known threshold, so the lack of activation does not mean that no activity occurs at that site. For this reason, and to obtain further evidence on the convergence between performance methods and neural activation methods, it is useful to study priming of visual word forms separately from semantic priming. This is, of course, very easy to do using standard priming methods (Posner, Sandson, Dhawan, & Shulman, 1989). When the standard lexical decision task for visual words is combined with the task of shadowing auditory words aloud (Posner et al., 1989), there is no interference of shadowing on the degree of repetition priming, but a very substantial reduction of semantic priming.

It appears that the development of the visual word form is automatic in that it shows no dual-task interference. Semantic priming appears to have an automatic component as well, but, as would be surmised by cognitive studies, it tends to be small and variable. Although it may be possible to influence the visual word form to some degree by attention, both neural imaging and performance studies suggest that it usually does not require attention to activate these systems. On the other hand, the semantic system seems to work in very close correspondence with attention. This fits rather well with the feeling we frequently have that our understanding of words and ideas involves effort. The convergence of the neural and cognitive methods augurs well for a joint anatomical and cognitive approach, which we use.

Attentional Control

Despite the success of new concepts of semantic networks, such networks do not presently exhibit the flexibility that human thought does. Networks may not be able to do so without development of better ideas of how they are controlled. Most of the chapters in this volume appear to accept the idea that unconscious networks are interfaced to an executive system that may alter their output. Indeed, one of the book's central contributions is the point that networks may be subject to control by attention.

An important concept in cognitive psychology and in this volume is the idea of the executive system (Neisser, 1967; Shallice, 1972). The executive system is held to be capable of inhibiting and thus controlling automatic activation patterns, and is a way of dealing with the interface between thoughts structured by our past learning and those under the control of current intentions. Although this idea has always been and is currently controversial, two developments have enhanced its utility. For the first time, there are serious proposals about how the computations of complex networks may allow learned associations to compute new solutions to problems. The current interest in connectionist networks has led to a tremendous expansion of the traditional concept of association between ideas. In the past, allowing thought to be based on "associations" created difficulty in dealing with the fluid nature of human concepts, their ability to assimilate new instances, the possibility of rule-based inferences, and so on. The new connectionist networks have made serious and useful proposals about how multilevel networks can handle these difficult problems. Thus, for the first time, we have serious proposals about what might be the computational ability of semantic networks (Rumelhart & McClelland, 1986).

Within cognitive science, the problem of the control of semantic activation remains an issue of great dispute between connectionists (Rumelhart & McClelland, 1986), who have generally ignored problems of control (but see Mozur, 1988), and symbol processors (Newell & Simon, 1972), who have placed search strategies at the heart of the theory. Networks appear to be a useful conceptualization of perception and motor processes, but it is unclear to what extent executive control is needed in order to prevent conflict. Perhaps, as some connectionists have wanted to argue, symbolic thought is an artifact and all processes are carried on within networks, without any necessity for an external control system.

Within purely cognitive psychology, it is difficult to choose what ought to be the correct architecture. However, since connectionists themselves have noted the similarities of their networks to neural systems, it seems relevant to ask whether the brain respects the distinctions sometimes made between executive (self-regulation) and automatic (data-processing) systems. By "self-regulation," we mean here the control over reactivity that can be exercised through selective attention. Attention as we understand it is an integrated cognitive system with its own anatomical base, although the neural systems subserving selective attention are not fully known (Posner, 1988).

There is compelling evidence that attention is a strongly interacting system with cognitive operations carried out at different brain sites (Posner, 1988). The story of selective attention as a brain system has emerged from a variety of experimental techniques and methods and is too long to deal with in detail in this commentary, but the results provide dramatic evidence that chronometric studies of the type used in this volume provide an important window on the operations of a neural system.

Attention may serve a number of functions. Some functions proposed for attention are as follows: to conjoin features within and across modalities (Treisman, 1987); to govern access to awareness and to nonhabitual responding (Posner, 1978); to foster semantic processing and integration of input into unified propositions (Kintsch, 1988); and so on. To understand the mechanisms of selective attention, it is useful to have model systems allowing the study of attentional influence over very simple types of sensory and motor responding.

As we see it, a single attention system allocates to different sensory and motor analyzers the appropriate mechanisms to allow the performance of various complex mental operations. We call this view a "hierarchical distributed attentional network" (Posner, 1988). One of the major functions of this network is to give priority to operations according to the current goals of the person. Thus, sensory input may only have access to output when its processing is in accord with the current motives of the organism (Derryberry & Rothbart, 1984). The idea that higher brain systems exercise inhibitory control over lower ones is an old one in physiology (Sechenov, 1965). Recent research suggests that the system responsible for selective attention may influence even very elementary levels of information processing. For example, there is some evidence that the attention system affects simple unisynaptic reflex activity (Logan, Chapter 2, this volume).

Is there a distinction between an unconscious network-like semantic system and an attentional system in the underlying neurology? We interpret recent research findings (Posner, 1988; Posner, Petersen, et al., 1988) as indicating two separate attentional areas. A posterior attention system is closely related to the selection and integration of sensory information. The portion of the posterior system involved with the selection of information from visual location is currently the best understood. This attentional system is important in visual pattern recognition. A more general anterior attention system controls the posterior one and is involved with a variety of cognitive systems, including semantic memory and language as well as spatial attention. Using the same dual-task technique described in the preceding section, it has been possible to show that the anterior and posterior attention systems, although anatomically quite distinct, are functionally closely interconnected (Posner, et al., 1989). Thus, despite the continued ambiguity of the purely cognitive evidence for "executive function," we believe that the brain does have fundamentally different structures to subserve attention.

We can now return to some of the issues raised above in connection with automatic activation of possibly unbidden thoughts. It should be clear that such processes as stereotype formation can be viewed at two levels. At the level of the unconscious, they arise because of the inevitable limits of human thought that require us to make classifications, think by use of prototypes, and so forth (see Fiske's arguments in Chapter 8 of this volume). There is a sense in which we are victims of our past learning, as represented in the semantic structures such learning has created. Thus, our past learning may produce more fear when we are approached at a quiet subway stop by a poorly dressed male than by a well-dressed female. However, it nevertheless remains possible to avoid discriminatory acts based on these stereotyped categories. Indeed, one of the great values of the intense discussion of affirmative action, discrimination, and related topics is that it makes us more clearly aware of the discriminatory acts we might perform based on our unconscious categories. The fact that many levels influence our actions toward others does not reduce the difficulty of legal decisions of responsibility, but one can believe in the existence of unconscious classifications without suspending belief in personal responsibility for action.

AFFECT AND SOCIAL COGNITION

The advantage of the combined cognitive–neuroscience approach is probably most apparent when one tries to deal with the problem of affect, as in the chapters relating to stress (Pennebaker, Chapter 11) and depression (Tait & Silver, Chapter 12; Moretti & Shaw, Chapter 13). There has been a strong tendency in cognitive studies to deal with affect or emotion as one node in a complex semantic network (Bower, 1981). Both biological and developmental perspectives, however, make this a very doubtful proposition. Studies of cognition and affect in normal adults using neural imaging techniques suggest that the underlying neural systems are quite different (Reiman, Fusselman, Fox, & Raichle, 1989). Adults during a panic attack and normal subjects expecting a shock show strong activation in the tip of the temporal poles on both sides of the brain. These areas are not active during nonevaluative semantic tasks (Petersen et al., 1988). Such findings suggest that affect should not be seen as just another node within a cognitive network, but as a system with its own separate neural basis and rules of operation that comes to be integrated with cognitive operations during evaluation.

If one accepts this idea, it becomes useful to ask this question: What is the good of attention in these complex networks? Derryberry and Roth-bart (1988) have found a negative correlation between individuals' self-reported skill at focusing and shifting attention and their self-reported sus-ceptibility to negative affect. Moretti and Shaw's example in Chapter 13 of therapists encouraging depressed patients to analyze their negative idea-tion suggests a further possibility of attentional control. Nevertheless, Wegner and Schneider (Chapter 9) indicate that shifting of attention is not always effective in reducing negative ideation, and Pennebaker (Chapter 11) points out the health risks associated with a generally repressive cognitive style.

There has been a debate in the cognitive literature concerning the in-tegration of cognition and affect (see Isen & Diamond, Chapter 4, and Tait & Silver, Chapter 12). One view has been that emotional responses lead cognition (Zajonc, 1984), and another that emotions are the result of cognitive labels applied to arousal. Posner and Snyder (1975) showed why resolution of this problem is difficult. Subjects were asked to judge whether a word had been on a previous list and to give their answer as quickly as possible. Some of the lists included all positive words, others all negative words. Although subjects had not been asked to deal with the affective dimension, they showed better performance in giving "no" responses when the emotion of the word mismatched the emotion of the array than when it agreed. An effect for list size was also found, which was interpreted as indicating that there were two quite separate structures, one representing the names of the words on the list and the other representing the pooled affect. Each structure had its own output. When the list was small, output was faster, and subjects responded correctly and rapidly even when the emotion mismatched; as the list became longer, the time to check whether the name was on the stored list increased, while the pooled affect produced a decrease in time needed to check affect. Under these conditions, a mis-matching affect led to poor performance. Thus even a simple cognitive appreciation of whether a word was present on an immediately prior list depends on the list length and the strength of the evaluation. For short lists and weak evaluations, the presence judgment occurs first; for long lists and strong evaluations, affect is first and influences the cognitive search. There appear to be separate memories working in parallel to influence an overall judgment, and neither is logically prior.

According to the general cognitive approach, it is important to ex-amine the time dynamics of mental processes in terms of their component facilitations and inhibitions (Posner, 1978). Is it possible to think of the activity of emotional reactions in this way? Recently, Derryberry (1988) has developed a very interesting on-line assay of emotion. He has defined a reaction time criterion so that a subject must be faster than the criterion to be rewarded for success on a given trial. For a given trial, a cue indi-cates that the subject can either win points (if faster than the criterion and correct) or lose points (if slower than the criterion or incorrect). A neutral cue means that on this trial the subject can neither win nor lose points.

The cue is followed by a single target word, which can be positive, neutral, or negative, and the subject's task is to classify the word according to its affective tone. Following the classification, the subject gets feedback as to whether points were won or lost.

Derryberry's reasoning is that the incentive signal sets off a positive or negative expectancy. If the signal indicates the subject can win points, it sets a positive expectancy. If points can only be lost and not won, it sets a negative expectancy. Do these brief affective states induced by the cues influence performance? If one looks within a trial, the incentive cue interacts with the word, so that positive incentives make the processing of positive words more efficient and negative incentives make the processing of negative words more efficient. It is likely that this effect operates via attention, since there are both costs and benefits when compared with the neutral-incentive condition.

There are other interpretations of this within-trial effect. It could be that subjects bias their responses for cognitive rather than emotional reasons. However, the effect of the outcome of the preceding trial on performance on the next trial is less likely to be influenced by cognitive factors. The outcome of the preceding trial has no objective consequences for performance on the next trial, which is equally likely to have positive and negative incentives or words, irrespective of the overall performance. However, a very interesting effect is found on the subsequent trial. Positive outcomes on the previous trials make efficient the processing of negative words, whereas negative outcomes make efficient the processing of positive words. This combination of an effect within trials congruent with the cue, and an effect across trials incongruent with the mood induced by the trial's outcome, is reminiscent of attentional effects found in spatial attention. With spatial orienting, it is found that when a subject is cued to attend to a given location, there is increased efficiency in processing items at that location; on the next trial, however, the previously advantaged location is now disadvantaged (Posner & Cohen, 1984). Whether Derryberry's effects are similar to those found with spatial attention is a question requiring further research.

The results obtained by Derryberry (1988) argue clearly that affect may influence judgment through attention. There are very strong anatomical connections between the anterior attention system and limbic areas. However, the earlier work of Posner and Snyder (1975) can be seen as demonstrating a direct influence of affect on the semantic network without mediation by intention or awareness. It seems clear that a more accurate account of the role of attention in emotional influences on performance will have to await further data. The tight chronometric paradigms of Derryberry might be combined with neural imaging techniques to provide more evidence in the future.

There has been an effort to study the role of attention in controlling the negative ideation in depression. Negative thoughts seem potentiated in depressed individuals (see Moretti & Shaw, Chapter 13, this volume) and sometimes defy even well-conceived programs designed to provide cognitive control of them. The ability to control depression by drugs, together with successes from cognitive therapy, makes it clear that the issues are at once physiological and cognitive, and that a theory dealing with both levels is important.

A second area of mental illness where the cognitive–neuroscience approach appears to be providing a useful research strategy is the study of schizophrenia (Posner, Early, et al., 1988). Schizophrenia is a cognitive disorder that has been described both as involving attention and as being a brain disorder with its own anatomy. One important aspect of schizophrenia is the illusion of patients that their ideas are being controlled from outside the self. For some reason the patients, who are aware of their own ideation, do not make the attribution that it comes from inside. One remarkable aspect of this is that the auditory hallucinations frequently accompanying the disorder may in fact be real internal speech mistakenly attributed to an outside agent (Bick & Kinsbourne, 1987).

Our research has provided some evidence that schizophrenic patients have a disorder that involves the anterior attentional system (Posner, Early, et al., 1988). This system is modulated by the dopamine pathways arising in the ventral tegmental area, and thus fits with the often-cited dopamine abnormality in the disorder. Our data and those of other researchers also argue that the disorder is lateralized and largely involves the left hemisphere. Thus, schizophrenic patients have difficulty in orienting attention to stimuli arising in the right visual field, fixate the left part of figures more than the right, and tend to turn leftward more than rightward. We believe the disorder has an influence on the ability of attention to control semantic activation. This fits with both the rather bizarre semantic associations sometimes found in the disorder, and the patients' illusion of external control of thought and ideas.

Issues involving the ability to deal with unintended association and illusions of control are important aspects of the combined cognitive–neuroscience approach. This is not to say that all issues of automaticity and attention need be approached at both levels; however, some problems such as schizophrenia, depression, and the general relation of emotion and cognition can benefit greatly from consideration of results from both fields.

DEVELOPMENT OF CONTROL MECHANISMS

The last part of this book deals with the issue of self-regulation of cognition. We all have the feeling that we can gain control over our cognition and direct it, at least for short periods, in the service of problem solving. The limits to this kind of control are obvious. Computers work away until the problem is solved or they are turned off; we become fatigued, lose motivation, go out for coffee, or quit. The problem of self-regulation is raised in a strong way in issues of the "ghost in the machine" (see Wegner & Schneider, Chapter 9, this volume). Nonetheless, the ideas of executive control and of separate attentional mechanisms suggest that there are systems designed to control the activation patterns that make up our thought processes.

In the light of the critical role that early development plays in ideas about the unconscious (Freud, 1924), it is important that Higgins (Chapter 3) and Newman and Uleman (Chapter 5) discuss developmental issues in this volume. This seems of particular importance to us, because we believe that an understanding of the development of control mechanisms in childhood may be a key to understanding how we regulate our thoughts. Luria (1973) distinguishes between two attention systems with strong similarities to the anterior and posterior systems we have previously described. He says, "[I]t is well known to psychologists that those features of the most elementary involuntary attention of the type which is attracted by the most powerful or biologically significant stimuli can be observed very early on during the first few months of child development" (p. 258). Vygotsky and, following him, Luria have stressed that during the interaction between caregiver and child, a second, more voluntary attention system is developed. We believe that Luria's distinction between voluntary and involuntary attentional systems is similar to the anatomically based anterior and posterior systems we have described above. Whereas Luria has stressed the biological basis of involuntary attention and the social basis of the voluntary system, we believe, in accord with our general cognitive–neuroscience theme, that these systems can both be described in terms of their anatomy and their cognitive operations.

In our previous work (Posner & Rothbart, 1980), we have argued that the problem of early infancy is to develop control over the peripheral systems available as effectors. Because our data have argued that visual attention and eye position are functionally but not physiologically related, we see it as an achievement of early infancy to place the eye movement system in coordination with the mechanisms that will become the central (anterior) attentional system. Eye movements are already present even before birth; however, they probably do not reflect the interest or preferences of the infant, but rather are driven by biologically potent stimulation. Only over time do they come to be in the service of the developing central system.

This perspective makes a major achievement of infancy the control of reflex patterns by central systems, the very question that forms the basic issue of Part III of this volume. The view of infancy as the development of regulation over inborn patterns of reaction is, of course, more pervasive than our specific model of attentional control over eye movements (Bruner, 1968; Schneirla, 1965/1972). In general, the newborn can be viewed as

primarily reactive, and the period of infancy as involved in the development of control systems (Rothbart & Derryberry, 1981). Sperry (1988)
has argued that psychology's new mentalistic (cognitive) approach places
emphasis on the emergent properties of cognition and their downward
control over earlier-evolving neural mechanisms. Control of stimulus reactions by reward and punishment represent the earliest control systems
to evolve and the first type of modification to develop in infancy. Only at
7–9 months of age does one begin to see the more general inhibitory control of activation that we have argued represents one sign of attentional
regulation found in adults. This level allows for the central control over
reaching we describe below. Later still, with the development of language,
one begins to see the formation of the verbal and semantic controls that
represent the heart of this volume.

We believe that the relative simplicity of infant behavior provides an
excellent model for attempting to achieve an understanding of central control at both a neural and cognitive level. One of the advantages of the
infant model as an approach to problems of central control is the ability
to disentangle cognition and affect. Even before young infants have developed complex cognitions about objects, they show strong evaluative and
approach–avoidance tendencies. These tendencies suggest that our emotional responses and evaluation of objects and people have their roots in
neural systems that exist prior to and are different from the semantic systems so heavily influenced by language (Rothbart, in press).

Thus infant studies help to support the distinctions between cognition
and affect developed in the preceding section. We believe that study of the
development of temperament is essential to a full understanding of how
attention and other controls come to regulate affective states (Rothbart &
Posner, 1985). During the period of infancy, individual temperament is
revealed in a relatively pure form, before it can be influenced by extensive
experience or the development of conceptual systems. We expect some of
these temperamental predispositions to persist, and would suggest that a
temperamental predisposition to negative emotionality may be one factor
influencing individual differences in ruminations upon unpleasant events,
as discussed by Tait and Silver (Chapter 12).

During development, temperament becomes modified through the
maturation of self-regulatory systems in interaction with experience. One
model for the study of individual differences in reactivity and its modification by attention can be found in the study of control of the eye movement system. Posner and Cohen (1980) have identified a sign of retinal–
collicular control that is quite prominent in eye movements in the infant.
This sign is the tendency to turn toward the temporal direction when
equivalent stimuli are presented simultaneously on the nasal and temporal
sides of fixation. Newborns appear to show particularly strong signs of the
retinal–collicular pathway, even with unilateral stimuli. In adults, the influence of the retinal–collicular pathway can be demonstrated only when

there is genuine competition between the stimuli. These data are in agreement with the general outline of Bronson's (1974) view of a shift from midbrain to cortical control over the first 3 months of life.

Visually guided reaching is another model for the study of developing self-regulation. Visually guided reaching and grasping is well developed by 5–6 months of age, and it appears to have an obligatory quality in the sense that children will reach and grasp objects that can lead to distress (Rothbart, 1988). In addition, young infants will reach on the line of sight, even though a Plexiglass barrier prevents them from obtaining the sighted object, and the object can be readily retrieved if they will only detour from sight lines (Diamond, 1981). There is good reason to suppose that the development of frontal systems is closely related to children's ability to refrain from reaching along the line of sight. It has been known for some years that monkeys with frontal lesions have great trouble in the delayed-response task. Recently it has been found (Diamond & Goldman-Rakic, 1983) that such monkeys have great difficulty in any situation in which a dominant response tendency must be held in check in order for a correct response to be made. For example, the frontal-lesioned monkeys, like young infants, cannot seem to inhibit visually controlled reaching in order to guide the hand to an open aperture to extract a reward (Diamond, 1981).

The delayed-response task appears to be one in which a previously rewarded response gains dominance over the visually observed location with delay on a given trial. Thus animals who are unable to avoid the dominant response make erroneous responses with increased delays. Infants before a year of age appear to exhibit the same inability to inhibit dominant response tendencies as do monkeys. Our understanding of the basic neurobiology of frontal systems is undergoing rapid development (Goldman-Rakic, 1987), and there is a good prospect that the neural system that underlies this form of self-regulation will soon be better understood. It is clear, however, that frontal systems responsible for this kind of inhibitory control are part of the circuits that have strong relationships to the visual–spatial attention system of the parietal lobe. Thus, we can identify these systems with the anterior attentional command mechanisms that seem to play an important role in controlling covert spatial orienting. These systems appear to continue to develop for some years, and may thus relate to other forms of self-regulation that we have described as occurring later in childhood (Rothbart & Posner, 1985).

CONCLUSION

The social-psychological approach to attention and automaticity adds new dimensions to our understanding of the topic gained from neuroscience, cognition, and development. In particular, it shows how automatic and attended processes are mixed together in everyday cognitions about people and events. This volume also illustrates that disentangling the roles of awareness, intention, and volition is not an easy process. However, experimental methods and theoretical concepts within cognitive psychology have clearly and usefully been adopted in this enterprise. In our commentary, we have attempted to show how cognitive concepts are becoming more closely linked to underlying neurology, and how the joint constraints of mind and brain may help in developing new approaches to such disorders as depression and schizophrenia and to normally developing controls over emotion and action.

ACKNOWLEDGMENTS

The research necessary for these comments was supported in part by Grant No. 43361 from the National Institute of Mental Health. We are grateful to the editors of this volume for inviting us to comment on its chapters.

REFERENCES

Bick, J., & Kinsbourne, M. (1987). Auditory illusions and subvocal speech in schizophrenic subjects. *American Journal of Psychiatry, 139*–166.

Bower, G. H. (1981). Mood and memory. *American Psychologist, 36*, 130–148.

Bronson, G. (1984). The postnatal growth of visual capacity. *Child Development, 45*, 873–890.

Bruner, J. (1968). *Processes of cognitive growth in infancy.* Waltham, MA: Clark University Press.

Collins, A. M., & Loftus, E. F. (1975). A spreading-activation theory of semantic processing. *Psychological Review, 82*, 407–428.

Derryberry, D. (1988). Emotional influences on evaluative judgments: Roles of arousal, attention and spreading activation. *Motivation and Emotion, 12*, 23–48.

Derryberry, D., & Rothbart, M. K. (1984). Emotion, attention, and temperament. In C. E. Izard, J. Kagan, & R. Zajonc (Eds.), *Emotion, cognition and behavior* (pp. 132–166). New York: Cambridge University Press.

Derryberry, D., & Rothbart, M. K. (1988). Arousal, affect and attention as components of temperament. *Journal of Personality and Social Psychology, 55*, 958–966).

Diamond, A. (1981). *Retrieval of an object from an open box.* Paper presented at the meeting of the Society for Research in Child Development, Boston.

Diamond, A., & Goldman-Rakic, P. S. (1983). Comparison of performances in a Piagetian object permanence task in human infants and rhesus monkeys: Evidence for involvement of prefrontal cortex. *Society for Neuroscience Abstracts, 9*, 641.

Freud, S. (1924). *General introduction to psychoanalysis* (J. Riviere, Trans.). New York: Berg & Liveright.

Gazzaniga, M. S. (1985). *The social brain.* New York: Basic Books.

Goldman-Rakic, P. S. (1987). Circuitry of primate prefrontal cortex and regulation of behavior by representational analysis. In F. Plum & V. Mountcastle (Eds.), *Handbook of physiology: Section 1. The nervous system. Vol. 5. Higher cortical function* (pp. 373–417). Bethesda, MD. American Physiological Society.

Keele, S. (1973). *Attention and human performance.* Pacific Palisades, CA: Goodyear.

Kihlstrom, J. F. (1987). The cognitive unconscious. *Science, 238,* 1445–1452.

Kintsch, W. A. (1988). The role of knowledge in discourse comprehension: A construction–integration model. *Psychological Review, 95,* 163–182.

Luria, A. R. (1973). *The working brain: An introduction to neuropsychology.* New York: Basic Books.

McLean, J. P., & Shulman, G. L. (1978). On the construction and maintenance of expectancies. *Quarterly Journal of Experimental Psychology, 30,* 441–454.

Milberg, W., & Blumstein, S. E. (1981). Lexical decision and aphasia: Evidence for semantic processing. *Brain and Language, 14,* 371–385.

Morton, J. (1969). Interaction of information in word recognition. *Psychological Review, 76,* 165–178.

Mozur, M. (1988). A connectionist model of selective attention in visual perception. *Proceedings of the Cognitive Science Society, 9,* 198–201.

Neisser, U. (1967). *Cognitive psychology.* New York: Appleton-Century-Crofts.

Neely, J. H. (1977). Semantic priming and retrieval from lexical memory. *Journal of Experimental Psychology: General, 106,* 226–254.

Newell, A., & Simon, H. A. (1972). *Human problem solving.* Englewood Cliffs, NJ: Prentice-Hall.

Petersen, S. E., Fox, P. T., Posner, M. I., Mintun, M., & Raichle, M. E. (1988). Positron emission tomographic studies of the cortical anatomy of single word processing. *Nature, 331,* 585–589.

Posner, M. I. (1978). *Chronometric explorations of mind.* Hillsdale, NJ: Erlbaum.

Posner, M. I. (1982). Cumulative development of attentional theory. *American Psychology, 37,* 168–179.

Posner, M. I. (1988). Structures and functions of selective attention. In T. Boll & B. K. Bryant (Eds.), *Clinical neuropsychology and brain function* (pp. 171–202). Washington, DC: American Psychological Association.

Posner, M. I., & Cohen, Y. (1980). Attention and the control of movements. In G. E. Stelmach & J. Requin (Eds.), *Tutorials in motor behavior* (pp. 243–250). Amsterdam: North-Holland.

Posner, M. I., & Cohen, Y. (1984). Components of attention. In H. Bouma & D. Bowhuis (Eds.), *Attention and performance X* (pp. 531–556). Hillsdale, NJ: Erlbaum.

Posner, M. I., Early, T. S., Reiman, E. M., Pardo, J., & Dhawan, M. (1988). Asymmetries in hemispheric control of attention in schizophrenia. *Archives of General Psychiatry, 45,* 814–821.

Posner, M. I., Petersen, S. E., Fox, P. T., & Raichle, M. E. (1988). Localization of cognitive function in the human brain. *Science, 240,* 1627–1631.

Posner, M. I., & Rothbart, M. K. (1980). The development of attentional mechanisms. In J. H. Flowers (Ed.), *Nebraska Symposium on Motivation* (Vol. 28, pp. 1–52). Lincoln: University of Nebraska Press.

Posner, M. I., Sandson, J., Dhawan, M., & Shulman, G. L. (1989). Is word recognition automatic: A cognitive anatomical approach. *Journal of Cognitive Neuroscience, 1,* 50–60.

Posner, M. I., & Snyder, C. R. R. (1975). Attention and cognitive control. In R. Solso (Ed.), *Information processing and cognition: The Loyola Symposium* (pp. 55–85). Hillsdale, NJ: Erlbaum.

Reiman, E. M., Fusselman, M. J., Fox, P. T., & Raichle, M. E. (1989). *Activation of temporopolar cortex in the production of anticipatory anxiety. Science, 243,* 1071–1074.

Rothbart, M. K. (1983). Cognition's search for emotion: Getting warmer? [Review of S. Clarke & S. Fiske (Eds.), *Affect and cognition.*] *Contemporary Psychology, 28,* 750–752.

Rothbart, M. K. (1988). Temperament and the development of inhibited approach. *Child Development, 59,* 1241–1250.

Rothbart, M. K. (in press). Temperament and development In G. Kohnstamm, J. Bates, & M. K. Rothbart (Eds.), *Temperament in childhood.* Chichester, England: Wiley.

Rothbart, M. K., & Derryberry, D. (1981). Development of individual differences in temperament. In M. E. Lamb & A. L. Brown (Eds.), *Advances in developmental psychology* (Vol. 1, pp. 37–86). Hillsdale, NJ: Erlbaum.

Rothbart, M. K., & Posner, M. I. (1985). Temperament and the development of self regulation. In L. C. Hartlage & C. F. Telzrow (Eds.), *The neuropsychology of individual differences: A developmental perspective* (pp. 93–123). New York: Plenum.

Rumelhart, D. H., & McClelland, J. (1986). *Parallel distributed processing* (Vols. 1 and 2). Cambridge, MA: MIT Press.

Schneirla, T. C. (1972). Aspects of stimulation and organization in approach–withdrawal processes underlying vertebrate behavior development. In L. R. Aronson, E. Tobach, D. S. Lehrman, & J. Rosenblatt (Eds.), *Selected writings of T. C. Schneirla* (pp. 344–412). San Francisco: W. H. Freeman. (Original work published 1965)

Sechenov, I. M. (1965). *Reflexes of the brain.* Cambridge, MA: MIT Press.

Shallice, T. (1972). Dual functions of consciousness. *Psychological Review, 79,* 383–393.

Sherrington, C. (1906). *The integrative action of the nervous system.* New Haven, CT: Yale University Press.

Simon, H. A. (1979). *Models of thought.* New Haven, CT: Yale University Press.

Sperry, R. W. (1988). Psychology's mentalist paradigm and the religion/science tension. *American Psychologist, 43,* 607–613.

Squire, L. R. (1986). Mechanisms of memory. *Science, 232,* 1612–1619.

Sulloway, F. (1979). *Freud, biologist of the mind.* New York: Basic Books.

Treisman, A. M. (1987). Features and objects in visual processing. *Scientific American, 16,* 114–125.

Tucker, D. M. (1985). What it means to feel. *Contemporary Psychology, 30,* 442–444.

Weizkrantz, L. (1977). Trying to build some neuropsychological bridges between monkey and man. *British Journal of Psychology, 68,* 431–445.

Weizkrantz, L. (1988). *Thought without language.* Oxford: Oxford University Press.

Zajonc, R. B. (1984). On the primacy of affect. *American Psychologist, 39,* 124–129.

Index